Electrocardiograms: Clinical Aspects

Electrocardiograms: Clinical Aspects

Edited by **Emma Fowler**

FOSTER
ACADEMICS

New Jersey

Published by Foster Academics,
61 Van Reypen Street,
Jersey City, NJ 07306, USA
www.fosteracademics.com

Electrocardiograms: Clinical Aspects
Edited by Emma Fowler

International Standard Book Number: 978-1-63242-122-7 (Hardback)

Printed in China.

Contents

Preface

The world is advancing at a fast pace like never before. Therefore, the need is to keep up with the latest developments. This book was an idea that came to fruition when the specialists in the area realized the need to coordinate together and document essential themes in the subject. That's when I was requested to be the editor. Editing this book has been an honour as it brings together diverse authors researching on different streams of the field. The book collates essential materials contributed by veterans in the area which can be utilized by students and researchers alike.

This book is an engaging exploration of electrocardiograms and its clinical aspects. Electrocardiograms are one of the most extensively used techniques for analyzing the structure-function relationships of the heart in physical conditions and disorders. This book discusses the technical aspects of the developments in electrocardiography. It is full of anatomical illustrations, electrocardiogram records, flow data and algorithms which demonstrate the contemporary aspects of electrocardiography. This book also elucidates how various technological impediments inherent to instrument-patient interfacing, recording and interpreting deviations in electrocardiogram time gaps and morphologies, etc. are overcome.

Each chapter is a sole-standing publication that reflects each author´s interpretation. Thus, the book displays a multi-facetted picture of our current understanding of application, resources and aspects of the field. I would like to thank the contributors of this book and my family for their endless support.

Editor

Part 1

Cardiac Structure and Function

1

Cardiac Anatomy

Augusta Pelosi[1] and Jack Rubinstein[2]
[1]*Michigan State University,*
[2]*University of Cincinnati*
USA

1. Introduction

The understanding of development and formation of normal anatomic structures is fundamental to comprehend electrocardiograms, conduction patterns and abnormalities. The aim of this chapter is to provide an overview of the cardiac chambers, the valves, the cardiac vasculature and the relation with the electrical conduction. The chapter will also review embryologic features of the cardiac structures.

2. Embryology

The heart develops in several sequential steps. The order and the completion of the entire process during fetal life are fundamental for having a post-birth functional and normally structured heart and conduction system. This section will review the basic steps of this process through the development of the cardiac chambers, the septa formation, the development of the major vessels, and the circulation before and after birth.
The heart is the first internal organ to form and become functional in the vertebrate development, (Srivastava, 2000) starting the first beats in humans by day 22 and the circulation by day 27-29. (Kelly, 2002, Pensky, 1992) Mesodermal cells migrate to an anterior and lateral position where they form bilateral primary heart fields (DeHaan 1963) which then coalesce to form two lateral endocardial tubes. (Harvey, 1999; Covin, 1998) The tubes fuse and merge into one endocardial tube surrounded by splanchnopleuric-derived myocardium. (Covin 1998) The cephalic and lateral folding of the embryo push the endocardial tube from a lateral position into the ventral midline. (Sherman, 2001) During the first month of gestation, the primitive, straight cardiac tube starts developing defined spaces with constrictions in series which will become the future cardiac structures: the *sinu-atrium* (most caudal), the *primitive ventricle*, the *bulbus cordis*, and the *truncus arteriosus* (most cephalad). (Abdulla, 2004; Angelini,1995) The primitive ventricle will eventually become the left ventricle whereas the right ventricle will develop from the proximal portion of the *bulbus cordis*. The distal portion of the right ventricle will form the outflow of both ventricles and the *truncus arteriosus* will form the root of the aorta and pulmonary arteries. (Abdulla, 2004) The linear heart tube becomes polarized with a posterior inflow pole (venous pole) and an anterior outflow pole (arterial). The *truncus arteriosus* is connected to the aortic sac and through the aortic arches to the dorsal aorta. (Pensky, 1992) Conversely, the *sinuatrium*, composted of the primitive atrium and the *sinus venosus*, receives the vitelline veins (from the yolk sac, also draining the gastrointestinal system and the portal circulation), the

common cardinal veins (draining the anterior cardinal vein coming from the anterior part of the embryo), the posterior cardinal vein (from the posterior part of the embryo), and the umbilical veins (from the primitive placenta).

Between day 22 and 28, the heart begins to fold and loop, as the epicardial cells start covering the outside layer of the heart tube. (Sherman, 2001) The heart tube loops because of intrinsic properties of the myocardium which encode for the initiation of the looping process, rather than due to asynchronous growth compared to the outside structures. (VanMierop, 1979) This process occurs prior to the formation of the chambers within the heart tube. By day 28, the atria move in a position higher than the ventricles, with the outside marks which refer to the *sinus venous, common atrial chamber, atrioventricular sulcus*, ventricular chamber, and *conotruncus* (outflow tracts). (Sherman, 2001) The *bulboventricular sulcus*, corresponding to the inner bulboventricular fold, starts to become visible from the outside. The heart assumes a U-shape where the *bulbus cordis* is located to the right and the primitive ventricle forms the left arm. The paired *sinus venosus* gives rise to the sinus horns. The two *sinus horns* are paired structures, which then fuse to form a transverse *sinus venosus*. (Abdulla, 2004) The entrance of the *sinus venosus* shifts rightward to enter into the right atrium. The right AV canal and right ventricle expand and align so that atria and ventricles are over each other, determining the alignment of the simultaneous left atrium and ventricle, and the proper alignment of the future aorta. (Sherman, 2001) The common atrioventricular junction changes into the atrioventricular canal, connecting the left side of the common atrium to the primitive ventricle. (Pensky, 1992) The inner surface is smooth except for the trabeculations, present at the level of the bulboventricular foramen. As the atrium grows, it pushes the bulbus cordis in the space between the two atria. (VanMierop, 1979) The symmetry in the development is lost by weeks 4-8 in the cardiac chambers and the aortic arches. (Kirby 2002) The cardiac neural crest, originating from the neural tube in the region of the three somites, starts migrating through the aortic arches 3, 4, and 6 into the developing outflow tract (week 5 and 6). These cells are responsible for septation of the outflow tract and ventricles, the anterior parasympathetic plexus, (Sherman, 2001) the leaflets of the atrioventricular valves, and the cardiac conduction system. (Hildreth, 2008; Poelman,1999)

2.1 Cardiac chambers and septation

Atria. The auricles of the right and left atria originate from the primitive atria, while the smooth sections come from the tissue originating from the venous blood vessels (*sinus venosus* on the right and pulmonary veins on the left). At day 35 an indentation provoked by the *bulbus cordis* and *truncus arteriosus* begins to create, on the inner surface of the common atrium, a wedge of tissue called *septum primum*, which extends into the common atrium separating it into a left and right compartment. (Steding, 1994) The *septum primum* allows a concave-shaped edge to form permitting shunting of blood from right to left. Apoptosis of cells in the superior edge of the *septum primum* forms a new foramen called the *ostium secundum*. (VanMierop, 1979) The endocardial cushions fuse with the *ostium primum* obliterating it. The *septum secundum* forms to the right of the *septum primum*. The septum is incomplete with a *foramen ovale* near the floor of the right atrium allowing passage of blood from right to left through the *foramen ovale*. (Abdulla, 2004; Angelini, 1995) Both *septum primum* and *secundum* fuse with the *septum intermedium* of the AV cushion.

Ventricles. The primary muscular ventricular septum begins to grow during the fifth week from the apex toward the atrioventricular valves. The initial growth is due to the growth of the two ventricles in the opposite direction. (Abdulla, 2004) The trabeculations from the inlet regions cause the formation of a septum which grows with a mildly different angle. This septum will meet the primary septum and provoke the primary septum to protrude into the right ventricular cavity forming the *trabeculae septomarginalis*. The high portion of the interventricular septum has a concave upper ridge which forms the *interventricular foramen*. The foramen closes at the end of week 7 by the posterior endocardial tissue, and the right and left bulbar ridges. (Abdulla, 2004) The majoriy of the muscular part of the septum is formed by the fusion of these septa. The outflow tract septum has grown down on the upper ridge of the muscular ventricular septum and onto the inferior endocardial cushion, separating the ventricular chambers.

2.2 Great vessels and arterial and venous development

Outlow tract septation. The mechanism of outflow septation is somewhat controversial. The proximal portion of the outflow tract septum septates by the fusion of the endocardial cushions and joints the atrioventricular endocardial cushion tissue and the ventricular septum. (Waldo 1998) The distal portion septates by intervention of the cardiac neural crest. (Kirby 2002). The septation of the outflow (conotruncus) is coordinated with the septation of the ventricles and atria. The septa fuse with the atrioventricular (AV) cushions dividing the left and right AV canals. Several theories for this process have been proposed. In general, three embryologic areas can be considered: the *conus*, the *truncus* and the aortopulmonary. (Abdulla, 2004) Each develops a ridge which is responsible for the formation of the septum between the fourth (future aortic arch) and the sixth (future pulmonary artery) arches. The *truncus* ridges form the septum between the ascending aorta and the main pulmonary artery, whereas the *conus* ridge forms the septation between the right and left outflow tract. (Abdulla, 2004)

Pulmonary arteries and veins. The main pulmonary artery develops from the *trunctus arteriosus*. The distal main and the right pulmonary artery develop from the ventral sixth aortic arch artery. The distal right and left have a different origin, deriving from the post branchial arteries. The *ductus arteriosus* develops from the left sixth aortic arch artery. The pulmonary venous system originates at the level of the left atrium, from a primitive vein sprout. These vessels anastomose with the veins extending from the bronchial bud. (Abdulla, 2004)

Systemic veins. The *sinus venosus* initially communicates with the common atrium, by week 7 the axis moves toward the right creating a connection between the right atrium and the *sinus venosus*. Around weeks 7-8 several changes occur to the venous system. The cardinal system is modified because the proximal left cardinal vein anastomoses with the right anterior cardinal vein via the left brachiocephalic vein creating the superior vena cava. The intermediate portion of the left cardinal vein degenerates and the portion close to the heart becomes the coronary sinus. (James, 2001) The left posterior cardinal vein degenerates, the right posterior cardinal vein becomes the azygous vein, and the left sinus horn contributes to the coronary sinus. The vitelline veins also undergo several changes: the right vitelline vein becomes the inferior vena cava. The course of the umbilical veins (coming from the placenta) is also modified by the degeneration of the left umbilical vein while the right umbilical vein connects to the right vitelline vein through the ductus venosus (derived from the vitelline veins). The veins draining into the left *sinus venosus* (left cardianal, umbilical, and vitelline) degenerate and the left *sinus venosus* becomes the *coronary sinus*, draining only the venous circulation of the heart. (Abdulla, 2004)

Aortic arches. The dorsal and ventral aorta are connected by six paired aortic arches. The first pair of aortic arches contributes to form the external carotid arteries. The second pairs regresses except a small portion forming the hyoid and stapedial arteries. The third pair forms the common and proximal part of the internal carotid arteries (the distal part is formed by the dorsal aorta). The left fourth arch forms the aortic arch maintaining the connection between the ventral to the dorsal aorta. The right fourth constitutes part of the right subclavian. The fifth pair regresses. The sixth evolves into the main and right pulmonary artery, whereas the distal portion forms the ductus arteriosus. (Abdulla, 2004)
Coronary arteries. The proepicardial organ surrounds the myocardium as the heart starts looping, forming the epicardium. (Komiyama, 1996) These cells form the coronary vasculature. These cells originate from an independent population of splanchnopleuric mesoderm cells and migrate into the primary heart tube. The coronary arteries (smooth muscle, endothelial, and connective tissue) form prior to migration into the heart tube. (Harvey, 1999; Mikawa, 1996).

2.3 Atrioventricular canal

The atrioventricular valves form during the 5th to 8th weeks. (Larsen, 1997) By the end of the 5th week, parts of the ventricles are visible and the left ventricle supports most of the circumference of the AV canal. The *endocardial cushion* starts from the sides of the atrioventricular junction with a superior and inferior cushion. They move toward the center of the canal forming the *septum intermedium* and the right and left atrioventricular orifices. (Snell, 2008) The cushion is also responsible for completing the closure of the interatrial communication at the level of the *septum primum*. (Van Mierop, 1979) Migration of the AV canal to the right and the ventricular septum to the left serves to align each ventricle with its appropriate AV valve. The formation of the valves starts with an asynchronous growth of the atria in comparison to the atrioventricular junction. The sulcus invaginates into the ventricular cavity with the formation of a hanging flap which is covered by the atrial and the ventricular tissue. (Abdulla, 2004)

2.4 Conduction system

The primary myocardium originates the contracting and the conducting tissue. The origin of the sinus and atrioventricular (AV) node is not well known. The cells seem to originate at the original connection of the sinus venosus with the right and left superior cardinal veins. These small groups of cells follow the cardinal veins as they move to their final destination. The right cardinal vein becomes the superior vena cava and maintains its connection to the sinus (SA) node. The left cardinal vein becomes the superior left vena cava and it is transformed into the coronary sinus, leaving sometimes a small vessel (the vein of Marshall). In general, the conducting system is formed by the accumulation of conduction myocardial tissue around the *bulboventricular foramen*. The dorsal portion becomes the bundle of His, whereas the lower tracts form the left and right bundle branches. Portions of this specialized tissue (*right atrioventricular ring* and the *retroaortic branch*) form but then disappear during normal development. (Abdulla, 2004)

2.5 Circulation

The fetal circulation is in parallel and dependent on the placenta because the lungs are not functional. The circulation in the adult becomes in series. There are several differences

between the two systems. The oxygenated blood, through the umbilical veins, reaches the heart of the fetus and flows away once deoxygenated , through the umbilical arteries. Once entered the fetal body, the blood bypasses the liver passing through the *ductus venosus* and enters the inferior vena cava to reach the right atrium. The position of the vena cava and the ligament of the inferior vena cava allow the blood to flow into the *foramen ovale* and into the left atrium. The foramen ovale appears like a valve formed by the foramen ovale and the *ostium secundum*. Part of the oxygenated blood in the right atrium mixes with the deoxygenated blood returning from the systemic circulation. From the left atrium, the blood follows the normal circulation and reaches the left ventricle, where it is pushed by the ventricular systole into the aorta. The venous return to the right atrium via superior vena cava follows the blood flow through the tricuspid valve into the pulmonary artery. Once the blood reaches the main pulmonary artery, it is diverted by the high pulmonary resistance into the *ductus arteriosus* at the level of the aortic isthmus. Only one-tenth of the right ventricular output reaches the lungs. The blood follows the descending aorta and returns to the placenta via the umbilical arteries. By the third month, the heart and major vessels are formed. However, the transition to the adult circulation occurs shortly after birth, when the umbilical cord is cut and the neonate takes the first breath. The lung expansion produces a drop in pulmonary resistance and increase in pressure inside the left atrium. Therefore, the pressure in the left atrium becomes mildly higher than the pressure on the right atrium, determining a closure of the valve flap associated with the *foramen ovale*, which transforms into a visible depression in the interatrial septum, called *fossa ovalis*. The increased concentration of prostaglandins, occurring with the parturition, results in the closure of the *ductus arteriosus*, which transforms into the *ligamentum arteriosum*. (Friedman, 1993)
The dramatic changes occurring with birth determine rapid transition toward the adult circulation with complete separation of the left and right compartments. The heart is functionally and anatomically divided into left and right. Each side has two chambers: atrium and ventricle, one major artery per side (aorta to the left and pulmonary artery to the right), and a venous return system (venae cavae to the right and pulmonary veins to the left). The deoxygenated blood returns to the right atrium from the systemic circulation through the venae cavae, and flows into the right ventricle through the tricuspid valve; it is then pushed into the lungs through the pulmonary valve and artery. The blood, now oxygenated, returns to the left atrium via the pulmonary veins, goes into the left ventricle through the mitral valve, and it is pushed to the rest of the body via the aorta.

3. Cardiac anatomy and thoracic cavity

The thoracic cavity can be divided into several compartments by imaginary lines. The mediastinum is divided into superior and inferior mediastinum by the *transverse thoracic plane*, which extends from the sternal angle to the space between the thoracic vertebrae T4 and T5. This line divides the thoracic cavity into **superior and inferior mediastinum**. The inferior mediastinum can be divided into an anterior, middle and posterior mediastinum. (Snell, 2008)
The **anterior mediastium** is bounded by a line crossing the thorax from the trachea to the xiphoid, just anterior to the pericardium. The **middle mediastinum** is the central part and contains the heart and the pericardium. The **posterior mediastinum** is contained between the pericardium anteriorly and the anterior surfaces of the bodies of the thoracic vertebrae (T5-T12). (Snell, 2008) Superiorly the thorax narrows as it enters the neck (1st ribs, the

manubrium and the 1st thoracic vertebra), and inferiorly the anatomic separation with the abdomen is well defined by the diaphragm. Along the midline, the mediastinum is responsible for the separation into two equal cavities, the left and the right pulmonary cavities.

The thoracic wall is formed of 12 ribs, the thoracic vertebrae, interventional discs, and the sternum. The ribs articulate with the thoracic vertebrae. The first 7 ribs are described as "true" because they articulate directly or indirectly with the sternum. The following ribs (8-10) are referred as "false" because they connect indirectly to the sternum. Ribs 11 and 12 are referred as "floating" ribs because they do not connect to the sternum. A posterior depression to the rib accommodates the intercostal neurovascular bundles, located between the internal and innermost intercostals layers. The sternum, formed by sternebrae, is a flat bone composed of three parts: the manubrium, body, and the xiphoid process. The muscles of the thoracic cavity play a fundamental role in respiration and movement of the thoracic cavity. The intercostal muscles are composed of three layers: the external, internal and innermost intercostals muscles. The diaphragm attaches to the upper lumbar vertebrae at the level of the right and left crura (lumbar vertebra 1 through 3). Laterally the diaphragm attaches to the abdominal wall musculature and to the xiphoid process. The diaphragmatic dome is formed by a muscular external portion and a central aponeurosis. It contributes to respiration by contracting during respiration. The central tendon contains the opening of the inferior vena cava. In the right crus the esophagus passes through the diaphragm, while the aorta passes from the thorax behind the diaphragm. The transit of these structures occurs at the level of the vertebrae 8, 10 and 12. (Netter, 2010)

The thoracic cavity contains the heart, lungs, great vessels, esophagus, trachea, thoracic duct, thymus and the autonomic innervations. The pleura covers the entire thoracic cavity.

The aortic arch moves from right to left as it enters the posterior mediastinum and becomes vertical as it crosses T4. Through the posterior mediastinum it moves to the middle at the level of T5. It crosses the diaphragm via the aortic hiatus and enters the abdomen at the level of T12. It gives off the posterior intercostal arteries and the subcostal artery, the bronchial and the esophageal branches. At the level of the aortic arch, three arteries branch off: the most anterior is the brachiocephalic artery, the left common carotid artery, and the left subclavian artery. The brachiocephalic artery bifurcates to become the right common carotid and the right subclavian arteries. The subclavian arteries form the axillary and brachial arteries. The subclavian artery gives off the internal thoracic arteries which reenter the superior mediastinum along the sternum. Occasionally there is an additional artery from the aortic arch. (Netter, 2010)

The internal jugular vein and the subclavian vein converge to form the brachiocephalic (or innominate) veins. These veins form two large trunks in either sides of the root of the neck and penetrate the superior mediastinum where they receive the contribution of the internal thoracic, inferior thyroid veins and the small pericardiophrenic veins, and the superior intercostal veins. The left crosses obliquely to join the right and form the superior vena cava. The superior vena cava enters the pericardial sac in the middle mediastinum to reach the right atrium from a superior position. The inferior vena cava enters from below. The azygous system consists of the azygous vein on the right and the hemiazygous and accessory hemiazygous vein on the left. The azygous and hemiazygous receives the blood from the abdomen and the subcostal vein. The azygous begins in the abdomen and enters the thorax via the aortic hiatus. It curves over the lung and drains into the superior vena cava. The hemiazygous crosses the diaphragm through the left crus and remains posterior the aorta, esophagus and thoracic duct before terminating into the azygous vein. The accessory hemiazygous vein either joins the azygous or terminates in the hemiazygous.

The pulmonary trunk arises from the right ventricle on the anterior surface of the heart directing to the left and posteriorly, passing anteriorly to the base of the aorta. The pulmonary artery bifurcates into the left and right pulmonary artery. The right enters the right lung passing under the aortic arch. The *ligamentum arteriosum* connects the left pulmonary artery to the aortic arch. (Netter, 2010)

The trachea terminates at the bifurcation into the bronchi at the level of the superior mediastinum. The esophagus descends behind the trachea at the level of the superior mediastinum, entering the abdominal cavity through the diaphragm at the level of T10. (Netter, 2010) The thymus is found in the anterior portion of the superior mediastinum. It is directly behind the manubrium and may extend into the anterior mediastinum It contacts the aorta, the left brachiocephalic vein and the trachea. The aortic arch is located to the left of the trachea and esophagus. The azygous vein crosses anteriorly to them and to the right. The thoracic duct enters into the posterior mediastinum through the aortic hiatus and travels between the thoracic aorta and the azygous vein behind the esophagus. It then drains into the left venous system close to the junction of the internal jugular and subclavian veins.

The superior mediastinum is crossed by the vagus and the phrenic nerve. The **phrenic nerves** originate from the ventral rami at the cervical levels 3, 4, 5. (Snell, 2008) They run along the neck, entering the thorax under the internal thoracic artery. The right nerve passes through the superior mediastinum, lateral to the right brachiocephalic vein and the superior vena cava. (Aquino, 2001) The left nerve passes lateral to the left subclavian artery and the aortic arch. Both nerves descend along the pericardium crossing through the middle mediastinum with the pericardiacphrenic artery (branch of the internal thoracic artery) and vein which empties into the subclavian vein. (Aquino, 2001) The **vagus nerves** leave the skull through the *jugular foramen* and descend along the carotid sheath. They give off cardiac branches in the neck (superior and inferior cardiac nerves) and a low number of small cardiac nerves in the superior mediastinum (thoracic cardiac branches), providing parasympathetic innervation to the heart via the cardiac nerve plexus. (Aquino, 2001; Snell, 2008) The right nerve descends between the lung and the trachea and it gives off the recurrent laryngeal nerve before entering the superior mediastinum (at the level of the right subclavian). (Aquino, 2001) It assists in the formation of the pulmonary plexus and then contributes to the formation of the esophageal plexus. (Snell, 2008) Conversely, the left descends between the carotid artery and the left subclavian artery and passes lateral to the aortic arch where it gives off the left recurrent laryngeal nerve, which passes under the arch just posterior to the ligamentum arteriosum. (Aquino, 2001) The left portion follows laterally the trachea and esophagus and ramifies into the esophageal plexus. (Aquino, 2001) Therefore the esophageal plexus, created by the right and left vagus in the middle mediastinum, forms the anterior and posterior vagal trunk which enters the abdomen through the esophageal hiatus. (Aquino, 2001) The **sympathetic innervation** is constituted by paired chains extending from the neck to the diaphram. (Aquino, 2001; Netter, 2010) The superior, middle, and inferior cardiac nerves provide postganglionic fibers to the heart providing sympathetic innervation. The thoracic ganglion and the inferior cervical ganglion form the "*stellate ganglion*" giving off the inferior cardiac nerve. (Snell, 2008) The cardiac plexus is a network of sympathetic and parasympathetic nerves primarily innervating the conduction system and the atria.

3.1 Heart in the thoracic cavity and external anatomy

The heart is located within the thoracic cavity in the middle of the inferior mediastinum, it occupies a large portion of this space. It is surrounded by the pericardium. The pericardium is a mesothelium formed by an external fibrous and an internal serous surface. The external parietal surface is composed of the two layers: an external thickened fibrous on the outside and an inner serous surface on the inside. (Snell, 2008) The two layers are adhered. The internal serous membrane presents a parietal and a visceral layer. The inner visceral layer covers the heart forming the epicardium. There is a potential space between the visceral and parietal layers containing small amount of fluid produced by the mesothelial cells. The parietal pericardium covers the aorta, pulmonary artery forming the *arterial reflections* and the superior, inferior vena cava and pulmonary veins forming the *venous reflections*. The oblique pericardial sinus is formed by the venous reflection of the inferior vena cava and pulmonary veins. The transverse pericardial sinus is formed between the arterial reflections and the venous reflections. Inferiorly, the parietal pericardium is attached to the diaphragm. Anteriorly, the superior and inferior *sternopericardiac ligaments* secure the parietal pericardium to the manubrium and the xiphoid process, respectively. (Netter, 2010)

Within the pericardium, the heart is a muscular four chamber organ connected to the rest of the thoracic cavity by two inflow and two outflow vessels. The orientation of the cardiac axis is oblique resulting in the apex being anterior and toward the left and a base located superior, posterior, and to the right of midline. The heartbeat is easily palpated between the 5th and 6th ribs. The left border is formed by the left ventricle and the right border by the right atrium. The right ventricle is located anteriorly while the left atrium is located posteriorly in front of the spine. The external separation between the left and right ventricle, highlighting the interventricular septum, is the **anterior interventricular sulcus (groove),** which contains the anterior interventricular descending branch of the left coronary artery and the **posterior interventricular sulcus (groove)**, containing the posterior interventricular (descending) artery and middle cardiac vein. The anatomical separation between the right atrium and right ventricle is provided by the **right atrioventricular sulcus (coronary groove)** in which the right coronary artery transits. The separation between the left atrium and left ventricle is highlighted by the **left atrioventricular sulcus (coronary sulcus)** containing the coronary sinus. The plane of this sulcus also contains the cardiac skeleton and the valves. The interatrial septum posteriorly is called the atrial sulcus. The intersection of the atrial sulcus and the posterior interventricular sulcus with the perpendicular coronary sulcus forms a cross shape on the posterior surface, called the **crux cordis.** (Netter, 2010)

4. Anatomy of the cardiac chambers, valves, and major vessels

The cardiac skeleton provides a scaffold for the attachment of the atrial and ventricular myocardium, the four valves and electrically insulates the atria from the ventricle. The fibrous structure present four rings for the opening of the aortic semilunar valve in the center and the other opening attached to it. The center is triangular shaped, called right fibrous trigone or central fibrous body, and it is included among the rings of the aortic semilunar valve, the medial parts of the tricuspid and mitral valve. The smallest left trigone is formed between the aortic semilunar valve and the anterior cusp of the mitral valve. The fibroelastic tissue from the right and left trigone partially encircle the AV opening to form the *tricuspid and mitral annulus* or *annulus fibrosus*. (Iaizzo, 2005) The annuli provide attachment to the myocardium and the AV leaflets. Strong collagen tissue from the right and left trigone also encircles the semilunar rings. The membranous septum provides support to the medial cusps of the aortic valve and continues superiorly to form the atrial septum. The *tendon of Todaro* is a fibrous extension of the membranous septum that is continuous with the *Eustachian valve of the inferior vena cava.* (Netter, 2010)

4.1 Right atrium and tricuspid valve

The interior of the right atrium has three distinct parts. The **posterior portion** of the right atrium has a smooth wall and is referred as the *sinus venarum* (the embryologic right horn of the sinus venosus). (Netter, 2010) The smooth posterior wall receives the superior and the inferior venae cavae and the coronary sinus. The **anterior portion** is very thin-walled but along its walls run the muscle bundles called *pectinate muscles.* (Snell, 2008) The physical separation between the anterior and posterior parts is a ridge of muscle, the *crista terminalis.* (Snell, 2008) In the embryo, the crista terminalis separates the sinus venosus and the primitive atrium. (Abdulla, 2004) This prominence corresponds to the external *sulcus terminalis.* (Snell, 2008) It is more prominent on the side of the superior venae cava and then fades out toward the inferior vena cava. The pectinate muscles continue into the **right auricle**, a triangular-shaped space on the superior portion of the right atrium. (Snell, 2008) The right auricle is broad and blunt. It extends from the superior vena cava almost to the inferior vena cava. (Netter, 2010) The inferior border of the right atrium contains the ostium of the vena cava and the ostium of the coronary sinus. The ostium of the vena cava opens anteriorly with a fold of tissue, the *inferior vena cava Eustachian valve* (fetal remnant). It is sometimes absent, but when present, it may appear with several openings, called *network of Chiari*. The coronary sinus opening is located anteriorly and inferiorly to the orifice of the inferior vena cava. It is sometimes guarded by a valve-like structure, called the *coronary-sinus Thebesian valve*. These two venous valves insert into a prominent ridge, the *Eustachian ridge* (sinus septum) which runs medial-lateral across the inferior border of the atrium and separates the os of the coronary sinus and inferior vena cava. Both valves originate from a large embryonic right venous valve. The **interatrial septum** forms the posteromedial wall of the right atrium. The interatrial septum has an interatrial and an atrioventricular part. It originates from the embryologic septum primum and septum secundum. It is muscular except for a central fibrous depression, called *fossa ovalis* resulting from the foramen ovale. It is surrounded by the *limbus fossae ovalis*, a muscular ridge surrounding the depression. The *fossa ovalis* is positioned anterior and superior to the ostia of both the inferior vena cava and the coronary sinus. A tendinous structure, the *tendon of Todaro*, connects the valve of the inferior vena cava to the central fibrous body of the cardiac skeleton. It appears as a fibrous extension of the membranous portion of the interventricular septum. It moves obliquely within the *Eustachian ridge* and separates the *fossa ovalis* from the coronary sinus below. This tendon has a structural role to support the inferior vena cava and is a useful landmark to approximate the location of the AV node.The conduction system is also closely associated with the right atrium. The SA node is located between the myocardium and the epicardium in the superior portion of the right atrium. To localize the SA node, the intersection of the line passing through the sulcus terminalis, the lateral border of the superior vena cava and the superior border of the right auricle, identify the position of the SA node. To approximate the location of the AV node, it is necessary to identify the *triangle of Koch*: the base passes through the coronary sinus; the sides are the septal leaflets of the tricuspid valve and the *tendon of Todaro*.

The **tricuspid valve** annulus lies on the floor of the right atrium, attached to the membranous portion of the septum. The tricuspid valve apparatus and the atrioventricular valve, is formed by an annulus, leaflets, papillary muscles, and the chordae tendinae. The AV orifice is reinforced by the annulus fibrosus of the cardiac skeleton. The three leaflets are the anterior (superior), posterior (inferior), and medial (septal). The leaflets have a smooth surface on the atrial side presenting only small nodules from the edges, called the *noduli albini*. (Netter, 2010) These appear to be present mostly in children and assure complete coaptation of the valve upon closure. The atrial side of the the leaflet is smooth whereas the ventricular surface is more irregular and provides insertion of the chordae. The anterior leaflet of the valve is the largest and extends from the medial border of the ventricular septum to the anterior free wall. The posterior leaflet extends from the lateral free wall to the posterior portion of the ventricular septum. The septal leaflet extends from the annulus to the medial side of the interventricular septum.

The primary order of chordae connects the papillary muscle to the free edge of the leaflets with several fine strands, impeding the valve leaflets from inverting. The secondary order chordae connect the papillary muscle to a ventricular portion of the leaflet. They are stronger and less numerous, providing the major stability to the valve. The tertiary order connects the ventricular myocardium to the leaflet. They form bands which can contain muscles. The commissures connect the leaflets and they are named after the connected leaflets: anteroseptal, anteroposterior and posteroseptal. They never reach the annulus so they provide only incomplete separation of the leaflets. (Netter, 2010)

4.2 Right ventricle and pulmonic valve

The right ventricular cavity is separated into two sections: posteroinferior portion containing the inflow with the tricuspid valve, and the anterosuperior outflow portion, containing the pulmonary trunk. The separation between these two portions is formed by a small ridge of several muscular bands, the *crista supraventricularis*, the *septal trabeculae (septal band)*, and the *moderator band*. These muscle bundles form the *trabeculae septomarginalis*, which form a semicircular arch (delineation of the outflow tract). (Netter, 2010) The inflow portion is heavily trabeculated by coarse *trabeculae carneae*, the outflow portion is named *infundibulum* and contains only a few trabeculae, and the subpulmonic area has a smooth surface. (Snell, 2008) Several papillary muscles connect the walls to the leaflets via the chordae tendinae. The anterior and the medial papillary muscles are always present, while additional papillary muscles can be present in variable number. The medial papillary muscle is located where the *crista supraventricularis* meets the septal band. It provides attachment to the chordae tendinae to the posterior and septal leaflet of the tricuspid valve. (Rogers, 2009) It is small in the adult heart. The largest papillary muscle is the anterior papillary muscle, which receives the chordae from the anterior and posterior leaflets of the tricuspid valve (Rogers, 2009) and it is located at the apex of the right ventricle.(Netter, 2010) The other papillary muscles (posterior and septal) are small and attach via chordae to the posterior and medial leaflet.

The **outflow portion** originates superiorly in the right ventricle. The pulmonary trunk bifurcates into right and left pulmonary arteries. The *ligamentum arteriosus*, remnant of the fetal *ductus arteriosus*, connects the bifurcation of the pulmonary artery to the inferior surface of the aortic arch. The pulmonary valve, as the other semilunar valve, differs from the atrioventricular valves. There is not a defined annulus to support the valve. The first portion of the vessel expands to form three pouches, the sinus of Valsalva which are mildly developed in the pulmonary artery compared to the aorta. The valvular leaflets are smooth and thin with a small fibrous nodule (*nodulus Arantii*) at the center of the free edge. (Netter, 2010)

4.3 Left atrium and mitral valve

The left atrium has a smooth surface with a transverse axis larger than the vertical and sagittal axes. The internal surface of the left atrial vestibule is smooth because the pectinate muscles are confined within the auricle. The left auricle is a continuation of the upper anterior portion of the left atrium. It is located anteriorly over the atrioventricular sulcus. Its shape is variable but it tends to be narrowed and pointed. (Ho, 2002; Ho, 2009) Its inner surface is irregular by the pectinate muscles. The septal surface is mostly smooth except for the area of the foramen ovale. (Snell, 2008) The left atrium receives two or three pulmonary veins from the right and two pulmonary veins from the left lungs. (Netter, 2010)

The **mitral valve** apparatus, as the other atrioventricular valve, is formed by an annulus, leaflets, papillary muscles and the chordae tendinae. The annulus is reinforced by the annulus fibrosus of the cardiac skeleton, supporting the posterior and lateral two-thirds of the mitral annulus. At the level of the right and left fibrous trigone, the annulus is reinforced by fibrous tissue. On the medial side, the attachment of the fibrous support of the aortic semilunar valve provides additional support. The valve has two leaflets: the anterior, also called medial or aortic, and the posterior (inferior or mural). (VanMieghen, 2010) The shape of the anterior leaflet resembles a trapezoidal shape. (Netter, 2010) The posterior leaflet is quite narrow and it subdivided into an anterior, central and posterior shape. When the valve closes, there is significant overlap of the leaflets. (Bolling, 2006) The connection between the leaflets is provided by the commissures, anterolateral and posteromedial. They never reach the annulus so they provide only incomplete separation of the leaflets. The leaflets have a smooth surface on the atrial side presenting only small nodules from the edges, called the *noduli albini*. These appear to be present mostly in children and assure complete coaptation of the valve upon closure. (Netter, 2010) The ventricular surface is more irregular and provides insertion of the chordae. The primary order of chordae connects the papillary muscle to the free edge of the leaflets with several fine strands, impeding the valve leaflets from inverting. The secondary order connects the papillary muscle to a more ventricular portion of the leaflet. They are stronger and less numerous, providing the greatest stability to the valve. The tertiary order connects the ventricular myocardium to the leaflet. (Bolling, 2006; Netter, 2010) They form bands which can contain muscles. The primary and secondary orders are constituted partially by muscle in the mitral apparatus. This feature is indicative of the common embryologic origin of the papillary muscles, the chordae and most of the leaflets from the embryonic ventricular trabeculae, which were muscular in origin. (Netter, 2010)

4.4 Left ventricle and aortic valve

The left ventricle has two separate portions, the inflow and the outflow separated by a fibrous band which provides attachment to the anterior mitral leaflet and the left and posterior aortic valve leaflets. The left ventricle is physiologically thicker than the right ventricle. The *trabeculae carnae*, presents mostly toward the apex, from the wall of the left ventricle but the muscular ridges are finer and less coarse compared to the walls of the right

ventricle. (Snell, 2008) The wall of the basilar portion is smooth. The interventricular septum is muscular except in the area below the right and posterior aortic leaflets which is membranous. The separation between the muscular and membranous part is called *limbus marginalis.* (Netter, 2010) The membranous portion is divided into two parts by the origin of the medial leaflet of the tricuspid valve, creating an upper portion, the atrioventricular part (between the left ventricle and the right atrium) and the lower one, the interventricular part (between the left and right ventricle). Two major papillary muscles connect the wall to the atrioventricular valve. (VanMieghen, 2010) The anterior papillary muscle is larger than the posterior. Occasionally a third papillary muscle is present. (Netter, 2010)
The outflow portion leads to the aorta through the aortic valve. The aortic valve, as the other semilunar valve, differs from the atrioventricular valves. There is not a defined annulus to support the valve. The first portion of the vessel expands to form three pouches, the sinus of Valsalva which are very obvious in the aorta. The wall of the vessel in this region is thinner than the aorta. The valvular leaflets are smooth and thin with a small fibrous nodule (*nodulus Arantii*) at the center of the free edge. Parallel to the free edges, a small area (*lunula*) of fine striations is evident. (Netter, 2010)

4.5 Aorta and pulmonary artery

The **aortic semilunar valve** is composed of three symmetric, semilunar-shaped cusps containing a recess called sinus of Valsalva. The junction of the sinuses and the aorta is called the *sinotubular ridge* since it makes a circular ridge. (Netter, 2010) When open, the valve forms a U-shape. The cusps are named based on the direction: the left and right (face the pulmonary valve), and the posterior. (Snell, 2008) The left and right have ostium on the inner surface opening into the left and right coronary arteries. The ostia are located below the sinotubular junction with the ostium of the left coronary; mildly superior and posterior to the right coronary ostium.The skeleton provides support to the structure. There is a small thickening on the center of the free edge of each cusp, the *nodulus of Aramtius or Morgagni.* The function of this nodule is to ensure complete closure. (Netter, 2010) From the nodule a line follows the free edge of the cusp, this line is called *linea alba.* Because of the increase aortic pressure, the linea alba, also present in the pulmonary cusps, is thicker and more pronounced. The plane of the aortic valve is mildly tilted.
The **pulmonary valve** resembles the structure of the aortic valve with the three symmetric, semilunar-shaped cusps. The cusps are attached to the right ventricular infundibulum and the pulmonary trunk. (Netter, 2010)

4.6 Coronary blood flow

Variations to the described anatomy are common. (Snell, 2008) The **right coronary artery** emerges from the right anterior sinus of Valsalva and runs in the *right atrioventricular sulcus.* Along this path the right coronary artery gives off two branches: the conus arteriosus branch and the right atrial branches. The conus artery and the communicating arteries in the interventricular septum serve as an important collateral blood supply to the left ventricle, anterior regions and anterior two-thirds of the interventricular septum. The right atrial branch gives the SA nodal artery (50-73 % of hearts), (Anderson, 1998; Iaizzo, 2005; Cohn, 2008) which runs along the anterior right atrium to the superior vena cava, encircling the vessels before reaching the SA node. As the right coronary artery reaches the AV groove, it gives several branches to the right atrium and ventricle, including the right marginal branch, which supplies the right margin of the heart. (Snell, 2008; Netter, 2010) The right coronary artery follows the sulcus posteriorly, curves until it reaches the crux cordis). It branches downward to form the posterior interventricular (descending) artery in the *posterior interventricular sulcus*. It supplies the posterior free wall of the right ventricle and in 85-90 % branches into smaller arteries (posterior septal arteries) to supply the distal one-third of the interventricular septum. (Iaizzo, 2005) The atrioventricular nodal artery passes anteriorly to the base of the atrial septum and supplies the AV node (50-60 % of hearts), the proximal part of the bundles of His, and parts of the posterior interventricular septum. (Snell, 2008; Netter, 2010) The Kugel's artery originates from either the left or the right coronary and runs anterior to posterior toward the atrial septum, providing collateral connection from the anterior arteries to the AV node and the posterior arteries. (Saremi, 2008; Cohn, 2008)

The **left coronary artery** originates from the left sinus of Valsalva and emerges from the aorta between the pulmonary trunk and the left atrial appendage. Under the appendage the artery divides into the anterior interventricular (left anterior descending artery) and the left circumflex artery. The anterior interventricular (descending) artery follows the *anterior interventricular sulcus*, curves around the apex and anatomose with the posterior descending. It branches to give the anterior septal perforating arteries, which enter the septal myocardium and supply the anterior two-thirds of the interventricular septum. The first perforator reaches the AV conduction system, the second or third perforator is the longest of the septal arteries and the main septal artery. This artery reaches the middle portion of the interventricular septum and sends branches to the moderator band. The branches called the diagonal arteries, originating from the anterior descending artery, reach the anterior free wall of the left ventricle. These arteries are named in order of appearance (first diagonal, second diagonal etc). The anterior interventricular artery also supplies the right and left ventricular free walls. One branch meets the artery from the right coronary artery at the level of the conus artery to form the *circle of Vieussens*. (Snell, 2008; Netter, 2010) The circumflex branch of the left coronary artery runs in the *left atrioventricular sulcus* and supplies most of the left atrium, the posterior and lateral free walls of the left ventricle and the anterior papillary muscle of the mitral valve. It divides into several branches to supply the left ventricle. The terminal branch is the largest. It continues through the AV sulcus to supply the posterior wall of the left ventricle and the posterior papillary muscle of the mitral valve. The circumflex artery supplies the SA node in 40-50 % of cases. (Iaizzo, 2005) In 30-60 %, it is between the anterior and the circumflex artery, there are diagonal or intermediate arteries which extend toward the apex. (Iaizzo, 2005) In approximately 15% of patients the posterior descending artery also arises from the circumflex, while in 85% from the right coronary artery. Other variations to the normal pattern for both the left and the right coronary circulation are common in humans. (Snell, 2008; Netter, 2010)

The **venous circulation** is divided into three systems: 1. the cardiac venous tributaries forming the coronary sinus, 2. the anterior cardiac veins (anterior right ventricular), and 3. the smallest cardiac (Thebesian) venous system. The satellite venous system, formed by the great, middle and posterior (small) cardiac veins, converge to form the coronary sinus and drain 49 % of myocardial blood. (Iaizzo, 2005, Snell, 2008) The anterior interventricular vein runs along the anterior interventricular sulcus with the anterior interventricular artery. Near the bifurcation of the left coronary artery, it turns and becomes the great cardiac vein. The great vein is formed by small tributaries from the left and right ventricle, and the anterior portion of the interventricular septum, the left atrium and the left ventricle. It also receives the large marginal vein which is parallel to the left marginal artery. The point of the great coronary vein becoming the *coronary sinus* is identified by the *valve of Vieussens* (a typical venous valve to prevent backflow), the space between the entry points of the oblique vein of the left atrium (vein of Marshall), and the posterior vein of the left ventricle. The oblique vein of Marshall runs superior to inferior along the posterior side of the left atrium, providing venous drainage of the area. It drains into the coronary sinus next to the great vein. The posterior vein ascends to the coronary sinus from the inferior portion of the left ventricle and provides drainage of the area. The coronary sinus also receives the middle vein. The veins, draining the posterior left and right ventricle and the interventricular septum, form the middle cardiac vein. This vein runs on the posterior interventricular sulcus and it enters the coronary sinus just before the right atrium. The small cardiac vein originates from the antero-lateral right ventricular wall and follows a path parallel to the marginal branch of the right coronary artery until it reaches the *right atrioventricular sulcus*. It turns and enters the coronary sinus with the middle cardiac vein. The small cardiac vein may be absent in 60 % of the cases. In 50 % of the cases it enters the right atrium directly. (Iaizzo, 2005) The anterior cardiac veins drain 24 % of myocardial blood and form a separate circuit which does not drain into the coronary sinus. (Iaizzo, 2005) They drain into the anterior right ventricular wall and travel superiorly to cross the right AV sulcus to enter the right atrium directly. When present, the right marginal vein follows the right marginal artery and enters the right atrium. It is considered part of the anterior veins. The third system is composed of small intramural intramyocardial veins called Thebesian veins draining 17 % of myocardial blood. (Iaizzo, 2005) These very small vessels don't have valves. They drain within the cardiac chambers via the *Thebesian ostia* in both the atria and the ventricles, but most commonly into the atrial and ventricular septa. They are more prevalent on the right side. (Netter, 2010)

5. Anatomy of the conduction system

The cardiac impulse arises in the sinoatrial (SA) node, located near the entrance of the superior vena cava. Known as the cardiac pacemaker, it generates the fastest rate of impulse. The impulse spreads to the interatrial and internodal conduction pathways to reach the atrioventricular (AV) node. The conduction travels to the bundle of His and then divides into left and right branches. Each bundle branch terminates in a network of fibers called the Purkinje fibers, whose stimulus generates ventricular contraction.

Under normal physiologic conditions the dominant pacemaker is the SA node, which in the adult fires at rate of 60 to 100 beat per minute (bpm). The overdrive suppression impedes other cells capable of spontaneous depolarization to become the dominant pacemaker. The cells located in the AV node and the Purkinje cells have a normal physiologic rate lower than the SA mode ranging from 25 to 55 bpm. (Iaizzo, 2005) In pathologic conditions the myocardial tissue itself can also exhibit self excitability generating ectopic beats. The parasympathetic system dominates at rest and slows the sinoatrial rate.

5.1 Sinus node

The SA node is located on the roof of the right atrium at the junction of the right atrial appendage, the superior vena cava, and the *sulcus terminalis*. In the adult it is 1 mm below the epicardium, 10-20 mm long and 5 mm thick. The P cells within the node are capable of spontaneous depolarization and are therefore responsible for generating the normal cardiac rhythm. (James, 2001) Importantly, the frequency of this depolarization is modulated by several factors both sympathetic and parasympathetic efferent innervation being the most important.

5.2 Interatrial conduction

After initial sinoatrial nodal excitation, depolarization spreads throughout the atria. The mechanism of impulse conduction through the atria is controversial. (Anderson, 1998; James, 2001) Excitation spreads through the myocardial atrial tissue cell-to-cell using specialized connections between the cells called gap junctions. Additional specialized conduction cells may be organized in pathways and constitute the internodal and interatrial pathways. It is believed, however, that there are three anatomic conduction pathways originating within the nodal tissue of the SA node or in the proximity of the node. The internodal tracts include the anterior internodal tract which extends from the anterior regions of the sinus node, travels on the roof of the right atrial septum and bifurcates into the Bachman's bundle directed to the left atrium and a second tract descending to the AV node, along the anterior part of the interatrial septum. The middle internodal tract (or Wenckebach's pathway) descends within the septum anteriorly to the fossa ovalis and reaches the AV node. It is the most inconsistent and not well developed. The third tract is called posterior internodal tract (Thorel's), which passes along the crista terminalis through the Eustachian valve, posteriorly to the coronary sinus. (James, 2001)

5.3 Atrioventricular node and His bundle

The AV node, also called *node of Tawara,* is located on the floor of the right atrium included within the *triangle of Koch.* (Ho, 2006) The proximal AV bundle continues into the portions of the AV node: transitional zone and compact node. It continues with the penetrating distal AV bundle (His bundle). (Anderson, 1998) The excitation from the SA travels through the AV node tissue following two functional and anatomical pathways, the slow and the fast pathways. The slow pathway crosses the isthmus between the coronary sinus and the tricuspid annulus and has slower conduction velocity but a shorter effective refractory period. (Anderson, 1998) The fast pathway is located superiorly and the fibers enter the node transversally in the distal portion of the compact node. It has a shorter conduction but a longer effective refractory period. Normal conduction occurs along the fast pathways, however, premature beats and higher rates find the fast pathway during the refractory period and conduct along the slow pathway. This system is a protective mechanism. In normal conditions the AV node-His bundle represents the only communication between the atria and ventricle. However, direct connections to the ventricular myocardium through the fibrous skeleton have been found. They constitute accessory pathways. The *Mahaim fibers* connect the penetrating portion of the distal bundle and the AV node to the ventricular myocardium. An additional aberrant pathway is the *bundle of Kent.* (Iaizzo, 2005)

5.4 Bundle branches

The AV bundle from the AV node penetrates the central fibrous body and passes through the membranous septum as a common bundle and splits into left and right bundle branches at the apex of the muscular septum. The left bundle branch splits into fascicles as it travels into the left subendocardic portion of the interventricular septum. Midway to the apex of the left ventricle, the left bundle splits into two major divisions, the anterior and posterior branches or fascicles. The right bundle continues inferiorly as a continuation of the bundle of His in the subendocardic portion of the interventricular septum.(James, 2001; Snell, 2008)

5.5 Purkinje fibers

The Purkinje fibers constitute a network of conduction specialized fibers arising from both left and the right bundle branches. They are characterized by rapid conduction. The fibers extend within the myocardium and the trabeculation of the right and left ventricle. One of the most common conduction pathways is the moderator band, which contains Purkinje fibers from the right bundle branch. (Snell, 2008)

6. References

Anderson PAW. (2000). Developmental cardiac physiology and myocardial function. In: *Pediatric cardiovascular medicine*, Moller JH, Hoffman JIE, eds., pp. 35–57,. Churchill Livingstone, New York

Anderson RH, Cook AC. (2007) The structure and components of the atrial chambers. *Europace*, 9 Suppl 6:vi3-9

Anderson, RH, Ho, SY.(1998) The architecture of the sinus node, the atrioventricular conduction axis, and the internodal atrial myocardium, *J Cardiovasc Electrophysiol.*. 9(11), pp.1233-1248

Angelini, P (1995) Embryology and congenital heart disease. *Tex Heart Inst J.*, 22(1): 1–12

Aquino, SL • Gregory R. Duncan, MS • L. Anne Hayman, MD (2001). Nerves of the Thorax: Atlas of Normal and Pathologic Findings, *RadioGraphics*, 21, pp.1275-1281

Bolling SF (2006) Functional anatomy of the mitral valve, In: *Atlas of mitral valve surgery*, Savage EB, Bolling SF eds pp.7-10, Lippincott Williams & Wilkins, Philadelphia, US

Colvin EV (1998) Cardiac embryology. In: *The Science and Practice of Pediatric Cardiology* Garson AJr (Eds.), (2nd), pp 91–126, Williams & Wilkins, Baltimore

DeHaan RL. (1963). Organization of the cardiogenic plate in the early chick embryo. *Acta Embryol Morphol Exp*, 6, pp. 26–38

Friedman AH, Fahey JT. (1993) The transition from fetal to neonatal circulation: normal responses and implications for infants with heart disease. *Semin Perinatol.* 17(2):106-121

Harvey RP, Rosenthal N. (1999) *Heart development.* (1st). Academic Press, San Diego

Hildreth V, Webb S, Bradshaw L, Brown NA, Anderson RH,Henderson DJ. (2008). Cells migrating from the neural crest contribute to the innervation of the venous pole of the heart. *J Anat*, 212, pp. 1–11

Ho SY, Anderson RH, Sánchez-Quintana D. (2002) Atrial structure and fibres: morphologic bases of atrial conduction. *Cardiovasc Res.*, 54(2), pp. 325-336

Ho SY, Sánchez-Quintana D. (2009) The importance of atrial structure and fibers. *Clin Anat.*, 22(1), pp. 52-63

Iaizzo PA (Ed) (2009). *Handbook of Cardiac Anatomy, Physiology, and Device* (2nd) ISBN: 9781603273718, NY

James TN.(2001) The internodal pathways of the human heart. *Prog Cardiovasc Dis.*, 43(6), pp. 495-535

Jason H. Rogers, MD; Steven F. Bolling, MD The Tricuspid Valve Current Perspective and Evolving Management of Tricuspid Regurgitation. *Circulation*. 2009;119:2718-2725

Kelly RG, Buckingham ME. (2002). The anterior heart-forming field: Voyage to the arterial pole of the heart. *Trends Genet*, 18, pp. 210–216

Kirby ML. (2002). Molecular embryogenesis of the heart. *Pediatr Dev Pathol*, 23, pp. 537–544

Komiyama M, Ito K, Shimada Y. (1996) Origin and development of epicardium in the mouse embryo. *Anat Embryol*, 176, pp. 183–189

Larsen WJ (1997b) *Human Embryology*, (2nd), Churchill Livingstone, New York

McCarthy KP, Ring L, Rana BS. Anatomy of the mitral valve: understanding the mitral valve complex in mitral regurgitation.*Eur J Echocardiogr*. 2010 Dec;11(10):i3-9.

Michael R. Mill, Benson R. Wilcox, and Robert H. Anderson (2008) Surgical Anatomy of the Heart, In: *Cardiac surgery in the adult* (3rd), Cohn SH ed, pp.29-50, ISBN 0071391290, McGrawHilld Education

Mikawa T, Gourdie RG. (1996) Pericardial mesoderm generates a population of coronary smooth muscle cells migrating into the heart along with ingrowth of the epicardial organ. *Dev Biol*, 173, pp 221–232

Netter FH, (2010) Netter FH, Dalley AF, eds. *Atlas of human anatomy*. (5th). Navartis, East Hanover, NJ

Pensky B (1982) *Review of Medical Embryology*., McMillan, New York

Poelmann RE, Gittenberger-de Groot AC. (1999). A sub-population of apoptosis prone cardiac neural crest cells targets the venous pole: Multiple functions in heart development?, *Dev Biol*, 207, pp. 271–286

R. Abdulla, G. A. Blew, M.J., Holterman MJ (2004). Cardiovascular Embryology. *Pediatr Cardiol* 25, pp. 191–200

Rogers JH, Bolling SF.The tricuspid valve: current perspective and evolving management of tricuspid regurgitation. *Circulation*. 2009 May 26;119(20):2718-25.

Saremi F, Abolhoda A, Ashikyan O, Milliken JC, Narula J, Gurudevan SV, Kaushal K, Raney A (2008) Arterial supply to sinuatrial and atrioventricular nodes: imaging with multidetector CT. *Radiology*. 246(1), pp. 99-107

Sherman LS, Potter SS, Scott WJ, eds. (2001) *Human embryology*. (3rd). Churchill Livingstone, New York

Snell, RS.(2008) The thorax: part II-The thoracic cavity, In *Clinical anatomy by regions*, pp. 77-130, ISBN 0781764041, Lippincott Williams & Wilkins, Philadelphia, US

Srivastava D, Olson EN. (2000). A genetic blueprint for cardiac development. *Nature*, 407, pp. 221-226

Steding G, Seidl W (1984) Cardiac septation in normal development. In: Nora JJ, Talao A(Eds.), *Congenital Heart Disease: Causes and Processes*. pp 481–500, Futura, New York,

Van Mieghem NM, Piazza N, Anderson RH, Tzikas A, Nieman K, De Laat LE, McGhie JS, Geleijnse ML, Feldman T, Serruys PW, de Jaegere PP. (2010) Anatomy of the mitral valvular complex and its implications for transcatheter interventions for mitral regurgitation. *J Am Coll Cardiol*. 17;56(8), pp 617-626

Van Mierop LHS (1979) Morphological development of the heart. In: Berne RM (Eds.), *Handbook of Physiology, the Cardiovascular System*. pp 1–28American Physiology Society, Bethesda, MD

Waldo K, Miyagawa-Tomita S, Kumiski D, Kirby ML. (1998) Cardiac neural crest cells provide new insight into septation of the cardiac outflow tract: Aortic sac to ventricular septal closure. *Dev Biol*, 196, pp. 129–144

Wessels, M.W.M. Markman, J.L.M. Vermeulen, R.H. Anderson, A.F.M. Moorman, W.H. Lamers (1996) The Development of the Atrioventricular Junction in the Human Heart *Circulation Research*. 78:110-117

Part 2

ECG Technique

2

Non Contact Heart Monitoring

Lorenzo Scalise
Dipartimento di Ingegneria Industriale e Scienze Matematiche,
Università Politecnica delle Marche,
Italy

1. Introduction

Heart rate is, among the many vital signs (respiration rate, blood oxygen saturation, arterial blood pressure, etc.), one of the most commonly measured and monitored. Whatever will be the sensing principle or the monitoring method used, data referred to the heart rate can be considered the primary vital sign information which is needed on a patient approach in both emergency and clinical situations. Heart rate data are used to measure anomalous rate or irregular pulse rate (arrhythmias) or heart block. The post-processing of the data can be used to verify trends or single events, providing precious elements to the patient diagnosis. Heart-rate variability (HRV) can be performed on recorded data in order to have an objective measure of eventual cardiac abnormalities (irregular beat-to-beat time is a prognostic factor for atrial fibrillation (Gorgas, 2004). Low HRV is also a known prognostic marker for several cardiovascular diseases. Other possible use of the heart rate data are related to the analysis of the circadian rhythm (sleep), temperature regulation, cardiac sympathetic nervous activity and synchronization with respiration rate.
Since the past centuries, observation of the electrophysiologic effects related to the heart beats are reported. In 1842, Carlo Matteucci, Professor of Physics at the University of Pisa, shows that an electric current accompanies each heart beat. In 1902 Einthoven publishes (Einthoven, 1902) the first electrocardiogram recorded on a string galvanometer, opening the way to the electrocardiography (ECG) era which is still, nowadays, the primary heart rate monitoring procedure.
To date, an enormous series of procedures, methods and devices for ECG monitoring are available on the market (Gorgels PM, 2007; Webster, 1988). The majority of these contributions are based on the need to place some electrodes on standard positions on the body surface (i.e. Einthoven's triangle), as depicted in fig. 1. ECG measurements can be divided into two types according to where electrodes are attached or fixed. The first type involves measurements with conventional "fixed-on-body" electrodes such as Ag - AgCl electrodes, and the other involves measurements using electrodes installed on appliances or furniture.
Even if fixed-on-body electrodes (fig. 2) are reliable and give good signal quality, they are inconvenient and inadequate for long-term, everyday measurements. Moreover the presence of cables (one for each of the electrodes placed) can considerably limit the patient mobility and comfort, forcing him to maintain the initial position (supine) for all the monitoring period of time or limiting his/her movements because of the cables length."

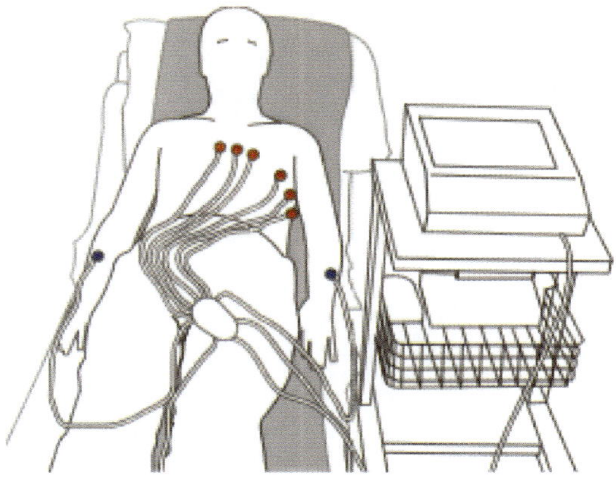

Fig. 1. Example of ECG electrodes placement and patient positioning for standard ECG monitoring.

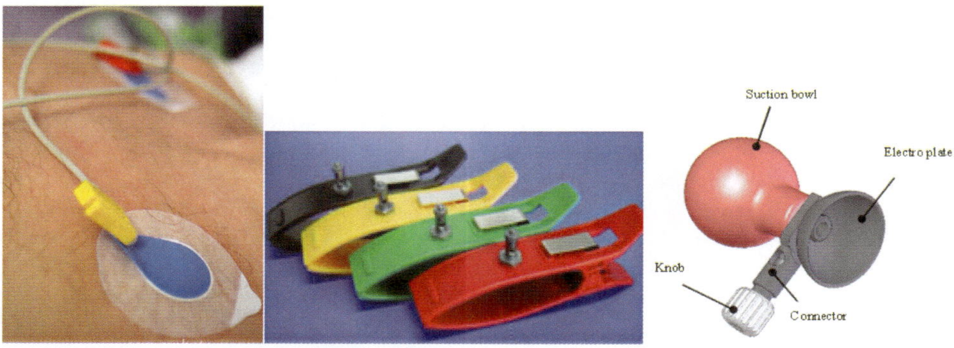

Fig. 2. Examples of ECG on-body electrodes commonly used for standard ECG: disposable, gel-impregnated, attachable electrodes (left), clamp reusable electrodes (center) and suction, reusable electrodes (right).

"Fixed-in-the-environment" electrodes are nonintrusive and more adequate for long-term monitoring, and even if they also present some shortcomings, the nonintrusive nature of fixed-in-the-environment electrodes makes them an attractive option for daily monitoring. The main limit is the requirement of maintaining direct contact between the bare skin of the subject and the electrodes which is fixed in the environment (chair, seats, etc.), which limits the application of fixed-in-the-environment electrodes to a few cases.

An alternative possibility for heart monitoring is phonocardiography, PCG (Webster, 1988; Dressier, 1970; Fowler, 1962; Durand and Pibarot, 1995) which consists essentially in recording/processing the acoustic waves produced by heartbeats and travelling through the body up to the skin. It was one of the first heart monitoring method developed and it is based on the observation that heart contractions produce acoustic waves travelling through the blood at the corresponding speed of sound. Therefore acoustic pick up of such waves can provide information on the periodic variation of pressure wave due to the heart pulsation , as well as other information related to the heart mechanics and valves dynamics (fig.3). The typical speed of dilatation pressure waves varies between 4 m/s to 10 m/s. Increasing stiffness of arteries and veins due to aging or cardiac diseases increases the speed of dilatation waves. Consequently, study of propagation of dilatation waves has a clear physiological and clinical interest. PCG can be considered a non-invasive method, but it still requires the contact between the high sensitivity acoustic transducer (typically a piezoelectric microphone) and the patient skin and therefore it can't be considered a solution to the problem of monitoring heart activity (in particular heart rate) without the direct contact between the device and the patient's skin.

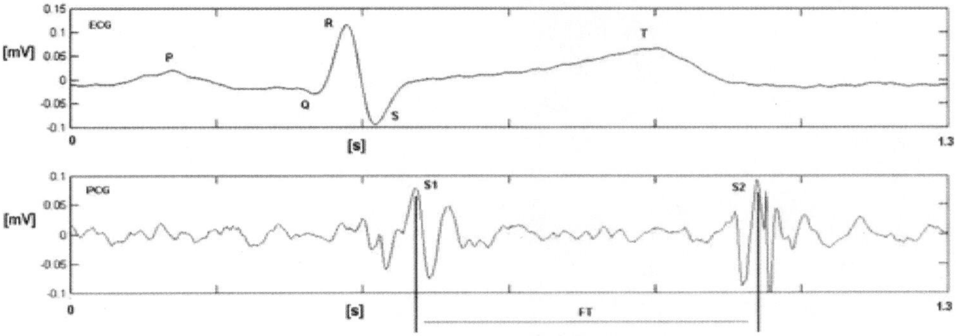

Fig. 3. Example of ECG II-lead trace (top) and simultaneous phonocardiogram (down) traces. S1 and S2 are the main signals measured during an heart cycle; (FT is the filling time).

A medical device frequently used to monitor patients pulse rate, is the pulse oximetry, PO (Webster, 1988; Alexander et al., 1989; Welch et al., 1990; Wahr et al., 1995). The device has been realized for the monitoring of oxygen saturation (percent of hemoglobin in the oxyhemoglobin configuration) in blood and is based on the different spectral absorption of hemoglobin and oxy-hemoglobin. In adults, PO's sensing elements are normally placed on the finger tip (or ear lobe) where the two emitting LEDs and the photodiode are placed (fig. 4). In addition to the digital read-out of O_2 saturation, most pulse oximeters display also a plethysmographic waveform as the blood micro-vessels under the skin expand and contract with every heart beat; from this trace, heart rate is automatically extracted.

As for the PCG microphone, the PO probe requires direct contact with the finger or ear lobe and it can't be considered a non contact method. The main drawback of PO is the sensitivity to motion artifacts which can generate repeated erroneous data and consequently activate false alarms signals.

In this chapter, the possibility to perform heart monitoring without physical contact with the subject is investigated and all available non contact methods are reviewed, trying also to predict the future trends of the technology. Before presenting such methods we will resume the motivations for such exploring the possibility of non contact monitoring of heart rate.

Non contact detection and monitoring of human cardiac activity without contact through bedding and clothing is a valuable tool in intensive care monitoring, long term-monitoring and home health care applications as well as in other non clinical fields such as the case of workers health monitoring (i.e. airplane pilots, firefighters, etc.). Patients with conditions

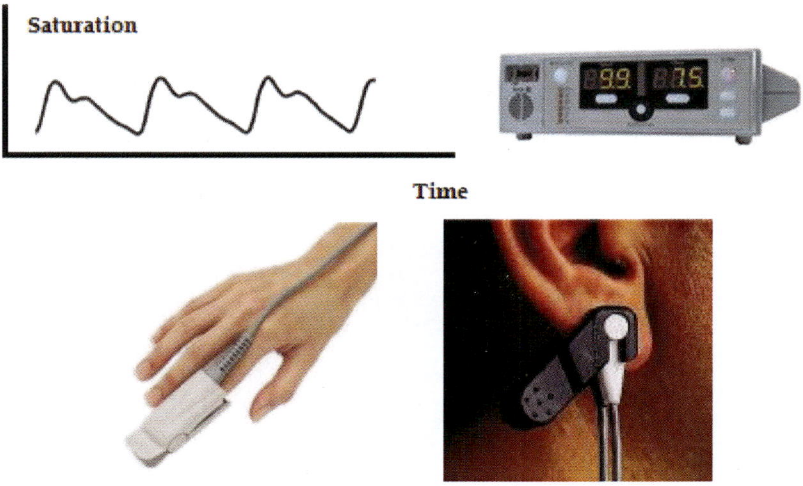

Fig. 4. Common pulsatile signal on a pulse oximeter (top, left); Oxymeter front panel reporting blood saturation and heart rate (top, right). Oxymeter probes: finger clip (down , left) and hear lob clip (down, right).

that can be perturbed or worsened by contact sensors include neonates (fig. 5), infants at risk of sudden infant death syndrome, and burn victims; a noncontact heart rate monitor provides a vital sign without affixed electrodes for these patients. Most alternatives to standard heart monitors need the application of electrodes or transducers (such as the case of thoracic belt) which often require accurate control or re-placement of electrodes/transducers during the monitoring period of time. Such aspect is sometimes critical and can also be impossible or undesirable in many situations.

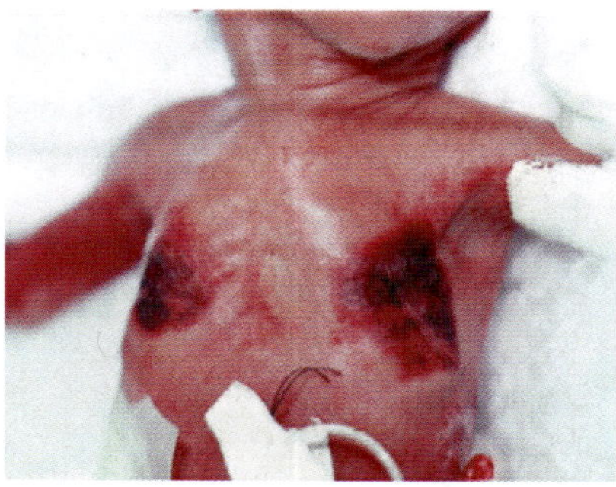

Fig. 5. Possible skin irritation effect on preterm infant due to prolonged use of skin ECG electrodes.

An important advantage associated to the possibility to have a non contact sensing of the heart rate, it should be recalled, is the intrinsic compliance with the safety recommendations concerning risk of electric hazards which are particularly strong with electromedical apparatus. Moreover the absence of contact is particularly important in specific cases such as security (hidden or suspected subjects identification), monitoring of contaminated patients, presence and conditions of live subjects in biologically and chemically contaminated environments, emergency (i.e. presence and conditions of subjects on a battle field, transport of patients), intensive care (pre-term infants, adults), long monitoring of vital signs as well as home monitoring especially of elderly adults (Abowd, 2002) and automatic activation emergency actions.

A first class of proposals in this field has been based on the usage of non conductivity electrodes for ECG recording for example with electrodes embedded in the bed or the chair (Ishijima, 1993; Matsuda et al., 2008; Lim et al., 2006 and 2007), or have been based on techniques such as the ballistocardiography (Pollock, 1957; Morris, 1954) where the sensing part is installed into the bed, chair or wheelchair, in furniture or is directly based on the vibration monitoring of the skin, such as for seismocardiography (Salerno and Zanetti, 1990; Poliac et al., 1991; Sandham et al., 1998).

More recently a laser-based, single point, non contact measurement method, named vibrocardiography (VCG), for the heart rate (HR) monitoring and the heart rate variability (HRV) assessment has been proposed. First studies using optical vibrometry (laser Doppler vibrometry) has been reported for the identification of the arterial pressure waves (Tomasini et al. in 1998). While a novel method, called vibrocardiography (VCG), has been later proposed to measure the velocity of displacement of the skin in correspondence of the chest wall (Scalise et al., 2005a;2005b;2006; Morbiducci et al., 2006; Scalise and Morbiducci, 2008). VCG has been demonstrated to be valid for the assessment of the cardiac frequency and variability and in Cardiac Resinchronization Theraphy as support in pacemaker programming after installation (Bocconcelli et al., 2006). The same laser-based optical approach has also been explored to have HR data correlated to the emotional state of the subject without the need of a physical contact (Rohrbaugh et al., 2007) as well as for the evaluation of biometric capabilities (Chen et al., 2010).

Other non contact methods, based on electromagnetic (EM) approaches for heart and respiration monitoring, have also been proposed. The first microwave system (a microwave Doppler radar) was firstly proposed in early 1970s (Lin, 1975) for respiration detection and was based on bulky, heavy and expensive components; today many solutions have been proposed demonstrating the possibility of compact, lightweight and inexpensive mass-producible solutions (Staderini, 2002; Matsui et al., 2004a and 2004b; Kim et al., 2007; Droitcour et al., 2001). The interest on the use of EM heart monitoring are based on the possibility to have data from the subject without the necessity of the direct contact with the skin or just the visibility of the skin (electromagnetic waves at certain frequencies can pass through the tissues). A series of different laboratory solutions as well as market available monitoring systems (see web references) have been already proposed. Finally HR monitoring based on image-based methods (Da Costa, 1995; Poh, 2010; Takano and Ohta, 2007; Garbey et al., 2007), electrical impedance (Ischijima, 1993; Harland et al., 2002), acoustic and ultrasound (Tanaka et al., 2002) approaches have also been reported as valid principles for non contact heart rate monitoring.

2. Non contact methods for heart monitoring

Non contact detection and monitoring of human cardiac activity through bedding and clothing would be a valuable tool in intensive care monitoring and home health care applications. Patients with conditions that can be perturbed or worsened by contact sensors include neonates, infants at risk of sudden infant death syndrome, and burn victims; a noncontact heart and respiration rate monitor could provide vital signs monitoring without affixed electrodes for these patients. Most alternatives to standard heart monitors need leads and contacts and often require accurate control or placement; this may be impossible or undesirable in many situations

In this chapter, the non contact methods for heart monitoring proposed in the last years have been divided in four categories, based on the working principle:

- Electromagnetic-based monitoring systems
- Laser-based monitoring systems
- Image-based monitoring systems
- Other methods

The common characteristic for all the methods, presented in the following, is that they aim to measure the surface (skin) displacement taking place because of the heart muscles contractions: change in the volume of the heart and consequently displacement of the external heart walls during systole move the tissues under the ribs and the soft intercostals tissues, causing the well perceived "beat" that everyone can experience simply putting the finger tip on the left-upper part of the thorax. Specific studies - carried out with optical methods - report that the maximum displacement takes place in the correspondence of the heart apex and it is reported to be in the order of about 600 μm (Aubert et al., 1984; Ramachadran and Singh, 1989). It must, anyway, be remarked that the motion of the surface due to the heartbeat, which is indeed detectable also from the right part of the thorax, is largely influenced by the subject health conditions and position (supine, prone or on a side), by the gender, by age and by body shape.

2.1 Electromagnetic-based monitoring methods

The basic principle of radar is to transmit a microwave (radio) signal towards a target. The strength of the backscattered signal is measured. There are two variants of radar sensing used for heart rate monitoring: continuous-wave (CW) and wide band pulsed radar (UWB).

Constant wave (CW) radar emits a continuous stream of electro-magnetic radiation. An antenna is used as transmitter and it radiates a signal to a target, the energy reflected from the target is detected by an antenna (it can be the same antenna used for transmission) and a mixer diode provides a tension proportional to the phase between the transmitted and received signal (which is related to the target movement). A filter section is needed to separate heartbeat from the respiration; valid measurements could be taken at a range exceeding 10 m. Microwave apexcardiography was demonstrated firstly with a continuous-wave 2 GHz antenna placed in correspondence to the apex and precordial motions were detected (Lin et al., 1979). In general, CW radar methods, reported in literature, appear simpler respect to UWB radar, but it presents problems when multiple reflections, due to scattering characteristics of the surrounding environment, are present. With CW radar, the phase of the received signal is containing the information on the displacement of the target $x(t)$ and, if we report the transmitted signal $T(t)$ as:

$$T(t) = A\cos(2\pi ft + \phi(t)) \tag{1}$$

Where, f is the frequency of the transmitted signal and $\Phi(t)$ is its phase; then, the received signal $R(t)$ can be approximated, as:

$$R(t) = KA\cos\left(2\pi ft - \frac{4\pi d_0}{\lambda} - \frac{4\pi x(t)}{\lambda} + \phi\left(t - \frac{2d_0}{c}\right) + \theta_0\right) \quad (2)$$

where, K is the reduction of the amplitude A of the originally transmitted signal, θ_0 is the phase shift due to the reflection at the surface, d_0 is the distance between system and the skin surface. When the phase of $R(t)$ is demodulated a signal proportional to the chest displacement (about ±1cm max, caused by the respiration activity and ± 0.6 mm, max caused by heart activity) can be inferred. The CW radar monitoring principle is reported in figure 6.

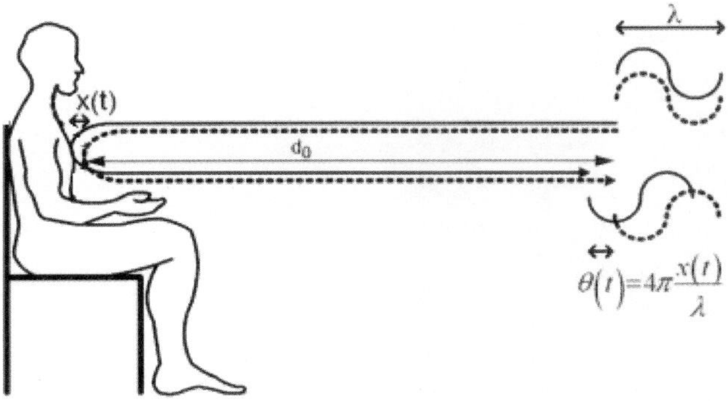

Fig. 6. Principle of CW radar monitoring of the chest movement: phase shift $\theta(t)$ caused on the reflected wave by the chest displacement x(t).

CW microwave reflectometers typically have a phase resolution of 1/200 fringe which corresponds to a spatial resolution of λ/ 400, where λ is the incident wavelength (Tateischi et al., 2007). For example, if a CW system working at a carrier frequency of 10 GHz is used (λ=3.0 cm) is used, the spatial resolution becomes 75 μm, allowing a full detection of the heartbeats. A typical technique used to extract from the detected signal the part due to the heart rate, is by use of an high-pass filter with a cut-off frequency of 0.7 Hz. Nevertheless, most of the authors propose specific signal processing in order to enhance the SNR of the heart beat signal and for the removal of residual motion artifacts (Nagae & Mase, 2010). With opportune filtering and signal processing, it was demonstrated that heart rate and respiration rate can simultaneously be detected by the same microwave apparatus (Chan et al., 1987). Particular measuring conditions taking into consideration the presence of persons in rubble (Chuang et al., 1990), athletes (Greneker et al., 1997) and persons behind walls (Chen et al., 2000) were explored, demonstrating that the approach is robust and mature for a wide employment on different scenarios. An example of a possible laboratory set-up using CW microwave reflectometry to detect respiratory and heart rate activities is reported in figure 7 (Scalise et al., 2011).

Experimental unfiltered phase signals acquired with the measurement system reported in fig. 7 (emitted signal at 6 GHz, 1 mW) are reported in fig. 8, for the case of a volunteer sitting on a chair and normally breathing (left) and holding the breath (right).

For HR monitoring scope, the direct comparison between phase variation, as detected using the CW set-up reported in figure 7 and the simultaneously acquired ECG trace of the subject are reported (fig.9), putting in evidence the high time correlation between the two signals.

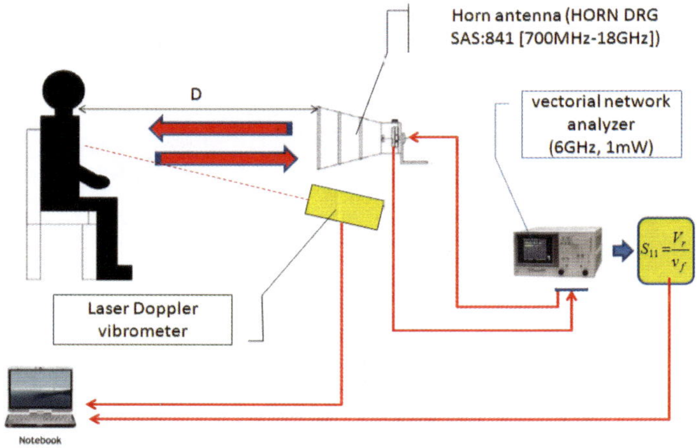

Fig. 7. Laboratory set-up for CW microwave reflectometry for respiratory and heart rate activities monitoring.

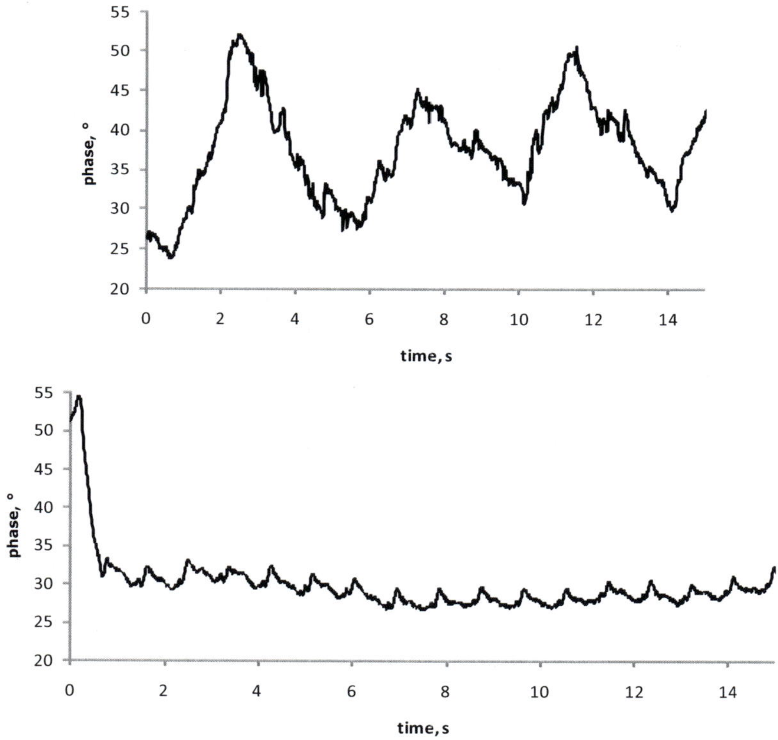

Fig. 8. CW microwave reflectometry: Respiratory and heart beat activities (top) and only cardiac activity (bottom).

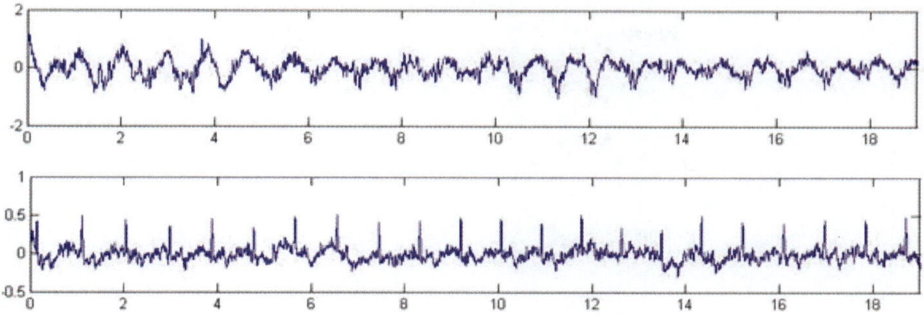

Fig. 9. Phase variation (normalized data respect to the max phase value, top) and ECG trace (down).

HRV analysis with a 24 GHz CW microwave system monitoring a volunteer from the back of a sitting subject at a distance of 34 mm, showed a strong correlation of the HRV measures from the microwave system with that from the ECG system in 2-minute recordings in rest and during simple arithmetic task. Comparison of 5 min recordings demonstrated also that there were no significant differences in the temporal, frequency domains and in non-linear dynamic analysis of HRV measures derived from heartbeat and ECG, which suggested this technique may used as practical alternative to ECG for HRV analysis. (Lu et al., 2009).

The second possible approach to the radar monitoring of the heart activity is based on the use of pulse radar (Staderini, 2002; Chia et al., 2005; Immorev & Tao, 2008) which are in the majority of the cases ultra wide band pulsed (UWB) radar. Unlike narrowband systems, which transmit continuous waveforms at a specific frequency, ultra-wideband (UWB) systems transmit narrow impulse-like signals that span a broad frequency range. The pulse width of such system is typically within a range of 100's of ps to several ns, with rise times as fast as 50 ps, corresponding to a frequency range that can span several GHz. Since the energy of the pulse is distributed across a frequency band, the power spectral density is much lower in magnitude than a narrowband system reducing also the eventual interferences with other RF or MW apparatus.

UWB application used to be limited mainly in military areas, however, since 2002, FCC has gradually allowed the commercial usage of these bandwidths (frequency for the UWB technique is 3.1-0.6 GHz in USA and 3.4-4.8 GHz and 6-8.5 GHz, in Europe) The power radiation requirement of UWB is strict and it usually it does not disturb the other equipments because UWB's spectrum is normally very low. Emitted pulses are spread over a wide frequency spectrum having a very short time duration (in the order of ns or sub-nano seconds of duration); the main advantage of such type of radar appears to be the low energy consumption due to the short pulses. Pulse radars make use of a pulse generator to allow the e.m. pulse transmission from the antenna and simultaneously the activate a so-called delay line used for controlling the sampling of the received echoes. Time duration between emitted and received echo is proportional to the target distance; the receiver can be activated at very short time intervals triggered by the delay-line (range gating). Thus, the length of the delay-line ensures that only pulses back-scattered from a certain distance are received. UWB is ideal in range measurement but can present some ambiguity in both range and velocity measurements. A typical set-up using a UWB-radar system is reported in figure 10.

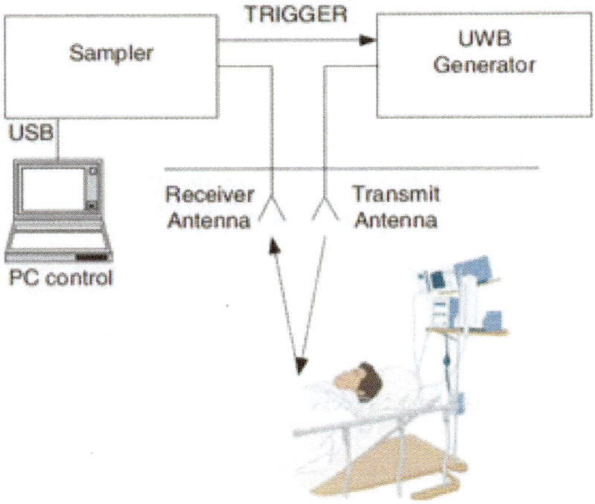

Fig. 10. Laboratory set-up for UWB-radar sensing of heart rate.

As for the case of CW systems, also UWB have been used to prove their capability in vital signs assessment. For example, data from 40 human volunteers at Walter Reed Army Institute of Research were collected using a micro-power impulse radar range finding prototype (Paulson et al., 2005). Readings from an ECG and pulse oximeter were captured simultaneously with MIR readings (Azevedo, 1996). MIR sensor readings were collected from each volunteer in four different body positions: standing upright, lying face up, lying on the right side, and lying face down. Since the readings of the MIR range finder prototype correspond to reflections off of tissue interfaces, rather than electrical impulses as in the ECG, body position was expected to be an important factor. Fixed range radar signals were compared to ECG, cardiac impedance, and acoustic heart signals showing well correlated relation among standard contact techniques (ECG) and the UWB-pulsed radar.

UWB's venture into the commercial domain of medical industry is now becoming a reality. Several vendors have been working on this technology to develop high value products aimed at the low-end and mid-range market segments in the patient monitoring and medical imaging markets (i.e. VSM, LifeWave and PAM™3000, see references). Some UWB systems are now available on the market allowing the check of occupancy of the bed and the vital signs monitoring of patients (primary elderly). In particular, if the at-risk patient should leave the bed without control or needed assistance, the UWB system, placed underneath the patient mattress, will detect it and send the alarm. Moreover the system is designed to wirelessly transfer heart rate and respiration rate data to the patient monitor or the nursering station. In figure 11, some example of market-available sytems are reported.

As against several imaging and patient monitoring modalities, UWB based medical technologies are expected to be impacted by the positive regulatory policies by European governments. In the United States, Federal Communication Commission (FCC) has mandated the use of UWB technology within the vast bandwidth of 3.1 to 10.6 GHz at power levels of -41 dB/MHz. On the other hand, there are no strict regulations mandating the use of certain frequency bandwidths for UWB devices for medical applications. In February 2007, the European Commission (EC) suggested that the use of UWB technology without mitigation is within the bandwidth of 4.2 to 4.8 GHz. It also accepted that in terms

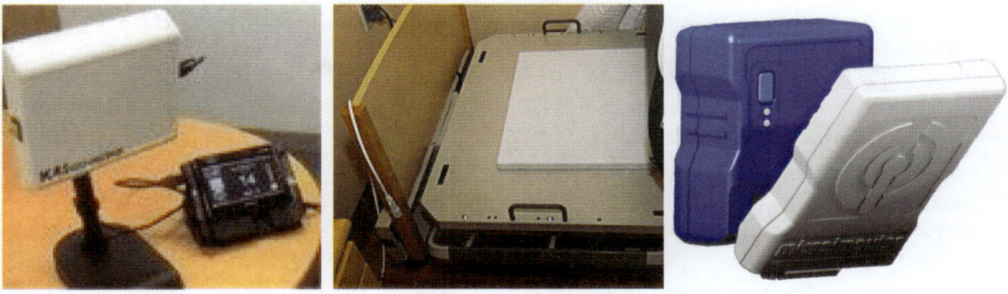

Fig. 11. Kai Sensors' technology platform enables wireless monitoring of vital signs (left); Wireless2000 (center), Microimpulse's VSM (right).

of the global use of this technology for medical as well as communication purposes, all UWB based devices shall operate above 6 GHz. Europe is likely to conform to this regulation by 2011. Furthermore, since most hospital devices operate at frequencies much lower than UWB, the possibility of electromagnetic interference caused by such devices is also minimal. This is likely to allow vendors convince the end users about the safety and utility of such devices, thereby easing the route to market entry.

2.2 Laser-based monitoring methods

In the 90's the first studies of skin deflections due to arterial blood pulses appeared; these were conducted with optical measurement systems (mostly laser interferometers), which, in those years, started to be available on the market. By means of a bulky, fiber-optic, Michelson interferometer, pulsatile movement of the artery (arterial wall) were firstly measured near a stenotic lesion in an embedded vessel, the maximum gradient of skin displacement has been shown to be proportional to the time derivative of the blood pressure profile within the underlying vasculature (Hong & Fox, 1997). Data were taken firstly on a phantom, then at eight different sites for manual palpation of rhythm and strength of arterial pulse, radial, brachial, carotid, temporal, popliteal, femoral, posterior tibial, and dorsalis pedis. Three cardiac auscultation points were also assessed by stethoscope: pulmonary (second left intercostal), tricuspid (lower left sternal border), and mitral valves (fifth intercostal space at the midclavicular line). This attempt was consider extremely promising, but still possible only in a laboratory environment were the optical interferometer can operate correctly. Nevertheless the fiber-optical probe used in this approach was placed over the skin by means of a skin adapter using a stethoscope bell placed on the distal side of the fiber (measurement side) need in order to minimize unwanted signal artifacts due to body movement. The authors observe that further research may be necessary to see whether this stretches or alters the skin at the sensing site, thus perturbing the natural skin surface vibration effect. This approach must therefore be considered (minimally) invasive and with contact.

The possibility to detect the skin deflection due to the pressure pulse and correlate with the carotid pulse was firstly demonstrated (Tomasini et al., 1998) using a laser Doppler vibrometer (Castellini et al., 2006); in this case, the observation was carried out without any physical contact with a distance between the sensing head and the volunteers of about 1.5 m. The set-up proposed was based on the use of a single point Laser Doppler Vibrometer (LDVi) aiming to the volunteer neck in correspondence to the skin overlaying the carotid. Some years after, researchers from the same group started an extensive and systematic analysis of the opportunities offered by the use of the LDVi as a non contact method (named vibrocardiography, VCG) to measure heart beat (Scalise et al., 2005, 2006 and 2008; Morbiducci et al., 2006), as well as the respiration activity (Scalise et al., 2011), the heart mechanics (Bocconcelli et al., 2006) and the artery stiffness (De Melis et al., 2008). Typically (Scalise et al., 2005), VCG, is used to monitor superficial chest displacement due to the heart activity (fig. 12).

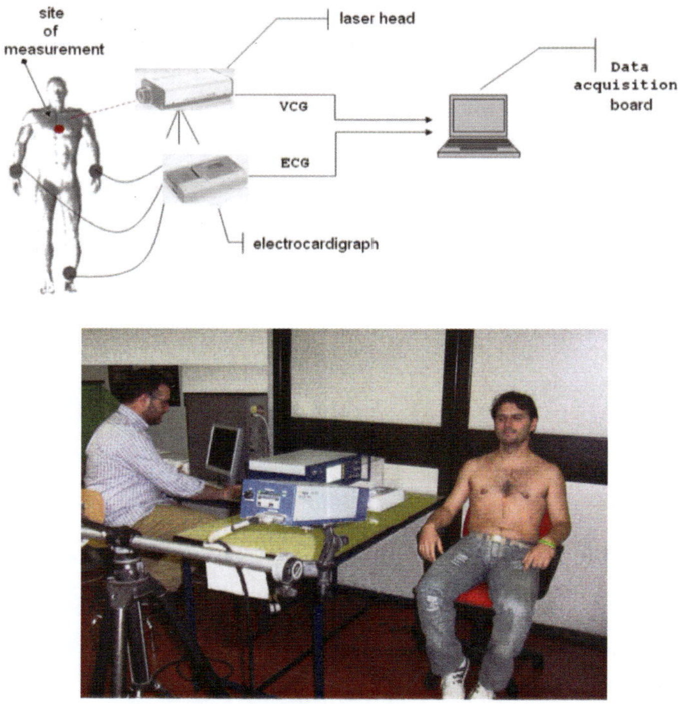

Fig. 12. Vibrocardiography set-up; Top: block diagram of the experimental set-up with the reference instrument (ECG); Bottom: Image of a test session.

Examples of typical signals, measured on two subjects (one male and one female), are reported in figure 13 with synchronous data acquisition from ECG reported for direct comparison.
Very high shore have been obtained with heart rate variability (HRV) carried out using the VCG (Morbiducci et al., 2006; Scalise and Morbiducci, 2008). Scatter plot of the HR measured by VCG and standard instrument (ECG) on the previously examined subjects, are reported in figure 14; the time series (fig. 15) built up from the time intervals between consecutive R peaks (RR), and VCG time intervals from the thorax (VV). Right side depicts a detail (50 beats) to show the close relationship of the two time series.
From results reported (Morbiducci et al., 2006; Scalise and Morbiducci, 2008), the results of the test of Bland-Altman put in evidence that significant differences are not present, from a clinical viewpoint. In fact, results showed mean percent differences of VCG derived descriptors, with respect to ECG ones, that do not threshold the 4.80% (3.03% mean value) for the LF/HF index and even lower for the other standard HRV parameters .

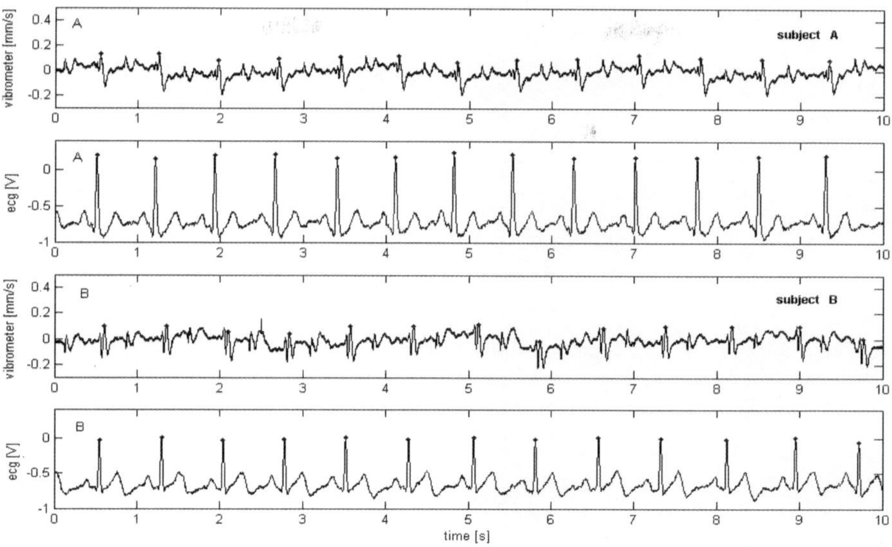

Fig. 13. Chest wall vibration (velocity) and ECG traces synchronously acquired, measured on two subjects (subject A: male, subject B: female).

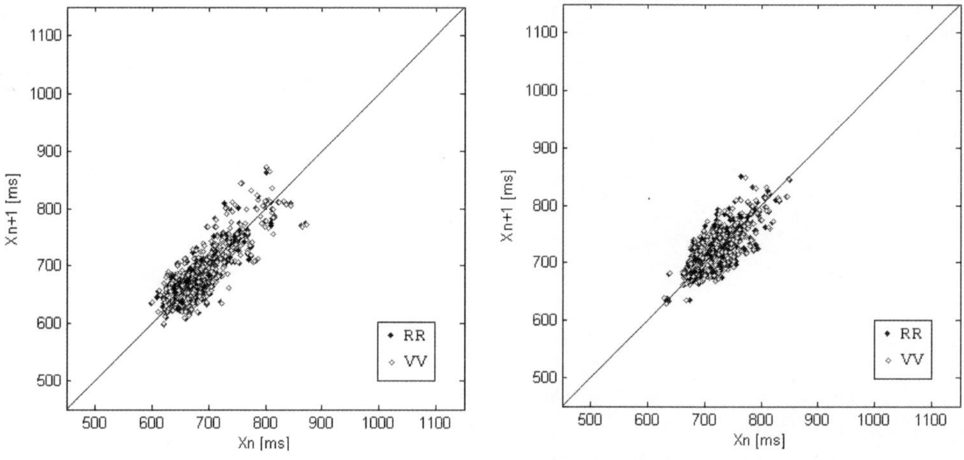

Fig. 14. Scatter plot of the heart rate measured by VCG (VV data) vs HR measured by ECG (RR).

The possibility to access the heart rate data from a different site respect to the chest wall was demonstrated (Scalise and Morbiducci, 2008) using the neck region (carotid site) as measurement site. High quality results are obtainable (fig. 16) and like for optical VCG signals measured in different sites of the chest wall (Morbiducci et al., 2006; Scalise et al., 2006), common morphologic features in the traces measured on the neck were observed,

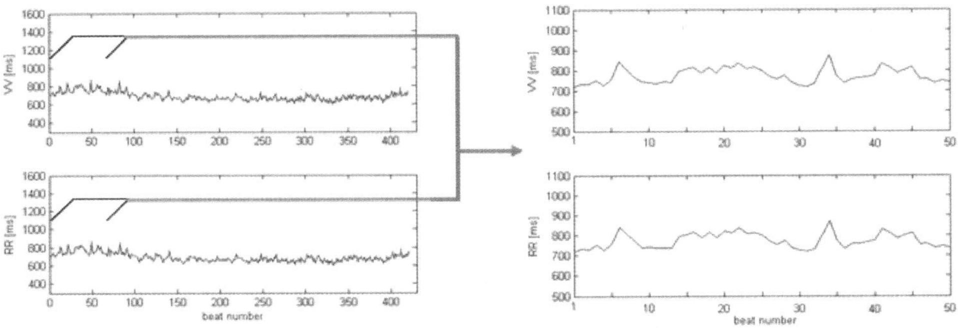

Fig. 15. Time series (relative to subject A and B of fig. 13) built up from the time intervals between consecutive R peaks (RR), and VCG time intervals from the thorax (VV). Right side depicts a detail (50 beats) to show the close relationship of the two time series.

with only inter-subject minor differences. HRV analysis, performed using VCG on the neck, agrees with the one derived from ECG with mean percent differences of VCG derived descriptors, with respect to ECG ones, < 2.94%. (relative to RMSSD) for the time domain and the 3.12% (relative to the sympatho-vagal balance LF/HF) for the frequency domain.

A very interesting comparison among ECG, phonocardiography (PCG) and VCG traces have been carried out in order to demonstrate the possibility to identify events of the cardiac mechanics, correlating the heart sounds relative to the closure of the mitral valve, and the following closure of the aortic and pulmonary valve with characteristic deflections identifiable on VCG traces (De Melis et al., 2007). Simultaneous acquisition of cardiac acoustic sounds, II-lead ECG trace and VCG are reported in figure 17, with indicated the S_1-S_2 and W_1-W_2 intervals (differences < 1.4 ms).

VCG was also explored (De Melis et al., 2008) as an alternative fully non contact method for the assessment of carotid-femoral pulse wave velocity (PWV), which is considered a gold standard method for assessing the stiffness of large arteries (high PWV values have been demonstrated to be associated with increased cardiovascular morbidity and mortality), and pulse transit time (PTT). With a simple approach (fig. 18), PWV and PTT were accurately measured with a mean PTTs of 75.85± 8.61 ms and 74.86± 8.63 ms for applanation tonometry (reference method) and VCG, respectively. A non contact method like optical VCG for the evaluation of large artery stiffness is considered of great interest because it could overcome limitations inherent to a contact method like arterial tonometry (based on contact piezo transducers manually kept in place), for which the debate on the influence of the contact of the probe over the skin on the measurements is still open in the scientific community.

A recent application of VCG has been reported as preliminary study for the cardiac resinchronization of patient using pacing devices (Bocconcelli et al., 2006). In figure 19, an example of simultaneous VCG and ECG beat monitoring is reported and compared with the same data acquired on a patient with weak ventricular depolarisation. Authors demonstrated the feasibility of VCG to provide data needed for a correct setting of the cardiac stimulator in order to provide optimal cardiac re-synchronization.

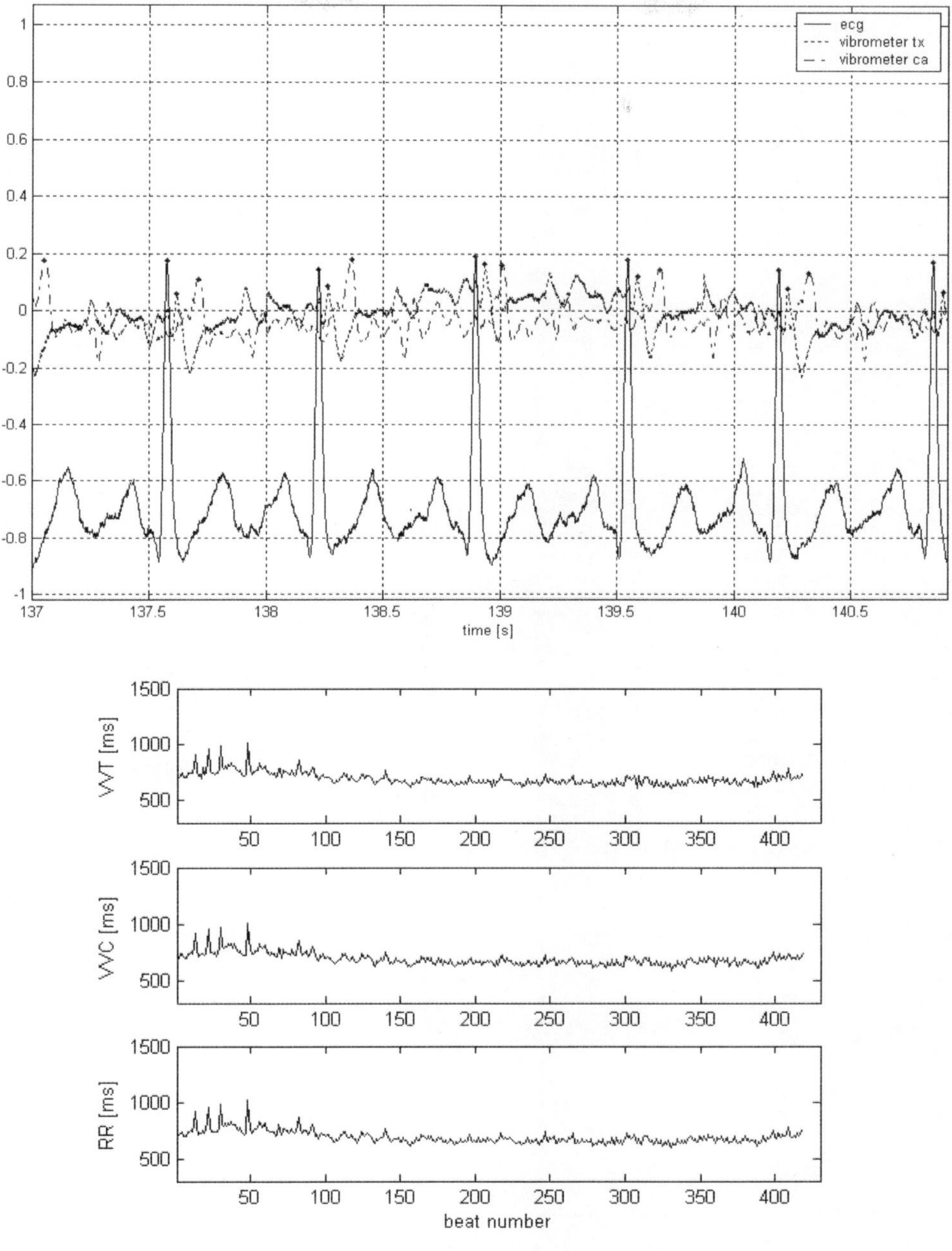

Fig. 16. ECG monitoring (in V) on a volunteer and simultaneous VCG trace (in mm/s) from chest wall and from carotid site (top);

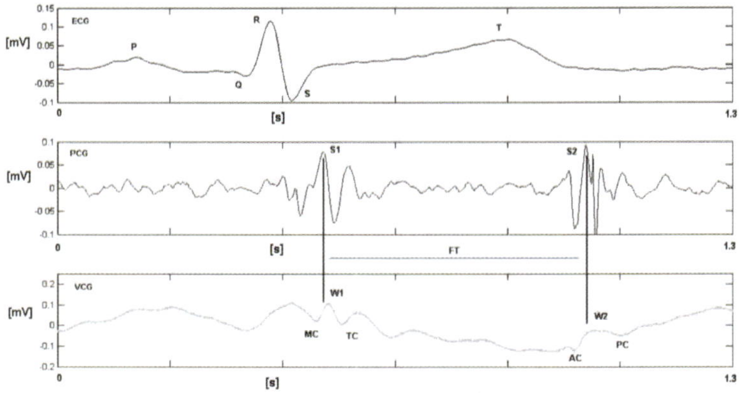

Fig. 17. Example of one beat recordings from VCG and PCG with II lead ECG compared with a gold standard vital signs representation.

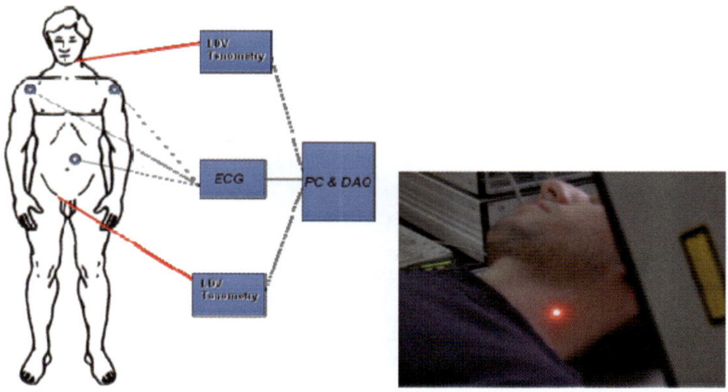

Fig. 18. Sketch of the measurement setup (left) and picture of measurement site (carotid artery).

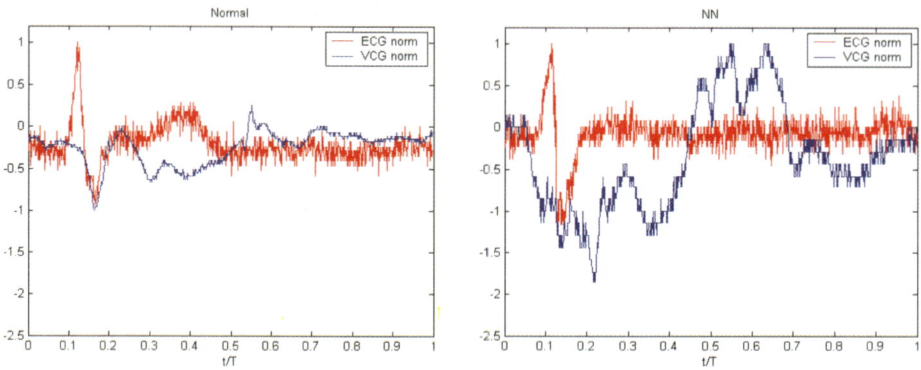

Fig. 19. ECG (in V) and VCG traces (in mm/s) for an healthy subject (left) and for a patient (right).

Very promising use of laser Doppler vibrometry have been proposed in the field of biometrics where the measure of cardiovascular activity as biometric marker appear to be promising (Chen et al., 2010; Rohrbaugh et al., 2007). In contrast to the traditional, contact ECG approach for cardiac activity monitoring, the signal examined is derived from movements of the skin associated with the blood pressure pulse in the underlying carotid artery using LDVi. The varied structure of the skin surface displacements (including some in the submicrometer range) comprising the LDVi signal would seem nearly impossible to mimic. Our studies confirm that the LDVi pulse signal is sufficiently textured to support a high level of discriminability among individuals. The signal changes in appearance somewhat from one occasion to the next, and is affected by factors such as physical exercise and mental stress. Data collected from 285 individuals showed good performance of LDVi and of the data processing method described especially on data collected within the same session; the discriminability characteristic of the LDV pulse is well maintained across an individual 5-min session. The increasing match error of the intersession tests may be due to time-varying factors.
Another field of application for laser-based heart rate monitoring methods has been proposed for distance monitoring of vital signs in risk environments. Proper functioning of the heart ensures the performance of the human body as well as sustenance of life, it can be used as a forward-looking indicator for assessing the performance limits of warfighters and athletes, prognosis of various health conditions, as well as for the determination of life signs in certain situations like triaging and battlefield management. Thus, in principle, detecting surface vibrations from the human subject allows information retrieval regarding the functionality and performance of the human heart. A novel laser-based vibrometer whose optical speckle-tolerant nature makes it ideal for assessing the surface vibration characteristics of, for example, human subjects whose surface quality is far from optically flat, is reported (Wang et al., 2010). The combination of excellent surface vibration detection sensitivity and optical speckle tolerance makes the novel pulsed laser vibrometer an ideal candidate for standoff monitoring and assessment of a human subject's cardiac activity and functionality. At the moment only preliminary, qualitative results are reported for laboratory tests with this special experimental set-up which seems to be extremely powerful allowing life signs detection in non-ideal measurement conditions (such as the case of directly on skin or directly on specific part of the body).

2.3 Image-based monitoring methods

The application of image-based methods for heart rate monitoring is based on the observation that the deflection of a human vessels due to heartbeats can be visually observed from the consequent deflection that the skin surrounding an important vase. One of the first use of image-based methods for HR monitoring (Da Costa, 1995; Parra & Da Costa, 2001) proposes to video acquire the deflections proposing two methods (fig. 20). In the first the skin is illuminated by a 2 mW HeNe laser beam in the neighborhood of the vein. The reflected speckle pattern is acquired, digitized and a specifically developed code, based on speckle image processing, is used to evaluate the skin displacement caused by the mechanical deflection produced by the arterial wall deflections due to the systolic pressure wave travelling along the vascular tree. In the second method a small mirror glued to the skin is illuminated by the laser beam. The position of the light spot resulting from intersection of the reflected beam with an opaque observation plane is recorded and plotted

as a function of time. Both the methods proposed allows the remote sensing of the heartbeats the later being (minimally) invasive requiring the need to glue a mirror on the subject skin.
Both the approach proposed don't report quantitative results; only a graph is reported and non correlations with reference signals (i.e. simultaneous ECG) are reported. Therefore, even if the solutions proposed were promising at the time when were presented, they can't be transferred to a real clinical environment or anyway can't be operated out of controlled conditions usual in laboratories of optics in the reported form. In fact, full filed digital speckle image experimental set-up, as well as laser reflection systems, need to have precise and accurate control of the subject to the set-up relative positions in order to isolate any artifact/vibration disturbance to the measurement data.

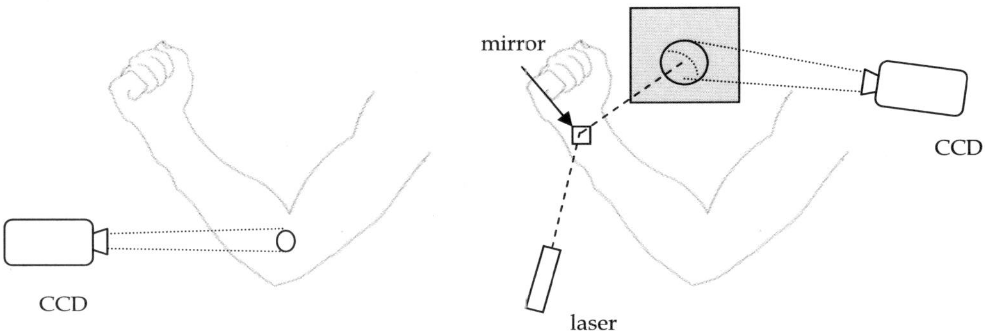

Fig. 20. Speckle image acquisition of skin surface deflections due to the systolic pressure wave (left) and laser reflectormetry of the mirror glued in correspondence of a large vase (right).

More recently (Takano & Ohta, 2007), it has been proposed a new device combining a time-lapse image from a handy video camera and image processing on a PC, and found that it could measure the 30s average heart and respiratory rates based on the changes in the brightness of the ROI set around the cheek of the unrestricted subject. Measurements were successfully conducted for subjects with or without facial cosmetics and that the system tended to detect the pulse rate more clearly around typical palpation points such as the common carotid artery and ulnar artery. Correlation coefficients of 0.90 has been obtained with respect heart rate measured with a pulse oxymeter.
One of the most recent and promising application of image-based techniques is the "cardiocam", as it has been named by its authors, which is a low-cost, non contact technology for measurement of physiological signals such as heart rate and breathing rate using a basic digital imaging device such as a webcam (Poh et al., 2010; Poh et al, 2011). The ability to perform remote measurements of vital signs is promising for enhancing the delivery of primary health care. It has been reported (Poh et al., 2011) Pearson's correlation coefficients among reference sensor and the web-camera-based system of r=1 for heart rate detection and of r=0.92 for HF and LF (common heart rate variability analysis parameters); the root-mean-squared error of the HR was 1.24 beats/min. In particular the system, developed at the Affective Computing research group at MIT laboratory, is suited for home applications and particularly for telemedicine, in fact the only sensing element utilised for heart rate monitoring is a standard web-camera which could be easily integrated on already

existing home furniture or home components such as mirrors or also utilising already existing camera such as the one integrated in most of the modern notebook or mobile phones. Despite these definitely promising advantage, still the robustness of the system and the efficiency of the procedure on large scale need to be demonstrated and improvement on the frame rate is required for adequate heart rate variability's analysis.

Finally another image-based system has been developed in collaboration with Philips Research Laboratory (Van Rooijen et al., 2010; Wieringa et al., 2005) mainly addressed for optical pletismography using non contact reflection mode imaging at three wavelengths. Respiration rate as well as heart rate mean values were very well correlated over a 50s window. A prototype of a small battery operated heart rate monitoring camera has been realised and demonstrated on professional swimmers for unrestrained heart rate measurement (Van Rooijen et al., 2010). Nevertheless at the moment further investigation need to be carried out for investigating the influence of factors such as movement artifacts, subcutaneous fat, skin thickness, skin pigmentation and blood pressure have not yet been investigated.

2.4 Other methods

An interesting application for non contact monitoring of heart (and lung) activity, has been demonstrated using magnetic induction (Steffen & Leonhardt, 2007). The physical principle demonstrated is that the mechanical actions of heart, diaphragm and thorax move blood and air through the body; by impedance point of view, this is a movement of well-conducting (blood) and poor conducting (air) matter inside the chest region. Inducing eddy currents into the tissue and measuring the re-inducted magnetic field externally, these impedance changes can be used as signals easily monitored. This is done using a simple arrangement based on one simple coil where excitation and measurement are performed. The proposed system assures a non contact monitoring (even if the coil needs to be placed sufficiently close to the thorax) and could be also integrated into textiles or integrated into bed. An high sensitivity to relative movements between coil and body is reported as the main limit of the technique.

The capacitive coupling method was also investigated for heartbeat detection through the subject's undergarments or an insulator (Kurita K, 2011). The potential of an electrode is measured against the body surface, thus, the capacitive coupling method enables detection of the human heartbeat under *in situ* conditions for a subject who is wearing clothing The capacitance is measured between the human body and an electrode that is isolated from the human body by a dielectric such as clothing. The experimental set-up used to demonstrate the principle is based on an electrode which is placed at a few centimeters from the subject' s chest, and the electrostatic induction current (on the order of pA) flowing through the electrode is measured. In such a scenario, we can express the induced current I flowing through the measurement electrode which is related to the electrostatically induced current generated because of the human heartbeat. The proposed method requires the use of a detection electrode (about 5 cm of radius) placed at 3 cm from the subject's chest. The method appears promising even if the sensitivity to external induction currents (common in non-laboratory and hospitals environments), the necessity to use filters and the very low amplitude of the sensing currents (<pA) appear to be the weak points of this method.

A different approach, reported in literature, is based on the pressure oscillations sensed from a sensing mat placed under a pillow (Zhu et al., 2006; Chen et al., 2005). The method is here reported because it is a non contact method even if it requires the use of a system (pillow) through which the pulse rate (and the respiration rhythm) is detected. Real-time implementation is conducted using a pressure sensors sensing trough catheters an air-free water-filled vinyl tube under a pillow during sleep. Data reported are very sensitive to body movements and to sensor placement below the pillow, which makes the proposed method needing further improvement before the use on large scale.

A simpler approach is reported for measuring the physiological parameters, using an ultrasonic sensing of heart and respiration rate and movement behavior, developed for elderly people which are in bed. Bed structure oscillations due to the respiration and heart pulses are detected using an ultrasonic transmitter and an ultrasonic receiver installed in both sides of the bed rail (Mukai et al., 2009). When a person is lying in any position, on any bed area, then his/her physiological parameters alter the shape of the mattress and amplitude modulate the received signal. When the person is out of bed, the amplitude does not change, so the system also monitors in/out of bed status, allowing the detecting if the patient has left the bed, which makes it useful for use on subject monitoring (especially for elderly).

3. Final remarks

People are not used to wearing sensors in contact with their body in everyday life and for prolonged period of time, thus, in general, the compliance with sensors, electrodes and devices is very low. Nevertheless, there is a growing interest in continuous monitoring of the physiological activity of patients and non patients in order to gain information on their health status. The ideal solution would consist of using sensing systems that do not require physical contact with the user: the subject is not touched by a sensor at all. Accordingly, the sensing process could be unobtrusive to the user. Heart rate or respiration rate, for example, could be continuously monitored and data transmitted for remote signal analysis and feature extraction, allowing recognition of possible anomalous behavior or worsening of vital signs.

As an important part of the pervasive health care systems are the sensing units, the computation units and the communication units that are directly related with the implementation costs of these kind of systems, but also with the easy acceptance by the users. Referring to the sensing units, the non-invasive and the unobtrusive characteristics are important requirements taking into account the acceptance from the user. In the past, different solutions have been proposed for improving the acceptance of such systems: the use of non conductivity electrodes for ECG recording, where the electrodes are embedded on the chair, ballistocardiography sensing, where the sensing part is embedded in bed, chair or wheelchair, in furniture and photoplethismography using oxymeters. Sensing units, as part of ubiquitous systems, which work without mechanical and electrical contact with the subject represent a big challenge.

A possible field of application of new non contact method for heart rate monitoring is the heart rate variability (HRV) which has been shown to be a predictor of mortality after myocardial infarction and it is also associated with congestive heart failure, diabetic neuropathy, depression post-cardiac transplant, susceptibility to SIDS and poor survival in premature babies. HRV studies have also been used to examine autonomic function in the context of bodily pain. In recent years, the stress evaluation technique using the heart rate variability (HRV) has been recognized widely as an advanced diagnostic tool to prevent the stress syndrome, for example, sleep sign while driving in a car, etc. HRV is typically carried out by means of long ECG analysis (more then 5/6 min).The HRV is obtained calculating RR intervals, however, evaluation of stress by ECG is not well suited for long-time monitoring due to the fact that several electrodes must be attached directly to a human body to acquire the ECG data. For this application non contact heart rate monitoring technique appear to be extremely interesting, especially for out of the hospital applications where application of electrodes are not feasible.

Another interesting field of application is represented by the need of HR monitoring of subjects during MRI; in such case, in fact, it is not recommended the presence of any metallic object which could create a serious risk for the patient (due to the presence of very high RF field). In such a case the laser-based as well as the image-based method reported are very encouraging avoiding heart rate (as well as respiration rate) monitoring without the need of metallic or conductive electrodes and reducing the possible interference effects.

A second important field of application where all the non contact heart rate monitoring technique could find important success is when the patient (or subject) can't be easily accesses (subject buried under building ruins), can't be safely accessed (contaminated subject) or it represents a risk for the operators to apply traditional monitoring procedures (such as the case of suspected victims). Remote sensing opportunities offered by laser-based, image based or electromagnetic-base techniques are extremely promising for those applications and have been demonstrated (at list in laboratory conditions) able to operate in such difficult conditions.

Nowadays, the electromagnetic-based systems are more advanced respect to the other non contact methods; the developments in the area of Doppler radar permit to develop unobtrusive cardiac and respiratory activity measurements that satisfied the above mentioned requirements. Doppler radars in continuous wave (CW) and pulsed radar (UWB) have, recently, been introduced to various applications, including home monitoring, research and rescue operations. As final remarks, it can be observed as the RF or MW based monitoring techniques appear to be among the most close to be ready for commercial distribution (first systems are already available, as seen in paragraph 2.1). Very interesting are the possibility to monitor from distance and to allow the monitoring also trough layers of different materials (tissues, clothes, wall, etc) which solve the problem of a direct access to the subject skin as it is for the laser-based methods. The aspects related to the exposition to electromagnetic fields are resolved considering the very low power density used for the cited applications (typically $< 1mW/cm^2$). Nevertheless, among the many papers published in this field, it appears necessary to act in a direction of a deep analysis of the phenomenon (interaction between RF wave and target, scattering from the target and the other environment objects, effect on the signal of the beam and of the antenna characteristics, etc.) using numerical simulation or developing specific codes in order to allow an optimal design of the RF monitoring system based not on empirical base, but on model based data of the many possible situations.

There are three benefits comparing MW sensing with ECG recording system. First, the subject will feel comfortable and relaxed without any physical and psychological burden, which the waveforms of the heartbeat will more objective. Second, the heartbeat can be detected at a distance of several meters by penetrating the clothing, thus the microwave sensor can be attached to the ceiling of a room or somewhere can not be seen by the subject. The procedure of the setup will be easier than the 3-lead ECG recording system, which needs the professional person to operate it. Finally, the microwave sensor can be easily integrated in unobtrusive healthcare systems.

However, two aspects limit electromagnetic-based systems the current use in ambulatory recording: e.m systems are susceptible to significant motion artifacts and the propagation loss in free space. Advanced signal processing represents a possible solution for the reduction of motion artifacts overlapped with the heartbeat signal, which might enable the sensors to be effectively used for long-term recording in mobile patients. Another aspect is that the propagation loss of the microwave sensor in free space should be taken into consideration during the recording and when the distance is increased, the transmitted power should be increased as well. Finally with the development of the integrated circuits, high gain and narrow side-lobe antenna in tiny size, the electromagnetic sensors can be made very small in size.
In reality, however, detecting human heartbeat at standoff via surface vibration monitoring poses a number of major technical hurdles. First of all, while physicians routinely monitor patient's heartbeat by accessing specific areas of the human body like the chest, carotid, and temples where surface displacement caused by heartbeat is most profound, it is to be noted that such accessibility can be very difficult, if not impossible, to achieve in situations where manipulation of the human subject's body is next to impossible for e.m. based systems, while feasible for laser-based methods. These situations include the inspection and evaluation of wounded, immobilized war fighters in the battlefield, real-time, standoff monitoring of astronauts operating inside space suits, as well as the monitoring of burn patients. The second technical challenge is the fact that while human body conducts acoustic vibrations relatively well, significant attenuation in the vibration strength excited by the heartbeat can be caused by the clothing, equipment, and other gears that the human subject might be wearing. As such, the surface vibrations that the human subject exhibits at the body parts accessible by the standoff interrogation technology can be greatly diminished, leading to the requirement of highly sensitive detection technologies in order to decipher such minute surface vibrations. Another technical hurdle relates specifically to laser based technologies which employ laser beams to conduct standoff monitoring of human subjects. Just like most of the objects we encounter in our daily lives, the surface quality of the human subject is far from optically flat, leading to the presence of optical speckles in the back-scattered light beam. Such optical speckles cause conventional coherent detection sensors to fail due to the random nature of phase fluctuations in the optical speckles, leading to erroneous output readings and mis-information. As human subject's body surface could be contaminated with sweat, grease, dirt, and even blood, it is safe to assume that abundant speckles exist in the laser light beam back-scattered from human subject's surface. Thus, whatever laser based technology is to be used to monitor the surface vibration of human subjects, it is vital that they be highly tolerant to the presence of speckles in the light beams so as to minimize the output of erroneous information in analyzing the cardiac functionality of the subject under standoff interrogation.
Image-based and the other methods reported appear to be promising for the simplicity of the hardware, the high degree of integration and the (probably) final cost, even if they need to be more deeply investigated in order to demonstrate they feasibility.
Finally it is important to evaluate the possible scenarios for the future use of noncontact electromagnetic system for the detection of heart rate. With several potential medical applications and ready-to-launch UWB radar based monitoring products, the medical device industry is likely to observe significant changes. One of the biggest advantages for the UWB based medical sensing products is the low cost associated with them (this is not still to be proven for the laser-based systems as well as fort the others techniques here

proposed). With budgetary concerns being a perennial challenge for both the European and US medical device markets, these devices are likely to find ready acceptance. However, whether these technologies shall gradually cannibalize the conventional vital signs monitoring devices market is yet to be ascertained. Most of These technologies are likely to target unconventional end user groups (including home care, low acuity areas in hospitals and the military sector) instead of the conventional high-end hospital market and this seems to prospect the possibility to create a niche market segment for itself instead of penetrating into the conventional markets. Amongst all the UWB based medical devices, it is likely that the vital signs monitoring device to hit the market first. The progress of this niche market segment shall be observed carefully by other global vendors selling vital signs and patient monitoring devices. It is likely that many of the new entrants could get acquired by the leading patient monitoring vendors who do not have a significant presence in the home care or low acuity care market segments. This will help them diversify to new markets and ensure that their existing market shares are sustained, if not increased.

4. References

Abowd G., Bobick A., Essa I., Mynatt E., and Rogers W (2002). The Aware Home: Developing Technologies for Successful Aging. In *AAAI Workshop and Automation as Care giver.*

Alexander CM, Teller LE, Gross JB (1989). Principles of pulse oximetry: theoretical and practical considerations. *Anesth Analg.*;68:368-376.

Aubert AE, Welkenhuysen L, Montald J, de Wolf L, Geivers H, Minten J, Kesteloot H, Geest H (1984). Laser method for recording displacement of the heart and chest wall, *J Biom Eng,* (2), 134-40.

Azevedo SG, McEwan TE (1996), Micropower Impulse Radar. *Science and Technology Review,* UCRL-52000-96-1/2.

Bocconcelli P, Pierantozzi A, Scalise L, Morbiducci U, De Melis M, Corbucci G (2006). Una nuova tecnologia senza per la valutazione della meccanica cardiaca nei pazienti scompensati: la vibrometria laser. 6° Congresso Nazionale Associazione Italiana Aritmologia e Cardiostimolazione (AIAC), 30 Marzo - 1 Aprile 2006.

Castellini P, Martarelli M, Tomasini EP (2006). Laser Doppler Vibrometry: Development of advanced solutions answering to technology's needs. *Mech Syst Sig Proc,* 20(6):1265-1285.

Chan KH, Lin JC. (1987). Microprocessor-based cardiopulmonary rate monitor. *Medical and Biological Engineering and Computing,* 25(1):41-44.

Chen M, O'Sullivan JA, Singla N, Sirevaag EJ, Kristjansson SD, Lai PH, Kaplan AD, Rohrbaugh JW (2010). Laser Doppler vibrometry measures of physiological function: Evaluation of biometric capabilities. *IEEE Transactions on Information Forensics and Security,* 5(3):449-60,.

Chen W, Zhu X, Nemoto T, Kanemitsu Y, Kitamura K, Yamakoshi K (2005). Unconstrained detection of respiration rhythm and pulse rate with one under-pillow sensor during sleep. *Med Biol Eng Comp,* 43(2):306–312.

Chia MY, Leong SW, Sim CK, Chan KM (2005). Through-wall UWB radar operating within FCC's mask for sensing heart beat and breathing rate. *IEEE European Microwave Conf. 2005,* 3(14).

Da Costa (1995). Optical remote sensing of heartbeats. *Optics Communications,* 117(5-6):395-98.

Daisuke Nagae and Atsushi Mase(2010). Measurement of heart rate variability and stress evaluation by using microwave reflectometric vital signal sensing. *Rev Sci Instrum* 81, 094301.

De Melis M, Morbiducci U, Scalise L, Tomasini EP, Delbeke D, Baets R, Van Bortel LM, Segers P (2008). A non contact approach for the evaluation of large artery stiffness: a preliminary study., *Am J Hyp*, 21:1280-83.

Dressier W (1970)., *Clinical aids in cardiac diagnosis* . Grune & Stratton.

Droitcour A, Lubecke V, Lin J, Boric-Lubecke O(1995). A microwave radio for Doppler radar sensing of vital signs, *IEEE MTT-S Int. Microw. Symp. Dig.*, 175.

Durand LG, Pibarot P (1995). Digital signal processing of the phonocardiogram: review of the most recent advancements. *Crit Rev Biomed Eng.*

Einthoven W (1902). Galvanometrische registratie van het menselijk electrocardiogram [Galvanometric registration of the human electrogram]. In: Herinneringsbundel Prof. S.S. Rosenstern Leiden, the Netherlands: Eduard Ijdo; 1902; 101–106.

Fowler NO (1962). *Physical diagnosis of heart disease*. Macmillan, New York.

Garbey M, Sun N, Merla A and Pavlidis I (2007). Contact-free measurement of cardiac pulse based on the analysis of thermal imagery, *IEEE Trans. Biomed. Eng.* 54(8), 1418–1426.

Gorgas, DL (2004). *Vital signs and patient monitoring techniques*, Clinical Procedures in Emergency Medicine 4th ed (JR Roberts and JR Hedges, Eds) Sauders, Philadelphia, USA.

Gorgels APM (2007). *Chapter 3 Electrocardiography*. In: Willerson JT, Cohn JN, Wellens HJJ, Holmes DR Jr, eds. Cardiovascular Medicine, 3d ed. Springer, London, UK.

Harland CJ, Clark TD and Prance RJ (2002). Electric potential probes-new directions in the remote sensing of the human body, *Meas. Sci. Technol.*, 13:163–169.

Hein JJ, Wellens MD, Gorgels AP (2004). The Electrocardiogram 102 Years After Einthoven. *Circulation*, 109:562-64.

Hong H and Fox M (1997). Noninvasive detection of cardiovascular pulsations by optical doppler techniques. *J of Biomedical Optics*, 2(4):382-390.
http://lifewaveinc.com/
http://www.microimpulse.no
http://www.wireless2000.com

Immoreev I, Tao TH (2008). UWB radar for patient monitoring, *Aerospace and Electronic Systems Magazine*, 11(18).

Ishijima M (1993). Monitoring of electrocardiograms in bed without utilizing body surface electrodes, *IEEE Trans. Biomed. Eng.*, 40(6):593–594.

Kim HJ, Kim KH, Hong YS and Choi Jj (2007). Measurement of human heartbeat and respiration signals using phase detection radar, *Rev Sci Instrum*, 78, 04703-1.

Kurita K (2011). Note: Human heartbeat measurement on the basis of current generated by electrostatic induction. *Rev Sci Inst* 82, 026105.

Lim YG, Kim KK and Park KS (2006). ECG measurement on a chair without conductive contact", *IEEE Trans. Biomed. Eng* ,53:956.

Lim YG, Ko Keun Park, Kwang Suk (2007).ECG Recording on a Bed During Sleep Without Direct Skin-Contact, *IEEE Transactions on Biomedical Engineering*, 54(4):718.

Lin, J. C. (1975). Noninvasive microwave measurement of respiration. *Proc. IEEE*, p. 1430.

Lin J C, Kiernicki J, Kiernicki M, Wollschlaeger PB (1979). Microwave Apexcardiography. *IEEE Transactions on Microwave Theory and Techniques*, 27(6): 618-620.

Lu G, Yang F, Tian Y, Jing X, Wang J (2009). Contact-free Measurement of Heart Rate Variability via a Microwave Sensor. *Sensors*. 9(12):9572-9581.

Matsuda, Toshiyuki, Makikawa, Masaaki (2008). ECG monitoring of a car driver using capacitively-coupled electrodes, *Engineering in Medicine and Biology Society, 2008. EMBS 2008. 30th Annual International Conference of the IEEE,*: 1315 - 1318, 20-25 Aug. 2008

Matsui T, Hagisawa K, Ishizuka T et al (2004) A novel method to prevent secondary exposure of medical and rescue personnel to toxic materials under biochemical hazard conditions using microwave radar and infrared thermography. *IEEE Trans Biomed Eng* 51:2184–2188.

Matsui T, Ishizuka T, Takase B et al (2004) Non contact determination of vital sign alterations in hypovolemic states induced by massive hemorrhage: an experimental attempt to monitor the condition of injured persons behind barriers or under disaster rubble. *Med Biol Eng Comput* 42:807–811

Mei C, O'Sullivan JA, Singla N., Sirevaag EJ, Kristjansson SD, Po-Hsiang L, Kaplan AD, Rohrbaugh JW(2010). Laser Doppler Vibrometry Measures of Physiological Function: Evaluation of Biometric Capabilities. *IEEE Transactions on Information Forensics and Security archive*, 5(3).

Morbiducci U, Scalise L, De Melis M, Grigioni M (2006). Optical vibrocardiography: a novel tool for optical monitoring of cardiac activity. *Annals of Biomedical Engineering* 35(1):45-58.

Morris, G. M. (1954). A review of ballistocardiography. *Journal of the American Medical Womens Association* 1972, 9(12), 391-393.

Mukai K, Yonezawa Y, Ogawa H, Maki H and Caldwell MW (2009). A remote monitor of bed patient cardiac vibration, respiration and movement. *31st Ann Int Conf IEEE EMBS* Minneapolis, Minnesota, USA, September 2-6.

Parra, JE, Da Costa, G (2001). Optical remote sensing of heartbeats. *Proceedings of SPIE - The International Society for Optical Engineering*, 4368, 113-121.

Paulson CN, Chang JT, Romero CE, Watson J, Pearce FJ, Levin N (2005). Ultra-wideband Radar Methods and Techniques of Medical Sensing and Imaging. *SPIE International Symposium on Optics East* Boston, USA, Oct. 23-25.

Poh, MZ, McDuff, DJ, Picard, RW (2011). Advancements in Non contact, Multiparameter Physiological Measurements Using a Webcam, *IEEE Transactions on Biomedical Engineering*, 58(1):7-11.

Poh, M.Z., McDuff, D.J., Picard, R.W. (2010). Non contact, Automated Cardiac Pulse Measurements Using Video Imaging and Blind Source Separation, *Optics Express*, 18(10):10762-10774.

Poliac MO, Zanetti J, Salerno DM, Wilcox GL (1991). Seismocardiogram (SCG) interpretation using neural networks. *4th IEEE Symp Computer-based Medical Systems*.

Pollock, P (1957). Ballistocardiography: A Clinical Review. *Canadian Medical Association Journal*, 76(9), 778-783.

Ramachandran G, Singh M (1989). Three-dimensional reconstruction of cardiac displacement patterns on the chest wall during the P, QRS and T-segments of the ECG by laser speckle interferometry. *Med Biol Eng* 27(5).

Rohrbaugh JW et al. (2007). The Physiology of Threat: Remote Assessment Using Laser Doppler Vibrometry . *The Journal of Credibility Assessment, and Witness Psychology*, 7(2):17-19.

Salerno DM, Zanetti J (1990). Seismocardiography: A new technique for recording cardiac vibration. Concept, method and initial observations. *J Cardiov Tech*, 9:2.

Sandham W et al. (1998). Multiresolution wavelet decomposition of the seismocardiogram. *IEEE Tr Signal Processing*, 46:9.

Scalise L. et al. (2005a). Optical monitoring of heart rate variability. *Laser in Medical Science*, 20, s25.

Scalise L et al. (2005b). Optical monitoring of heart beat. In *Modelling in Medicine and Biology*, WIT press, 181-190.

Scalise L et al. (2006)A laser Doppler approach to cardiac motion monitoring: Effects of surface and measurement position. *Proc SPIE 7th Int Conf on Vibration Measurements by Laser Techniques: Advances and Applications*, Ancona.

Scalise L , Morbiducci U (2008). Non contact monitoring from carotid artery using optical vibrocardiography. *Med Eng & Phy*, 30(4): 490-97.

Scalise L, Ercoli I, Marchionni P, Tomasini E P (2011). Measurement of Respiration Rate in Preterm Infants by Laser Doppler Vibrometry. *Proc. 2011 IEEE International Symposium on Medical Measurements and Applications (MeMeA 2011)*, 418-422.

Staderini E M. (2002). UWB radars in medicine. *IEEE Aerosp. Electron. Syst. Mag.*, p.13.

Steffen M, Aleksandrowicz A, Leonhardt S (2007). Mobile Noncontact Monitoring of Heart and Lung Activity. *IEEE Transactions on Biomedical Circuits and Systems*, 4(1):250-57.

Takano C, Y Ohta (2007). Heart rate measurement based on a time-lapse image. *Med Eng & Phy*, 29(8):853-857.

Tanaka S, Matsumoto Y, Wakimoto K (2002) Unconstrained and non-invasive measurement of heart-beat and respiration periods using a phonocardiographic sensor. *Med Biol Eng Comput* 40:246–252

Tateishi N., Mase A., Bruskin L., Kogi Y., Ito N., Shirakata T., and Yoshida S. (2007). Microwave Measurement of Heart Beat and Analysis Using Wavelet Transform. *Proceedings of the 2007 Asia Pacific Microwave Conference*, Bangkok, 2007, pp. 2151–2153.

Tomasini EP et al. (1998). Carotid artery pulse wave measured by a laser vibrometer. *Proc SPIE of the 3rd Int Conf on Vibration Measurements by Laser Techniques: Advances and Applications (3411*), Ancona, 1998;: 611-616.

Van Rooijen V, de Voogd-Claessen L, Lauche K, Jeanne V, van der Vliet R (2010). Development of a new product for unrestrained heart rate measurement in swimming: a user centered design approach. *Procedia Engineering* , vol. 2, no. 2, pp. 2693-2699.

Wahr JA, Tremper KK, Diab M (1995). Pulse oximetry. *Respiratory Care Clinics of North America*.1:77-105.

Wang C,Trivedi S, Rodriguez P, Jin F,Kutcher S, Swaminathan V, Nagaraj S, Quoraishee S, Prasad N (2010). Non contact Human Cardiac Functionality Assessment Using a High Sensitivity Pulsed Laser Vibrometer. Proceedings of *27th Annual Army Science Conference*, Orlando, Fla., Nov. 29 - Dec. 2. , 2010.

Webster J.B. (1988). *Encyclopedia of medical devices and instrumentation*, Vol. 4, Wiley, New York, USA.

Welch JP, DeCesare R, Hess D (1990). Pulse oximetry: instrumentation and clinical applications. *Respiratory Care*. 35:584-601.

Wieringa FP, Mastik F and van der Steen AFW (2005). Contactless Multiple Wavelength Photoplethysmographic Imaging: A First Step Toward SpO2 Camera Technology. *Annals of Biomedical Engineering* 33(8), 1034-1041.

Zhu X, Chen W, Nemoto T, Kanemitsu Y, Kitamura K, Yamakoshi K and Wei D (2006). Real-Time Monitoring of Respiration Rhythm and Pulse Rate During Sleep. *IEEE Transactions on Biomedical Engineering*, 53(12):2553-2564.

3

Low-Frequency Response and the Skin-Electrode Interface in Dry-Electrode Electrocardiography

Cédric Assambo and Martin J. Burke
University of Dublin, Trinity College
Ireland

1. Introduction

In recent years, there has been a growing interest in the area of ambulatory electrocardiogram (ECG) recording using dry or unjelled electrodes for long-term physiological monitoring. The key advantage of dry electrodes is the elimination of allergic reactions or other forms of skin irritation, commonly associated with electrolyte gels. It results in the improvement of patient comfort and compliance, allowing the recording technique to cater for a wider range of users such as elderly, the long-term ill, cardiac rehabilitation patients, paediatrics and neonates. Furthermore, dry-electrode recording does not require preparation of the electrodes before or after application apart from cleaning and they can be re-used almost indefinitely. The durability of dry electrodes over gel-based ones permits their shelf-life to be extended and considerably increases the length of time for which they can be worn, allowing long-term ambulatory ECG recording at much lower cost. Embedded in remote telemetry systems, dry-electrode ECG recording can thus contribute to the improvement of health care delivery.
The investigation of the use of dry electrodes for ECG monitoring has led to the development of several pasteless electrode systems which overcome the disadvantages associated with traditional approaches employing wet electrodes. The following question however was immediately raised: how should the recording amplifier be adapted to the high source impedance commonly associated with dry electrodes? Optimised designs of the amplifier front-end have usually involved measuring the impedance of the skin-electrode interface (Burke & Gleeson, 2000; Chang et al., 2010; Ko et al., 1970; Mühlsteff & Such, 2004; Valverde et al., 2004). Some solutions have then inserted resistors in series with unbalanced electrodes to match the effective impedance seen at each input of the recording amplifier (Lee et al., 2006). Others have fabricated dry electrodes having impedances lower in magnitude than those of conventional Ag/AgCl wet electrodes (Chang et al., 2010; Wolfe & Reinhold, 1974). Commercial dry-electrode Holter monitors providing diagnostic quality ECGs are however not available to date. The recent development in 2009 of a wearable two-channel dry-electrode ECG system called *care.mon* has shown some prospects in the realisation of long-term telemetric application in the near future (Fuhrhop et al., 2009). The designers have admitted, however, that their prototype cannot get a signal of the same quality as that of a standard electrode Holter system.
A critical source of error was soon identified as low-frequency distortion introduced at the amplifier's front-end. In this chapter, the authors show how high-pass filtering can affect the quality of the recorded ECG waveform and demonstrate that the risk of distortion is

exacerbated by the presence of a frequency dependent skin-electrode impedance. New approaches for the determination of the model parameters of the skin-electrode interface and new input impedance requirements for dry-electrode ECG recording are then presented.

2. Importance of the recorder's low-frequency response in diagnostic quality electrocardiography

To ensure that the electrocardiograph's output signal is an accurate representation of the physiological input waveform, the amplifier must faithfully reproduce all frequency components of the ECG signal. Out-of-band high frequency interfering signals are normally removed from the preamplifier's output by implementing linear-phase low-pass filters. However, distortion introduced by an inadequate low-frequency response cannot generally be corrected in real time by simple filtering in the subsequent amplification stages (Tayler & Vincent, 1983). The quality of the recorder's low-frequency response relies therefore on the performance of the preamplifier's front-end. To prevent recording error caused by the electrocardiograph, the preamplifier must preserve the ECG signal by providing flat amplitude response and linear or zero phase within the ECG bandwidth (Berson & Pipberger, 1966; Tayler & Vincent, 1983). Failure to fulfil these requirements can have serious clinical implications.

2.1 Diagnostic implications of a poor low-frequency response

Berson & Pipberger have demonstrated that ECG preamplifiers implementing high-pass filters with a poor low-frequency amplitude response are a potential source of recording error that may lead to misdiagnosis of serious cardiac conditions (Berson & Pipberger, 1966). They concluded that an increase of the filter's cutoff frequency above 0.05 Hz or a roll-off greater than 6 dB per octave causes distortion of the S-T segment and the T wave of the ECG waveform. Yet, accurate measurement of slow deflections, especially in the first quarter of the ST-T complex, is usually crucial for assessing the condition of the heart and its response to therapy (Symanski & Gettes, 1993). For example, acute myocardial infarction, commonly known as heart attack, is frequently accompanied by an elevation of the ST segment but inadequate low-frequency response reduces this elevation and can produce an inversion of the terminal part of the T wave, as shown in Fig. 1(a). In addition, it was reported that the ECG of patients who had suffered damage to the surface of the heart, referred to as an old infarct, usually shows a downward sloping S-T segment (Berson & Pipberger, 1966). Fig. 1(b) illustrates how poor high-pass filtering can modify the S-T segment by converting a downward slope into an upward slope, which has a different clinical interpretation.

It was found that low-frequency distortion is generally greater for abnormal than for normal ECG waveforms and for records having essentially monophasic QRS patterns than for those having biphasic QRS complexes. Besides, it was observed that the increase in heart rate associated with exercise can alter recording error in an unpredictable manner (Berson & Pipberger, 1966).

The works of Berson & Pipberger were followed by studies led by Tayler & Vincent on the low-frequency phase response of filters used in ECG recording (Tayler & Vincent, 1983). They concluded that phase nonlinearity is also a major source of recording error and misdiagnosis. For example, myocardial ischaemia is a disease that reduces the supply of blood to the heart muscle and normally manifests itself in the ECG record as elevation or depression of ST segments (Lynch et al., 1980). However, false ST segment shifts such as those depicted in Fig. 2(a) have been noted with ambulatory ECG recorders exhibiting a nonlinear phase

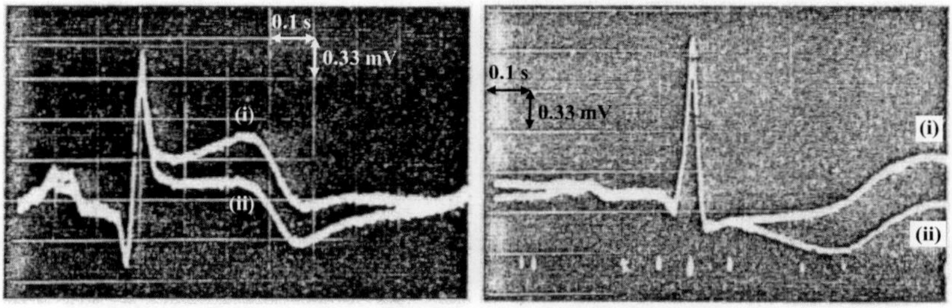

(a) Acute infarct record. (b) Old infarct record.

Fig. 1. Oscilloscope photographs of the electrocardiogram of patients suffering from (a) acute myocardial infarction and (b) an old infarct (from (Berson & Pipberger, 1966)). In both pictures, the upper record, labelled (i), is obtained with a simulated dc amplifier system while the lower record , (ii), is the output of a high-pass filter having a 0.5-Hz cutoff and 24-dB-per-octave roll-off.

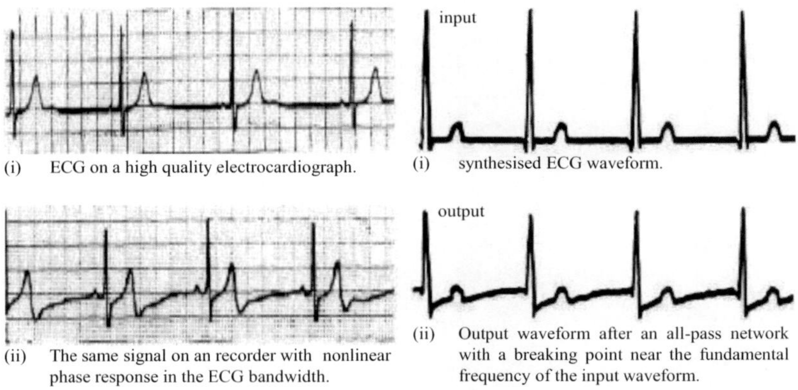

(a) Effect of phase distortion on a patient's ECG. (b) Effect of an all-pass network with nonlinear phase response.

Fig. 2. Electrocardiograms showing the effect of low-frequency distortion caused by nonlinear phase response in the bandwidth of the ECG signal from (a) a patient's record and (b) a synthesised ECG waveform (modified from (Tayler & Vincent, 1983)). In (b), the input waveform is filtered by an all-pass network with flat amplitude response from dc to 10 kHz ($\pm$ 1 dB), but a nonlinear phase response with a breaking point approaching the fundamental frequency of the input waveform.

response at low frequency. Results revealed that the ST segment is more readily affected by distortion when the point of maximum phase nonlinearity approaches the fundamental frequency of the ECG signal, as shown in Fig. 2(b). Once phase nonlinearity is introduced at the preamplifier front stage, its effects on the ST-T complex cannot be corrected subsequently without distorting other portions of the ECG waveform (Tayler & Vincent, 1983).

2.2 Low-frequency performance requirements of ECG recorders

The empirical findings reported in (Berson & Pipberger, 1966) and (Tayler & Vincent, 1983) have played a key role in defining the frequency response requirements of ECG recorders utilised today and can be considered as part of the classical publications in ECG signal conditioning. The traditional performance criteria have been enhanced by the addition of specifications in the time domain. The evolution of the low-frequency performance requirements in electrocardiography can be summarised as follows:

1. In the mid 1960s, to ensure that recording errors are kept under 50 μV in the early portion of the ST-T complex, Berson & Pipberger recommended that ECG preamplifiers provide a 0.05-Hz low-frequency cutoff with a 6-dB-per-octave roll-off (Berson & Pipberger, 1966), as achieved for example by a single-pole high-pass filter. The American Heart Association (AHA) has endorsed this low-frequency cutoff since 1967 (A.H.A., 1967) and added in 1985 that the amplitude response should be flat to within ± 6 % (0.5 dB) over the range 0.14 to 30 Hz (A.H.A., 1985), as shown in Fig. 3(a).
2. In the early 1980s, Tayler & Vincent recommended that phase linearity must be maintained down to the fundamental frequency of the physiological signal to allow high fidelity in the reproduction of the ECG waveform (Tayler & Vincent, 1983). The AHA has adopted this recommendation since 1985 by specifying that the phase shift introduced by the amplifier should not be greater than that introduced by a 0.05-Hz, single-pole high-pass filter (A.H.A., 1985), as depicted in Fig. 3(b).
3. In more recent years, specification of the low-frequency performance of electrocardiographs based on the system's impulse response have been introduced. The International Electrotechnical Committee (IEC) and the American National Standard Institute (ANSI) have indicated that a 300-μVs impulse shall not yield an undershoot on the ECG record from the isoelectric line of greater than 100 μV, and shall not produce a recovery slope of greater than 300 μVs^{-1} following the end of the impulse (Berson et al., 2007; I.E.C., 2001), as illustrated in Fig. 4.

2.3 The effect of high-pass filtering on the ECG signal

The performance requirements can be explained from a simple mathematical model of the physiological signal and the recording system. From a signal viewpoint, the ECG waveform may be regarded as a periodic time function represented by the following Fourier series:

$$f(t) = \sum_{n=0}^{\infty} \left[\alpha_n cos\left(\frac{2\pi nt}{T_{R-R}}\right) + \beta_n sin\left(\frac{2\pi nt}{T_{R-R}}\right) \right] \tag{1}$$

where T_{R-R} is the $R - R$ interval or cardiac cycle time and α_n and β_n are the Fourier coefficients. The fundamental frequency of the ECG signal is therefore determined by $1/T_{R-R}$ and defines the heart rate while its dc component is given by α_0.

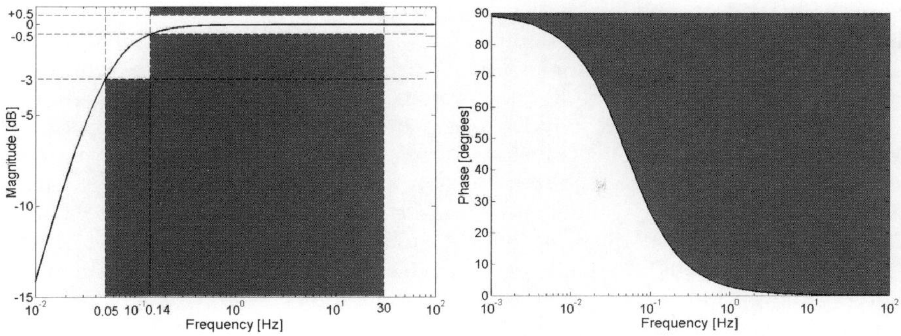

(a) Amplitude response criterion (b) Phase response criterion

Fig. 3. Plots of the low-frequency (a) amplitude and (b) phase criteria illustrated with a 0.05-Hz single-pole high-pass filter. The shaded areas indicate the "forbidden" areas as specified by the AHA (A.H.A., 1985).

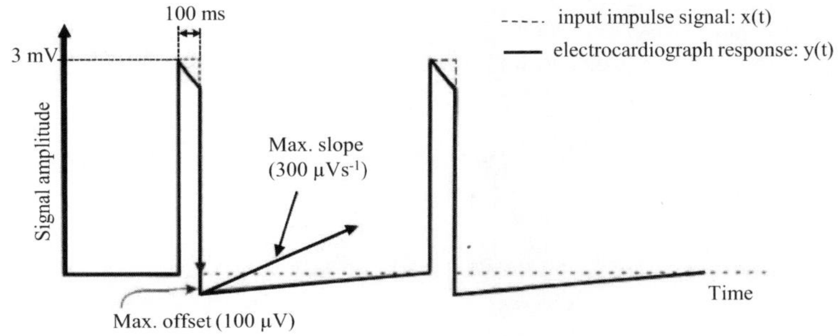

Fig. 4. Plots of the impulse response requirements (from (Berson et al., 2007; I.E.C., 2001)).

If $A(s)$ represents the preamplifier's transfer function, its response to the ECG signal defined in eq. (1) can then be modelled in the Laplace domain by the following product:

$$V_{out}(s) = A(s) \int_0^{\infty} f(t) e^{-st}\, dt \quad (2)$$

$V_{out}(t)$, the preamplifier's response to $f(t)$ in the time domain, is obtained from the inverse Laplace transform of eq. (2) by convolution once $A(s)$ is known.
Taking $s = j\omega$, the preamplifier response may also be specified in the frequency domain as follows:

$$A(j\omega) = |G(\omega)|\, e^{j\theta(\omega)} \quad (3)$$

with $|G(\omega)|$ its amplitude response and $\theta(\omega)$ its phase response. An ideal amplitude response is achieved when $|G(\omega)|$ is frequency-independent, which in practice would require the ECG recorder to be dc-coupled to the source signal. This approach is, however, inadvisable due to excessive base-line wander and artefacts commonly associated with dc-coupled recording equipment. In addition, the large dc offset inherently present with dry electrodes would quickly limit the obtainable gain of the amplification stages due to saturation. AC-coupling is

therefore unavoidable in diagnostic quality ECG recording but it comes at the cost of potential amplitude and phase distortion as outlined by (Berson & Pipberger, 1966) and (Tayler & Vincent, 1983). Because of phase nonlinearity, a non-constant group delay is introduced into the ECG waveform. Consequently the low-frequency components of the QRS complex are affected by a greater time delay than its high-frequency components and can therefore become superimposed on the ST complex (Tayler & Vincent, 1983). Low-frequency phase distortion is avoided if the phase shift or the group delay is made negligible. For example, the phase shift introduced by a first order high-pass filter is less than 6° from a decade above the cutoff frequency, f_c. Therefore, if frequencies in the vicinity of the fundamental ECG frequency are to be reproduced, the 3-dB low-frequency point must be about 10 times lower than $1/T_{R-R}$. Considering a lower limit heart rate of 30 beats per minute gives $1/T_{R-R} = 0.5$ Hz and thus $f_c = 0.05$ Hz.
The impulse response requirements complement the frequency response specifications to ensure that the fast varying signals in the ECG, such as the QRS complex and P wave, do not generate noticeable depressions as result of filtering. A visible undershoot could, in fact, be misinterpreted as an additional ECG component. The Common Standards for Quantitative Electrocardiography (CSE) issued by the European Union defines the presence of a QRS deflection as a waveform having an amplitude greater than or equal to 20 μV and a duration greater than or equal to 6 ms (Berson et al., 2007). Moreover, the slope of the response after the end of the input impulse must be minimised to preserve base line stability and allow accurate amplitude measurement of the P wave and the QRS complex.

3. Effect of the skin-electrode interface on the low-frequency performance of ECG recording systems

High pass-filtering is commonly achieved in dry-electrode ECG recording by inserting a dc-blocking capacitor, C_{in}, in series with each sensing electrode as shown in Fig. 5. Z_s simulates the skin-electrode impedance and R_{in} is the input impedance of the recording amplifier. Two electrical models of have been principal used to simulate the skin-electrode interface at the preamplifier's input: a simple single-time-constant RC network and a more complete double-time-constant model.

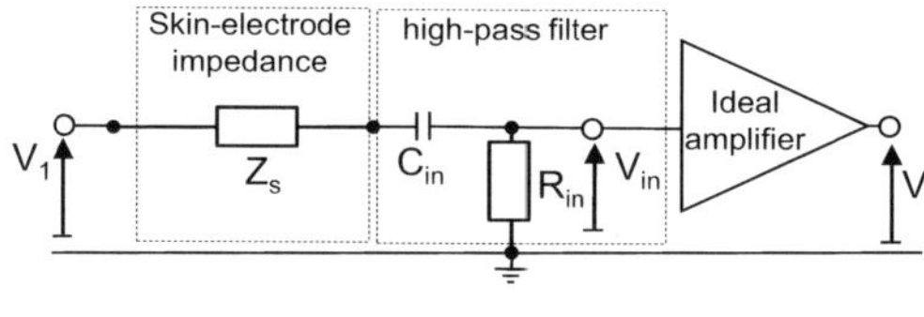

Fig. 5. Schematic representation of a simple high-pass filter at the amplifier's front-end. AC-coupling achieved this way allows dc offset voltages associated with polarisation effects at the skin-electrode interface to be blocked from the amplifier input.

3.1 A single-time-constant model of the skin-electrode interface

Fig. 6 shows the general form of the single-time-constant skin-electrode model which represents the impedance of the electrode with a resistor, R_e, in parallel with a capacitor, C_e, while the lumped resistance of the skin and body tissue is simulated by a resistor, R_s. However, because of its relatively low value, R_s is often omitted. The electrode polarisation potential is modelled with a dc voltage source, V_{DC}.

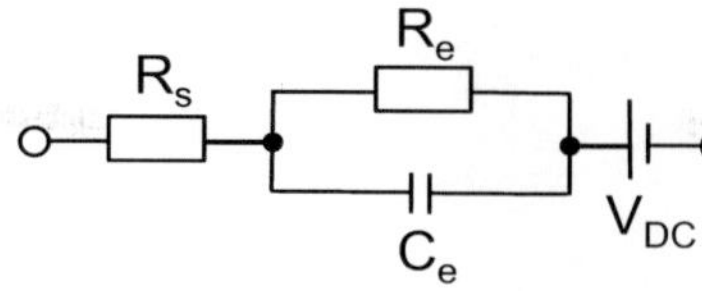

Fig. 6. A standard single-time-constant representation of the skin-electrode interface. The half-cell potential, V_{DC}, introduces a dc offset but does not contribute to the ac impedance of the interface.

The parameter values stipulated in international standards issued by both IEC and ANSI are R_e =0.62 MΩ and C_e=4.7 nF (Berson et al., 2007; Bruce et al., 2007; I.E.C., 2001; 2005). In all standards it is stated that the skin-electrode impedance in series with any patient-electrode connection must not result in a signal reduction of more than 6% of that obtained without the simulated impedance. The standards specify that the preamplifier must provide an input impedance of at least 10 MΩ at 10 Hz, since the magnitude of the simulated source impedance would be equal to 0.6 MΩ at this frequency. In addition, a low-frequency cutoff at 0.05 Hz or lower must be achieved by the amplifier, with the simulated skin-electrode impedance disconnected. Given R_{in} = 10 MΩ, an input capacitance C_{in} = 0.33 μF is required to implement a 0.05-Hz single-pole high-pass filter at the amplifier input. It must be noted, however, that the input impedance specification does not take into account phase response, impulse response or attenuation below 10 Hz.

In 2004, considering the amplitude and phase criteria recommended by the AHA (A.H.A., 1990), the relationship between input impedance requirement and source impedance was analytically studied by Valverde et al (Valverde et al., 2004) who suggested that for frequencies below 100 Hz, the interface can be approximated by the electrode resistance, R_e. It was concluded that an amplifier having a low-frequency input impedance $R_{in} > 17R_e$ would not cause more than 6% attenuation at 0.14 Hz nor introduce a phase shift of greater than 6° at 0.5 Hz. Based on electrode resistance R_e = 150 kΩ, R_{in} was estimated at 2.4 MΩ at 0.14 Hz and the dc-blocking capacitor was chosen as C_{in} = 2.2 μF.

In 2000, Burke & Gleeson (Burke & Gleeson, 2000) estimated the component values of the skin-electrode interface as R_s = 10 kΩ, R_e = 1.4 MΩ and C_e= 20 nF. The preamplifier front-end was designed so that its input impedance would be significantly larger than that of the skin-electrode impedance to minimise interference caused by motion artefact and unwanted common-mode voltages. It was reported that the attenuation caused by R_s is limited to 1% for $R_{in} > 100R_s$ and the phase shift introduced by R_e and C_e is kept below 1° in the bandwidth of the ECG signal for $R_{in} > 60R_e$. The designed low-power preamplifier achieved an input impedance of 260 MΩ and was coupled with a 1 μF dc-blocking capacitor. Emphasis must be placed on the fact that input impedance requirements have not traditionally included impulse response criteria. The authors have therefore evaluated the performance of simulated high-pass filters based on the models outlined above to assess whether or not amplitude, phase and impulse response criteria would be simultaneously met when the electrode impedance is taken into account. A program was written in *MATLAB* to determine and plot the low-frequency response of the skin-electrode-amplifier networks based on the provided skin-electrode model and the amplifier's front-end design. Plots of the simulated amplitude, phase and impulse responses, together with the recovery slope are shown in Fig. 7. Results are compared with the response of a 0.05-Hz single-pole high-pass filter equivalent to the amplifier operating with a dc-blocking capacitor but omitting the skin-electrode impedance. A summary is given in Table 1.

	max. magitude 0.14-30 Hz [dB]	phase @ 0.5 Hz [°]	max. undershoot after impulse [mV]	max. slope after impulse $[mVs^{-1}]$
specification limit	-0.5	6	-0.1	0.3
0.5-Hz single-pole high-pass filter	-0.5	5.8	-0.093	0.03
IEC min. input impedance requirement	**−0.96**	5.3	**−0.25**	**53.6**
solution proposed by Valverde et al	-0.5	4.1	**−0.11**	**0.49**
solution proposed by Burke & Gleeson	-0.05	0.1	-0.02	**0.55**

Table 1. Low-frequency performance of simulated skin-electrode-amplifier networks compared to that of a single-pole 0.05-Hz high-pass filter. Bold case indicates that performance requirement is not met.

Columns 2 and 3 indicate the maximum attenuation in the frequency range 0.14 to 30 Hz and the phase shift at 0.5 Hz, respectively. Plots of the frequency response are presented in Figs. 7(a) and 7(b), which suggest that the amplitude and phase criteria would not be met if the IEC minimum input impedance requirement was applied with the electrodes used in international standards. It can be observed that the capacitive component of the simulated skin-electrode introduces additional phase shift into the signal for frequencies above 10 Hz. However, these criteria are fulfilled in the case of designs suggested by Valverde et al. and Burke & Gleeson. Plots of the time response of the systems to a 300-mVs input impulse are presented in Fig. 7(c). The fourth column of Table 1 gives the maximum value of the undershoot following the input impulse. It can be seen that the simulated impulse response using the minimum input impedance specified by the IEC or Valverde's solution would result in undershoots greater than the specified limit. The threshold is however respected for the simulated system based on the design proposed by Burke & Gleeson. Fig. 7(d) shows the corresponding recovery slope and the last column of Table 1 gives its maximum value that must be limited in magnitude to 0.3 mVs^{-1} to meet requirements. Results indicate that all three simulated skin-electrode-amplifier networks would exceed the specified maximum recovery slope. The recovery slope is significantly high when the IEC minimum input impedance requirement is followed since it is expected to reach a maximum of 55.6 mVs^{-1}, about 185 times the specification limit.

These results demonstrate that amplitude, phase and impulse response criteria are not met if the minimum IEC input impedance requirement is applied. In addition, an unsatisfactory recovery slope is exhibited by electrocardiographs despite following the amplitude and phase recommendations. The results also demonstrate that the risk of signal distortion can only be assessed with accuracy when the skin-electrode impedance is taken into account.

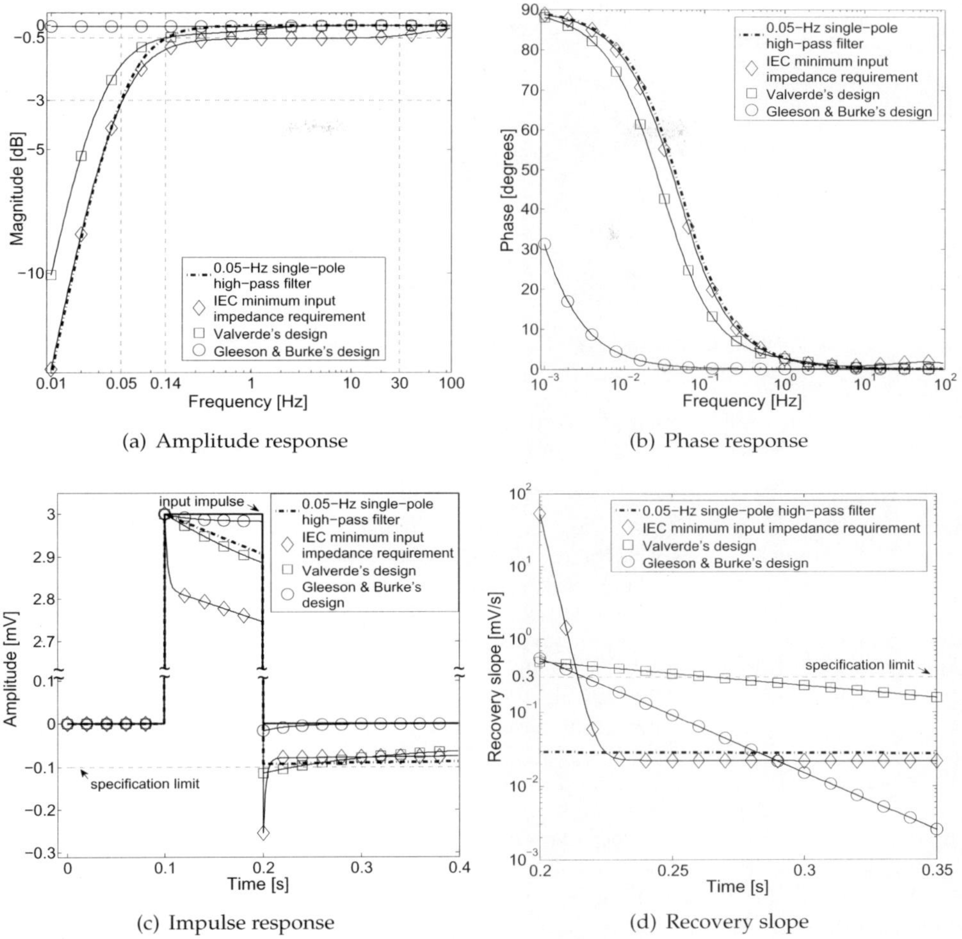

(a) Amplitude response

(b) Phase response

(c) Impulse response

(d) Recovery slope

Fig. 7. Plots of (a) the amplitude response, (b) phase response, (c) impulse response and (d) recovery slope of the simulated skin-electrode-amplifier networks compared to that of a single-pole 0.05-Hz high-pass filter.

3.2 A double-time-constant model of the skin-electrode interface

Using the double-time-constant model depicted in Fig. 8(a), Mühlsteff et al. investigated in 2004 the complex impedance of the skin-electrode interface of silicone rubber dry electrodes (Mühlsteff & Such, 2004). Measurements, taken in the frequency range 0.1 to 1000 Hz indicated that the ac behaviour of the skin-electrode contact interface is not accurately simulated by a single parallel RC-model. They proposed a double RC model with parameter values in equilibrium estimated as: $R_{1s} + R_{3e} = 8\ \mathrm{k\Omega}$, $R_{2s} = 140\ \mathrm{k\Omega}$, $C_{2s} = 3\mu\mathrm{F}$, $R_{4e} = 150\mathrm{k\Omega}$ and $C_{4e} = 180$ nF.

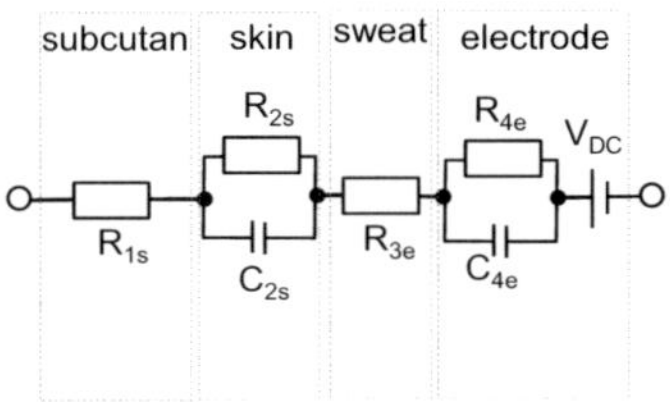

(a) A double-time-constant model of the skin-electrode interface.

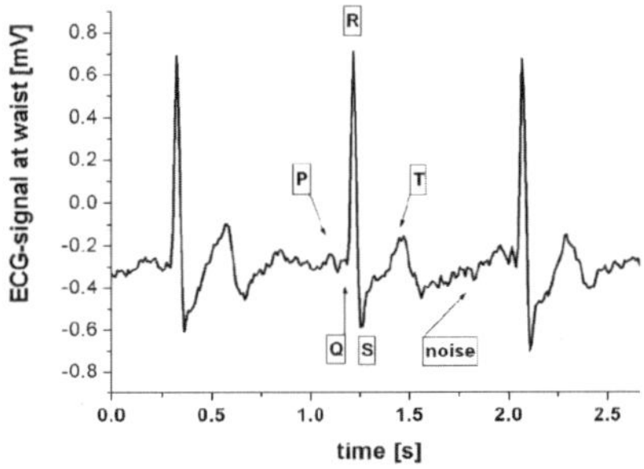

(b) Sample ECG recording with dry electrodes in equilibrium.

Fig. 8. Figures showing (a) the equivalent electrical representation of the skin-electrode assumed by Mühlsteff et al and (b) a sample ECG recording (from (Mühlsteff & Such, 2004)).

An instrumentation amplifier having 10 MΩ input impedance was then used for recording the ECG shown in Fig. 8(b). The record clearly displays the QRS complex and the T wave. The P wave can also be identified despite its low amplitude. However, it can be observed that the baseline is not horizontal, especially immediately following abrupt voltage variations associated with the QRS complex and the T wave. Such effects can be attributed to low-frequency distortion similar to that reported by Tayler & Vincent (Tayler & Vincent, 1983). The authors have investigated the origin of the observed distortion by reproducing the low-frequency response of the dry-electrode design suggested Mühlsteff et al. Several different input capacitance values available in non-electrolytic form were used, ranging from 0.33 to 3.3 μF. Given $R_{in} = 10$ MΩ, the 3-dB point of the simulated high-pass filters varies between 0.05 and 0.005 Hz, and therefore meets AHA recommendations. This allows assessment of whether or not the low-frequency distortion suspected on the ECG recording of Fig. 8(b) might be caused by a degradation of the frequency response due to the presence of the double-time-constant skin-electrode interface. Results are presented in Fig. 9 and Table 2. Results from the simulated skin-electrode-amplifier network using the double-time-constant model indicate that for $R_{in} = 10$ MΩ, a cutoff frequency of about 0.03 Hz or lower is needed to fulfil both amplitude and phase requirements ($C_{in} \geq 0.47$ μF). It suggests that the presence of the modelled skin-electrode interface impedance has increased the effective 3-dB point of the skin-electrode-amplifier network. However, this increase alone cannot explain the level of distortion observed on the ECG of Fig. 8(b). Frequency response plots shown in Figs. 9(a) and 9(b) suggest that the amplitude and phase response would remain very close to that of a 0.05-Hz single-pole high-pass filter if C_{in} was equal to 0.33 μF.
Fig. 9(c) gives plots of the systems' response to a 3-mV pulse of 100-ms duration. As R_{in} remains constant, the offset following the input impulse is less than 0.1 mV for $C_{in} \geq 1$ μF, suggesting that in the presence of the skin-electrode impedance defined above, a lower 3-dB point of about 16 mHz is needed to meet the requirement of maximum undershoot. Fig. 9(d) is a graph of the recovery slope after the 300-mVs input impulse. The maximum slope of the response immediately after the impulse is about 1.6 mVs^{-1}, five times the allowed limit, and shows little variation when C_{in} is increased from 0.33 μF to 3.3 μF. In comparison, the recovery slope exhibited by a 0.05 Hz high-pass filter is not greater than 0.03 mVs^{-1}. Consequently, the

slope of the impulse response is not satisfactory for the range of input capacitances simulated. Excessively high recovery slope can therefore explain why the baseline of the ECG recording of Fig. 8(b) is not horizontal, immediately following abrupt voltage variations.

These results confirm that amplitude and phase requirements provide necessary conditions for the reproduction of low-frequency components of the ECG but they are not sufficient to prevent distortion and possible clinical misinterpretation of the waveform.

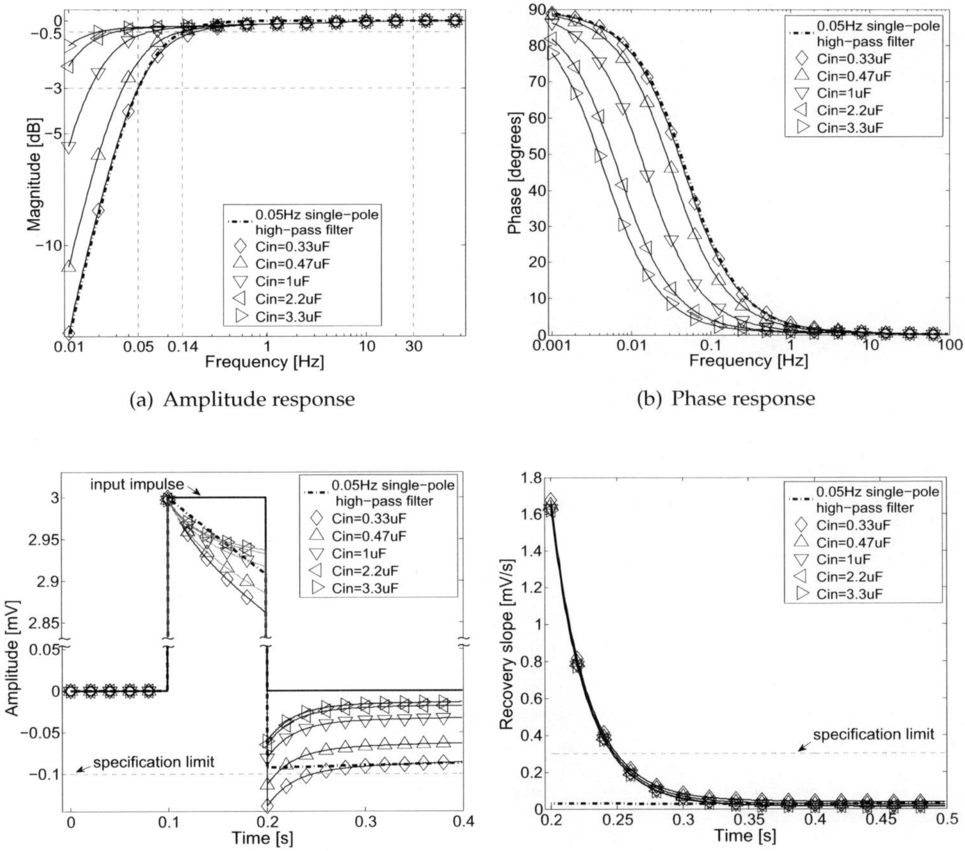

(a) Amplitude response (b) Phase response

(c) Impulse response (d) Recovery slope

Fig. 9. Plots of (a) the amplitude response, (b) phase response, (c) impulse response and (d) recovery slope of simulated transfer functions based on the design suggested by Mühlsteff et al. compared to that of a 0.05-Hz single-pole high-pass filter.

	max. magnitude 0.14-30 Hz [dB]	phase @ 0.5 Hz [°]	max. undershoot after impulse [mV]	max. slope [mVs^{-1}]
specification limit	-0.5	6	-0.1	0.3
0.5-Hz single-pole high-pass filter	-0.5	5.8	-0.093	0.03
C_{in}=0.33 μF	**−0.72**	5.9	**−0.14**	**1.68**
C_{in}=0.47 μF	-0.49	4.3	**−0.11**	**1.65**
C_{in}=1 μF	-0.29	2.3	-0.08	**1.63**
C_{in}=2.2 μF	-0.25	1.3	-0.07	**1.62**
C_{in}=3.3 μF	-0.25	1	-0.06	**1.62**

Table 2. Low-frequency performance of simulated transfer functions based on the design model by Mühlsteff et al. compared to that of a single-pole 0.05-Hz high-pass filter: $R_{in} = 10$ MΩ, $R_{1s} + R_{3e} = 8$ kΩ, $R_{2s} = 140$ kΩ, $C_{2s} = 3$ μF, $C_{4e} = 0.18$ μF. Bold case indicates that the requirement is not met.

3.3 Discussion

Simulation results have shown that the input impedance specification stated in international standards is not consistent with the accompanying low-frequency performance requirements. In addition, despite fulfilling both amplitude and phase criteria, some designs may fall short of meeting the impulse response requirements when the skin-electrode impedance is taken into account for dry-electrode recording. For the range of input capacitance values used, simulations based on the double-time-constant skin-electrode model indicate that the recovery slope is not significantly affected by a change of C_{in}. This can be explained by the presence of capacitive elements as small as 0.18 μF in the skin-electrode interface. The reactance of the electrode impedance is therefore considerably greater than that of C_{in} and dominates the reactance of the skin-electrode-amplifier network. It can therefore be concluded that:

1. Impulse response considerations must be included as an inherent part of the design strategy of new dry-electrode preamplifiers.
2. A complete characterisation of the skin-electrode interface is fundamental for the appropriate design of the amplifier front-end.
3. Meeting the impulse response specifications implies tighter requirements than compliance with the amplitude and phase criteria when the electrode impedance is taken into account.
4. The optimum values of R_{in} and C_{in} must be determined in relation to the parameter values of the skin-electrode interface so that all low-frequency requirements are simultaneously fulfilled.

4. New methods of characterisation of the skin-electrode interface

Previous studies have demonstrated that measurement of the dc skin-electrode impedance does not provide sufficient information. Because of the capacitive components, corresponding to the epidermal layer and the electrode's permittivity, ac measurement is needed to obtain an accurate estimate of the skin-electrode impedance (Zepeda-Carapia et al., 2005). The research group of which the authors are members has attempted to measure the resistive and capacitive properties of wet and dry electrodes using two experimental approaches, namely frequency-domain based and time-domain based measurement. Several identification algorithms were also considered by the group: an asymptotic method requiring only five points extracted from the frequency response and curve fitting based on least squares error minimisation algorithms.

4.1 Instrumentation set-up

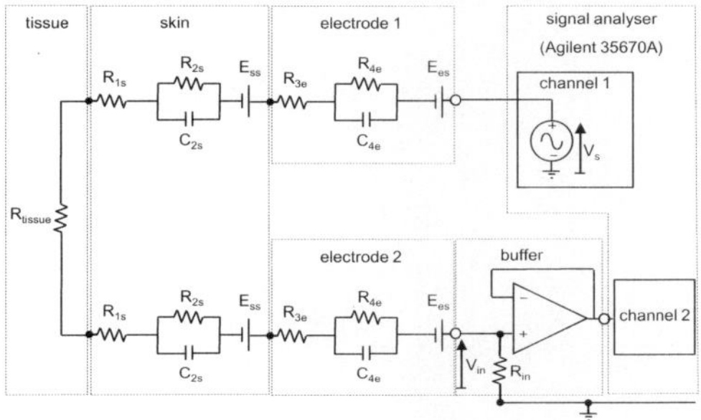

Fig. 10. Schematic representation of the measurement set-up assuming a double-time-constant model.

Impedance spectroscopy is generally the method applied to characterise the skin-electrode interface in the frequency range 0.05 Hz to 1 MHz (Burke & Gleeson, 2000; Chang et al., 2010; Gruetzmann et al., 2007; Ko et al., 1970; Mühlsteff & Such, 2004; Valverde et al., 2004; Zepeda-Carapia et al., 2005). The measured impedance is then fitted to an equivalent electrical model to identify the resistive and capacitive elements of the interface. Fig. 10 shows the instrumentation set-up considered by the authors for measuring the frequency response of the skin-electrode interface which consists of a dual electrode configuration connected to a resistive load, R_{in}. One electrode is fed with a sinusoidal voltage from a signal analyser (Agilent 35670A) and connected to the body. A second electrode is used to detect the resulting signal from the skin and feeds it to the input of the analyser. The selected signal analyser can generate sinusoidal signals in the frequency range 15 mHz to 51 kHz.

4.2 The proposed identification method

Fig. 11 shows the asymptotic bode diagram and the simulated frequency response of the interface based on the parameter values reported by Mühlsteff et al. ($R_{1s} + R_{3e} = 8$ kΩ, $R_{2s} = 140$ kΩ, $C_{2s} = 3$ μF, $R_{4e} = 150$ kΩ , $C_{4e} = 180$ nF and $R_{in} = 10$ MΩ) (Mühlsteff & Such, 2004). For the model provided, the phase response exhibits three local extrema at $f_1 = 0.45$ Hz, $f_2 = 1.40$ Hz and $f_3 = 5.26$ Hz. The authors have developed a novel method for the characterisation of the interface that relies upon knowledge of these three frequencies, and the attenuation introduced by the interface at low and high frequency. Taking $\tau_{2s} = R_{2s}C_{2s}$ and $\tau_{4e} = R_{4e}C_{4e}$, the phase measured at the amplifier input and its first derivative with respect to the angular frequency ω are given in eqs. (4) and (5) as:

$$\varphi(\omega) = tan^{-1}\left(\frac{\omega\frac{R_{2s}\tau_{2s}+R_{4e}\tau_{4e}}{R_{in}+2(R_{1s}+R_{2s}+R_{3e}+R_{4e})}+\omega^3\tau_{2s}\tau_{4e}\frac{R_{4e}\tau_2+R_{2s}\tau_{4e}}{R_{in}+2(R_{1s}+R_{2s}+R_{3e}+R_{4e})}}{1+\omega^2\frac{\tau_{2s}^2[R_{in}+2(R_{1s}+R_{3e}+R_{4e})]+\tau_{4e}^2[R_{in}+2(R_{1s}+R_{3e}+R_{4e})]}{R_{in}+2(R_{1s}+R_{2s}+R_{3e}+R_{4e})}+\omega^4\frac{[R_{in}+2(R_{1s}+R_{3e})]\tau_{2s}^2\tau_{4e}^2}{R_{in}+2(R_{1s}+R_{2s}+R_{3e}+R_{4e})}}\right) \quad (4)$$

$$\frac{d\varphi(\omega)}{d\omega} = \frac{1+a_1\omega^2+a_2\omega^4+a_3\omega^6}{\left[1+\left[\frac{\tau_{2s}^2[R_{in}+2(R_{1s}+R_{3e}+R_{4e})]+\tau_{4e}^2[R_{in}+2(R_{1s}+R_{2s}+R_{3e})]}{R_{in}+2(R_{1s}+R_{2s}+R_{3e}+R_{4e})}\right]\omega^2+\left[\frac{R_{in}+2(R_{1s}+R_{3e})}{R_{in}+2(R_{1s}+R_{2s}+R_{3e}+R_{4e})}\tau_{2s}^2\tau_{4e}^2\right]\omega^4\right]^2 + \left[\left[\frac{2R_{2s}\tau_{2s}+2R_{4e}\tau_{4e}}{R_{in}+2(R_{1s}+R_{2s}+R_{3e}+R_{4e})}\right]\omega+\left[\frac{2R_{2s}\tau_{4e}+2R_{4e}\tau_{2s}}{R_{in}+2(R_{1s}+R_{2s}+R_{3e}+R_{4e})}\tau_{2s}\tau_{4e}\right]\omega^3\right]^2} \quad (5)$$

where

$$a_1 = \frac{3\left(R_{4e}\tau_{2s}+R_{2s}\tau_{4e}\right)\tau_{2s}\tau_{4e}}{R_{2s}\tau_{2s}+R_{4e}\tau_{4e}} - \frac{\tau_{2s}^2\left[R_{in}+2\left(R_{1s}+R_{3e}+R_{4e}\right)\right]+\tau_{4e}^2\left[R_{in}+2\left(R_{1s}+R_{2s}+R_{4e}\right)\right]}{R_{in}+2\left(R_{1s}+R_{2s}+R_{3e}+R_{4e}\right)} \quad (6)$$

$$a_2 = \frac{\tau_{2s}\tau_{4e}\left[\tau_{2s}^2\left[R_{in}+2\left(R_{1s}+R_{3e}+R_{4e}\right)\right]+\tau_{4e}^2\left[R_{in}+2\left(R_{1s}+R_{2s}+R_{3e}\right)\right]\right]\left(\tau_{2s}R_{4e}+\tau_{4e}R_{2s}\right)}{\left[R_{in}+2\left(R_{1s}+R_{2s}+R_{3e}+R_{4e}\right)\right]\left(R_{2s}\tau_{2s}+R_{4e}\tau_{4e}\right)} - \frac{3\tau_{2s}^2\tau_{4e}^2\left[R_{in}+2\left(R_{1s}+R_{3e}\right)\right]}{R_{in}+2\left(R_{1s}+R_{2s}+R_{3e}+R_{4e}\right)} \quad (7)$$

$$a_3 = -\frac{\tau_{2s}^3\tau_{4e}^3\left[R_{in}+2\left(R_{1s}+R_{3e}+R_{4e}\right)\right]\left(R_{4e}\tau_{2s}+R_{2s}\tau_{4e}\right)}{\left[R_{in}+2\left(R_{1s}+R_{2s}+R_{3e}+R_{4e}\right)\right]\left(R_{2s}\tau_{2s}+R_{4e}\tau_{4e}\right)} \quad (8)$$

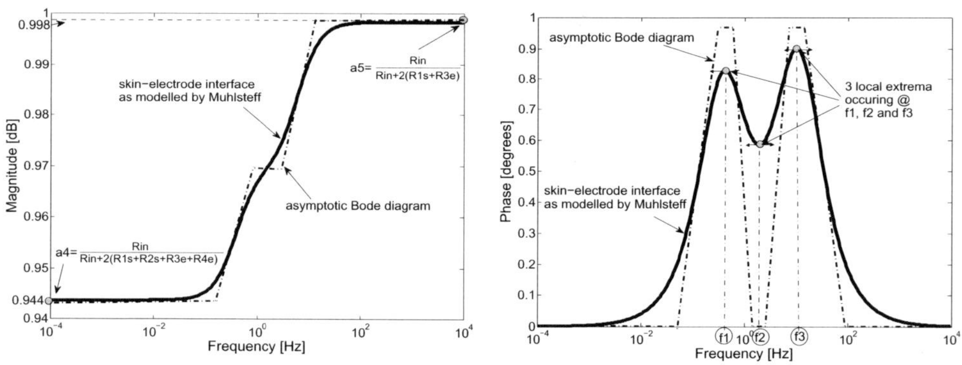

(a) Amplitude response (b) Phase response

Fig. 11. Plots of (a) the magnitude response and (b) the phase response of the skin-electrode interface as defined by Mühlsteff et al. for $R_{in} = 10\ \mathrm{M}\Omega$.

The three frequencies f_1, f_2 and f_3 identified in Fig. 11(b) are associated with three angular frequencies $\omega_1 = 2\pi f_1$, $\omega_2 = 2\pi f_2$ and $\omega_3 = 2\pi f_3$ that correspond to the positive and real solutions of $\frac{d\varphi(\omega)}{d\omega} = 0$. The following system of equations is then obtained:

$$\begin{cases} 1+a_1\omega_1^2+a_2\omega_1^4+a_3\omega_1^6 = 0 & (9) \\ 1+a_1\omega_2^2+a_2\omega_2^4+a_3\omega_2^6 = 0 & (10) \\ 1+a_1\omega_3^2+a_2\omega_3^4+a_3\omega_3^6 = 0 & (11) \end{cases}$$

It can be shown that the system defined in eqs. (9) to (11) can be rearranged to give the coefficients as:

$$\begin{cases} a_1 = -\frac{1}{\omega_1^2} - \frac{1}{\omega_2^2} - \frac{1}{\omega_3^2} & (12) \\ a_2 = \frac{\omega_1^2 + \omega_2^2 + \omega_3^2}{\omega_1^2\omega_2^2\omega_3^2} & (13) \\ a_3 = -\frac{1}{\omega_1^2\omega_2^2\omega_3^2} & (14) \end{cases}$$

In addition, the magnitude response shown in Fig. 11(a) exhibits two asymptotes at low and high frequency corresponding to:

$$a_4 = \lim_{\omega \to 0} \left| \frac{V_{in}(\omega)}{V_s(\omega)} \right| = \frac{R_{in}}{R_{in} + 2\left(R_{1s} + R_{2s} + R_{3e} + R_{4e}\right)} \tag{15}$$

and

$$a_5 = \lim_{\omega \to \infty} \left| \frac{V_{in}(\omega)}{V_s(\omega)} \right| = \frac{R_{in}}{R_{in} + 2\left(R_{1s} + R_{3e}\right)} \tag{16}$$

It can be noted that the magnitude response reaches more than 99.99% of its asymptotic values at 15 mHz and 1 kHz, giving good estimates of a_4 and a_5. The coefficients defined in eqs. (12) to (16) provide sufficient information for the identification of $q = \tau_{2s}\tau_{4e}$ as the positive and real solution of the following polynomial equation:

$$-\frac{3a_3^2a_5^2}{a_4^2} - \frac{a_1a_3a_5}{a_4^2}q^2 + \frac{a_2}{a_4}q^4 + \frac{3}{a_5}q^6 = 0 \tag{17}$$

After solving eq. (17), the time constants are obtained from the positive solutions of the following equation:

$$1 + \frac{\left(a_1a_4q^2 + 3a_3a_5\right)\left(a_3a_5 - a_4q^3\right)a_5 - \left(a_4 - a_5\right)q^3\left(a_4q^3 + a_3a_5\right)a_4}{a_4\left(a_3a_5^2 - a_4^2q^3\right)q^4}\tau^2 + \frac{1}{q^2}\tau^4 = 0 \tag{18}$$

Two valid solutions are then available for τ. In previous literature the skin contribution is considered to be dominant, therefore the larger of the two solutions can be allocated to τ_{2s}, the second one being τ_{4e}. Eqs. (12) to (18) are then utilised to determine the model parameters as:

$$R_{4e} = \frac{R_{in}}{2}\frac{\left(a_5 - a_4\right)\left(a_4q^4 + a_5a_3\tau_{2s}^2\right)}{\left(a_3a_5 - a_4q^3\right)a_4a_5\left(\tau_{2s}^2 - q\right)} \tag{19}$$

$$R_{2s} = \frac{R_{in}}{2}\frac{\left(a_5 - a_4\right)}{a_4a_5} - R_{4e} \tag{20}$$

$$C_{2s} = \frac{\tau_{2s}}{R_{2s}} \tag{21}$$

$$C_{4e} = \frac{q}{\tau_{2s} R_{4e}} \tag{22}$$

$$R_{1s} + R_{3e} = \frac{R_{in}}{2} \frac{(1 - a_5)}{a_5} \tag{23}$$

Only solutions that are real and positive are relevant for the purpose of parameter identification. For example, the five reference points indicated in the bode plot of Fig. 11 suggest the following coefficient values:

$$a_1 = -0.14 \mathrm{s}^2 \mathrm{rad}^{-2} \tag{24}$$

$$a_2 = 1.7 \mathrm{s}^2 \mathrm{rad}^{-2} \tag{25}$$

$$a_3 = -1.48 \mathrm{s}^2 \mathrm{rad}^{-2} \tag{26}$$

$$a_4 = 0.998 \tag{27}$$

$$a_5 = 0.944 \tag{28}$$

Applying theses values to eq. (17) yields:

$$-7.78 \text{ x } 10^{-12} - 2.30 \text{ x } 10^{-7} q^2 + 1.8 \text{ x } 10^{-3} q^4 + 3q^6 = 0 \tag{29}$$

Eq. (29) has a unique positive real solution at $q = \tau_{2s}\tau_{4e} = 0.0114$ s^2. This value is then inserted into eq. (18) to solve the following equation:

$$1 - 1.39 \text{ x } 10^3 \tau^2 + 7.71 \text{ x } 10^3 \tau^4 = 0 \tag{30}$$

The two positive solutions are: $\tau_{2s} = 0.423$ s and $\tau_{4e} = 0.027$ s. Taking $R_{in} = 10$ MΩ, the model parameters can then be deduced from eqs. (19) to (23) as:

$R_{4e} \simeq 148$ kΩ, $R_{2s} \simeq 139$ kΩ, $C_{2s} \simeq 3$ µF, $C_{4e} \simeq 182$ nF and $R_{1s} + R_{3e} \simeq 10$ kΩ.

The small discrepancy observed between the estimated values and the simulated parameters is due to floating point approximation error in solving eqs. (17) and (18) and the limited precision with which a_4 and a_5 can be measured. The resolution method is described in more detail by the authors in (Assambo et al., 2006).

4.3 Measurement results

A hardware model of the skin-electrode interface was constructed using actual resistors and capacitors, based on the model provided by Mühlsteff et al. to assess the ability of the signal analyser to reproduce the simulated results shown in Fig. 11. A pair of 3.3-µF and 220-nF multi-layer ceramic capacitors simulated the effects of C_{2s} and C_{4e}, respectively, the original capacitance values (3 µF and 180 nF) being unavailable. Fig. 12 compares the measurement of magnitude and phase to that obtained as a result of the new identification method. Raw measurement data are filtered to remove measurement noise and to facilitate the detection of the two peaks and the trough in the phase response. The frequency of the three local extrema in the phase response and the two extremum values in the magnitude response allow the five coefficients to be estimated and and the frequency response of the network to be simulated. A theoretical curve is included to assess the precision of the measurement and the accuracy of the fitted model.

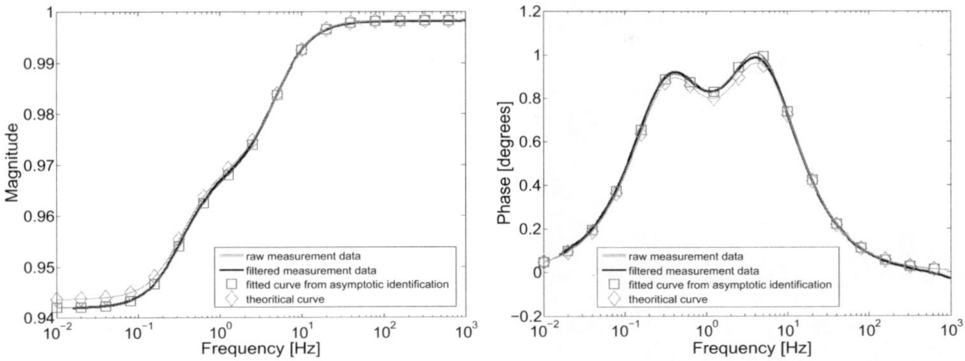

(a) Amplitude response

(b) Phase response

Fig. 12. Comparison between the measured data ((a) magnitude and (b) phase) and data obtained as a result of the novel identification procedure for a constructed hardware model defined in Table 3.

The accuracy of the method can be appreciated from the results shown in Table 3, which suggest that if the skin-electrode interface in equilibrium behaves in a similar way as that measured by Mühlsteff et al., the proposed method would then provide a fast and accurate identification tool.

	actual component value	estimated value	% error
$R_{1s} + R_{3e}$ [kΩ]	8.20	8.47	+3.3 %
R_{2s} [kΩ]	140.00	141.21	+0.9%
R_{4e} [kΩ]	150.45	157.99	+5.1 %
C_{2s} [μF]	3.340	3.395	+1.6%
C_{4e} [μF]	0.219	0.218	-0.4 %

Table 3. Accuracy of the new identification method assessed from a constructed hardware model.

Fig. 13 shows measurements obtained in vivo with wet and dry electrodes which are significantly different than the results obtained with the hardware model.
It was observed that very often the phase response did not display two distinct peaks but only a single peak as shown in Fig. 13(a). This means that the polynomial $p(\omega) = 1 + a_1\omega^2 + a_2\omega^4 + a_3\omega^6$ has one real and positive root (ω_i), one real and negative root ($-\omega_i$) and four complex conjugate roots (ω_j, ω_j^*, $-\omega_j$ and $-\omega_j^*$). Similar results have been obtained from simulation when the time constant τ_{2s} and τ_{4e} differ by less than one order of magnitude, as shown in Fig. 14.

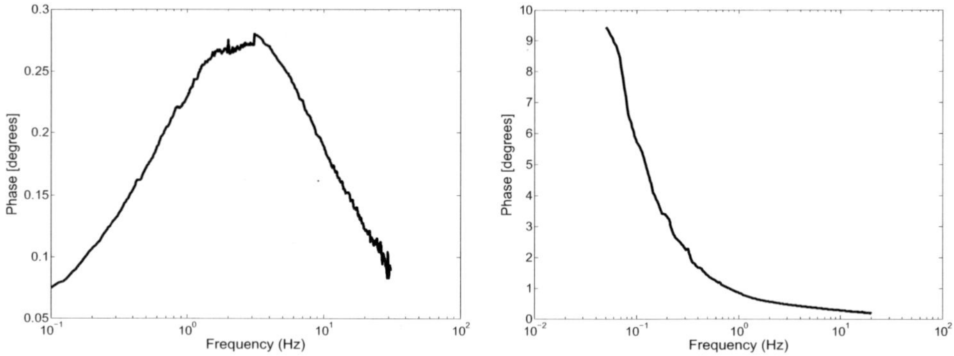

(a) wet electrodes (Wandy, E-50mm Hydrogel). (b) dry electrodes (Wandy, E-45).

Fig. 13. Typical phase response measurements obtained in vivo from (a) wet electrodes and (b) dry electrodes on the same subject.

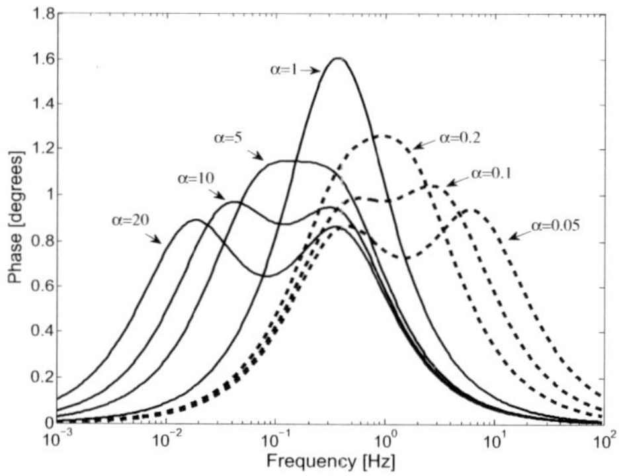

Fig. 14. Plot of the phase against frequency for different values of the ratio $\alpha = \frac{\tau_{2s}}{\tau_{4e}}$ when $R_{in} = 10\ \text{M}\Omega$, $R_{1s} + R_{3e} = 8\ \text{k}\Omega$, $R_{2s} = 140\ \text{k}\Omega$ and $R_{4e} = 150\ \text{k}\Omega$.

4.4 Alternative approaches

Alternative approaches have been investigated to solve the parameter estimation problem in situations where the phase response does not display the expected double-peak behaviour. Dozio and Baba considered different fitting algorithms and measurement set-ups and concluded that time-domain measurements combined with least squares error minimisation were the most appropriate (Assambo et al., 2006; Baba & Burke, 2008; Dozio et al., 2007).

4.4.1 Fitting magnitude and phase

Dozio et al. first developed a least squares error minimisation program for fitting both the magnitude and phase response (Assambo et al., 2006). The algorithm successfully converged when applied to a pair of adhesive electrodes (Wandy, E-50mm Hydrogel) placed on the lower abdomen and returned the the following model parameters:

$$R_{1s} + R_{3e} = 3.6\ \text{k}\Omega,\ R_{2s} = 35.2\ \text{k}\Omega,\ C_{2s} = 0.9\ \mu\text{F},\ R_{4e} = 29.5\ \text{k}\Omega,\ C_{4e} = 5.8\ \mu\text{F}.$$

The experiment also confirmed that a simple 3-parameter model is not suitable for describing the skin-electrode impedance. The curve fitting algorithm did not however converge in the case of dry, pasteless electrodes (WANDY, W-45) for which the phase response exhibited no peak in the frequency range 0.05 to 30 Hz, as shown in Fig. 13(b). This was thought to be because the peak existed at a frequency below the minimum range of the analyser.

4.4.2 Time-based measurement

Frequency-based measurements have been unsuccessful when applied to dry electrodes since the characteristic frequencies are too low to allow reliable steady state measurement. To overcome this limitation time-based measurements have been developed. Baba et al. implemented a novel measurement technique that relies upon the time response of the skin-electrode interface to a current source (Assambo et al., 2006; Baba & Burke, 2008; Dozio et al., 2007). A constant current is fed through the body while measuring the skin-electrode impedance and a high-frequency sine wave input current is used to determine $R_{1s} + R_{3e}$. The knowledge of $R_{1s} + R_{3e}$ reduces the complexity of the fitting procedure to only four parameters and improves the accuracy of the results. Measurements were taken on seven subjects, using seven different types of dry electrodes, under variable conditions of contact pressure, electrode settling time and current level. Dozio developed a curve fitting program for the time-based data acquired. The time-domain measurement procedure and the results obtained are discussed in detail in (Baba & Burke, 2008).

Table 4 gives a summary of values for each component, measured across all subjects, electrodes, locations and contact pressures as published by Baba & Burke (Baba & Burke, 2008). The identification of the skin-electrode interface model parameters from two hundred and sixty eight measurements returned values of resistance ranging from 640 Ω to 2.54 MΩ and of capacitance ranging from 0.01 μF to 432.35 μF, while values of the time constants $\tau_{2s} = C_{2s}R_{2s}$ and $\tau_{4e} = C_{4e}R_{4e}$ varied from 0.02 s to 31.29 s. It was also discovered that there were substantial differences in the component values and the time constants between the rise and the fall phases in the step response of the skin-electrode interface. Worst-case parameter values obtained can now be used in the design of the input differential amplifier in ECG recording equipment to prevent low-frequency distortion of the ECG signal.

	Current rise phase		Current fall phase	
	min.	max.	min.	max.
$R_{1s} + R_{3e}$ [kΩ]	0.64	12	0.64	12
R_{2s} [kΩ]	4.94	1760.24	23.87	2540.93
R_{4e} [kΩ]	23.26	1840.52	84.78	1380.00
C_{2s} [μF]	0.01	21.51	0.04	21.88
C_{4e} [μF]	0.10	432.35	0.69	65.15
$R_{1s} + R_{2s} + R_{3e} + R_{4e}$ [kΩ]	161.24	3616.83	125.82	3326.10
τ_{2s} [s]	0.02	1.84	0.06	1.17
τ_{4e} [s]	0.18	31.29	0.77	7.19

Table 4. Summary of dry electrode parameter values published by Baba & Burke from 268 measurements (Baba & Burke, 2008).

5. New amplifier input impedance requirements for dry-electrode ECG recording

As seen in previous sections, the front-end amplifier plays a crucial role in the ability of the ECG recorder to preserve the low-frequency components of the signal. The low-frequency performance achieved by the amplifier in the presence of the electrode impedance is principally determined by the magnitude of the input impedance of the recording system. Fig. 15 shows the equivalent impedance seen at the amplifier input when skin-electrode interface, current limiting resistor (R_1) and the dc-blocking capacitors (C_{in}) are taken into account.

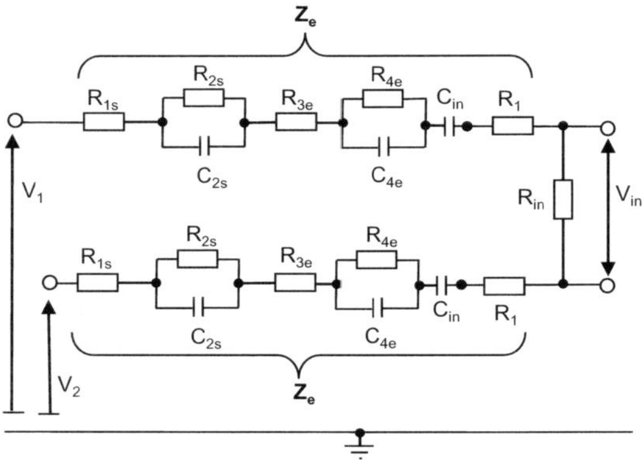

Fig. 15. Schematic representation of the equivalent impedance seen at the amplifier input.

The transfer function of the skin-electrode-amplifier network in this configuration is defined as follows:

$$H_d(s) = \frac{V_{in}(s)}{V_1(s) - V_2(s)} = R_{in}\frac{C_{in}}{2}\left[\frac{\tau_{2s}\tau_{4e}s^3 + (\tau_{2s} + \tau_{4e})\,s^2 + s}{d_3s^3 + d_2s^2 + d_1s + 1}\right] \tag{31}$$

where:

$$d_1 = [R_{in} + 2\,(R_1 + R_{1s} + R_{2s} + R_{3e} + R_{4e})]\,\frac{C_{in}}{2} + \tau_{2s} + \tau_{4e} \tag{32}$$

$$d_2 = [[R_{in} + 2\,(R_1 + R_{1s} + R_{3e})]\,(\tau_{2s} + \tau_{4e}) + 2R_{2s}\tau_{4e} + 2R_{4e}\tau_{2s}]\,\frac{C_{in}}{2} + \tau_{2s}\tau_{4e} \tag{33}$$

$$d_3 = [R_{in} + 2\,(R_1 + R_{1s} + R_{3e})]\,\frac{C_{in}}{2}\tau_{2s}\tau_{4e} \tag{34}$$

In the following sections, the authors establish new input impedance requirements for use in dry-electrode ECG recording.

5.1 Frequency response criteria

5.1.1 Amplitude response

The equivalent skin-electrode impedance, shown in Fig. 15, is responsible for a reduction in the signal amplitude before reaching the amplifier input. Minimum attenuation is obtained at high frequencies for which the impedance of capacitive elements in the electrode impedance tends toward zero, ensuring:

$$|H_d(\omega)| < \frac{R_{in}}{R_{in} + 2\,(R_1 + R_{1s} + R_{3e})} < 1 \tag{35}$$

At low frequencies, the source impedance is given by:

$$Z_e(\omega) = R_{1s} + R_{3s} + \frac{R_{2s}}{1 + j\omega R_{2s}C_{2s}} + \frac{R_{4e}}{1 + j\omega R_{4e}C_{4e}} + \frac{1}{j\omega C_1} + R_1 \tag{36}$$

The AHA recommends a maximum attenuation of 0.5 dB (or 6%) at 0.14 Hz, which establishes the requirement:

$$\frac{R_{in}}{|R_{in} + 2Z_e(\omega_{0.14})|} > 0.94 \tag{37}$$

where $\omega_{0.14} = 0.28\pi$.
It can be shown that the condition specified in eq. (37) implies the following relationship between R_{in} and the parameters of the skin-electrode interface:

$$\begin{aligned} R_{in}^2 \frac{1-0.94^2}{0.94^2} &- 4R_{in}\left[R_1 + R_{1s} + R_{3e} + \frac{R_{2s}}{1+\tau_{2s}^2\omega_{0.14}^2} + \frac{R_{4e}}{1+\tau_{4e}^2\omega_{0.14}^2}\right] \\ &- 4\left[R_1 + R_{1s} + R_{3e} + \frac{R_{2s}\tau_{2s}\omega_{0.14}}{1+\tau_{2s}^2\omega_{0.14}^2} + \frac{R_{4e}\tau_{4e}\omega_{0.14}}{1+\tau_{4e}^2\omega_{0.14}^2} + \frac{1}{\omega_{0.14}C_{in}}\right]^2 \\ &- 4\left[R_1 + R_{1s} + R_{3e} + \frac{R_{2s}}{1+\tau_{2s}^2\omega_{0.14}^2} + \frac{R_{4e}}{1+\tau_{4e}^2\omega_{0.14}^2}\right]^2 > 0 \end{aligned} \tag{38}$$

The amplitude response criterion is then fulfilled for R_{in} selected as follows:

$$\begin{aligned} R_{in} > \frac{2*0.94^2}{1-0.94^2} &\sqrt{\begin{aligned} &\left(R_1 + R_{1s} + R_{3e} + \tfrac{R_{2s}}{1+\tau_{2s}^2\omega_{0.14}^2} + \tfrac{R_{4e}}{1+\tau_{4e}^2\omega_{0.14}^2}\right)^2 \\ &+ (1-0.94^2)\left(R_1 + R_{1s} + R_{3e} + \tfrac{R_{2s}\tau_{2s}\omega_{0.14}}{1+\tau_{2s}^2\omega_{0.14}^2} + \tfrac{R_{4e}\tau_{4e}\omega_{0.14}}{1+\tau_{4e}^2\omega_{0.14}^2} + \tfrac{1}{\omega_{0.14}C_{in}}\right)^2 \end{aligned}} \\ &+ \frac{2*0.94^2}{1-0.94^2}\left(R_1 + R_{1s} + R_{3e} + \frac{R_{2s}}{1+\tau_{2s}^2\omega_{0.14}^2} + \frac{R_{4e}}{1+\tau_{4e}^2\omega_{0.14}^2}\right) \end{aligned} \tag{39}$$

5.1.2 Phase response

The transfer function defined in eq. (31) can be rearranged so that real and imaginary parts are more easily identified:

$$H_d(\omega) = R_{in}\frac{C_{in}}{2}\left[\frac{\begin{array}{c}[(d_1 - \tau_{2s} - \tau_{4e})\,\omega^2 + [d_2(\tau_{2s}+\tau_{4e}) - d_3]\,\omega^4 + d_1 d_3 \tau_{2s}\tau_{4e}\omega^6] \\ +j\,[\omega + (d_1\tau_{2s} + d_1\tau_{4e} - \tau_{2s}\tau_{4e})\,\omega^3 + [d_2\tau_{2s}\tau_{4e} - d_3(\tau_{2s}+\tau_{4e})]\,\omega^5]\end{array}}{(1-d_2\omega^2)^2 + (d_1\omega - d_3\omega^3)^2}\right] \tag{40}$$

Replacing d_1, d_2 and d_3 by their expressions as given in eq.(32) to (34) yields the following:

$$H_d(\omega) = R_{in}\frac{C_{in}}{2}\omega \left[\frac{\begin{array}{l} R_T\frac{C_{in}}{2}\omega + \left[R_T\frac{C_{in}}{2}\left(\tau_{2s}^2+\tau_{4e}^2\right) + 2\tau_{2s}\tau_{4e}\left(R_{2s}+R_{4e}\right)\frac{C_{in}}{2}\right]\omega^3 \\ +R_{13}\frac{C_{in}}{2}\tau_{2s}^2\tau_{4e}^2\omega^5 \\ +j[1+\left[2\left(R_{2s}\tau_{2s}+R_{4e}\tau_{4e}\right)\frac{C_{in}}{2}+\tau_{2s}^2+\tau_{4s}^2\right]\omega^2] \\ +j[\tau_{2s}\tau_{4e}\left[2\left(R_{2s}\tau_{4e}+R_{4e}\tau_{2s}\right)\frac{C_{in}}{2}+\tau_{2s}\tau_{4e}\right]\omega^4] \end{array}}{\begin{array}{l} \left[1-\left[\left[R_{13}\left(\tau_{2s}+\tau_{4e}\right)+2R_{2s}\tau_{4e}+2R_{4e}\tau_{2s}\right]\frac{C_{in}}{2}+\tau_{2s}\tau_{4e}\right]\omega^2\right]^2 \\ +\left[\left(R_T\frac{C_{in}}{2}+\tau_{2s}+\tau_{4e}\right)\omega - R_{13}\frac{C_{in}}{2}\tau_{2s}\tau_{4e}\omega^3\right]^2 \end{array}} \right] \tag{41}$$

where

$$R_T = R_{in} + 2\left(R_1 + R_{1s} + R_{2s} + R_{3e} + R_{4e}\right) \tag{42}$$

and

$$R_{13} = R_{in} + 2\left(R_1 + R_{1s} + R_{3e}\right) \tag{43}$$

Since both imaginary and real parts of $H_d(\omega)$ are positive, an expression for the phase response can then be extracted from (41) as:

$$\varphi_d(\omega) = tan^{-1}\left(\frac{1+\left[\left(R_{2s}\tau_{2s}+R_{4e}\tau_{4e}\right)C_{in}+\tau_{2s}^2+\tau_{4s}^2\right]\omega^2+\tau_{2s}\tau_{4e}\left[\left(R_{2s}\tau_{4e}+R_{4e}\tau_{2s}\right)C_{in}+\tau_{2s}\tau_{4e}\right]\omega^4}{R_T\frac{C_{in}}{2}\omega+\left[R_T\frac{C_{in}}{2}\left(\tau_{2s}^2+\tau_{4e}^2\right)+\tau_{2s}\tau_{4e}\left(R_{2s}+R_{4e}\right)C_{in}\right]\omega^3+R_{13}\frac{C_{in}}{2}\tau_{2s}^2\tau_{4e}^2\omega^5}\right) \tag{44}$$

Eq. (44) indicates that:

$$0 < \varphi_d(\omega) < 90^\circ, \forall\omega \in \Re^{+*} \tag{45}$$

The phase introduced by a single-pole high-pass filter having a cutoff frequency f_c is given by:

$$\Phi(\omega) = tan^{-1}\left(\frac{2\pi f_c}{\omega}\right) \tag{46}$$

The AHA recommends that the amplifier should introduce no more phase shift into the signal than that which would be introduced by a linear 0.05-Hz, single-pole filter. This condition is respected for $\varphi_d(\omega) < \Phi(\omega)$.

Both phase shifts belong to the interval $]0, \frac{\pi}{2}[$, in which the function *tan* is strictly increasing. The phase criterion is therefore equivalent to:

$$\frac{1+\left[\left(R_{2s}\tau_{2s}+R_{4e}\tau_{4e}\right)C_{in}+\tau_{2s}^2+\tau_{4s}^2\right]\omega^2+\tau_{2s}\tau_{4e}\left[\left(R_{2s}\tau_{4e}+R_{4e}\tau_{2s}\right)C_{in}+\tau_{2s}\tau_{4e}\right]\omega^4}{R_T\frac{C_{in}}{2}\omega+\left[R_T\frac{C_{in}}{2}\left(\tau_{2s}^2+\tau_{4e}^2\right)+\tau_{2s}\tau_{4e}\left(R_{2s}+R_{4e}\right)C_{in}\right]\omega^3+R_{13}\frac{C_{in}}{2}\tau_{2s}^2\tau_{4e}^2\omega^5} < \frac{2\pi f_c}{\omega} \tag{47}$$

Taking $\omega_c = 2\pi f_c$, the condition specified in eq. (47) is met for:

$$\left[\omega_c R_{13}\frac{C_{in}}{2}\tau_{2s}^2\tau_{4e}^2 - \tau_{2s}\tau_{4e}\left[\left(R_{2s}\tau_{4e} + R_{4e}\tau_{2s}\right)C_{in} + \tau_{2s}\tau_{4e}\right]\right]\omega^4$$
$$+\left[\omega_c\left[R_T\frac{C_{in}}{2}\left(\tau_{2s}^2 + \tau_{4e}^2\right) + \tau_{2s}\tau_{4e}\left(R_{2s} + R_{4e}\right)C_{in}\right] - \left[\left(R_{2s}\tau_{2s} + R_{4e}\tau_{4e}\right)C_{in} + \tau_{2s}^2 + \tau_{4s}^2\right]\right]\omega^2$$
$$+\omega_c R_T\frac{C_{in}}{2} - 1 > 0 \quad (48)$$

The polynomial function of eq. (48) is positive when two conditions are satisfied: (i) the coefficient of the highest power of ω is positive and (ii) there is no positive root. All roots must therefore be negative or complex. Both conditions are simultaneously met when:

$$\begin{cases} \omega_c R_{13}\frac{C_{in}}{2}\tau_{2s}^2\tau_{4e}^2 - \tau_{2s}\tau_{4e}\left[\left(R_{2s}\tau_{4e} + R_{4e}\tau_{2s}\right)C_{in} + \tau_{2s}\tau_{4e}\right] > 0 & (49) \\ \omega_c R_T\frac{C_{in}}{2} - 1 > 0 & (50) \end{cases}$$

Substituting $\tau_{2s} = R_{2s}C_{2s}$, $\tau_{4e} = R_{4e}C_{4e}$, $R_{13} = R_{in} + 2\left(R_1 + R_{1s} + R_{3e}\right)$ and $R_T = R_{13} + 2\left(R_{2s} + R_{4e}\right)$, eqs. (49) and (50) become:

$$\begin{cases} R_{in} > \frac{2}{\omega_c}\left(\frac{1}{C_{2s}} + \frac{1}{C_{4e}} + \frac{1}{C_{in}}\right) - 2\left(R_1 + R_{1s} + R_{3e}\right) & (51) \\ R_{in} > \frac{2}{C_{in}\omega_c} - 2\left(R_1 + R_{1s} + R_{2s} + R_{3e} + R_{4e}\right) & (52) \end{cases}$$

Eq. (52) establishes the phase criterion at low frequency, when the reactance of the capacitive effects in the skin-electrode interface tends towards infinity. At these frequencies C_{2s} and C_{4e} are equivalent to open switches making the skin-electrode impedance purely resistive. Phase shift is therefore solely introduced by the input capacitance C_{in}. This result is consistent with traditional design strategies which state that low-frequency distortion can be prevented if $R_{in}C_{in} > 1/\omega_c$, since other capacitive effects are neglected (Bergey et al., 1971; Valverde et al., 2004).

As frequency increases, the effects of C_{2s} and C_{4e} must be considered and eq. (51) ensures that the phase of the combined skin-electrode-amplifier network will not be greater than that introduced by a high-pass filter having a single pole at $f_c = \omega_c/2\pi$. Experience with insulated electrodes have shown that the effect of changing skin impedance can be minimised by making the coupling capacitance at least two orders of magnitude smaller than those of the skin. Coupling capacitance values ranging from 50 nF to 1 fF (f= 10^{-15}) have thus been used with buffer amplifiers having 10^8 to 10^{18} Ω input impedance (Ko et al., 1970; Prance et al., 2008; Taheri et al., 1994). Eq. (51) confirms that for $C_{in} << \{C_{2s}, C_{4e}\}$, the reactance of the skin-electrode interface can be neglected, and therefore selecting $R_{in}C_{in} > 1/\omega_c$ would prevent distortion. However, this approach involves the use of ultra-high input impedance amplifiers, whereas, the input impedance requirement can be relaxed if eq. (51) is applied instead.

With $f_c = 0.05$ Hz, the phase requirement is satisfied at all frequencies when the input impedance is chosen such that for the worst-case values of skin-electrode parameters:

$$R_{in} > \frac{20}{\pi}\left(\frac{1}{C_{2s}} + \frac{1}{C_{4e}} + \frac{1}{C_{in}}\right) \quad (53)$$

5.2 Impulse response requirements

In more recent years, the IEC have defined more precisely the low-frequency criteria for ECG signal reproduction in terms of the system impulse response. The response to a rectangular pulse $x(t)$ of amplitude V_m and duration T is limited to a maximum offset, ΔV_{max}, and a maximum slope, s_{max}. Fig. 16 shows in a generic form the impulse response requirement defined by international standards.

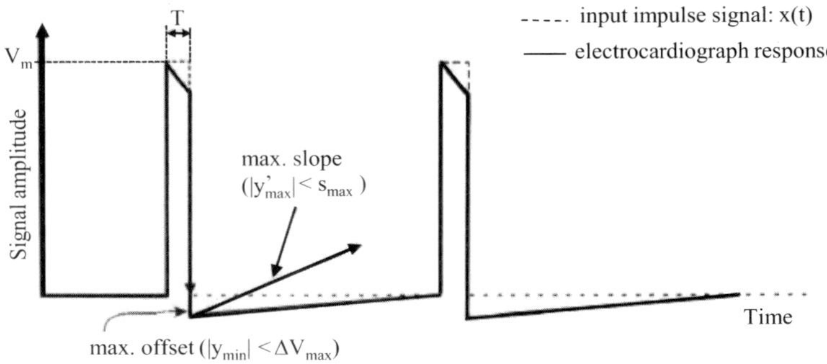

Fig. 16. Schematic illustrating the impulse response requirements.

The rectangular pulse $x(t)$ is ideally modelled using the Heaviside unit step function u as:

$$x(t) = V_m\left[u(t) - u(t-T)\right] \tag{54}$$

The Laplace transform of $x(t)$ is therefore given by:

$$X(s) = \frac{V_m}{s}\left(1 - e^{-Ts}\right) \tag{55}$$

Using the transfer function $H_d(s)$ defined in eq. (31), the frequency response $Y_d(s)$ of the skin-electrode-amplifier network to the pulse $X(s)$ is:

$$\begin{aligned} Y_d(s) = X(s)H_d(s) &= V_m\left(1 - e^{-Ts}\right) R_{in}\frac{C_{in}}{2}\left[\frac{\tau_{2s}\tau_{4e}s^2 + (\tau_{2s}+\tau_{4e})\,s + 1}{d_3s^3 + d_2s^2 + d_1s + 1}\right] \\ &= V_m\left(1 - e^{-Ts}\right) R_{in}\frac{C_{in}}{2}\tau_{2s}\tau_{4e}\left[\frac{\left(s+\frac{1}{\tau_{2s}}\right)\left(s+\frac{1}{\tau_{4e}}\right)}{d_3\,(s-p_1)\,(s-p_2)\,(s-p_3)}\right] \end{aligned} \tag{56}$$

where p_0, p_1 and p_2 are the poles of $H_d(s)$, and d_1, d_2 and d_3 are defined in eqs. (32) to (34). Substituting d_3 by its expression allows $Y_d(s)$ to be simplified as follows:

$$Y_d(s) = \frac{R_{in}}{R_{13}}V_m\left(1 - e^{-Ts}\right)\left[\frac{\left(s+\frac{1}{\tau_{2s}}\right)\left(s+\frac{1}{\tau_{4e}}\right)}{(s-p_1)\,(s-p_2)\,(s-p_3)}\right] \tag{57}$$

with R_{13} given in eq. (43). The impulse response can then be expanded by partial fractions as:

$$Y_d(s) = \frac{R_{in}}{R_{13}}V_m\left(1 - e^{-Ts}\right)\left[\frac{A_0}{(s-p_0)} + \frac{A_1}{(s-p_1)} + \frac{A_2}{(s-p_2)}\right] \tag{58}$$

where the three coefficients A_0, A_1 and A_2 are functions of the parameters of the skin-electrode-amplifier network. Eqs. (56) and (58) imply:

$$\begin{aligned} Y_d(s)(s-p_0) &= \frac{R_{in}}{R_{13}} V_m \left(1-e^{-Ts}\right)\left[A_0 + (s-p_0)\frac{A_1}{(s-p_1)} + (s-p_0)\frac{A_2}{(s-p_2)}\right] \\ &= \frac{R_{in}}{R_{13}} V_m \left(1-e^{-Ts}\right)\left[\frac{\left(s+\frac{1}{\tau_{2s}}\right)\left(s+\frac{1}{\tau_{4e}}\right)}{(s-p_1)(s-p_2)}\right] \end{aligned} \tag{59}$$

Taking $s = p_0$ yields:

$$A_0 = \frac{\left(p_0+\frac{1}{\tau_{2s}}\right)\left(p_0+\frac{1}{\tau_{4e}}\right)}{(p_0-p_1)(p_0-p_2)} \tag{60}$$

A similar approach leads to expressions for A_1 and A_2 as follows:

$$A_1 = \frac{\left(p_1+\frac{1}{\tau_{2s}}\right)\left(p_1+\frac{1}{\tau_{4e}}\right)}{(p_1-p_0)(p_1-p_2)} \tag{61}$$

$$A_2 = \frac{\left(p_2+\frac{1}{\tau_{2s}}\right)\left(p_2+\frac{1}{\tau_{4e}}\right)}{(p_2-p_0)(p_2-p_1)} \tag{62}$$

The inverse Laplace transform of $Y_d(s)$ gives the corresponding response in time $y_d(t)$ as:

$$\begin{aligned} y_d(t) = &\frac{R_{in}}{R_{13}} V_m \left(A_0 e^{p_0 t} + A_1 e^{p_1 t} + A_2 e^{p_2 t}\right) u(t) \\ &- \frac{R_{in}}{R_{13}} V_m \left(A_0 e^{p_0 (t-T)} + A_1 e^{p_1 (t-T)} + A_2 e^{p_2 (t-T)}\right) u(t-T) \end{aligned} \tag{63}$$

If $x(t)$ is an ideal pulse, the amplitude of the response following the end of the impulse is given by:

$$y_d(t)|_{t>T} = -\frac{R_{in}}{R_{13}} V_m \sum_{k=0}^{2}\left[A_k(e^{-p_k T}-1)e^{p_k t}\right] \tag{64}$$

The derivative of $y(t)$ at $t > T$ defines the slope of the impulse response following the impulse:

$$y'_d(t)|_{t>T} = \left.\frac{dy_d(t)}{dt}\right|_{t>T} = -\frac{R_{in}}{R_{13}} V_m \sum_{k=0}^{2}\left[p_k A_k(e^{-p_k T}-1)e^{p_k t}\right] \tag{65}$$

The poles p_0, p_1 and p_2 are obtained by solving the polynomial $d_3 s^3 + d_2 s^2 + d_1 s + 1 = 0$. Computing the equation with *Mathematica* returns the following solutions:

$$\begin{aligned} p_0 = &-\frac{d_2}{3d_3} - \frac{2^{1/3}\left(-d_2^2+3d_1d_3\right)}{3d_3\left[-2d_2^3+9d_1d_2d_3-27d_3^2+\sqrt{4\left(-d_2^2+3d_1d_3\right)^3+\left(-2d_2^3+9d_1d_2d_3-27d_3^2\right)^2}\right]^{1/3}} \\ &+ \frac{\left[-2d_2^3+9d_1d_2d_3-27d_3^2+\sqrt{4\left(-d_2^2+3d_1d_3\right)^3+\left(-2d_2^3+9d_1d_2d_3-27d_3^2\right)^2}\right]^{1/3}}{3 2^{1/3} d_3} \end{aligned} \tag{66}$$

$$p_1 = -\frac{d_2}{3d_3} - \frac{(1+j\sqrt{3})(-d_2^2+3d_1d_3)}{32^{1/3}d_3\left[-2d_2^3+9d_1d_2d_3-27d_3^2+\sqrt{4(-d_2^2+3d_1d_3)^3+(-2d_2^3+9d_1d_2d_3-27d_3^2)^2}\right]^{1/3}} - \frac{(1-j\sqrt{3})\left[-2d_2^3+9d_1d_2d_3-27d_3^2+\sqrt{4(-d_2^2+3d_1d_3)^3+(-2d_2^3+9d_1d_2d_3-27d_3^2)^2}\right]^{1/3}}{62^{1/3}d_3} \quad (67)$$

$$p_2 = -\frac{d_2}{3d_3} - \frac{(1-j\sqrt{3})(-d_2^2+3d_1d_3)}{32^{1/3}d_3\left[-2d_2^3+9d_1d_2d_3-27d_3^2+\sqrt{4(-d_2^2+3d_1d_3)^3+(-2d_2^3+9d_1d_2d_3-27d_3^2)^2}\right]^{1/3}} - \frac{(1+j\sqrt{3})\left[-2d_2^3+9d_1d_2d_3-27d_3^2+\sqrt{4(-d_2^2+3d_1d_3)^3+(-2d_2^3+9d_1d_2d_3-27d_3^2)^2}\right]^{1/3}}{62^{1/3}d_3} \quad (68)$$

The terms d_1, d_2 and d_3 may be substituted with their expressions given in eqs. (32) to (34) to evaluate p_0, p_1 and p_2. This would allow $y_d(t)$ and $y'_d(t)$ to be represented in terms of the parameters of the skin-electrode-amplifier network and the input impedance requirement to be identified. However, this method involves solving non-linear functions in the complex domain for which analytical solutions are not available. An alternative approach consists of implementing a numerical algorithm to find the minimum value of R_{in} for which the recording system meets the impulse response requirements. An algorithm was developed in *MATLAB* to test the maximum undershoot and recovery slope for a range of values of R_{in}.

5.3 Results

Data collected from two hundred and sixty eight measurements of the skin-electrode interface are analysed using the proposed methods. Measurements were taken on seven subjects, using seven different types of dry electrodes, under variable conditions of contact pressure, electrode settling time and current level. As for simulations referred to in Section 2.1, the input capacitance is initially set at $C_{in} = 0.33$ µF. The current limiting resistor was chosen as $R_1 = 100$ kΩ, as recommended in previous literature (Burke & Gleeson, 2000).

5.3.1 Amplitude and phase criteria

Fig. 17(a) shows the frequency response of the skin-electrode-amplifier network when the input impedance is selected following the amplitude response criterion defined in eq. (39). For all measurements, the minimum input impedance that fulfils the amplitude response recommendation varies from 21 MΩ to 115 MΩ. Fig. 17(b) gives the corresponding results when the front-end is designed according to the phase response requirement indicated in eq. (53). Meeting the phase criterion requires an input impedance between 21 MΩ and 750 MΩ.

5.3.2 Impulse response criteria

Results from the analysis of the impulse response for all measurements are presented in Fig. 17. A rectangular wave of amplitude 3 mV and duration 100 ms is used as input. The response is analysed over a 2 s period. Fig. 17(c) shows a plot of the maximum undershoot produced for a range of input impedance values between 10 MΩ and 10 GΩ. In Fig. 17(d), the maximum absolute values of the slope of the responses following the impulse are shown over the same range of input impedance values. With $C_{in} = 0.33$ µF, the required minimum input impedance varies between 20 MΩ and 2 GΩ.

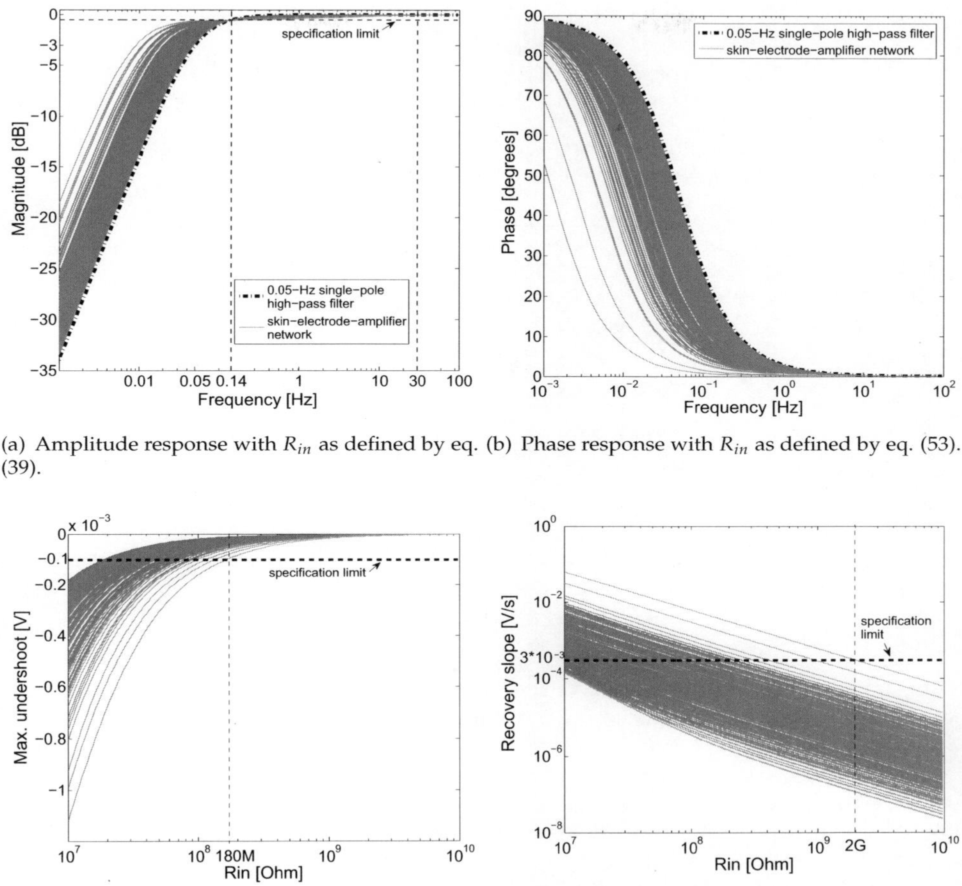

(a) Amplitude response with R_{in} as defined by eq. (39).

(b) Phase response with R_{in} as defined by eq. (53).

(c) Maximum undershoot vs. R_{in}.

(d) Maximum slope absolute value vs. R_{in}.

Fig. 17. Plots of (a) the amplitude response, (b) phase response, (c) the maximum undershoot and (d) the maximum recovery slope for 268 measurements of skin-electrode interface impedance with $C_{in} = 0.33\mu F$ and $R_1 = 100\ k\Omega$.

5.3.3 Influence of the coupling capacitance

Tables 5 and 6 compare the values of input impedance suggested by the frequency response and impulse response criteria. The values of R_{in} are given in both tables for a range of non-electrolytic capacitance values of C_{in} varying from 0.1 μF to 3.3 μF, available in multilayer ceramic forms. Table 5 gives the maximum values of input impedance suggested by all measurements. When one pair of outlying values is removed from the results, the requirements suggested by 99.2% of the data are shown in Table 6.

C_{in} [μF]	0.1	0.22	0.33	0.47	1	2.2	3.3
amplitude response: R_{in} [MΩ]	139	119	115	114	112	112	112
phase response: R_{in} [MΩ]	764	730	720	714	707	704	703
impulse response: R_{in} [MΩ]	2040	2040	2040	2040	2040	2040	2040

Table 5. Worst-case input impedance requirements as a function of the capacitance of the dc-blocking capacitor C_{in} for all 268 measurements.

C_{in} [μF]	0.1	0.22	0.33	0.47	1	2.2	3.3
amplitude response: R_{in} [MΩ]	120	96	91	89	87	86	86
phase response: R_{in} [MΩ]	236	201	192	185	180	175	174
impulse response: R_{in} [MΩ]	429	429	429	429	429	429	429

Table 6. Worst-case input impedance requirements as a function of the capacitance of the dc-blocking capacitor C_{in} for 99.2% of measurements.

Results for both tables indicate that the value of R_{in} levels out at around a value of $C_{in} = 1$ μF. As suggested by eq. (53), with increasing dc-blocking capacitance value, the parameters of the skin-electrode interface become the limiting factor. All results confirm that meeting the impulse response involves the highest values of input impedance, which are selected as the target design value. This is seen to be 2 GΩ, well above the IEC specification value of 10 MΩ. This again highlights the inappropriateness of this impedance specification for dry electrodes.

6. Conclusion

In this chapter, poor low-frequency response was shown to be a primary source of measurement error that jeopardises the ability of the ECG recording to provide reliable diagnostic clinical information. Despite being necessary to prevent base line wander, high-pass filtering can cause distortion in the ECG signal if implemented inadequately. A numerical tool was developed by the authors to assess the performance of passive high-pass filters up to fourth order against standards requirements. Simulation results have highlighted the lack of consistency between minimum input impedance requirement and low-frequency specifications in ECG standards. It was also demonstrated that the input impulse criteria imply more stringent requirements than the traditional amplitude and phase specifications. In particular, it was shown that recording systems for which the impulse response exhibits an unsatisfactory recovery slope may distort the ECG waveform despite providing acceptable amplitude and phase characteristics in the signal bandwidth. The need for new input impedance requirements that rely upon a complete characterisation of the skin-electrode interface was therefore identified.

Different approaches have been undertaken to model the skin-electrode interface. Experiences with self-adhesive electrodes confirmed that an early model which describes the interface as a single-time-constant RC network is inadequate. A model involving two time constants proves more accurate. Based on the latter model, an algorithm has been implemented to identify the parameters of any double-time-constant system the phase response of which displays a double-peak. Simulations returned highly accurate results when the two time constants forming the system are in a ratio of greater than 10 to 1. The method reaches its limits, however, when the time constants are close to each other and the difference in the phase of the two peaks in the response becomes too small to be accurately measured by the instruments available. Time-domain measurements were employed to obtain parameter values for dry, pasteless electrodes. The fitting procedure converged when the rise and fall phases of the response were analysed separately, producing two estimates of the model parameters. The authors have then derived, using a combination of analytical and numerical methods, a set of input impedance requirements which ensure that performance specifications are met in dry-electrode recording. The minimum requirement for the input resistance of the amplifier is determined as 2 GΩ over a range of electrodes, measurement conditions and the value of dc-blocking capacitors used. However, 99.2% of measurements suggested that a value of R_{in} of 500 MΩ would meet requirements.

7. References

A.H.A. (1967). Recommendations for standardization of leads and of specifications for instruments in electrocardiography and vectorcardiography, *Circulation* 35: 583 – 602.

A.H.A. (1985). Aha special reports: Recommendations for standards of instrumentation and practice in the use of ambulatory electrocardiography, *Circulation* 71: 626A – 636A.

A.H.A. (1990). Recommendations for standardization and specifications in automated electrocardiography: bandwidth and digital signal processing. a report for health professionals by an ad hoc writing group of the committee on electrocardiography and cardiac electrophysiology of the council on clinical cardiology, american heart association, *Circulation* 81: 730 – 739.

Assambo, C., Baba, A., Dozio, R. & Burke, M. J. (2006). Parameter estimation of the skin-electrode interface model for high-impedance bio-electrodes, *WSEAS Transactions on Biology and Biomedicine* 3: 573 – 580.

Baba, A. & Burke, M. J. (2008). Electrical characterisation of dry electrodes for ecg recording, *Proceedings of the 12th WSEAS International Conference in Circuits Systems Communications and Computers*, Crete, Greece, pp. 591 – 596.

Bergey, G. E., Aquires, R. D. & Sipple, W. C. (1971). Electrocardiogram recording with pasteless electrodes, *IEEE Transactions on Bio-medical Engineering* BME-18: 206 – 211.

Berson, A. S., Galen, P., Adams, W. O., Adan, M., Berson, A. S., Briller, S. A., Daleo, S., Daly, D. L., Dobbins, J., Fink, M. N., Galen, P., Geselowitz, D., Gupte, P. M., Hernke, D., Klement, H., Milsap, J. P., Rutishauser, K., Smirles, W. J., Webster, J. G., Brown, D., Cangelosi, R., Charbonnier, F., Kutik, M. J. & Rowlandson, I. (2007). *ANSI/AAMI EC11:1991/(R)2001/(R)2007: Diagnostic electrocardiographic devices.*

Berson, S. & Pipberger, H. V. (1966). The low frequency response of electrocardiographs, a frequent source of recording errors, *Amererican Heart Journal* 71(6): 779 – 789.

Bruce, R. E., Moody, G., Bruce, R. E., Deedwania, P. C., Richard Gregg, P. M., Ho, C., Moody, G., Murray, W., Rutishauser, K., Sajadi, A., Sunderl, R. A., Young, B. J., Eloff, B. C., Marinello, S. A., Schneider, M. & Wang, J. (2007). *ANSI/AAMI EC38:2007: Medical electrical equipment - Part 2-47: Particular requirements for the safety, including essential performance, of ambulatory electrocardiographic systems.*

Burke, M. J. & Gleeson, D. T. (2000). A micropower dry-electrode ecg preamplifier, *IEEE Transactions on Biomedical Engineering* 47.

Chang, C.-L., Chang, C.-W., Huang, H.-Y., Hsu, C.-M., Huang, C.-H., Chiou, J.-C. & Luo, C.-H. (2010). A power-efficient bio-potential acquisition device with ds-mde sensors for long-term healthcare monitoring applications, *Sensors* 10: 4778 – 4793.

Dozio, R., Baba, A., Assambo, C. & Burke, M. J. (2007). Time based measurement of the impedance of the skin-electrode interface for dry electrode ecg recording, *Proceedings of the 29th Annual International Conference of the IEEE Engineering in Medicine and Biology Society*, Lyon, France, pp. 5001 – 5004.

Fuhrhop, S., Lamparth, S., Kirst, M., Wagner, G. & Ottenbacher, J. (2009). Ambulant ecg recording with wet and dry electrodes: A direct comparison of two systems, *in* O. Dossel & W. C. Schlegel (eds), *IFMBE proceedings of the 2009 World Congress on Medical Physics and Biomedical Engineering*, Vol. 25 / V, Munich, Germany, pp. 305 – 307.

Gruetzmann, A., Hansen, S. & Müller, J. (2007). Novel dry electrodes for ecg monitoring, *Physiological Measurement* 28: 1375 – 1390.

I.E.C. (2001). *Medical electrical equipment Part 2-47: Particular requirements for the safety, including essential performance, of ambulatory electrocardiographic systems (IEC 60601-2-47:2001)*, 2nd edn.

I.E.C. (2005). *Medical electrical equipment Part 2-27: Particular requirements for the safety, including essential performance, of electrocardiographic monitoring equipment (IEC 60601-2-27:2005)*.

Ko, W. H., Neuman, M. R., Wolfson, R. N. & Yon, E. T. (1970). Insulated active electrodes, *IEEE Transactions on Industrial Electronics and Control Instrumentation* IECI-17: 195 – 198.

Lee, K.-H., Lee, J.-W., Jung, W.-C., Kim, K.-S., Jun, J.-H. & Kim, D.-J. (2006). Asymmetric skin-to-electrode impedance characterisation of concentric circular ring electrode for monitoring of electrical activity of the heart, *Proceedings of the SICE-ICASE International Joint Conference*, pp. 1135 – 1136.

Lynch, P., Dargie, H., Krickler, S. & Krickler, D. (1980). Objective assessment of anti-anginal treatment: A double blind comparison of propranolol, nifedipine, and their combination, *British Medical Journal* pp. 184 – 187.

Mühlsteff, J. & Such, O. (2004). Dry electrodes for monitoring of vital signs in functional textiles, *Proceedings of the 26th Annual International Conference of the IEEE EMBS*, San Francisco, CA, USA, pp. 2212 – 2215.

Prance, R. J., Beardsmore-Rst, S., Aydin, A., Harland, C. J. & Prance, H. (2008). Biological and medical applications of a new electric field sensor, *Proceedings of the ESA Annual Meeting on Electrostatics*.

Symanski, J. D. & Gettes, L. S. (1993). Drug effects on the electrocardiogram: a review of their clinical importance, *Drugs* 46: 219 – 248.

Taheri, B. A., Knight, R. T. & Smith, R. L. (1994). A dry electrode for eeg recording, *Electroencelography and Clinical Neurophysiology* 90: 376 – 383.

Tayler, D. & Vincent, R. (1983). Signal distortion in the electrocardiogram due to inadequate phase response, *IEEE Trans. Biomed. Eng.* 30(6): 352 – 356.

Valverde, E. R., Arini, P. D., Bertran, G. C., Biagetti, M. O. & Quinteiro, R. A. (2004). Effect of electrode impedance in improved buffer amplifier for bioelectric recordings, *Journal of Medical Engineering and Technology* 28: 217 – 222.

Wolfe, A. & Reinhold, H. (1974). *A Flexible, quick application ECG electrode system, in Biomedical Electrode Technology*, 1st edn, Academic Press, chapter 2, pp. 183 – 192.

Zepeda-Carapia, I., Marquez-espionaza, A. & Alvarado-Serrano, C. (2005). Measurement of the skin-electrode impedance for a 12-lead electrocardiogram, *Proceedings of the 2nd International Conference on Electronics Engineering and XI Conference on Electrical Engineering*, pp. 193 – 195.

4

Implantation Techniques of Leads for Left Ventricular Pacing in Cardiac Resynchronization Therapy and Electrocardiographic Consequences of the Stimulation Site

Michael Scheffer[1] and Berry M. van Gelder[2]
[1]Maasstad Hospital, Rotterdam
[2]Catharina Hospital, Eindhoven
The Netherlands

1. Introduction

The first descriptions of beneficial effects of left ventricular (LV) or simultaneous LV and right ventricular (RV) pacing were published more than 35 years ago (Vagnini et al.,1967; Tyers et al.,1970; Gibson et al.,1971). In 1994 Cazeau published the first successful cases of biventricular pacing in patients with severe congestive heart failure (CHF) and no conventional indication for cardiac pacing (Cazeau et al.,1994). At the same time Bakker and colleagues reported their experiences (Bakker et al.,2000), with epicardial LV pacing by thoracotomy. The transvenous approach via the coronary sinus (CS) tributaries was first published by Daubert in 1998 and was an important contribution in the application of cardiac resynchronization therapy (Daubert et al.,1998) (Fig 1).
The transvenous approach has been more and more developed and has become the implantation technique of choice. CRT is recently categorized as class I level of evidence A in the European Society of Cardiology guidelines in patients with a dyssynchronous failing heart (Swedberg et al.,2005). In case of unsuccessful transvenous implantation, surgical LV lead placement can be achieved under direct visualization. Another approach for LV lead placement, when neither CS placement nor surgical options are available, is a trans-atrial septal puncture to pass the LV lead via the left atrium through the mitral valve and screw into the LV lateral wall (Leclercq et al.,1999; Jaïs et al.,1998; van Gelder et al.,2007), or by apical insertion of the LV lead (Kassaï et al.,2009).

2. Venous access

Venous access can be obtained by subclavian or axillary vein puncture or by the cephalic vein cut down method.
The subclavian puncture is most frequently used for transvenous pacing leads. After the puncture is performed, a guide wire is passed into the subclavian vein and a dilator with a splitable sheath is advanced over the guide wire into the vein. The guide wire and the

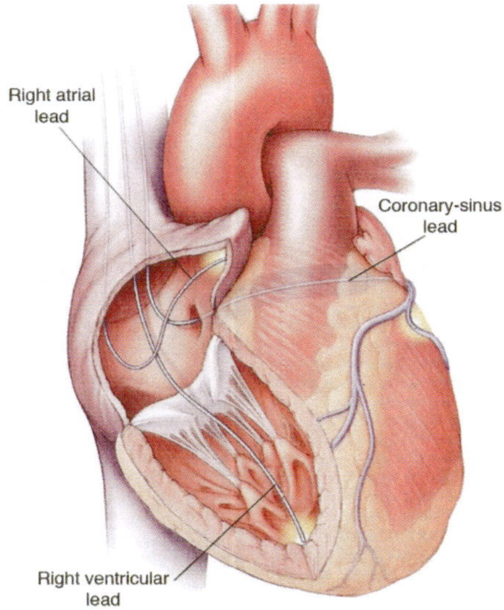

Fig. 1. The transvenous approach to CRT.
Right atrial lead placed in the right atrial appendage. Right ventricular lead placed in the apex of the right ventricle. The left ventricular lead is advanced through the coronary sinus in one of the venous side branches running along the left postero-lateral wall of the left ventricle to allow synchronous activation of the left ventricle through continuous stimulation of left and right ventricular leads in a simultaneous or sequential way with an adjusted V-V interval.

dilator are removed and the sheath is left in the vein for passage of the pacing lead. This technique is referred to as the Seldinger technique. With a single puncture both RA and RV leads can be introduced. The RV lead is placed in the right ventricle leaving the guide wire alongside the lead. The sheath is withdrawn and the retained wire is used to introduce a second sheath for the RA lead. A separate puncture is advisable to introduce the LV lead.

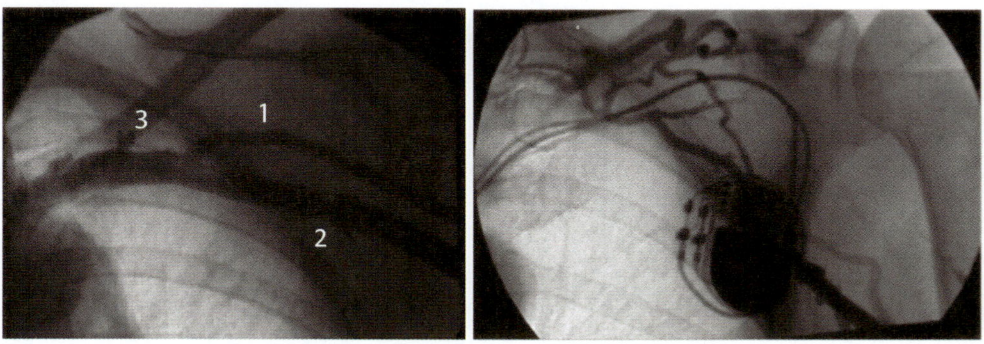

Fig. 2. Venous contrast injection showing the cephalic vein (1), axillary vein (2) and the subclavian vein (3) running under the clavicle. (left panel) Complete occlusion of the axillary and subclavian vein before an upgrading of a DDD pacemaker to a biventricular pacemaker (right panel).

As an alternative the cephalic vein can be located and cannulated in the deltopectoral groove to introduce one or more pacing leads. Usually this approach is combined with the puncture method, because the cephalic vein is often too small to insert three leads.
In our institution we prefer to start the implantation procedure with a contrast injection of 20 cc in the peripheral vein of the arm to visualize the cephalic, axillary and subclavian vein (Fig 2).
After the venography an image hold can help in case of a difficult puncture and RA and RV lead choice can be made depending on the size of the vessels and cardiac anatomy. If an upgrade to CRT is necessary subclavian thrombosis or severe stenosis is present in up to 15 % of the patients and with a planned venography needless effort can be prevented and a desirable strategy can be determined.
The left shoulder is the preferred implantation site, because it provides a more natural curve for the guiding catheter to enter the CS from the superior vena cava and right atrium. For implantation of a biventricular implantable cardioverter defibrillator (CRT-D) the left side is also preferable because of lower defibrillation threshold from this side. The cephalic vein cut down is used for both RA and RV leads and a separate puncture of the subclavian vein or axillary vein is used for the LV lead. This facilitates removal of the guiding delivery catheter for the LV lead with the slitting method.
In case of an absent cephalic vein double or triple puncture of the subclavian or axillary vein is used to introduce separate sheaths for the three leads. The RV lead is first implanted to provide backup pacing in case of traumatizing the right bundle in patients with preexisting left bundle branch block or due to traumatic atrioventricular block with introduction of the guiding catheter in the CS, which occur in 1-4% of cases (Abraham et al.,2002; Kautzner et al.,2004) (Fig 3).

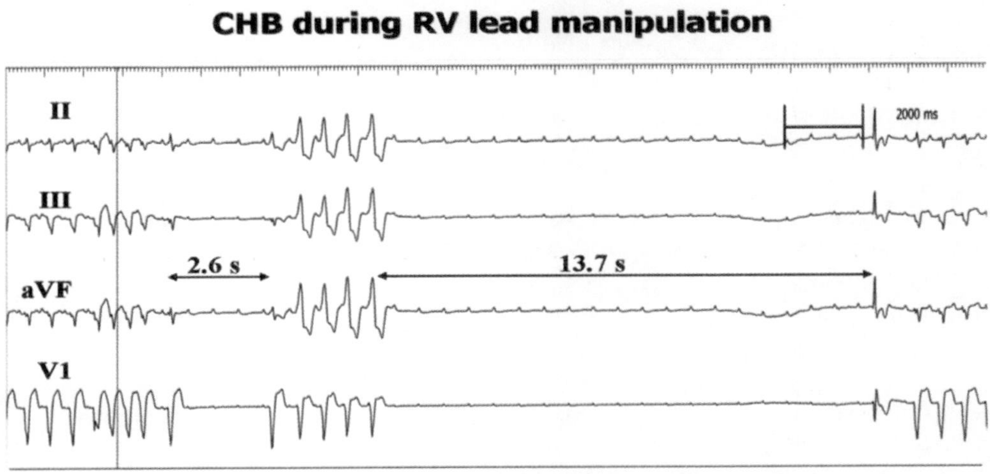

Fig. 3. During manipulation of the right ventricular lead complete heart block can occur due to traumatizing the right bundle as shown above. After a non sustained VT a pause of 2.6 seconds is followed by another non sustained VT and a second pause of 13.7 seconds in which only P waves are seen.

The RV lead can be screwed in the RV septum or placed in the RV apex. Although not proven is the mid septum position the best position to create an optimal separation between the RV and LV lead, which should be positioned in the postero-lateral wall.
The RA lead is positioned in the right atrial appendage or in case of interatrial conduction time delay of more than 120 ms in the interatrial septum to synchronize both atria. Interatrial conduction time delay can be measured beforehand with echocardiography using the Doppler signal from the tricuspid and mitral inflow and the p wave on the electrocardiogram, which gives the interatrial mechanical delay (Fig 4).

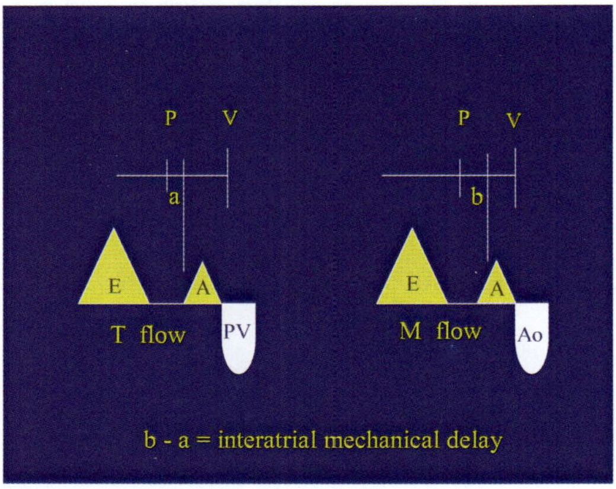

Fig. 4. Interatrial mechanical delay. With the use of echo-Doppler the inflow over the tricuspid and mitral valve can be obtained after which the difference between the electrical and mechanical activation of the right and left atrium can be measured. In the figure appointed as **a** for the right atrium and **b** for the left atrium. The difference between both gives the interatrial mechanical delay.

3. How to insert the left ventricular lead

3.1 Finding the coronary sinus

The key step in the implantation procedure for resynchronization therapy is finding the entrance to the CS. The CS ostium measures 5-15 mm in diameter and is located on the posterior interatrial septum anterior to the Eustachian ridge and valve and posterior to the tricuspid annulus (Fig 5).

Anatomy of the right atrium

The Thebesian valve frequently covers a part of the ostium, but can as a fenestrated valve completely occlude the ostium. Other valves found in the CS, like the Vieussens, sometimes seen at the ostium of the primary postero-lateral vein, opposite to the vein of Marshall and the non Vieussens valve at the ostium of the middle cardiac vein. Understanding the anatomy of the right atrium in the failing heart helps to successful access the CS. Non invasive imaging of the coronary venous anatomy has shown that the relationship between the RA and the CS in patients with congestive heart failure is quite different from that in patients with normal hearts (Chan et al.,2004). Due to the enlargement of the failing heart, the heart will rotate, causing the ostium of the CS to move to a low and posterior position in the right atrium (León et al.,2005). Other landmarks seen with fluoroscopy can be used to identify the CS, such as calcifications of the right coronary artery, or the lucent adipose pad overlying the atrial-ventricular groove that marks the course of the CS.

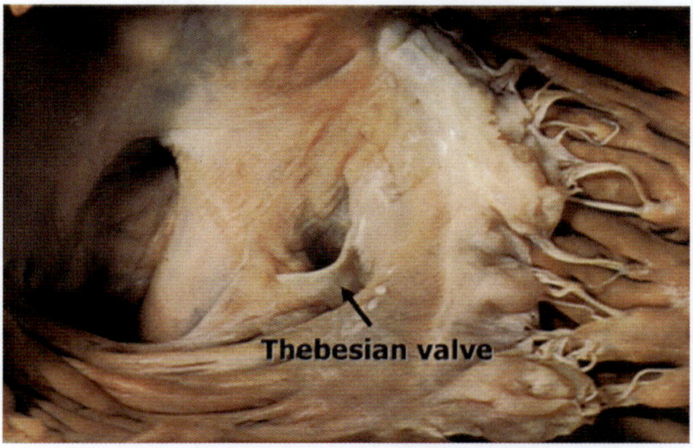

Fig. 5. The right atrium with the Thebesian valve partly covering the ostium of the coronary sinus.

Cannulation of the CS is done with preshaped guiding delivery sheaths, which are available in many different models (Fig 6). The main purpose of the guiding delivery sheath is to provide stability and pushability of the LV lead during cannulation of one of the tributes of the CS and it also offers the possibility the make a venogram with the balloon catheter.

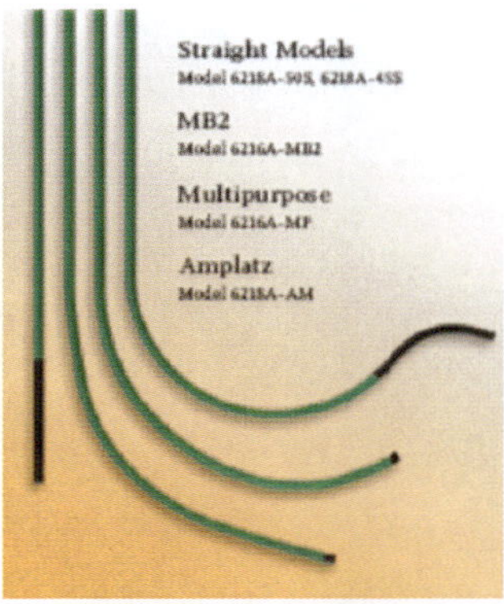

Fig. 6. Several types of guiding delivery sheaths used for cannulation of the coronary sinus. The type used depends on the side of implantation, enlargement of the right atrium and angulation of the CS and stability given by the provided guiding delivery sheath.

The guiding delivery sheath is brought into the subclavian vein through a 9 French sheath, so the guiding delivery catheter can move easily. The left anterior oblique (LAO) 30°-45° projection best guides CS access, because the CS runs toward the spine in a posterior direction to encircle the mitral annulus in that view.

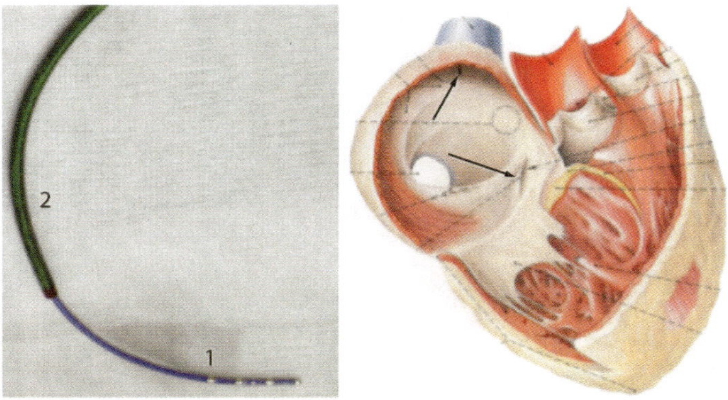

Fig. 7. The TORQR (1) is inside the guiding delivery sheath (2), left panel. Both catheters are brought into the roof of the right atrium (upper arrow), where the guiding delivery sheath is kept and the TORQR is advanced to cannulate the coronary sinus (lower arrow), right panel.

The guiding delivery sheath is brought in the roof of the right atrium after which the EP catheter is advanced in the floor of the right atrium and pulled up with counterclockwise torque to direct it posterior to the ostium of the CS. (Fig 7, right panel)

Another way is to maneuver the EP catheter into the right ventricle and then slowly withdrawn with counterclockwise torque towards the right atrium to engage the CS. Engagement of the CS ostium results in a characteristic rocking motion of the catheter due to systolic movement of the AV groove. The guiding delivery catheter is then pushed over the EP catheter as a railing system inside the CS to a distal position to prevent dislodgement.

When numerous attempts fail to locate the ostium of the CS, coronary angiography catheters like the Amplatz L2-L3 can be used for contrast injections near the ostium of the CS or a guidewire (0.035″ J wire) is introduced to explore the lower right atrium for the ostium of the CS. If this also fails a selective coronary angiography of the left coronary artery in the LAO 30°-45° projection will disclose the CS if the venous passage of contrast is visualized. Otherwise visualization with intra cardiac echocardiography has been proposed, but this technique is relatively expensive and experience is limited.

After a learning curve the CS can be cannulated within several minutes, but even in experienced hands a failure rate to cannulate the CS is reported in the range of 1-3%.

A rare case of failure is an anatomical aberrancy in which the CS has no communication with the RA. In this situation the CS drains into the venous circulation through a persistent left superior caval vein. This aberrancy is encountered in 3 out of 500 CS implants (Gelder et al.,2003).

Once the CS is successfully cannulated the electrophysiology catheter can be exchanged for a balloon catheter to perform an occlusive CS venography in two projections LAO and RAO 30°-45°.

3.2 Retrograde coronary venography

The use of venography of the CS is necessary to facilitate LV lead implantation. The balloon catheter is loaded with a PCI wire and the balloon catheter is advanced to the end of the guiding delivery sheath under fluoroscopy. The 0.014 PCI wire is pushed out the balloon catheter and advanced into the CS. This will prevent dissection from the CS by the balloon catheter.

The PCI wire will be pulled back to allow a retrograde contrast injection after balloon occlusion of the CS (Fig 8). This is done with a 10 cc syringe hand injection of contrast diluted with saline 0,9 %.

Retrograde injection of contrast opacifies all potential target veins, valves, structures, collateral connections and specific anatomic details of the target veins that will help to make the right choice for the LV lead (Fig 9). It is desirable to make a long cine sequence to visualize collaterals or side branches occluded by the balloon. To avoid occlusion of side branches by the balloon catheter or if no side branches are visualized, contrast injections must be repeated at several levels in the CS.

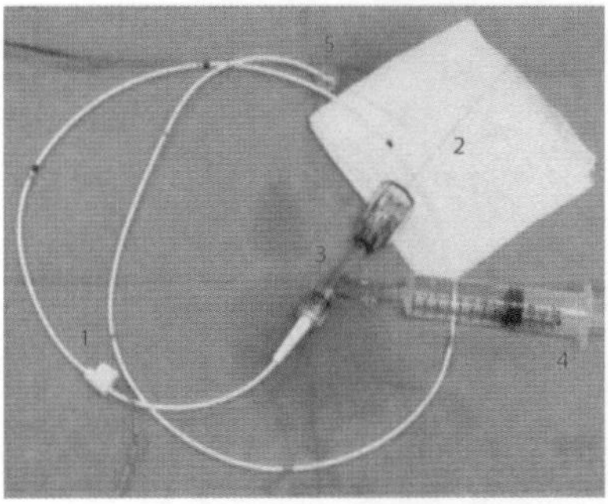

Fig. 8. Balloon catheter (1) with the PCI wire (2) and Y connector (3) together with a contrast syringe (4) to the side port. The balloon catheter is advanced in the CS with the PCI wire running before the balloon catheter to prevent dissection of the CS. After the PCI wire is pulled back a retrograde injection in the CS is made after balloon inflation (5).

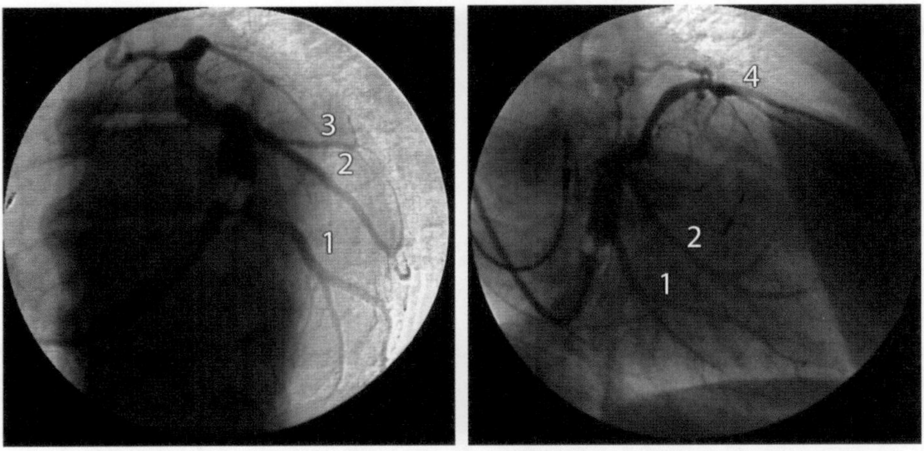

Fig. 9. Retrograde coronary venography of the coronary sinus. On the left panel the LAO projection shows the coronary sinus with two large postero-lateral branches (1 and 2) and a small lateral branch (3). The right side shows the RAO projection. In this projection we see again both postero-lateral branches (1 and 2) with second order branches and the great cardiac vein running over the anterior wall (4).

The PCI wire can be left in the balloon catheter to steer it into the selected vein. Position can be checked by contrast injection through the Y connector.

LV pacing from the lateral, postero-lateral or antero-lateral cardiac vein provides the optimal result of the CRT device (Butter et al.,2001). (Fig 10). Successful implantation also depends on the inclusion criteria, which should include mechanical dyssynchrony to provide responders to CRT (Scheffer et al.,2010; Yu et al.,2002; Bax et al.,2003). Stimulation at the LV site with the latest mechanical activation measured with TDI will provide the highest cardiac output (Ansalone et al.,2002).

Storing digitally acquired images in two radiographic views (RAO 30°and LAO 30-45°) offer a reference for advancing PCI wires and LV pacing leads in the target branch of the CS.

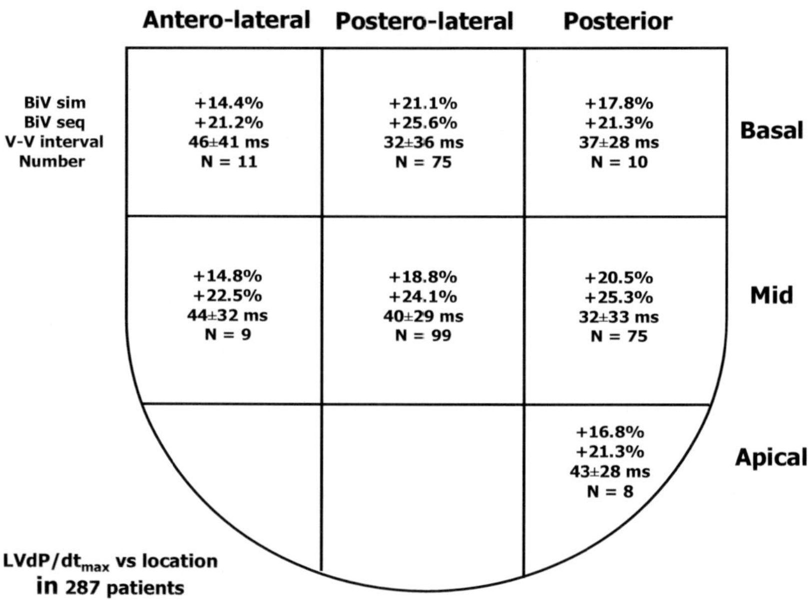

Fig. 10. Diagram of LV lead positions of 287 patients implanted with a CRT device combined figures from the Catharina Hospital, Eindhoven, The Netherlands and Maasstad Hospital Rotterdam in three years. Percentages indicate the rise in LV dP/dt compared to baseline. The preferred position is the basal lateral or mid lateral position measured with LV dp/dt immediately after implantation of a CRT device. These locations are also found by others to be the preferred position for optimal CRT.

3.3 Accessibility of side branches

Side branches too small for lead placement or complete absence of the side branches are a rare phenomenon, but can occasionally occur. Visualization of the middle cardiac vein can help to find a way to a lateral position for the LV lead. After coronary artery bypass surgery pericardial fibrosis or severe stenosis of the target vein may complicate the placement of the

LV lead. Coronary venoplasty or stenting is used in those patients to overcome these problems (Hansky et al.,2002; van Gelder et al.,2003) (fig 11).

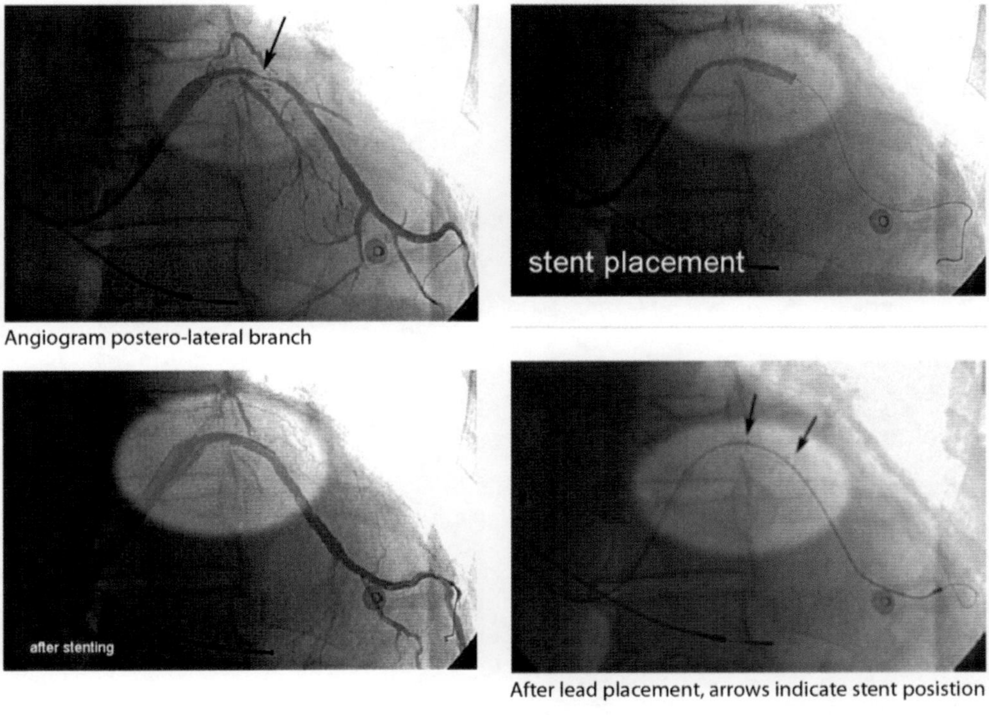

Fig. 11. Severe stenosis of a postero-lateral branch could be conquered with stenting after which the LV lead could be simply introduced.

Sometimes there are no tributes found in the CS and just a small part of the entry of the target vein is shown on the retrograde venography of the CS. Totally occluded target veins can be opened with the use of PCI wires and balloon dilatation (Fig 12).

With the knowledge of the retrograde venography of the CS the LV lead can be chosen, depending on the diameter and tortuosity of the target vein. Considerable advancements in LV lead design have led to numerous different unipolar, bipolar and multipolar LV leads. The LV leads can be used stylet driven or over the wire (OTW) similar to percutaneous coronary intervention.

In general the stylet driven LV leads are larger in diameter and used for larger veins, but some can also be used OTW and are called hybrids. Advancement of these stylet driven leads is performed by bending the distal 1-2 cm of the stylet at an angle corresponding to the angle of entry of the target vein into the CS. With the use of the bended stylet the LV lead can be steered into the target vein and exchanged for a soft, straight stylet to push the lead inside the vein. Lead advancement is often facilitated by clockwise rotation and repeated pushing of the lead with slight retraction of the stylet.

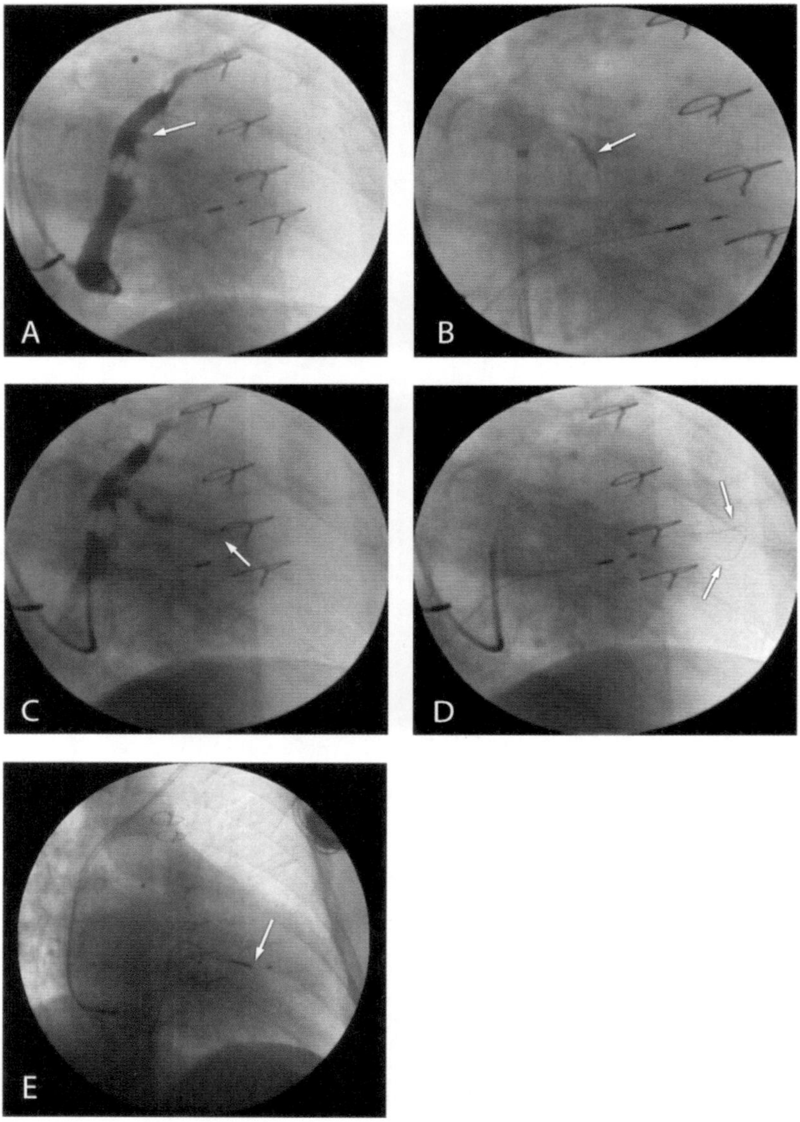

Fig. 12. a: coronary sinus projected in the RAO view with a total occluded posterolateral branch. (arrow pointing to occlusion)
b: showing a balloon dilatation after a PCI wire crossed this total occlusion.
c: slight filling of the postero-lateral branch.
d: buddy wire technique to cross the difficulties in this narrowed vessel. (two arrows pointing to both PCI wires)
e: Successful placements of the LV lead in the postero-lateral wall. (arrow)

3.4 The Over The Wire (OTW) technique

The OTW technique is different and provides access of the PCI wire to the target vein. First the LV lead is loaded with a PCI wire. The distal 5 mm of the PCI wire is slightly bended (Fig 13) and the LV lead combined with the PCI wire is brought into the CS through the guiding delivery sheath near the target vein.

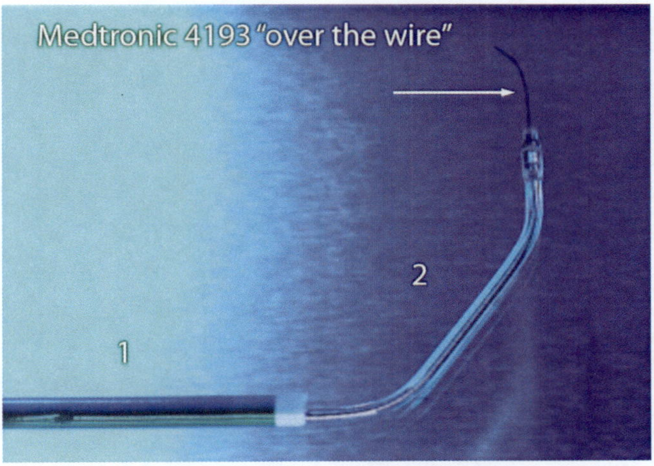

Fig. 13. Over the wire technique showing the guiding delivery sheath (1) with the LV lead (2) pushed out of the guiding delivery catheter and the PCI wire going ahead to advance into the side branch of the CS. The slight bend in the PCI wire (arrow) makes it possible to steer the PCI wire in the desired direction.

The PCI wire is advanced out the LV lead and with the ease of a torque steered in the desired vein. The PCI wire is advanced as distally as possible into the vein to provide a track for the lead. Subsequently the LV lead is pushed over the PCI wire into the vein, while the PCI wire is fixed or slightly retracted until the tip of the LV lead wedges or has a stable position. The OTW technique enables the pacing lead to go into secondary veins or to maneuver the LV lead to the optimal position.

Several problems can come across why the PCI wire will not enter the target vein: valves at the entrance of the target vein, severe angulated proximal segments, very tortuous segments or a very small caliber of the vein. When the PCI wire cannot be advanced from the CS into the first branch, because there is an acute angle, a guide catheter is used. For this purpose special Attain catheters with different curves and soft tips are made (Fig 14 a, b) to cannulate the target vein. Instead standard coronary angiography catheters can be used.

Depending on the angle of the ostium of the target vein an Attain Select catheter or a coronary angiography catheter can be used. This catheter introduced into the guiding delivery sheath and used as a telescoping catheter to hook on to the target vein enabling to give selective contrast injections to facilitate cannulation. Once the catheter engages the target vein a PCI wire is passed through the catheter and the PCI wire is advanced as distally as possible into the vein. Under continuous fluoroscopy the catheter is withdrawn while keeping the PCI wire in place. Thereafter the LV lead is frontloaded (not all LV leads can be frontloaded) with the PCI wire and the LV lead is advanced while retracting the PCI wire like a rail system to the desired site. Occasionally the LV lead cannot be advanced because the PCI wire has not straightened the acute angle or tortuous segment and a stiffer guidewire can be helpful. If this will not work the use of a buddy wire or telescopic sheaths may be the last resort to bring the lead transvenous to the desired place.

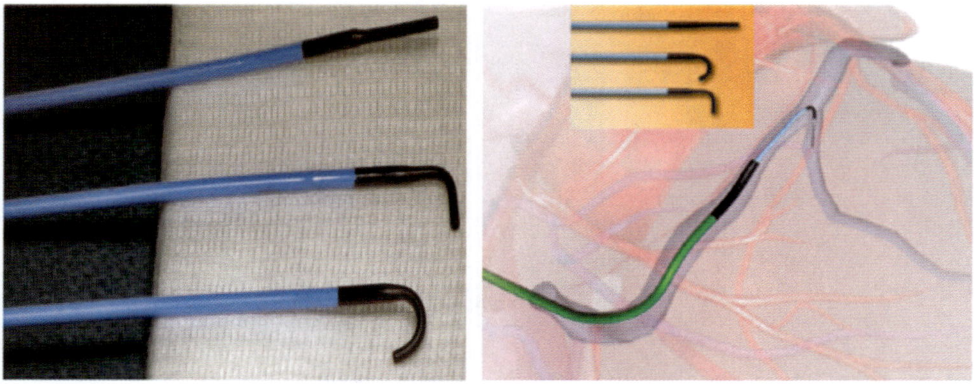

Fig. 14. Three Attain Select catheters (Medtronic) specially designed with a soft tip to cannulate side branches with sharp take off from the coronary sinus (left panel). The Attain Select catheters can be loaded with PCI wires to engage the target vessel or to give contrast injections in the tributary to visualize the peripheral part (right panel).

3.5 Special techniques or solutions for LV lead advancement

The buddy wire technique refers to the placement of one or more PCI wires alongside the first wire to optimal straighten the vein and allow passage of the LV lead. (Fig 12 d)

The telescoping sheath technique can only be used in larger diameter target veins, because the risk of perforation exists. The CS guiding delivery sheath must be at least 9 French and the target vein is cannulated with a heavy weight PCI wire. Over the PCI wire into the CS delivery guiding sheath is brought a smaller diameter straight CS sheath with a soft tip. On this CS catheter a Y connector is fastened to inject contrast if needed and allow visualization of the encroachment of the CS catheter into the target vein and dissection or perforation can be avoided. Sometimes even with the PCI wire in place the straightened CS sheath will not advance. The PCI wire is then replaced by an Attain Select catheter or coronary artery catheter that resembles the shape of the target vein and with manipulation of the tip the difficulties can be conquered.

The straightened soft CS sheath is advanced over the Attain Select or coronary artery catheter and the latest is withdrawn, so a stylet driven LV lead can pass through. In large diameter veins it is not always possible to obtain a stable LV lead position and new designed LV leads can solve this problem (Fig 15).

With the LV lead in place two new problems can be encountered, high left ventricular stimulation thresholds and phrenic nerve stimulation. Another more intriguing problem is ongoing mechanical dyssynchrony after implantation. This topic will be addressed in par.6.

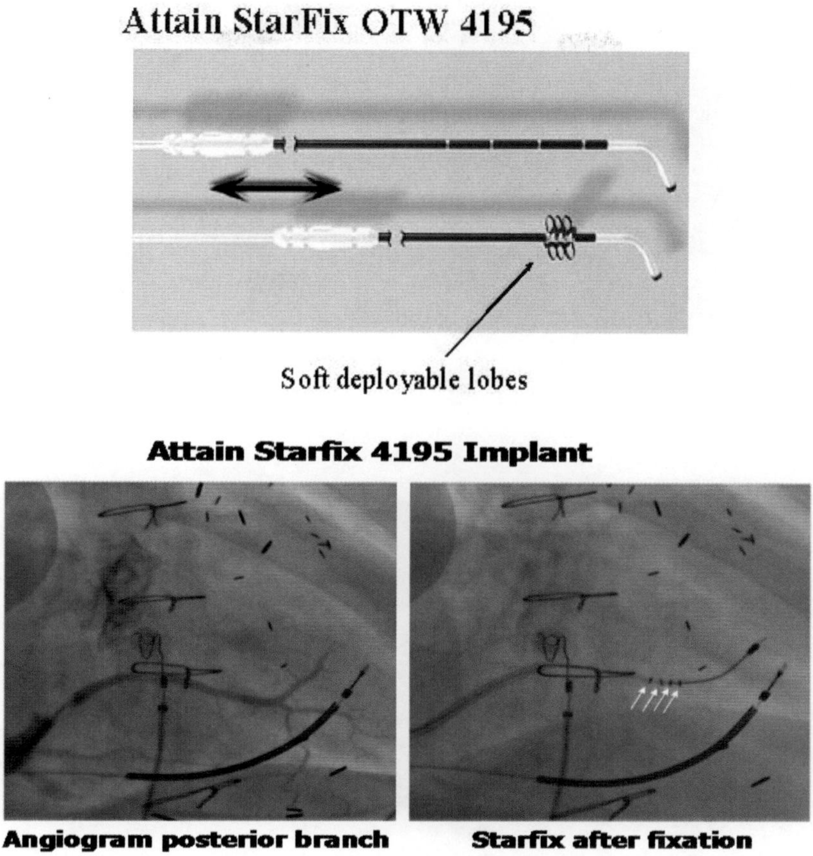

Fig. 15. The Starfix lead (Medtronic) with deployable lobes. By pushing up the redundant blue tube, which covers the lead at the proximal part of the lead, the distal part of the tube will show deployment of three lobes. In this way the lead will fix itself in the target vein. The two lower pictures shows the Starfix lead brought in position in a large postero-lateral vein under fluoroscopy.

4. The ECG in cardiac resynchronization therapy

4.1 Electrocardiographic consequences of different stimulation sites

Bi-ventricular pacing systems for ventricular resynchronization in the treatment of heart failure patients with a QRS complex > 120 ms and LBBB configuration have been employed for over 10 years. In these systems the ventricular stimulus is applied both to a left ventricular lead, positioned in one of the lateral, postero-lateral or posterior branches of the coronary sinus, and a right ventricular lead, positioned in an apical, septal or outflow tract position. Output on both leads can be programmed separately. In a normally functioning biventricular pacing system capture is obtained from both sites and the QRS morphology has a fusion pattern of right and left ventricular pacing.

The paced morphology of the QRS complex is dependent on the anatomical position of the right and left ventricular lead and a number of additional factors. Factors that determine the final morphology are

1. Location of the right and left ventricular lead.
2. Presence of anodal capture
3. The programmed AV interval
4. The programmed VV interval
5. Intrinsic AV conduction

An interaction between some of these factors also can contribute to the final morphology, like for instance the programmed AV interval and the intrinsic AV conduction, which may lead to fusion between paced an intrinsic ventricular activation.

4.2 The ECG in right ventricular pacing

The morphology for right ventricular pacing can be divided in pacing from the right ventricular apex, right ventricular septum and right ventricular outflow tract. In the following ECG stimulation from these sites in the same patient are demonstrated in figure 16.

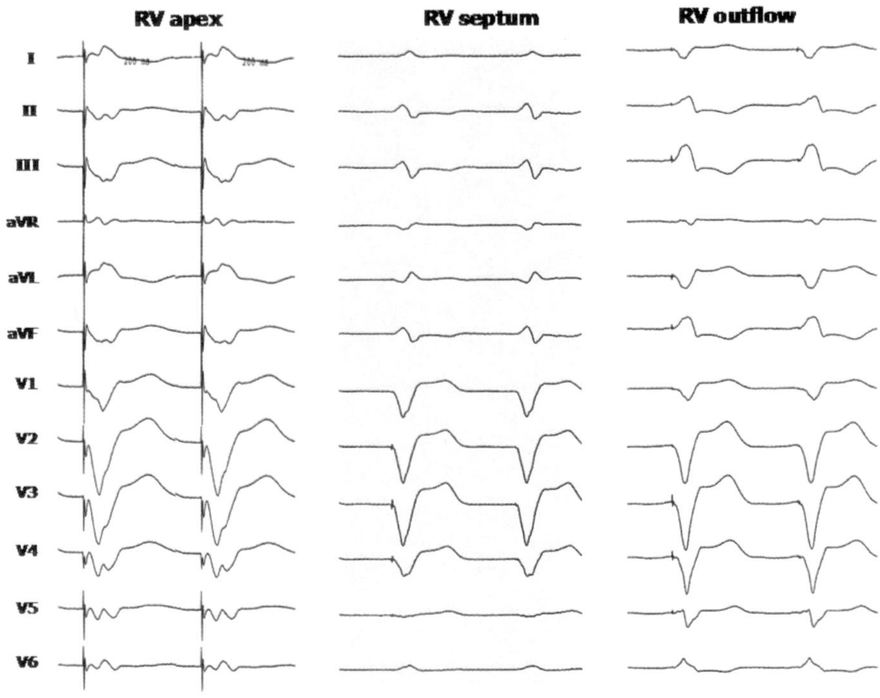

Fig. 16. ECG's from RV apex, RV septum and RV outflow tract.

The difference between the 3 locations is best appreciated from the frontal leads II and III that have a negative deflection during apex pacing (inferior to superior activation), a biphasic configuration during septum pacing indication interior to superior and superior to inferior activation, and a positive configuration during outflow tract pacing (superior to

inferior activation). The precordial leads show a LBBB pattern more or less similar for all locations.
Figure 17 illustrates the effect of location of the RV lead combined with left ventricular pacing from the postero-lateral area.

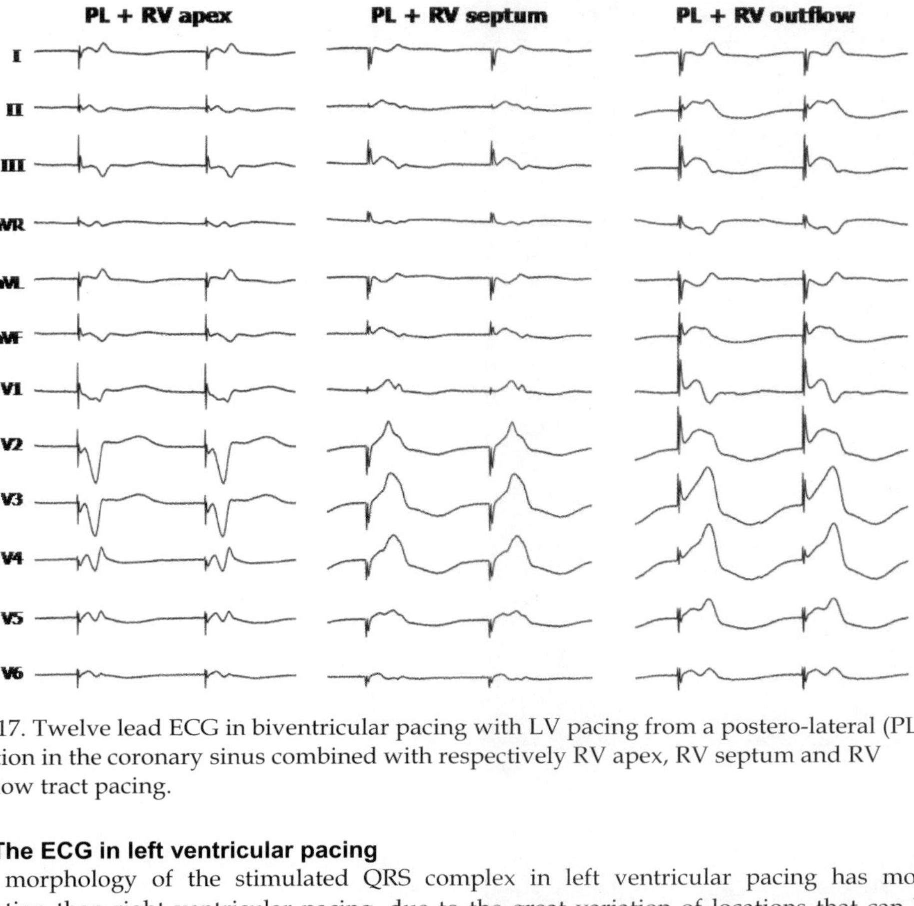

Fig. 17. Twelve lead ECG in biventricular pacing with LV pacing from a postero-lateral (PL) location in the coronary sinus combined with respectively RV apex, RV septum and RV outflow tract pacing.

4.3 The ECG in left ventricular pacing

The morphology of the stimulated QRS complex in left ventricular pacing has more variation than right ventricular pacing, due to the great variation of locations that can be obtained from the coronary venous anatomy. In a cross-section of the left ventricle, the segments can be divided in a posterior, postero-lateral, lateral, antero-lateral and anterior segment. In a longitudinal direction the left ventricle can be divided in 3 segments, the basal, the mid ventricular and apical segment.
Recognition of the longitudinal segment is relatively easy. The basal location will result in activation from superior to inferior, which is best reflected in the frontal plane of the ECG in the lead II and III. Similar an apical location will result in a negative QRS complex in the leads II and III, due to the activation travelling from inferior to superior. A mid segment location will result in a biphasic configuration in the leads II and III.

For the traverse segments during LV pacing the precordial leads are mandatory. For the postero-lateral area the QRS complex in the precordial leads will be positive from V1 to V4-5. For the posterior position the positive morphology will be limited to the leads V1-V3. In the lateral and antero-lateral positions there will a decrease in the positive amplitude in the pre-cordial leads which will gradually change to a negative deflection in the precordial leads. The closer the left ventricular stimulation electrode is located towards the intraventricular septum, the more resemblance there is with the morphology of right ventricular pacing characterized by a left bundle branch block pattern in the pre-cordial leads.
The morphology during left ventricular pacing and the location of the stimulation electrode is illustrated in the ECG represented in figure 18.

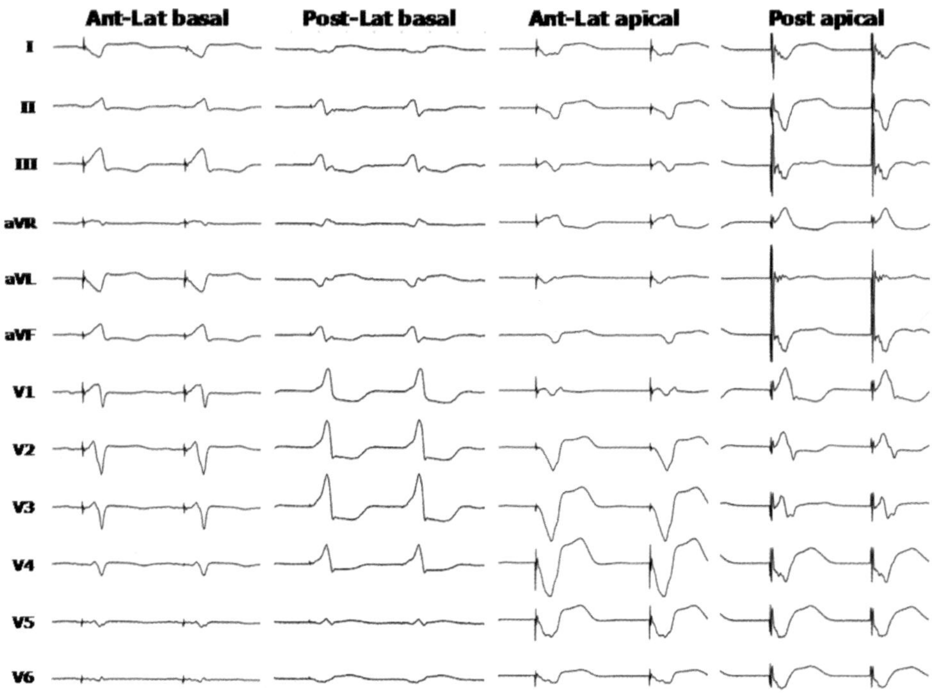

Fig. 18. Twelve lead ECG's from different LV epicardial locations (coronary sinus) illustrating the relationship between QRS morphology and stimulation site. See text for further explanation.

For the determination of the stimulation site with respect to the QRS morphology it is mandatory that left ventricular pacing is pure left ventricular pacing, not associated with any form of fusion with intrinsic activation. When pacing is performed in an atrial synchronous mode in patients with intrinsic AV conduction, the value of the programmed AV interval and the intrinsic AV conduction will determine the presence and degree of fusion (van Gelder et al. 2005). This is illustrated in figure 19.

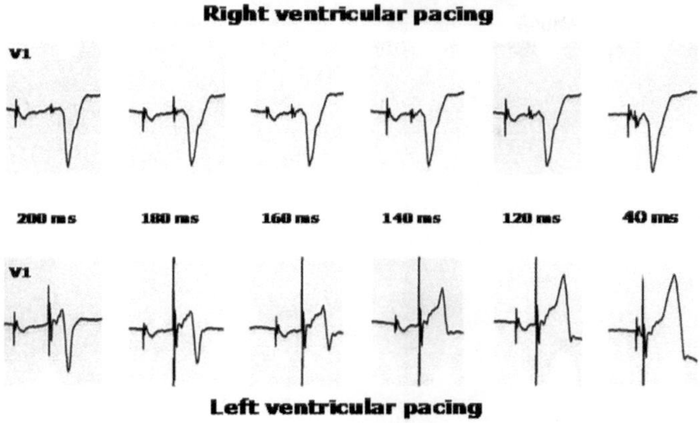

Fig. 19. Right and left ventricular pacing in the same patient with intrinsic AV conduction. Right and left ventricular pacing are performed with varying AV intervals. The RV pacing morphology is not affected by the AV interval. For LV pacing the degree of fusion determines the variation in the QRS morphology.

From this recording it is clearly demonstrated that for obtaining pure LV pacing, when pacing in an atrial synchronous mode, the AV interval should programmed to the shortest paced AV interval. Pacing in an atrial asynchronous mode (VVI) is no guarantee that fusion is excluded. Fusion can still be present when coincidentally LV pacing occurs simultaneous with intrinsic activation.

4.4 Anodal stimulation in cardiac resynchronization therapy

Primarily LV coronary sinus leads had a unipolar configuration. Therefore the can of the device was used as the positive anodal electrode for LV pacing. In case of pectoral muscle stimulation the pacing configuration could be changed from the LV electrode to the ring electrode of the right ventricular lead. However, in this configuration RV anodal stimulation could be initiated by LV pacing, which resulted in simultaneous pacing from the left and right ventricle (van Gelder et al. 2001). This phenomenon is illustrated in figure 20.

An effective way of avoiding anodal stimulation is programming the device in the unipolar configuration using the can of the device as the anodal electrode (van Gelder et al., 2001). This is illustrated in figure 21, where changing the V-V interval is changing the morphology of the QRS for every value, so V-V programming is not hindered by anodal capture. When however, the LV configuration is changed from LVtip to RVring, in the presence of anodal capture the morphology doesn't changing when changing the V-V interval from 80 to 60 and 40 ms. However, when the V-V interval was changed from 40 to 20 ms and subsequently 0 ms changes in the QRS morphology were observed.

This change in morphology is caused by triple site stimulation. When BiV pacing with a V-V interval of 40 ms or more is initiated, the LV stimulus captures LV (cathodal) as well as RV (anodal). This implies that the RV stimulus, which is delivered 40 to 80 ms later, is ineffective because the myocardial tissue is already refractory at the time of delivery of the RV stimulus. The myocardial tissue around the RV tip electrode is not immediately

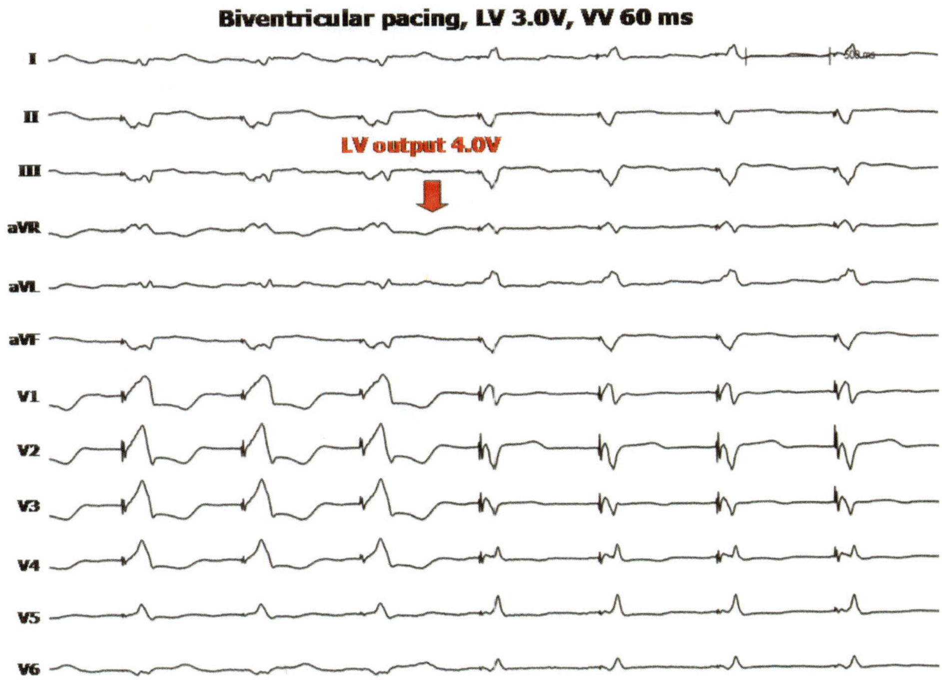

Fig. 20. Twelve lead ECG initially programmed in BiV pacing with LV pacing preceding RV pacing with 60 ms (V-V 60 ms). Because of this programmed value LV pacing dominates ventricular activation (R wave V1-5). But after programming LV output to 4.0V RV anodal capture occurs changing the QRS morphology due to simultaneous biventricular pacing.

refractory when anodal stimulation from the ring electrode occurs. It takes a short time for the anodal RV activation to reach the surrounding tissue of the RV tip electrode. Refractoriness of the myocardial tissue at the time of delivery of the RV stimulus depends on the distance between the ring and tip electrode of the RV lead, the time difference between LV and RV stimulation (V-V interval), and the conduction velocity of the myocardium (van Gelder et al., 2005, Fig. 22).

Anodal stimulation will not be present in configurations where the LV electrode is combined with the coil electrode of an ICD lead as anodal electrode, because of the surface area of this electrode which is around 500 mm^2. The current density is too low to evoke anodal capture. However, when a true bipolar ICD lead (e.g. Medtronic) is combined with a device of a company that standard uses integrated bipolar (e.g. BostonScientific), programming LVtip to RV coil leads to stimulation between LV tip and RV ring with the potential possibility of anodal capture (van Gelder et al., 2008).

4.5 The lead I paradox

Follow-up is often performed using ECG monitoring with the limb leads, implicating that lead I is the most important indicator for recognition of right or left ventricular activation. We reported on the paradoxical morphology of the QRS complex in lead I, showing a

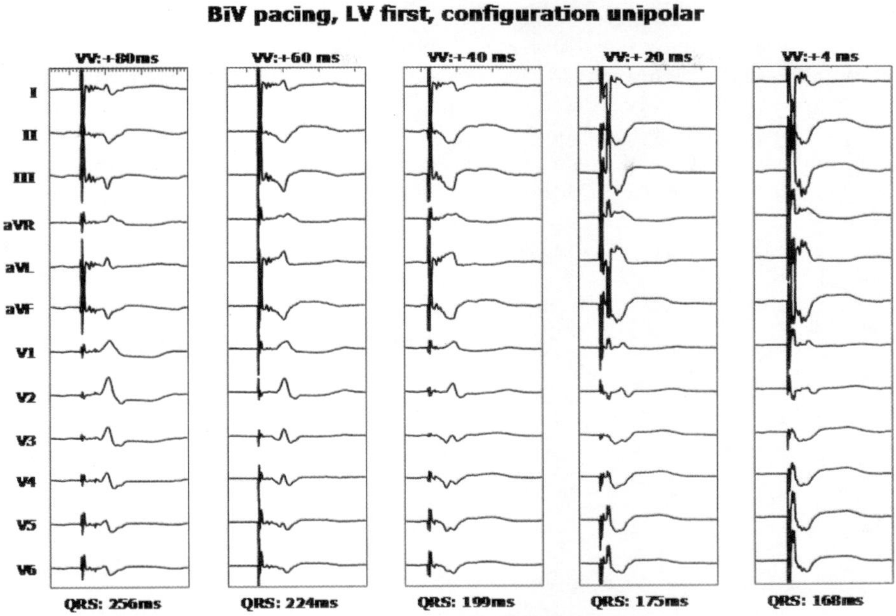

Fig. 21. Changing of V-V interval changes the QRS morphology. See text.

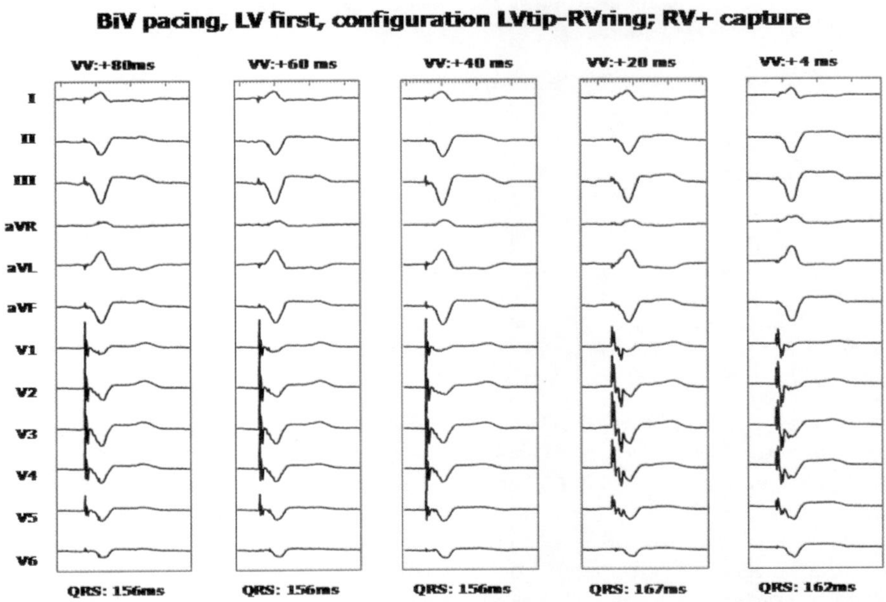

Fig. 22. No change in QRS morphology during anodal capture when programming V-V interval from 80 to 40, but changes are observed after programming V-V interval below 24 ms.

negative complex during right ventricular (RV) pacing and positive during left ventricular (LV) pacing in the same patient (van Gelder et al. 2008).

During stimulation at the high septal site of the RV a negative QRS complex in lead I can be recorded. On the other hand a basal position of the LV lead in one of the posterior or postero-lateral veins may result in a positive deflection in lead I. When both phenomenon are present in the same patient, the configuration is in contradiction with the general finding of a positive QRS complex in lead I during RV pacing and negative during LV pacing and was called the lead I paradox. This paradoxical behavior might be an argument to record a precordial ECG lead (preferably V1) in the follow-up of patients with biventricular pacing systems (Fig. 23).

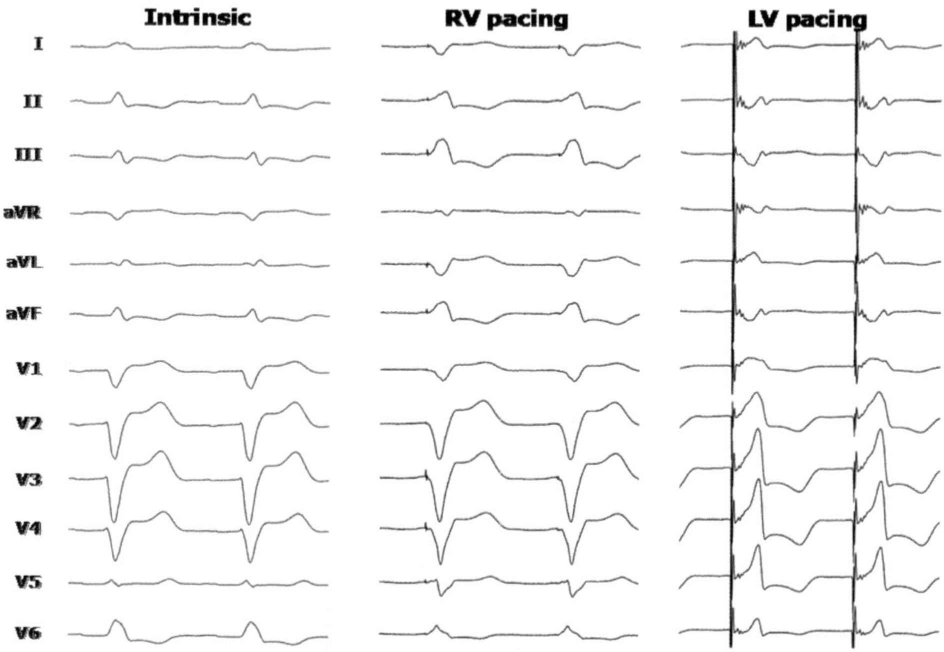

Fig. 23. Twelve-lead ECG of patient 2 showing the paradoxical presentation in lead I of RV and LV pacing. However,in the precordial leads a LBBB pattern is observed during RV pacing and a RBBB pattern during LV pacing.

The paradox in lead I has no relation to each other: a negative QRS complex in lead I during RV pacing has no effect on the positive QRS complex during LV pacing and vice versa. The negative QRS complex in lead I during RV high septal pacing is a known observation described during ventricular tachycardia arising from the RV outflow tract. A more anterior oriented position of the lead in the septum is more prone to this pattern due to the amount of ventricular myocardium depolarized from left to right, which is higher than with a posterior position of the lead. The presence of a preexisting right axis deviation with a negative QRS complex in lead I with fusion or pseudo fusion was ruled out as a cause by programming a short AV interval.

A positive QRS complex in lead I during LV pacing could be explained by the basal position of the LV lead combined with a more horizontal anatomical position of the long axis of the left ventricle or rotation of the left ventricle. Under these conditions, the ventricular myocardium is mainly depolarized in a right to left direction, thus giving rise to a negative QRS complex in lead I. Preexistence of an intrinsic positive QRS complex in lead I could be an explanation for the positive QRS complex during LV pacing due to fusion, which was ruled out as stated before. A positive QRS complex in lead I during LV pacing is also described by Kistler et al. (2003), but in their patient the LV lead was positioned in the great cardiac vein, close to the interventricular septum, whereas in all our patients CS leads were implanted in the postero-lateral area of the left ventricle (Fig. 24). A positive QRS complex during LV pacing can also be observed when anodal stimulation from the RV ring electrode occurs. This RV activation might dominate in the "biventricular" activation resulting in a positive QRS complex. In our patients RV anodal stimulation was ruled out during LV pacing. The presence of scar tissue affecting QRS morphology in these patients was unlikely because the indication was dilated cardiomyopathy in the majority.

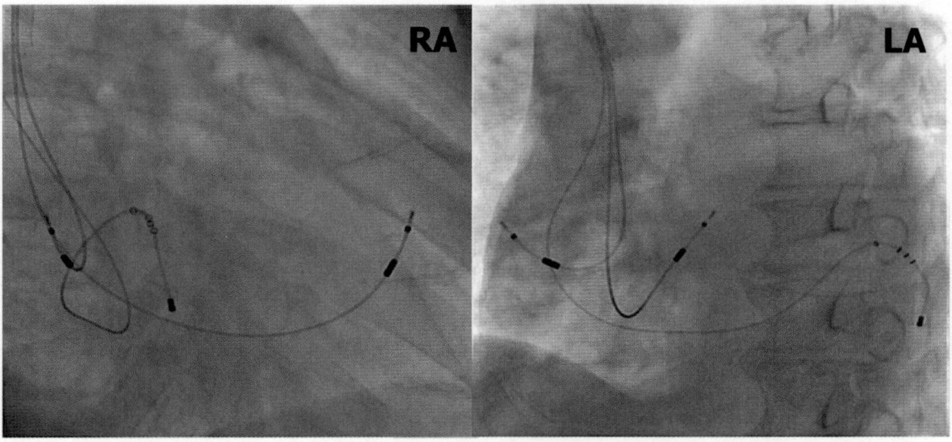

Fig. 24. X rays showing the lead positions in right anterior oblique (RAO) view and left anterior oblique view(LAO) of a patient showing the Lead I paradox, see also figure 23.

4.6 Electrode configuration in coronary sinus leads

The over the wire leads addressed in the previous paragraph all had a unipolar configuration. This implies that LV pacing is delivered between the distal electrode of the CS lead and the can of the device or the anodal electrode of the RV lead. In case of an ICD lead, the coil electrode will serve as the anodal electrode in the majority of cases. One of the drawbacks of this configuration is anodal capture that can occur when a RV ring electrode is used as the anodal electrode. Anodal capture results in simultaneous LV and RV activation, even when a V-V interval with LV pacing preceding RV pacing is programmed, so V-V timing can be deregulated by anodal capture.

Anodal RV capture can easily be prevented by the use of bipolar CS leads (e.g. Medtronic 4194). In this lead the ring electrode has an electrode surface area of 38 mm^2, but even in spite of this large surface area stimulation threshold is lower when the coil electrode of an ICD lead, with a surface area of approximately 500 mm^2 is used as anodal electrode.

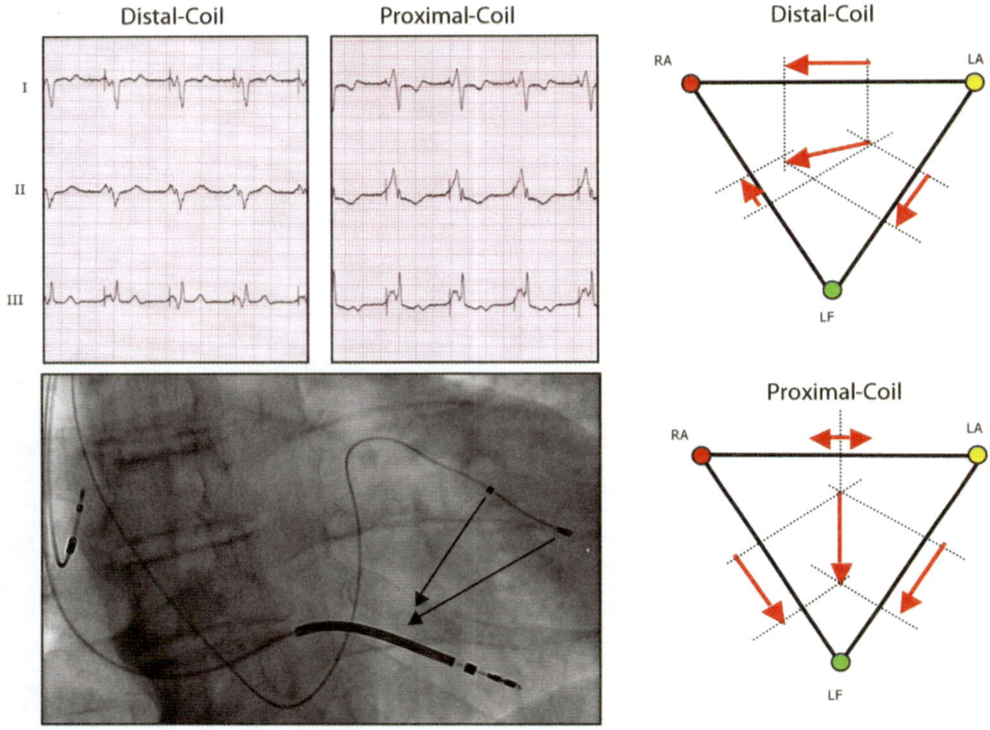

Fig. 25. Dual unipolar lead Medtronic 4196 implanted in a postero-lateral branch of the coronary sinus with the corresponding ECG's from pacing from proximal and distal electrode.

More recently bipolar CS leads are introduced, in which the proximal electrode has a surface area approximately equal to the surface area of the distal electrode (e.g. Guidant Easytrak 2, Medtronic 4196). These leads are far from ideal when used in a bipolar configuration, because the small surface area at the proximal electrode gives a rise in lead impedance without an increase of current efficiency. The idea behind the lead is that the stimulating electrode can be switched from distal to proximal in a unipolar configuration, in which the coil of the ICD lead is used as anodal electrode.

This option creates the possibility of changing non-invasively the pacing configuration, which can be useful in case of phrenic nerve stimulation or high stimulation threshold. The name "dual unipolar" or "dual cathodal lead" better covers the lead options than simply calling it a bipolar lead. In case of acceptable cathodal threshold from both electrodes a selection can be made based on the optimal hemodynamic effect. Figure 25 demonstrates the position of such a lead (Medtronic 4194) with corresponding ECG during LV pacing from the distal and proximal electrode.

Because of the difference in location of the pacing electrodes in the LVtip-can and LVring-can configuration the QRS complex during LV paving also differs and also the hemodynamic effect can be changed by the choice of the stimulation electrode. Since the tip and ring electrode has an equal surface area the bipolar pacing configuration (LVtip-ring) can easily result in dual site pacing due to anodal capture at the ring electrode. This is illustrated in figure 26.

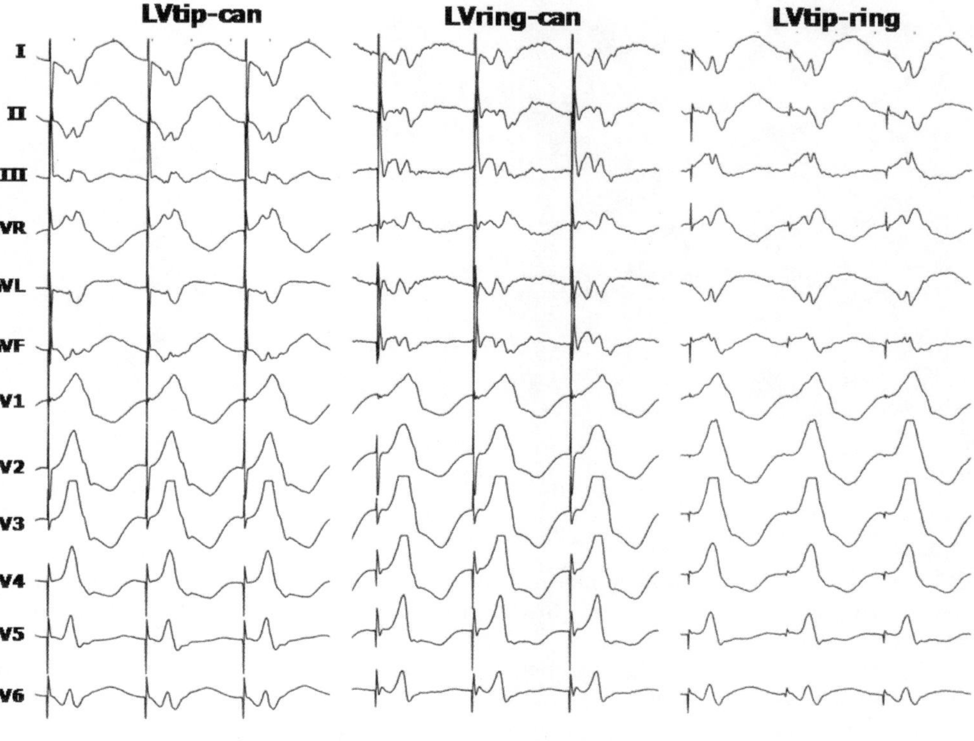

Fig. 26. Twelve lead ECG with unipolar stimulation from tip and ring electrode,(LVtip-can and LVring -can). The morphology of the QRS complex during LVtip-ring pacing has a different morphology from both other configuration indicating dual site LV pacing by anodal capture.

The hemodynamic effect of single and dual site LV paving is demonstrated in figure 27. From our initial experience it is clear that this example is representative for this lead with an inter-electrode distance of 21 mm. The single site best result does not become better by dual site pacing.

In future developments quadripolar CS leads will be employed, which increase the number of pacing vectors thus increasing the possibilities to handle phrenic nerve stimulation or elevated stimulation threshold. However, if this option has also hemodynamic consequences still has to be investigated.

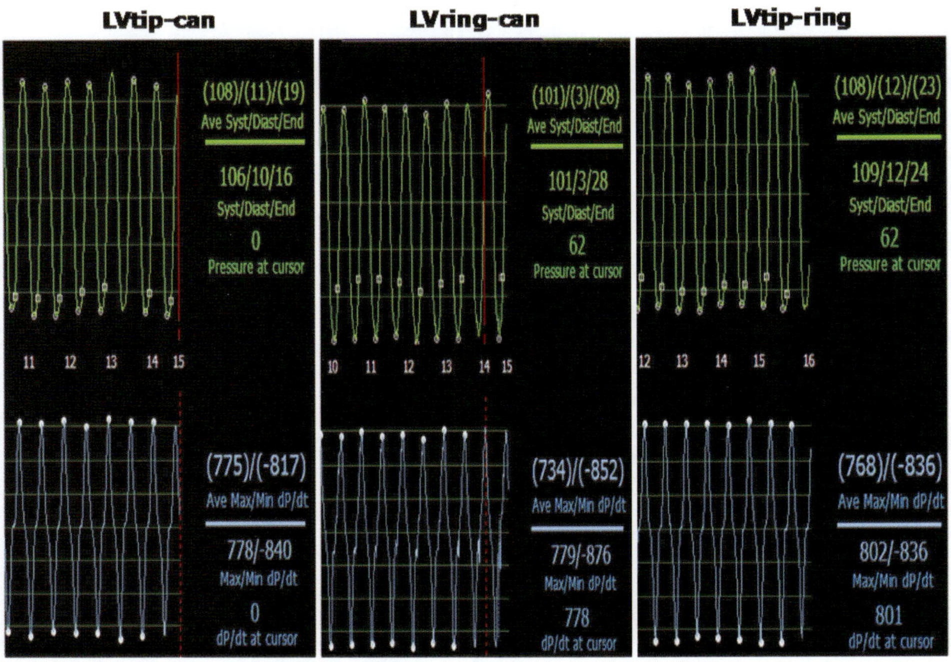

Fig. 27. Hemodynamic effect of single site (*LV tip and LV ring) and dual site LV pacing (LV tip-ring).

5. Slitting or cutting the guiding delivery catheter

The last step during the implantation procedure is the removal of the guiding delivery sheath. This is challenging because dislodgement of the LV lead is frustrating after a fatiguing implantation procedure.

The LV lead is kept in place with a finishing stylet provided with the LV lead. A special cutting device is attached to the lead and the guiding delivery catheter is removed by longitudinal slitting. The guiding delivery sheath is withdrawn in one continuous smooth motion under continuous fluoroscopic observation. Another technique is the use of long finishing stylet to keep the LV lead in place and use the traditional break and peel-away method.

With both techniques the long stylet or the cutting tool must be fixed in place, else redundancy of the LV lead introduces dislodgement, especially at the point the delivery sheath reaches the ostium of the CS. Advancing the finishing stylet or the LV lead at that point into the venous system paradoxically giving too much slack of the LV lead in the right atrium and the LV lead will drop out of the CS. Slight backward traction will prevent dislodgement by straightening the LV lead. Repositioning the LV lead without the back-up of the delivery sheath is occasionally achievable, but generally a new delivery sheath is needed to provide support for the renewed placement of the LV lead.

In case habitual dislodgement occurs the Star-fix LV lead (Medtronic) can be inserted and fixed in the target vein to ensure a supplementary steady position. The finishing wire is drawn back and the LV lead must be secured with tight sewing collars around the sleeve of the LV lead. The same is done with RA and RV lead and all three leads are attached to the CRT device and the implantation procedure is finished.

6. Problems after LV lead placement

High left ventricular stimulation threshold can be due to the presence of scar tissue, however the place for the LV lead is dictated by the native coronary venous anatomy and sometimes thresholds up to 3.5 Volt at 0.5-msec pulse duration are accepted.

The other problem is left phrenic nerve stimulation causing diaphragmatic contraction. The left phrenic nerve is located anywhere along the lateral wall of the heart as multiple side branches of the phrenic nerve crosses broad areas of the pericardium. Phrenic nerve stimulation is not tolerated by the patient and repositioning of the LV lead is advisable even if pacing at outputs above 5 Volts with acceptable stimulation threshold stimulate the diaphragm. The patient is in a supine position during implantation and after the procedure the diaphragmatic threshold may drop and/or the LV lead threshold may rise with body changes and repositioning the LV lead to a tertiary branch or more proximal in the target vein can prevent a re-intervention with lead repositioning.

The use of bipolar leads does not prevent left phrenic nerve stimulation.

Special LV leads can be used with two electrodes that permit stimulation between one of the two electrodes and the anodal electrode of the RV lead, or coil electrode of the shock lead. Altering the LV-RV pacing vector may prevent left phrenic nerve stimulation. If left phrenic nerve stimulation persists one should go to surgical LV lead placement.

A third problem one can encounter after implantation is ongoing mechanical dyssynchrony despite optimization of the CRT device. This is mostly due to inappropriate LV lead placement and sometimes a second LV lead to recruit more of the left ventricular wall is needed to gain mechanical synchrony. In such a case both LV leads are coupled to a Y-splitter and attached in the LV port of the pacemaker (Fig 28)

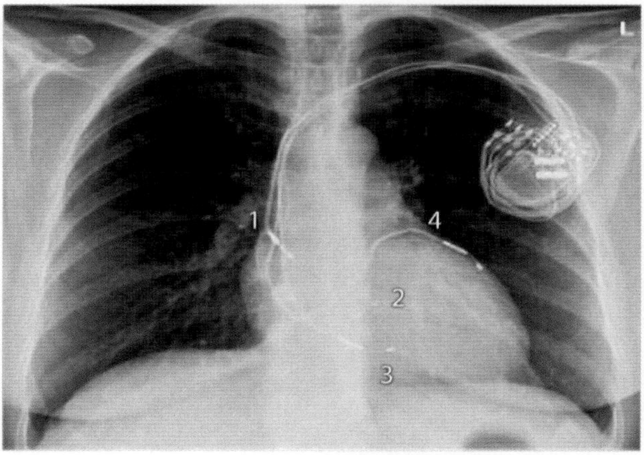

Fig. 28. X-ray of the chest showing a CRT device with a RA lead (1), RV lead screwed in the RVS (2) and two LV leads. The first LV lead (3) is positioned in a posterior branch. Because no mechanical resynchronization could be obtained a second lead (4) was placed afterwards in an antero-lateral branch, after which mechanical synchrony was achieved.

7. Concluding remarks

The implantation of a LV lead in patients with congestive heart failure is technically a rather complex procedure. Implantation training for CRT has a significant learning curve. Duration of implantation and fluoroscopic time will greatly reduce with experience (Kautzner et al.,2004).Implantation failure is due to inability to intubate the CS, unstable guiding delivery catheter, absence of suitable side branches in the postero-lateral region, coronary vein stenosis or occlusion, lead instability, high stimulation threshold, phrenic nerve stimulation or a combination of the above (Bentkover et al.,2003; Gras et al.,2002).
Success depends on multiple factors including operator's experience and technique, individual anatomy of the CS, threshold and phrenic nerve stimulation regions and available instrumentation and leads. With advanced materials and experienced operators up to 92 % of LV leads are successful via the transvenous approach (León et al.,2005). Complications inherent to LV lead implantation include CS dissection, intimal dissection of the target vein sometimes combined with acute thrombotic occlusion, hematoma in the wall of the target vessel, which can contribute to venous thrombosis and a life threatening complication due to wire exit is coronary venous perforation. Peri-implantation mortality risk is reported 0.4 % from ten pooled studies including 3,223 patients. Re-implantation occurs in 6-8% of patients within 6 months due to LV lead dislodgement, exit block or phrenic nerve stimulation (Greenberg et al.,2003). Further post-implantation risks are similar to conventional pacing. However if placement of a LV lead or the re-implantation fails one should consider surgical placement of an epicardial LV lead, which also can be performed with robotic assistance (DeRose et al.,2005) to provide the patient the benefit of CRT. In case surgery is contraindicated transseptal or transapical approaches with endocardial LV lead should be considered.

8. References

Abraham WT, Fisher WG, Smith AL et al. For the MIRACLE Study Group. Cardiac resynchronization in chronic heart failure. N Eng J Med 2002; 346:1845-1853.

Ansalone G, Giannantoni P, Ricci R et al. Doppler myocardial imaging to evaluate the effectiveness of pacing sites in patients receiving biventricular pacing. J Am Coll Cardiol 2002 106; 39:489-499.

Bakker P, Meijburg H, De Vries JW et al. Biventricular pacing in end stage heart failure improves functional capacity and left ventricular function. J Interv Card Electrophysiol 2000; 4:395-404.

Bax JJ, Molhoek SG, Erven van L, et al. Usefulness of myocardial tissue Doppler echocardiography to evaluate left ventricular dyssynchrony before and after biventricular pacing in patients with idiopathic dilated cardiomyopathy. Am J Cardiol 2003;91:94-97.

Bentkover JD, Stewart EJ, Ignaszewski A et al. New technologies and potential cost savings related to morbidity and mortality reduction in class III/IV heart failure patients in Canada. Int J Cardiol 2003;88:33-41.

Butter C, Auricchio A, Stellbrink et al. Effect of resynchronization therapy stimulation site on the systolic function of the heart failure patients. Circulation 2001;104:3026-3029.

Cazeau S, Ritter P, Bakdach S et al. Four chamber pacing in dilated cardiomyopathy. PACE 1994; 17:1974-1979.

Chan FP, Napoli A, Narayan G et al. Anatomy of the coronary venous system in patients with left heart failure. Hearth Rhythm 2004; 1: S-29.

Daubert JC, Ritter P, Le Breton H et al. Permanent left ventricular pacing with transvenous leads inserted into the coronary veins. PACE 1998; 21:239-245.

DeRose JJ, Ashton RC, Balaram S et al. Robotically assisted left ventricular epicardial lead implantation for biventricular pacing. J Am Coll Cardiol 2005;46:2358-2359.

Gelder B van, Bracke F, Meijer A. The effect of anodal stimulation on V-V timing at varying V-V intervals. Pacing and Clin Electrophysiol 2005;8:771 – 776.

Gelder van B, Scheffer M, Meijer A et al. Transseptal endocardial left ventricular pacing : An alternative technique for coronary sinus lead placement in cardiac resynchronization therapy. Heart Rhythm 2007; 4:454-460.

Gelder van BM, Elders J, Bracke FA, et al. Implantation of a biventricular pacing system in a patient with a coronary sinus not communicating with the right atrium. PACE 2003;26:1294-1296.

Gelder van BM, Meijer A, Bastings P et al. Successful implantation of a coronary sinus leads after stenting of a coronary vein stenosis. Pace 2003;26:1904-1907.

Gelder van BM, Bracke FA, Meijer A and Pijls NHJ The Hemodynamic Effect of Intrinsic Conduction During Left Ventricular Pacing as Compared to Biventricular Pacing JACC 2005; 46: 2305-2310

Gelder van BM, Bracke, FA, Meijer A, Pilmeijer A. Triple-site ventricular pacing in a biventricular pacing system. Pacing and Clin Electrophysiol 2001;24:1165-1167

Gelder van BM and Bracke FA. The ECG Lead I paradox in cardiac resynchronization therapy. Pacing Clin Electrophysiol 2008;31: 1519-1521

Gibson DG, Chamberlain DA, Colart DJ et al. Effect of changes in ventricular activation on cardiac haemodynamics in man. Comparison of right ventricular, left ventricular and simultaneous pacing of both ventricles. Br Heart J 1971: 33:397-400.

Gras D, Leclercq C, Tang AS et al. Cardiac resynchronization therapy in advanced heart failure : the multicenter inSync clinical study. Eur J Heart Fail 2002;4:311-320.

Greenberg JM, Mera FV, Delurgio DB et al. Safety of implantation of cardiac resynchronization devices: A review of major biventricular pacing trials. PACE 2003;26:952.

Hansky B, Lamp B, Minami K et al. Coronary vein balloon angioplasty for left ventricular pacemaker lead implantation. J Am Coll Cardiol 2002; 40:2144-2149.

Jaïs P, Douard H, Shah DC et al. Endocardial biventricular pacing. PACE 1998 ; 21 :2128-2131.

Kassai I, Foldesi C, Szekely A,, Szili-Torok T. Alternative method for cardiac resynchronization. Transapical lead implantation. Ann Thoracic Surg 2009;87(2):650-652.

Kautzner J, Riedlbauchová L, Čihák R et al. Technical aspects of LV lead for cardiac resynchronization therapy in chronic heart failure. PACE 2004;27:783-790.

Kistler PM, Mond HG, Corcoran SJM. Biventricular pacing: It isn't always as it seems. Pacing Clin Electrophysiol 2003; 26:2185–2187

Leclercq F, Hager FX, Macia JC et al. Left ventricular lead insertion using a modified transseptal catheterization technique: a totally endocardial approach for permanent biventricular pacing in end-stage heart failure. PACE 1999; 22:1570-1575.

León AR, Delurgio DB, Mera F. Practical approach to implanting left ventricular pacing leads for cardiac resynchronization. J Cardiovasc Electrophysiol 2005;16:100-105.

Leon AR, Abraham WT, Curtis AB et al. Safety of transvenous cardiac resynchronization system implantation in patients with chronic heart failure: combined results of over 2000 patients from a multicenter study program. J Am Coll Cardiol 2005;46:2348-2356.

Scheffer M, Dessel van PFHM, Gelder van B, et al. Peak longitudinal strain delay is superior to TDI in the selection of patients for resynchronization therapy. Neth Heart J 2010;18:574-582.

Swedberg K, Cleland JG, Dargie H et al. Guidelines for the diagnosis and treatment of chronic heart failure: executive summary (update 2005). Task Force for the diagnosis and treatment of Chronic Heart Failure of the European Society of Cardiology. Eur Heart J 2005; 26:1115-1140.

Tyers GF. Comparison of effect on cardiac function of single-site and simultaneous multiple-site ventricular stimulation after A-V block. J Thorac Cardiovasc Surg 1970; 59:211-217.

Vagnini FJ, Gourin , Antell HI et al. Implantation sides of cardiac pacemaker electrodes and myocardial contractility. Ann Thorac Surg 1967; 4:431-439.

Yu CM, Sanderson JE, Fan K, et al. Tissue Doppler echocardiographic evidence of reverse remodeling and improved synchronicity by simultaneously delaying regional contraction after biventricular pacing therapy in heart failure. Circulation 2002;105:438-445.

5

Automated Selection of Optimal ECG Lead Using Heart Instantaneous Frequency During Sleep

Yeon-Sik Noh, Ja-Woong Yoon and Hyung-Ro Yoon
Dept. of Biomedical Engineering, Yonsei University
Republic of Korea

1. Introduction

The analysis of the breath signal during sleep provides key information for the revelatory analysis of the clinical symptoms of sleep diseases such as sleep apnea, etc which disturbs normal sleep and further on can become the potential cause of heart diseases. This information can be used importantly for such purposes as to remove change quantity by breathing not only for the system modeling of the cardiovascular system for the function analysis of the autonomic nervous system (ANS), which is generated in the human body during sleep, but also for the accurate analysis during the analysis of the frequency of the changing rate of heartbeats, and the classification of significant electrocardiogram (ECG), which includes an accurate breath signal during sleep which has immense meaning (Park et al., 2004).

In general, the methods measuring breath signals can be largely divided into a direct method and an indirect method. A direct method which measures changes of air temperature around the nose by breathing and using a spirometer suggests a standard in research and can have accurate breath signals (Cysarz et al., 2008). However, because of the disadvantage of cumbersome and inconvenient measurements, an indirect method, which can measure the breath of the examinee without binding and consciousness in a relatively simple measurement method, is more preferred. As these indirect methods, a method, which extracts breath by measuring the inductance and impedance changes of the thorax by breath or by measuring column changes of the thorax, and ECG-derived respiratory (EDR) method, which induces breath signals from ECG by using impacts of changes of impedance within the thorax on ECG according to the filling and exhausting of air within the lungs which accompanies it during breathing, have been suggested (Yi et al., 2006; Moody et al., 1985).

However, in the case of using a method measuring inductance or impedance changes of the thorax or column changes of the thorax for monitoring the breath during sleeping, it can disturb the normal sleeping of the examinee because the examinee has to be put on a belt or attach an electrode on the thorax. In addition, it may be difficult to detect accurate breath because lots of noise components accompany it according to the surrounding environment. Therefore, recently, the EDR method, which extracts breath signals from the ECG measured during sleep by using the conductive textile electrode, is utilized more for detecting breath with the minimum binding of the examinee (Park et al., 2008; Yi et al., 2006). The EDR method does not need additional hardware except the ECG measurement and in cases when there is no distortion in the QRS complex of the ECG even if noise by a power source or noise by external interference and motion (tossing) during sleep is generated, better breath signals than the existing indirect method can be extracted.

In existing early research using the EDR method, research extracting breathing forms were carried out based on amplitude changes (amplitude modulation, AM) of the R wave of the ECG, which are modulated by breathing, were implemented. As the most representative methods, there is method extracting breathing information listed on ECG with amplitude changes of the R wave of ECG and a method extracting breath through changes of the axle of heart activity by using arctangent ratio of amplitude of QRS complex between the two leads which cross at right angles using multi-leads (Mazzant et al., 2003; Behbehani et al., 2002; Travaglini et al., 1998; Correa et al., 2008). However, in cases when applying these methods actually during sleep, there are disadvantages that its characteristic can deteriorate compared to the EDR through a single lead because aspects for breathing to modulate this ECG are different according to the breathing method, the location of hearts and the level of the spinning of an axle of each individual examinee and lead I and lead III do not orthogonal actually (Park et al., 2008).

However, breathing affects other cardiovascular functions as well as on the amplitude of the ECG with impedance changes within the thorax (Noh et al., 2007). The frequency modulation method of the ECG, which changed besides the amplitude of the ECG, also began to be studied because the EDR which extracted by the amplitude modulation due to breathing can include the wrong information under sensitive situations to motion like during sleep. The frequency modulation (FM) method was developed by using respiratory sinus arrhythmia (RSA) which causes the changes of heart activity due to breathing. RSA was first discovered in 1847 as Ludwig had observed breathing, the synchronized number of the heartbeat and the vibration of the artery blood pressure in dogs. The RSA, which is the physiological mutual interaction of respiratory quotient and circulatory system, is the change of breath and synchronized heart beat rate and interval of R peaks of the ECG becomes shortened during inhalation of the ECG and also becomes longer during exhalation (Eckberg, 1983; Hayano et al., 1996). The differences of the R-R intervals (RRIs) of these ECG can be considered to show respiratory sinus arrhythmia. RSA is generated by all of the reflective primary factors and centric primary factors and as reflective primary factors there are artery pressure reflection and lung and kidney reflection (Yi et al., 2006).

The EDR methods by the ECG amplitude modulation method and frequency modulation method were used broadly in lots of research for confirming breathing status during sleeping or walking. However, there exists a limit in extracting breathing only with simple EDR. The accurate measurement of the ECG is prioritized because these methods induce basically breathing signals through amplitude and R peak detection of the ECG. The reliability of the breathing information by these methods can be degraded if the ECG is distorted because the R peak detection of ECG is difficult due to the motions of the examinee. In particular, the algorithm for the deployment of electrodes and the lead selection of the significant optimum ECG became necessary because the changes of postures such as tossing during sleep can become very big obstacles in the acquisition of a significant ECG. Therefore, research to classify a significant ECG by judging whether the measured ECG reflects breathing signals well or not was implemented and Park et al estimated instantaneous frequency based on the Hilbert Transform and had suggested a new algorithm which selects optimum lead in which it possible to extract significant breathing signals by perceiving the point that the instantaneous frequency of the breathing signals with inappropriate lead show big frequency changes (Park et al., 2008). However, this method has a limit like selecting the wrong lead in cases when instantaneous frequency is changed by instantaneous motions or external noises, which can be generated during sleep because it selects optimum lead by judging with only the changed width of the instantaneous frequency.

So, Noh et al attempted to verify that the correlation of the power spectrum in HF (high frequency) range, which is a breathing related frequency range in the frequency analysis of the breathing signals and heart rate variability (HRV) induced from the ECG and also tried to classify significant data by using this fact (Noh et al., 2006). However, these elements require high electricity consumption in the system because it must be measured in the high sampling rate of the ECG over 500Hz for obtaining HRV signals and also a re-sampling course is required for the analysis between interpolation and the frequency following the R peak detection. Therefore, Noh et al had attempted the classification of the ECG signals including significant breathing signals during sleep by introducing the heart instantaneous frequency (HIF) concept which can efficiently replace HRV in a ubiquitous healthcare environment (Noh et al., 2007). But, this study has disadvantages as it is impossible to acquire a significant ECG in cases when the ECG signals become distorted by the motions of the human body or external interference noises generated during sleep because only the measured ECG under one lead during sleep was evaluated.

Therefore, in this study, we tried to automatically classify signals by evaluating respectively based on HIF signals whether the ECG measured in two ECG leads (I and III) possible to measure during sleep is a significant ECG which reflects sound breathing signals and consequently, we have selected a significant ECG lead.

We first explain correlation between the autonomic nervous system and breathing and intend to introduce HIF which can effectively replace correlation between the HRV representing the autonomic nervous system and breathing and HRV. And we explain the signal processing method used in this study and finally, we introduce the ECG classification algorithm based on HIF.

2. Autonomic nervous system and respiration

2.1 Autonomic nervous system

The human body is adjusted by the autonomic nervous system which maintains the balance of the internal environment with regards to changes of the internal and external environment. This is directly operated for enjoying healthy life by maintaining life preservation activity and homeostasis within the human body. The autonomic nervous system involves in functions which cannot be controlled consciously just like metabolism such as digestion, breathing and sweat. The autonomic nervous system is anatomically divided again into the two nervous systems of sympathetic nervous system and parasympathetic nervous system and these two are controlled through antagonism, which is a method that another one is suppressed if one becomes active. The sympathetic nervous system becomes active when physical or mental stress becomes immense while generating various reactions of physical constitutions for the homeostasis maintenance of the human body and in preparation for emergency situations. Reactions required for responding to these stresses due to the activation of the sympathetic nervous system and the supply of energy appears and consequently, blood pressure and the number of heartbeats increases, the pupils expand and gooseflesh is generated. On the contrary to operations of this sympathetic nervous system, the parasympathetic nervous system becomes activated if one's status is comfortable. The parasympathetic nerve is distributed within the internal organs of the human body and maintains a smooth function by adjusting the internal organ functions. If the parasympathetic nervous system is activated, the number of heartbeats and blood pressure decreases and the whole body is operated directionally to secure energy as the digestive enzyme secretion becomes active with lots of blood circulation in digestive organs. The parasympathetic nerve is very local and impacts rippling into the whole body are little compared to the influence of the sympathetic nerve but it plays a very important role in the homeostasis adjustment mechanism. However, these two do not always operate in the opposite direction and operate in cooperation according to some organs.

A method, which judges the most accurate autonomic nervous system of the human body, is the way to evaluating by analyzing the nerve transmission material of the autonomic nervous system in blood, but it is difficult to evaluate realistically because the metabolism hours of the transmission materials of the autonomic nerve are very short and it must be measured in invasion. In addition, the electric physiological inspection regarding the autonomic nerve has a limit which is difficult to directly apply to the human body because it must be carried out by surgical operation such as severance of nerve, etc (Park et al., 2004). Therefore, recently, an indirect method, which observes the activity of the autonomic nervous system through the activity of the cardiopulmonary vascular system reflecting the best autonomic nervous system, is used broadly. Evaluating the autonomic nervous system by extracting activity information of the autonomic nerve from signals of the cardiopulmonary vascular system can be regarded as very significant because a method measuring activity of the cardiopulmonary vascular system is very convenient and used broadly compared to other methods.

2.2 Relationship between breathing and the autonomic nervous system

The operation of breathing is basically the operation of the somatic nervous system of the musculoskeletal system. Breathing can adjust coughing quickly and slowly if we want by using the somatic nervous system. We implement these adjustments by commanding orders to lower the motor neuron at the back of the cerebrum cortex. If we want to use the diaphragm quietly and deliberately when we breathe the axon signals are delivered to the diaphragm through the diaphragm nerve by commanding orders to lower the motor neuron.

The autonomic nervous system has a mutual interaction relation with the somatic nervous system. Let's review from the viewpoint of breathing. When the human body is active in physical sports and exercises, the number of heartbeats increase due to the autonomic nervous system and the output quantity of the heartbeats also increases, and at this time, breathing is adjusted as the autonomic nervous system sends signals to the somatic nervous system for fulfilling the oxygen quantity required for the human body. The adjustment of breathing immediately provides impacts on the autonomic nervous system after the completion of sports and exercises and the parasympathetic nerve is activated to operate the human body to reach a stable status. This operates in the same method when people take sleep. The somatic nervous system induces the most stable breathing when taking sleep. At this time, induced breathing is deeply involved in the activity of the parasympathetic nervous system of the autonomic nervous system (Song and Lehrer, 2003).

2.3 Autonomic nervous system and heart rate variability

The heartbeat change rate does not mean changes of the maximum or minimum number of heartbeat per minute appearing on the ECG recorder, but is to measure the variation from one heart cycle to the next heart cycle. That is, the HRV signals mean the level of the variation of the heartbeats and we can obtain information from a finer variation from one heart cycle to the next heart cycle. The heartbeat change rate represents the cardiovascular control mechanism, which changes endlessly, and quantifies the changing trend of heartbeats (Noh et al, 2008).

The heartbeat change rate changes every moment by the homeostasis mechanism which is adjusted by the autonomic nervous system. We judge the status of the human body only with these changes and we judge that there is a problem in the adjustment mechanism of the autonomic nervous system if there is almost no change during the stable period and on the contrary, we can judge that it is in a healthy status if changes are active.

The autonomic nervous system evaluation by the heartbeat change rate can be divided into a method using parameters in the time domain, a method using the parameters in the frequency domain and a method, which uses these in both domains. A method using parameters in the time domain evaluates the autonomic nervous system based on the hourly statistical data of the degree of the changes of heartbeats and also evaluates with the component size of the section by obtaining a power spectrum density (PSD) at signals of intervals between R

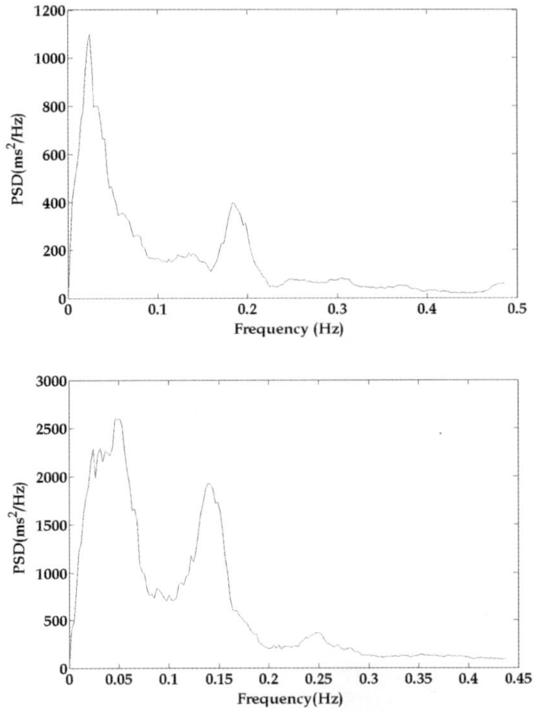

Fig. 1. HRV PSD (upper) in normal daily life and HRV PSD during deep sleep (lower)

peaks within a fixed times (typically 5 min) in the the frequency domain. In particular, in the the frequency domain, activities of the sympathetic nervous system and parasympathetic nervous system can be directly evaluated by using PSD (Task Force of the ESC & NASPE, 1996).

If we observe the the frequency domain of the HRV signals, we can observe through the activity of the parasympathetic nervous system range by breathing because breathing signals receive the impacts of the parasympathetic nervous system of the autonomic nervous system. Breathing provides impacts on the high frequency (HF) range in the the frequency domain of HRV signals and it appears, in general, in 0.15 ~ 0.4 Hz. However, in recent research, the necessity to observe in a lower frequency range was emphasized because there is almost no new volume activity and it is in a very stable status during sleep. As seen in Fig. 1, actual sleep breathing signals are much lower and stable than breathing frequency in normal daily life. So, in this study, the level of activation is evaluated through the PSD of 0.1 ~ 0.4 Hz section. If we compare the HF range section among the HF range of the HRV and the frequency range of the EDR extracted from the ECG, we can evaluate how a well measured ECG reflects breathing signals (Aysin and Aysin, 2006; Choi et al., 1999; Cammann and Michel, 2002).

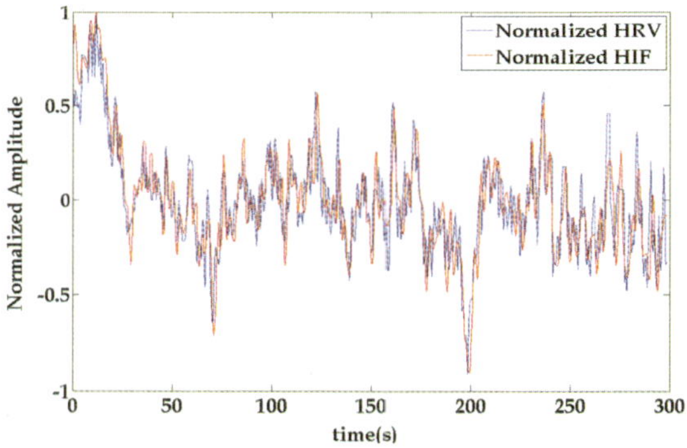

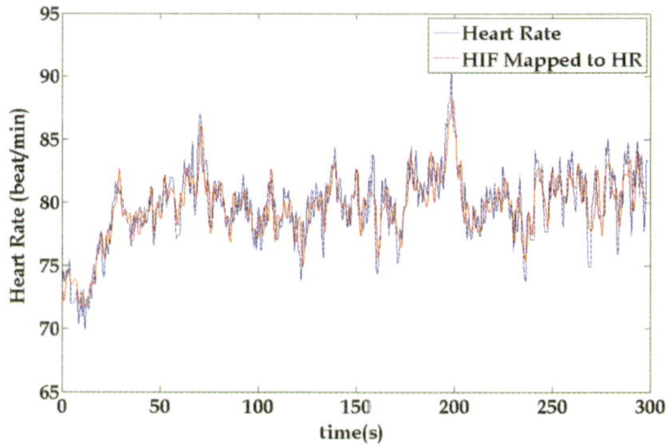

Fig. 2. HRV PSD(upper) in normal daily life and HRV PSD during deep sleep (lower)

2.4 Relationship between heart rate variability and heart instantaneous frequency

HRV and HIF extracted from the ECG are the same signals basically. It is because the modulation frequency, which is generated while intervals between each R peak is changed due to heartbeats, forms a fundamental frequency owned by the ECG and the HIF is the expression by finding out at every moment the maximum value of the fundamental frequency band changing every moment. In particular, HIF extracts the instantaneous frequency response of heart activity and was reported to have close correlation with HRV signals (Barros and Ohnishi, 2001). The HIF signals acquired from the ECG have the same form of time series of HRV and HIF can also provide the autonomic nervous system information which HRV provides. In addition, it can become the efficient alternative plan of the HRV in a ubiquitous healthcare environment because it can be extracted in time-frequency analysis base without a stage to detect R peak in ECG signals and has a much lower sampling rate and little signal processing courses than the HRV (Noh et al., 2008). Figure 2 and 3 are in comparison by obtaining each HRV and HIF regarding the ECG during the stable period. If we compare after normalizing the two signals, it is possible to confirm that they are almost the same signals and it can be noticed that there is almost no difference even in the PSD analysis.

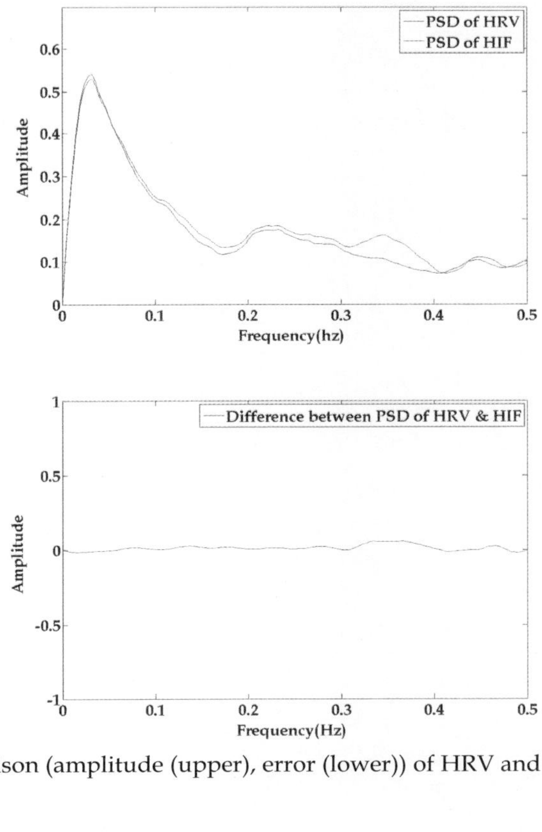

Fig. 3. PSD comparison (amplitude (upper), error (lower)) of HRV and HIF

3. Methodology

3.1 ECG measurement system using textile electrode

ECG lead I and lead III were measured by using the conductive textile electrode for measuring the ECG during sleep without consciousness and binding. The motions of the human body during sleep can be largely divided into lying left/right, lying supine and lying on one's front and the ECG lead, which can efficiently respond to these, was judged as I and III. Each ECG is measured continuously during sleep and the quality of breathing information is judged by calculating EDR and HIF with 5 minutes of data measured every 5 minutes. As seen in Fig. 4, electrodes (75cm × 41cm) of lead I are positioned on both shoulders for measurement and electrodes of lead III are measured through the neck electrode(103 cm × 50 cm) in the form of a pillow and the electrode (149 cm × 41 cm) of both legs. The conductive textile electrodes used in the test were coated with silver (Ag) and was selected in material property which does not aggravate users during sleep. And, the data was collected by additionally installing a thorax belt breath measurement device (AD instruments Powerlab, AUS) for comparison with actual breathing. The ECG signals are measured for 6 hours during a night and actually use 4 hours of data after subtracting one hour at the start and one at the end. This was carried out for using data during sufficiently deep sleep. ECG and breathing signals were acquired with the sampling rate of 500Hz and the ECG was acquired through self-developed module. The ECG module transmits data real-time to an automated ECG classification system to be suggested in this study by connecting with PC and wireless (bluetooth) or cable (RS232) communication. The examinees who have been selected and implemented are healthy and without sleep apnea or respiratory quotient pain disease. The average age of them was 23.5 years old ± 2.59 (mean ± SD), height was 176.3 cm ± 5.75, body weight was 77.7 kg ± 10.55 and Body Mass Index (BMI) was 24.94 ± 2.81. It was arranged that all examinees slept wearing running shirts and shorts.

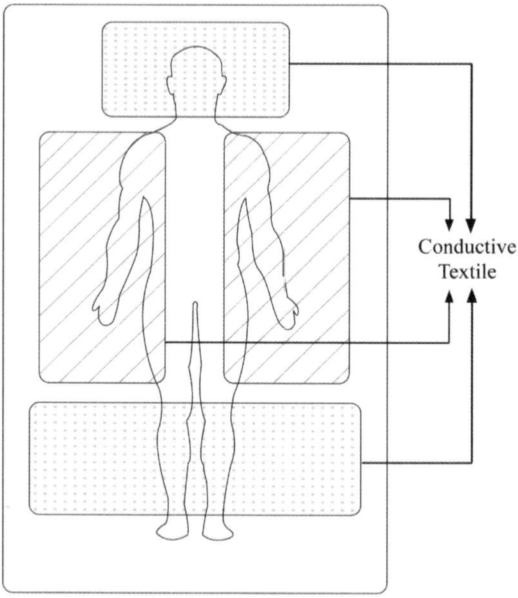

Fig. 4. Deployment map of conductive textile electrode

3.2 Extraction algorithm of ECG-derived respiration (EDR)

We use the EDR as it provides impacts on ECG, and which changes of impedance within the thorax according to the inflow and outflow of air in the breathing cycle are measured in electrodes contacted with the skin. Short period changes of thorax impedance indicate the filling and the exhausting of lungs and this phenomenon becomes the base of change records of impedance volume. Physical impacts of these breaths are appearing in changes of the amplitude of vibration in the ECG. In inhaling breath, the thorax impedance is increased as the volume is increased due to the inflow of air. The amplitude of the ECG to be measured by an electrode becomes smaller due to the impacts of the increased thorax impedance. On the contrary to this, in exhaling breath, thorax impedance is reduced as the volume is reduced due to the outflow of air. The amplitude of the ECG to be measured by an electrode becomes bigger due to the reduced thorax impedance.

However, as mentioned in the introduction, the breath generates RSA regarding heart activity in addition to size of the ECG. The number of heartbeats of a person is decided by the activity frequency of SA node with a cardiac pacemaker. This frequency is decided in balance of activities between the sympathetic nerve and the vagus nerve of the heart in SA node. In here, changes of breath are reflected in heart activity because the vagus nerve receives impacts with each breath. That is, during inhalation, R peak intervals of the ECG becomes short due to the reduction of activity of the vagus nerve and during exhalation, R peak intervals become longer due to the activity of vagus nerve. And it can be considered that the interval differences between the R peaks of the ECG due to inhalation and exhalation indicates RSA.

The most general method for inducing ECG-derived respiratory (EDR) is by using the size of the amplitude of vibration of the ECG is a method which goes through a ECG

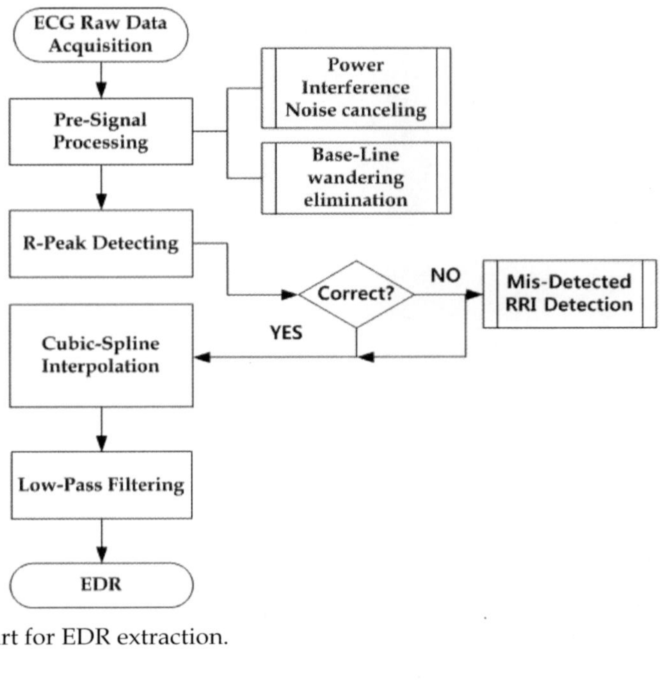

Fig. 5. Flow chart for EDR extraction.

measurement, a whole processing course removing baseline changes using median filtering, the ECG R peak detection and the QRS section area calculation, the movement average calculation of the obtained section area and cubic-spline interpolation, and the multi regression processing course to remove DC and low frequency components of finally induced signals. However, a method using the size of the amplitude of the vibration of the ECG can show a big error in the section area in cases when the ECG is distorted by motions, etc which can be generated during sleep. Therefore, in this study, a method obtaining amplitude or the QRS section area of the accurate R wave of the ECG was not used, but the frequency modulation based breath extraction method, which extracts EDR by using intervals between R peaks of the ECG receiving impacts by breathing, was used. If we can obtain only the R peak intervals in ECG to be measured in case of using this method, it has the possible advantage to extract breathing signals. Breathing signals were extracted through a baseline wandering removing course using the high pass filter, interval

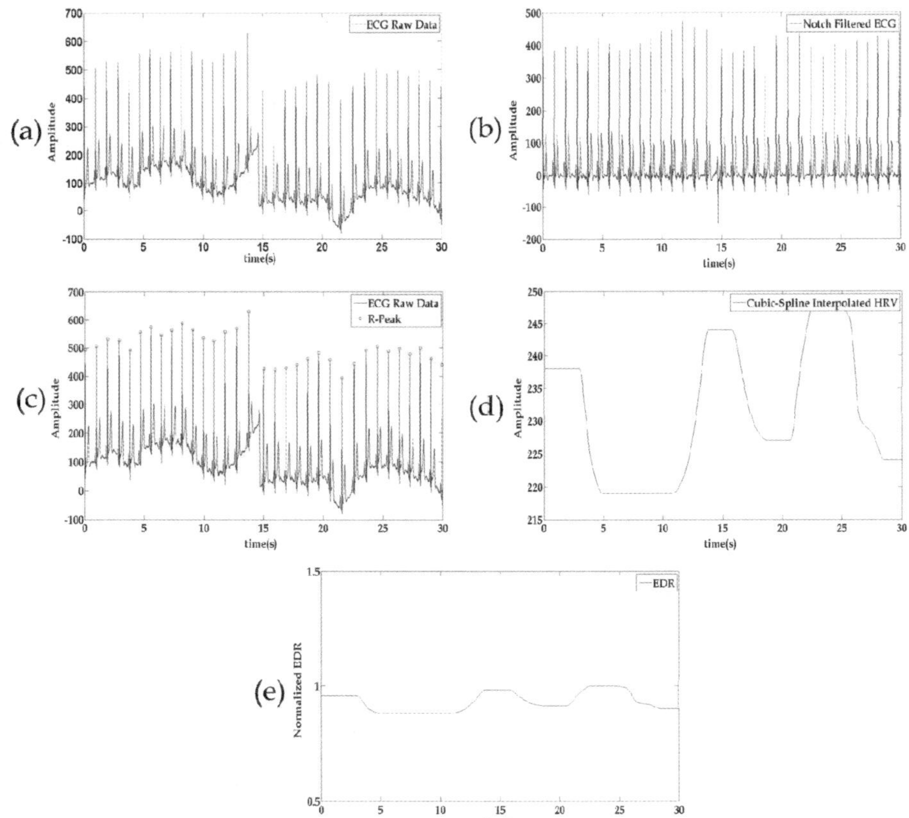

Fig. 6. Signal processing course extracting EDR. (a) ECG raw data, (b) The course of pre-signal processing (power interference noise cancelling & baseline wandering elimination), (c) The course of R-peak detection (Marked as red circle at ECG raw data), (d) The course of cubic-spline interpolation, and (e) The extracted EDR signal.

calculation between R waves through R wave detection and of course the band pass filter (0.2 ~ 0.8 Hz). Figure 5 shows the signal processing course and Figure 6 shows the signal processing result of each course.

3.3 Extraction algorithm of instantaneous heart frequency

A model having the basic frequency, which changes according to times, is necessary because the heart does not beat in a fixed ratio. For example, it is to make the heartbeat or heart frequency by changes of breathing through classifying the RSA, which modulates the ECG frequency according to changes of the breath. Under the given signal, each instantaneous angle frequency $w(t)$ is calculated by using the equation (1) and the equation (2). In here, $H[s(t)]$ is the Hilbert Transform value of the signal.

$$w(t) = \frac{d\Phi(t)}{dt} \tag{1}$$

$$\Phi(t) = \arctan\left(\frac{-H[s(t)]}{s(t)}\right) \tag{2}$$

The HIF signal is extracted from the spectrum response of the ECG. The ECG signal $z(t)$ must be effectively filtered from instantaneous frequency, which a new signal $s(t)$ with a basic frequency that is extracted, because it has multiple harmonics. Therefore, the filter characteristic for the fundamental frequency, which changes according to the times, must be changed properly in compliance to situations.

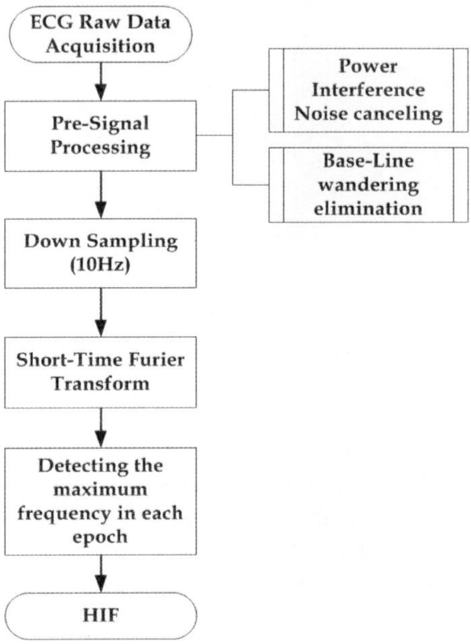

Fig. 7. Flow chart for HIF extraction

First, the extract course is an estimation of the spectrum graph. The spectrum graph of the ECG signal *z(t)* is defined in window function suggested in equation (3) according to the ECG signal *z(t)*.

$$P(t,f)=\frac{1}{2\pi}\left|\int e^{-2\pi f\tau}z(\tau)h(\tau-h)d\tau\right|^{2} \tag{3}$$

In second, we can be found the frequency values corresponding to the maximum values of *P(t,f)* of each point of time of frequency scope. When the founded value is considered $\delta(t)$, it can be expressed in equation (4).

$$\delta(t)=\underset{f}{\arg\max}\left[P(t,f)\right]_{\delta(t^{-})-\alpha}^{\delta(t^{-})+\alpha} \tag{4}$$

As a frequency value limiting scope in equation (4) it can be defined as α and $\delta(t^{-})$ is defined as $\delta(t)$ at t^{-}. In addition, equation (4) represents an algorithm finding the maximum value of *P(t,f)* along the frequency axle with intervals of $[\delta(t^{-})+a, \delta(t^{-})-a]$.

In third, instantaneous frequency can be calculated by using a band pass filter in the vicinity of the central frequency given at each point. In particular, the wavelet is used for the composition of filters. The basic wavelet is a little modification of the Gabor function, which is limited to all time and frequency domains. The equations are implemented according to the spectrum response movement of the filter at the central frequency. Therefore, the basic wavelet during short hour interval (Ω) is given like equation (5) and (6). The filtered signal in intervals Ω is given by equation (7).

Finally, the HIF signal can be obtained if it is calculated by substituting equation (7) in equation (1) and equation (2) (Barros and Ohnishi, 2001). Figure 7 shows the signal processing course for extracting HIF signals and Figure 8 shows the signal processing result for each course.

$$\psi(t)=\frac{1}{2\pi}\left[\exp\left(-\pi\left\{\frac{\overline{\delta(t)}t}{2}\right\}^{2}\right)\cos\left(2\pi\int_{\Omega}\delta(\tau)d\tau\right)\right] \tag{5}$$

$$\overline{\delta(t)}=\frac{1}{\Omega}\sum_{\Omega}\delta(t) \tag{6}$$

$$s_{\Omega}(t)=\int_{\Omega}z_{\Omega}(\tau)\psi(t-\tau)d\tau \tag{7}$$

4. Results and discussion

4.1 EDR evaluation

We have compared the EDR extracted from each lead with actual breathing. The purpose of this evaluation was to show that EDR extracted during sleeping is not always the same as actual breathing. EDR can show significant differences with actual breathing in case when the original ECG signals are not good as explained in the extraction course because it goes through the signal processing course between the R peak detection of the ECG and interpolation. In addition, as seen in Table 1, the actual respiratory quotient and the breathing of the EDR extracted from each lead appear in distribution of lead I and lead III without being concentrated on one lead. This means that the ECG of other lead has been distorted due to the motions of examinee and the external interference noises during sleep and it provides meaning to the necessity of the classification of a significant ECG suggested in this study.

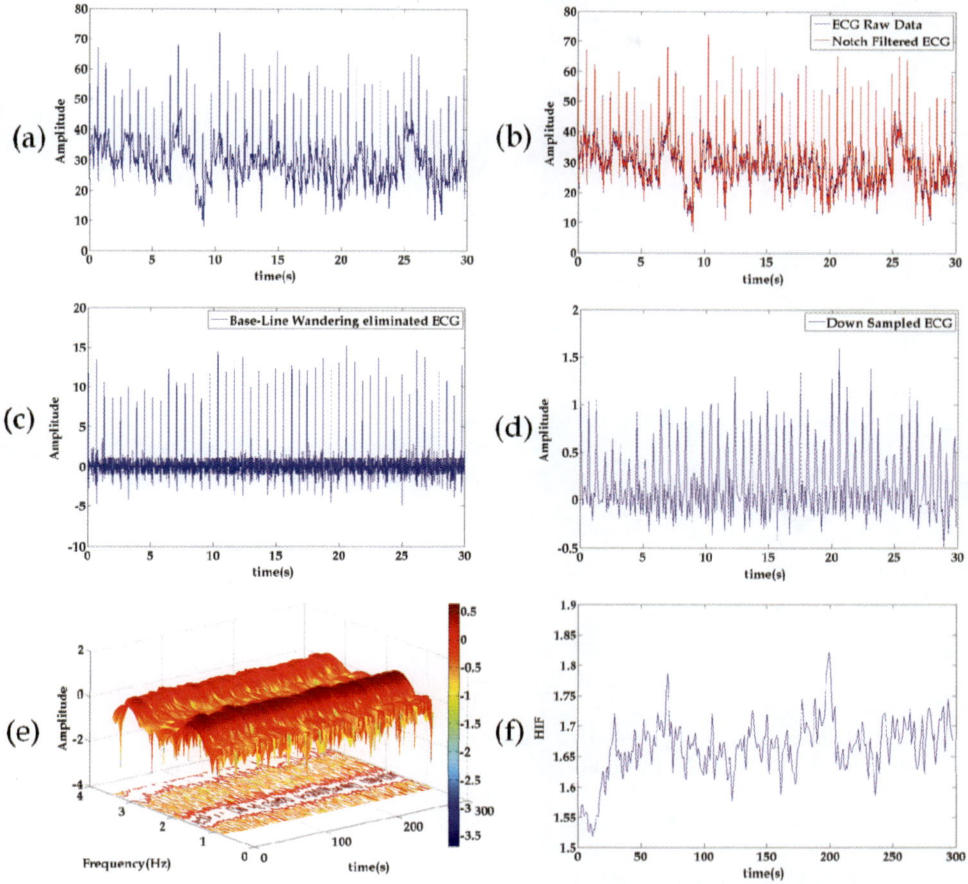

Fig. 8. Signal processing course for extracting HIF. (a) ECG raw data, (b) The course of pre-signal processing (power interference noise canceling), (c) The course of pre-signal processing (baseline wandering elimination), (d) The course of down sampling, (e) The course of Short time Fourier Transform (STFT) and (f) The extracted HIF signal.

We have analyzed a section of 4 hours when the examinee took a deep sleep and did not limit the sleeping habits of the examinee during sleep. We have evaluated the relativity with actual breathing based on the respiratory quotient and have confirmed the correlation between actual breathing in lead I and lead III under the unit of 1 hour and extracted the EDR regarding data during the sleep of each examinee.

Big differences of correlation coefficient between the leads per hour in the sleep information of several examinees (A, F, H, I and J) can be considered as they were basically the motions of the examinee during sleep. It mainly occurs when the conductive textile electrode forming each lead does not contact well with the skin according to changes of sleeping postures. In particular, in the case of examinee C, from the second hour, it noticed that the signal processing for extracting the EDR was not operated properly because the quality of the ECG signal from the electrode deteriorated.

Subjects	1st hour		2nd hour		3rd hour		4th hour	
	lead I	lead III	lead I	lead III	lead I	lead III	lead I	lead III
A	0.78	0.82	0.35	0.82	0.21	0.77	0.83	0.76
B	0.71	0.72	0.73	0.70	0.66	0.69	0.58	0.71
C	0.75	0.69	0.34	0.26	0.39	0.11	0.20	0.18
D	0.52	0.71	0.72	0.66	0.72	0.77	0.74	0.68
E	0.69	0.61	0.65	0.74	0.57	0.62	0.61	0.73
F	0.73	0.77	0.55	0.53	0.10	0.79	0.56	0.74
G	0.62	0.62	0.58	0.55	0.59	0.63	0.49	0.51
H	0.66	0.70	0.14	0.64	0.55	0.69	0.64	0.71
I	0.49	0.42	0.57	0.59	0.47	0.41	0.27	0.76
J	0.71	0.68	0.46	0.50	0.14	0.56	0.19	0.47

Table 1. Correlation coefficient comparison between actual breathing and the EDR of each extracted lead

4.2 Optimum ECG lead selection algorithm during sleep by using HIF

ECG data during actual sleep receive lots of impacts from the motions of the examinee and external interference noises. In particular, because the conductive textile electrode used as an electrode is not attached to the body of an examinee so it is possible to measure the ECG without binding and the consciousness of the examinee, but it is easily exposed to impacts from surrounding noise. So, we have developed an algorithm which can automatically classify the ECG including significant breath signals by evaluating each of the two leads measured during sleep.

The ECGs (lead I and lead III) measured during sleep apply the algorithm after an elapse of one hour from the start of sleeping. Each ECG data is divided into the unit of 5 minutes and classification work is implemented in real-time. 5 minutes unit ECG is measured in each ECG lead extracts EDR and HIF signals and transforms them again into a frequency range respectively. We select the optimum lead, which reflects breathing information well, by comparing the PSD of the two transformed signals and we classify and store them automatically. Figure 9 is the system screen which has realized the automatic selection algorithm of the ECG lead. The program was realized with LabVIEW 8.6 (National Instruments, USA).

Judgment standard analyzes how much high relativity does the PSD of EDR extracted in each lead have by comparing it to the PSD of HIF signals. HIF signals are not largely distorted by the motions of the examinee or external interference noises because it is based on instantaneous frequency component according to each time of information of measured ECG signals and also because it can be obtained without various courses required for HRV analysis or extracting EDR. Therefore, more stable and high reliability information can be obtained. So, in this study, we judge whether EDR extracted based on the standard of frequency analysis obtained from HIF signals has meaning or not and can classify the corresponding ECG as significant information. Figure 10 is a flow map of the algorithm for the automatic classification of the ECG leads suggested in this study.

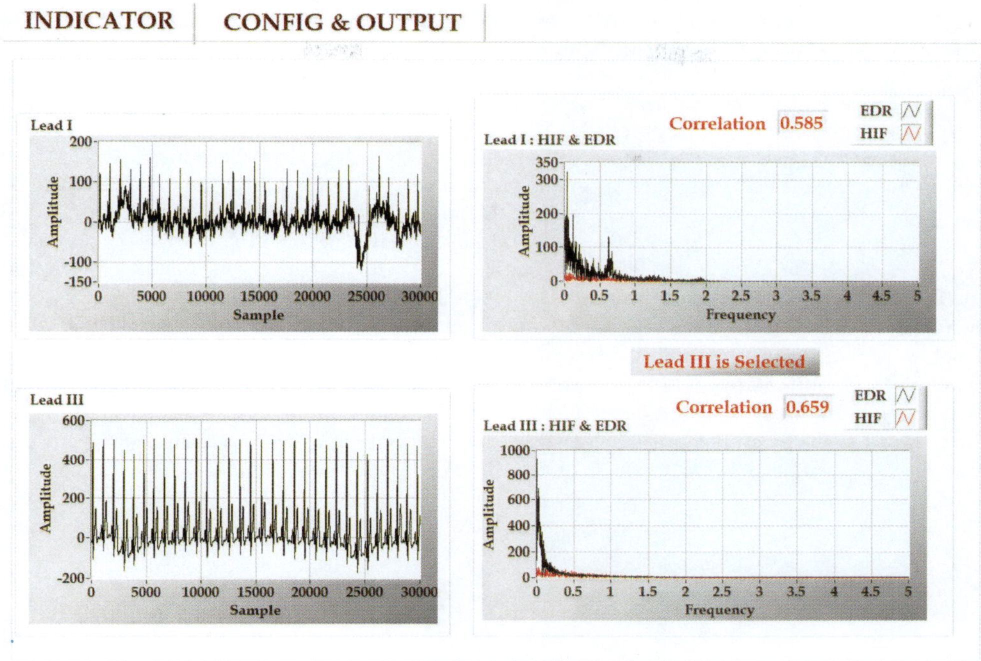

Fig. 9. Automatic classification system screen (LabVIEW)

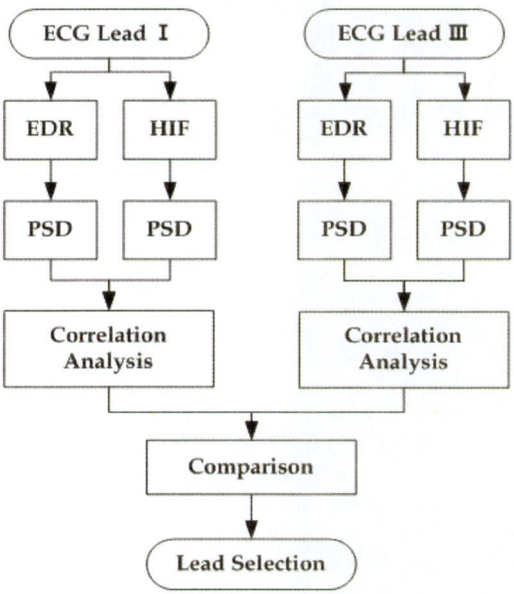

Fig. 10. Selection algorithm block diagram

In general HRV frequency analysis, shows the impacts of the parasympathetic nerve of the autonomic nervous system which includes breathing information appear mainly in the HF range of 0.15 ~ 0.4 Hz. However, as seen in Fig. 1, the intervals of breathing become larger and the quantity of one breath increases as a person becomes stabilized physically and mentally when the human body enters deep sleep. In reality, it can be activated in a much lower range than this one (Aysin and Aysin, 2006; Choi et al., 1999; Cammann and Michel, 2002). Therefore, in this study, it was evaluated by expanding the HF range into 0.1 ~ 0.4 Hz. Figure 11 shows the evaluation with regard to 1 hour(3rd) of examinee D in the unit of 5 minutes through the comparison of correlation between the PSD of HIF and the one of EDR. We have basically judged and selected that the ECG lead, which has a high correlation coefficient among the two leads, and includes actual breathing properly during sleep. However, even if it is a lead with relatively high correlation, if the correlation coefficient is below an absolute number (<0.5), the two leads are all judged as meaningless signals. Even though we store the ECG with relatively high correlation coefficient, we did not classify them as significant ECG signals. Figure 12 shows the signal processing status when the ECG was distorted due to the motions of the examinee during sleep and also when the ECG was measured stably. In this case, lead I was discarded and the ECG of lead III was classified and stored.

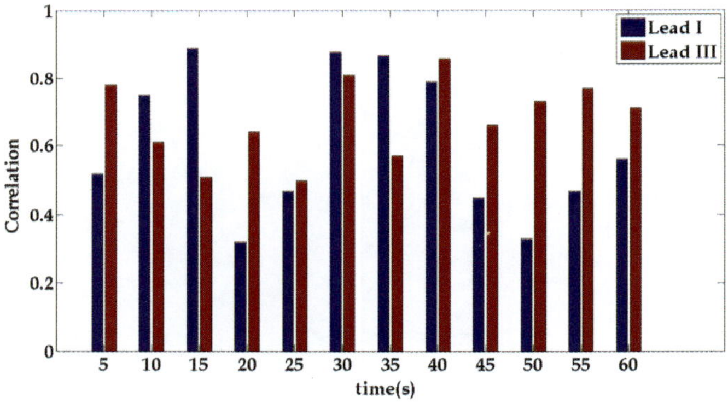

Fig. 11. Evaluation with regard to 1 hour(3rd) of examinee D in the unit of 5 minutes

5. Conclusion

HIF can provide frequency information like HRV, which is a biometric signal representing the best autonomic nervous system. Based on this fact, we can classify significant ECG signals which include accurate actual breathing information during sleep. We have developed algorithm which can automatically select and classify the significant ECG signals successively through PSD correlation analysis between the HIF signal and EDR which are acquired in the leads by acquiring the ECG with two leads (Lead I and III) in preparation for cases when the signal processing of the ECG is difficult due to motions or external interference noise, which can be generated during sleep. The continuous classification of the significant ECG acquired during sleep has a very important meaning and through the result of this study, it is believed that the very accurate and useful information can be provided to the sleep apnea symptom patients who need the accurate diagnosis or people who need breathing monitoring.

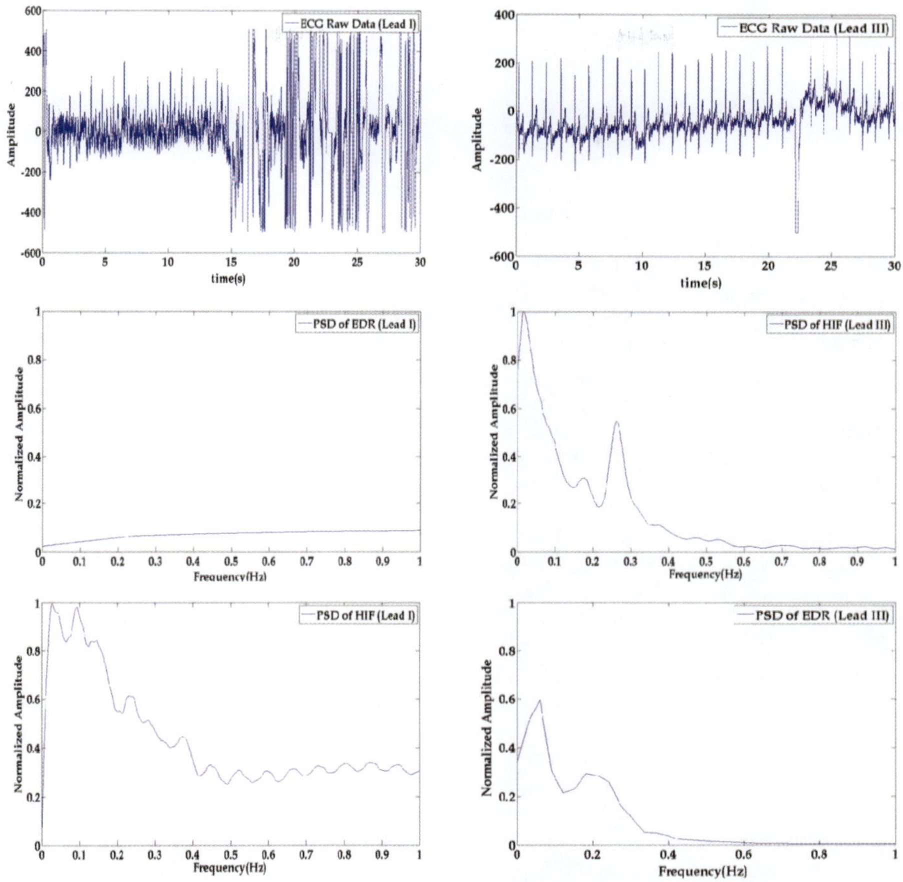

Fig. 12. Significant ECG lead (Right), and a lead which is not significant (Left)

6. Acknowledgment

We would like to thank Sung-Bin Park, Sung-Jun Park, Young-Myoun Han, and Jae-Hoon Jung. They provided a lot of support in the system configuration and signal processing for developing our algorithm. This study was supported by a grant of the Korea Health 21 R&D project, Ministry of Health & Welfare, Republic of Korea. (Grant No. A020602).

7. References

Park, SB.; Yi, KH.; Kim, KH. & Yoon, HR. (2004). An Improved Algorithm for Respriation Signal Extraction from Electrocardiogram Using Instantaneous Frequency Estimation based on Hilbert Transform, Trans. KIEE, Vol.53D, No.10, pp.733-740

Cysarz, D.; Zerm, R.; Bettermann, H.; Fruhwirth, M.; Moser, M. & Kroz, M. (2008). Comparison of Respiratory Rates Derived from Heart Rate Variability, ECG Amplitude, and Nasal/Oral Airflow. Annals of Biomedical Engineering, Vol.36, No.12, pp.2085-2094

Yi, KH.; Park, SB. & Yoon, HR. (2006). Real Time ECG Derived Respiratory Extraction from Heart Rate for Single Lead ECG Measurement using Conductive Textile Electrode, Trans. KIEE, Vol.55D, No.7, pp.335-343

Moody, GB.; Mark, RG.; Zoccola, A. & Mantero, S. (1985). Derivation of Respiratory Signals from Multi-lead ECGs, Computers in Cardiology, Vol.12, pp-113-116

Park, SB.; Noh, YS.; Park, SJ. & Yoon, HR. (2008). An improved algorithm for respiration signal extraction form electrocardiogram measured by conductive textile electrodes using instantaneous frequency estimation, Med Bio Eng Comput, Vol.46, pp.147-158

Mazzanti, B.; Lamberti, C. & Bie, J. (2003). Validation of an ECG-Derived Respiration Monitoring method, Computers in Cardiology, Vol.20, pp-613-616

Behbehani, K.; Vijendra, S.; Burk, JR. & Lucas, EA. (2002). An Investigation of The Mean Electrical Axis Angle and Respiration During Sleep, Proceedings of the Second Joint EMBS/BMES conference, pp.1550-1551, Houston, USA, Oct 23-26, 2002

Travaglini, A.; Lamberti, C.; DeBie, J. & Ferri, M. (1998). Respiratory Signal Derived from Eight-lead ECG, Computers in Cardiology, Vol.25, pp.65- 68

Correa, LS.; Laciar, E.; Torres, A. & Jane, R. (2008). Performance evaluation of three methods for respiratory signal estimation from the electrocardiogram, 30th Annual International IEEE EMBS conference, pp.4760-4763, Vancouver, British Columbia, Canada, Aug 20-24, 2008

Noh, YS.; Park, SJ.; Park, SB. & Yoon, HR. (2007). A Novel Approach to Classify Significant ECG Data Based on Heart Instantaneous Frequency and ECG-Derived Respiration using Conductive Textiles, Proceedings of the 29th Annual International Conference of the IEEE EMBS, pp.1503-1506, Cite Internationale, Lyon, France, Aug 23-26, 2007

Noh, YS.; Park, SB.; Hong, KS.; Yoon, YR & Yoon, HR. (2006). A Study of Significant data Classification between EDR extracted and frequency analysis of Heart Rate Variability from ECG using Conductive textile, World Congress 2006, pp.3958-3961, Seoul, Republic of Korea, Sep 28-30, 2006

Eckberg, DL. (1983). Human sinus arrhythmia as an index of vagal cardiac outflow, J Appl Physiol, Vol.54, No.4, pp.961-966

Hayano, J.; Yasuma, F.; Okada, A,; Mukai, S. & Fujinami, T. (1996). Respiratory Sinus Arrhythmia : A Phenomenon Improving Pulmonary Gas Exchange and Circulatory Efficiency, Circulation, Vol.94, pp.842-847

Noh, YS.; Park, SJ.; Park, SB. & Yoon, HR. (2008). Design of Real-Time Autonomic Nervous System Using Heart Instantaneous Frequency, Journal of Electrical Engineering & Technology, Vol.3, No.4, pp.576-583

Task Force of The European Society of Cardiology and The North American Society of Pacing and Electrophysiology. (1996). Heart rate variability (Standards of measurement, physiological interpretation, and clinical use), European Heart Journal, Vol.17, pp.354-381

Aysin, B. & Aysin, E. (2006). Effect of Respiration in Heart Rate Variability (HRV) Analysis, Proceedings of the 28th Annual International Conference of the IEEE EMBS, pp.1776-1779, New York City, USA, Aug 30 - Sep 3, 2006

Choi, HJ.; Jeong, KS.; Lee, BC.; Kim, YK.; Ahn, IS. & Joo, KS. (1999). Study on HRV Analysis in Sleep Stage Using Wavelet Transform, Korean J Med Phys, Vol.10, No.3, pp.141-149

Cammann, H. & Michel, J. (2002). How to avoid misinterpretation of heart rate variability power spectra?, Computer Methods and Programs in Biomedicine, Vol.68, pp.15-23

Song, HS. & Lehrer, PM. (2003). The Effects of Specific Respiratory Rates on Heart Rate and Heart Rate Variability, Applied Psychophysiology and Biofeedback, Vol.28, No.1, pp.13-23

Part 3

ECG Feature Analysis

6

QT Interval and QT Variability

Bojan Vrtovec and Gregor Poglajen
Department of Cardiology, University Medical Center Ljubljana, Slovenia

1. Introduction

Sudden cardiac death (SCD) is among the most common types of mortality in developed countries. It for more deaths each year than the total number of deaths from AIDS, breast cancer, lung cancer and stroke together. SCD accounts for approximately 50% of all deaths from cardiovascular diseases and 20% of total mortality (1). In the general population, SCD mostly occurs in individuals who are unrecognized to be at risk (2,3).

Although the causes of SCD are multiple, the majority (80–85%) of sudden cardiac deaths is caused by acute ventricular arrhythmias (4). Traditionally, the risk of ventricular arrhythmias has been evaluated based on the duration of QT interval on a standard surface ECG.

2. QT interval

QT interval is measured in milliseconds (ms) from the Q-top, the beginning of the QRS complex, until the end of the T wave and reflects the time between the initial fast depolarization of the left ventricle and its subsequent repolarization (5). Duration of the QT interval is highly dependent on T wave morphology, which is determined by the differences in the time course of repolarization of 3 predominant ventricular myocardial cell types (endocardial, epicardial, and M cells) (6).

The start of the T wave is caused by the more rapid rate of decline of the plateau or phase 2 of the epicardial action potential, creating a voltage gradient and electrotonic current flow across the wall. The gradient gradually increases as the epicardial action potential continues to repolarize, reaching a maximum with full repolarization of epicardium; this juncture marks the peak of the T wave. Divergence of the plateau of the endocardial AP from that of the M cell occurs soon after that of epicardium, causing a voltage gradient between endocardium and the M region and thus a current opposite to that generated by the voltage gradient that develops between epicardium and the M region. Under normal conditions, current flow between the M region and epicardium is greater than that between the M region and endocardium, resulting in the inscription of the ascending limb of the upright T wave. Once epicardium is fully repolarized, continued repolarization of endocardium leads to a progressively larger voltage gradient between endocardium and the M region, giving rise to the initial descending limb of the upright T wave. The last cells to repolarize are the M cells, contributing to the final segment of the T wave. Full repolarization of the M region marks the end of the T wave (7,8).

In the presence of cardiac disease, ventricular repolarization heterogeneity is increased, leading to QT interval prolongation (9). However, QT interval duration is also affected by various noncardiac factors, such as age, gender, inflammation, changes in autonomic nervous tone, and electrolyte disturbances (10), thereby limiting its use in the analysis of the electrophysiological properties of ventricular myocardium. Furthermore, QT interval duration is highly dependent on heart rate. Despite a variety of methods that have been proposed to derive a rate-corrected (QTc interval), which would allow the comparison of QT values obtained at different heart rates, no consensus has been reached so far (11). Since there is growing evidence that QT interval prolongation by itself cannot accurately predict the pro-arrhythmic potential, other ECG parameters are considered more reliable and have been investigated in pre-clinical and clinical studies.

3. Long QT syndrome

The long QT syndrome (LQTS) is characterized by the appearance of long QT intervals in the electrocardiogram, an atypical polymorphic ventricular tachycardia displaying features of torsade de pointes, and a high risk for sudden cardiac death (12). Congenital LQTS can be further subdivided into six genotypes distinguished by mutations in at least five different ion channel genes located on chromosomes 3, 7, 11, and 21 (13,14). These mutations result in defects in the sodium channel (SCN5A, LQT3), the rapidly activating delayed rectifier channel (I Kr) (HERG, LQT2 or KCNE2, LQT6), and the slowly activating delayed rectifier channel (I Ks) (KvLQT1, LQT1 or KCNE1, LQT5), respectively. Acquired LQTS is a term long reserved for a syndrome similar to that encountered in the congenital forms but caused by exposure to drugs that prolong the duration of the ventricular action potential (15) or to QT prolongation secondary to bradycardia, electrolyte imbalance or remodeling of the ventricular myocardium that accompanies dilated and hypertrophic cardiomyopathies (16,17).

Management of patients with long QT syndrome is strongly dependent of the genetic basis of the disease. The trigger for most of the episodes of life-threatening arrhythmias of long QT syndrome is represented by a sudden severe increase in sympathetic activity, which is largely mediated through left cardiac sympathetic nerves. (12) Therefore B-adrenergic blockade represents the first line of treatment in symptomatic patients with long QT syndrome. It has been shown that in LQT1 patients B-blockers significantly reduce life-threatening events and these patients seldom need more than antiadrenergic therapy. Compared to LQT1 patients, LQT2 and LQT 3 patients have more life-threatening events despite treatment with B-blockers. (18) In these patients additional therapies are needed. In patients who remain symptomatic despite treatment with B-blockers (minority of LQT1 and the majority of LQT2 and LQT3 patients) left cardiac sympathetic denervation (LCSD) is to be considered. Although moderately invasive (it requires surgical removal of first four thoracic ganglia) it has proven effective since it was shown that with LCSD we can achieve about 90% reduction in cardiac events and with this a dramatic improvement in patients' quality of life. (19). Regarding ICD therapy it is uniformly agreed that in case of documented cardiac arrest ICD should be implanted immediately. However, there are significant differences in opinion regarding the use of ICDs in patients without cardiac arrest. It should not be forgotten that ICD do not prevent the occurrence of malignant arrhythmias and that most of arrhythmias in patients with long QT syndrome are self terminated. Furthermore pain associated with shocks can in turn perpetuate malignant rhythm disturbances through massive catecholamine release. It is therefore of paramount importance to implant only to symptomatic patients since there to date no clear benefit of ICDs in asymptomatic patients with long QT syndrome has been demonstrated. (20)

4. Short QT syndrome

Short QT syndrome (SQTS) is an inheritable primary electrical disease of the heart, discovered in 1999. It is characterized by an abnormally short QT interval (<300 ms) and a propensity to atrial fibrillation and SCD (21). Like in the case of long QT syndrome there is more than one genetic mutation that can lead to a short QT interval in the ECG and so far gain-of-function mutations in KCNH2, KCNQ1, KCNJ2, encoding potassium channels and loss-of-function mutations in CACNA1C and CACNB2b, encoding L-type calcium channel subunits have been identified (22). Shortening of the effective refractory period combined with increased dispersion of repolarization is the likely substrate for re-entry and life threatening tachyarrhythmias (23). ICD is the therapy of choice in patients with a short QT syndrome. However, antiarrhythmic drug therapy may constitute a potential adjunct or even an alternative therapy in children and newborns, where ICD implantation is very challenging. To date several antiarrhythmic agents were tested in this patient population. Flecainide, sotalol and ibutilide (acting through blocking of the rapidly activating delayed rectifier potassium current) all failed to prolong the QT interval in patients with short QT syndrome.(24) In vitro electrophysiological studies showed that the mutation of the I_{Kr} channel led to a reduced ability of these antiarrhythmic agents to block the channel.(25) It was recently shown that quinidine, in contrast to flecainide, ibutilide and sotalol, can normalise the QT interval at resting heart rates. Additionally, quinidine also restored the heart rate dependence of QT interval towards an adaptation range of normal subjects.(26) Although studied extensively, the exact mechanism of its action for now remains incompletely understood. We have to keep in mind, however, that short QT interval can be a consequence of several gain- and loss-of-function mutations. Therefore for this patient population a uniform medical management currently cannot be recommended.

5. QT variability

Repolarization of the ventricular myocardium is a complex process that varies in duration from site to site and from beat to beat. The mechanisms that govern spatial heterogeneity in ventricular repolarization are well studied, and are largely related to variation in ion channel function and density from one myocardial region to another (27). Ventricular wall comprises of 3 cell types: epicardial, M and endocardial cells. Epicardial and M cell action potentials differ from endocardial cells with respect to the morphology of phase 1. These cells possess a prominent transient outward current mediated notch responsible for the 'spike and dome' morphology of the epicardial and M cell response. M cells are distinguished from the other cell types in that they display a smaller slowly activating delayed rectifier current, but a larger late sodium current and sodium-calcium exchange current. Because of these differences spatial heterogeneity in ventricular repolarization occurs.

The mechanisms responsible for temporal fluctuations in repolarization, however, are poorly understood. Several clinical studies over the past decade have examined beat-to-beat variability in QT interval of the surface electrocardiogram (ECG) as a means for quantifying temporal repolarization lability (28).

Recently, a PC-based electrocardiogram software program has been developed that in real time, acquires, analyzes, and displays QT variability in each of the 8 independent channels that constitute the 12-lead conventional electrocardiogram (29). The system also analyzes and displays the QT variability from QT-interval signals that are derived from multiple channels and from singular value decomposition such that the effect of noise and other artifacts on the QTV results are substantially reduced compared with existing single-channel methods.

When analysis begins, templates for the overall ECG signal in each channel are first formed. To construct the initial templates, the first 20 beats are collected into a single averaging bin. Then, the mode of the probability function of the R-R interval is created for those beats and its maximum determined. Finally, those 10 beats that are closest to the determined maximum are selected, and a template ECG wave for the same beats is then obtained by averaging the superimposed ECG signals based on the fiducial point of the QRS wave.

After the initial global templates have been constructed, breaking points called PQbreak (between the P wave and the QRS complex), QTbreak (between the QRS complex and the T wave), Tend (the final point of the T wave), and Pini (the initial point of the P wave) are used to construct individual templates for the 3 principal waveforms QRS, T, and P.

The principal steps of the algorithm used in analyzing QT variability are described in detail, as follows:

1. The template beat φ(n), where n is the sample number, is constructed from the selected beats using a signal averaging technique. Only those beats with shape similar to the template are selected for averaging. Because the program automatically determines the borders of each wave component (P, QRS, and T templates, as described previously) and therefore the time window for matching of waves, its remaining task is to shift the particular incoming wave component with respect to the template until obtaining an acceptable match. The matching algorithm is based on the least square deviation of the incoming wave vs the template.
2. The matching of waves is performed in 2 substeps. First, a broader time interval containing the complete wave component is used to reach the best fit. Second, each wave of any incoming beat is shifted to or from the trigger point to achieve the best alignment with the template in the appropriate time window. For this purpose, an error function of time shifting is defined as the sum of the squared differences between the template wave (P, QRS, or T) and the appropriate shifted version of the incoming beat.
3. The program uses the QT variability algorithm to generate, in real time, the time series of the QT interval along with that of the R-R interval. Time series are analyzed according to the recommendations of the Task Force of the European Society of Cardiology and the North American Society of Pacing and Clinical Electrophysiology (30) using specific indices such as the SD of normal-to-normal (NN) R-R and QT intervals (SDNN R-R and SDNN QT, respectively), the root mean square (RMS) of the successive interval difference (RMSSD R-R and RMSSD QT), and so on.

6. Clinical application

Although QT interval prolongation has been proposed as a risk factor for death in an apparently healthy population in patients after myocardial infarction in diabetic patients, and patients with advanced heart failure, its direct relation to pro-arrhythmic risk remains questionable (1,17).

While measuring subtle variation in QT interval duration is technically challenging, new methodology (28,29) has enabled investigators to study the effect of disease states on ventricular repolarization variability, and the prognostic value of the QT interval variability measurement. QT variability has been shown to be elevated in congestive heart failure (CHF) (28), ischemia (31), and some types of hypertrophic cardiomyopathy (26). Increased QT variability was also found to predict appropriate implantable cardioverter-defibrillator shocks in the MADIT-II (Multicenter Automatic Defibrillator Implantation Trial-II) study (33), as well as total mortality and sudden death in post-myocardial infarction patients without implantable cardioverter-defibrillators (34).

Based on the current clinical evidence it appears that although currently considered 'the golden standard' QT interval measurement will in the future be replaced by novel, more reproducible automated methods that will allow for better prediction of arrhythmic events in various clinical settings.

7. Pharmaceutical application

Pro-arrhythmic drug effects have been one of the most common reasons for withdrawal of drugs from the market in many therapeutic areas. Currently, the potential pro-arrrhytmic effects of drugs are addressed in accordance with The 'International Conference on Harmonization of Technical Requirements for Registration of Pharmaceuticals for Human Use' (ICH) E14 clinical guidance issued in May 2005. The centre-piece of the guidance is the 'thorough QT/QTc study' (TQT), which is a dedicated study with the primary objective to quantify the effect of a new molecular entity on the QT interval (35).

Although considered the 'golden standard', use of QT interval duration as a surrogate marker for the prediction of drug-induced arrhythmias has several pitfalls (36,37):

- Many drugs affect both QT interval duration and heart rate. Since all current heart rate correction methods are imperfect, it is difficult to distinguish the drug-related changes in QT interval from those caused by heart rate alterations.
- Since QT interval duration is dependent on several non-cardiac factors (e.g. inflammation, autonomic nervous system), the therapeutic effect of drugs on the underlying disease may mask the potential adverse drug effects on cardiac repolarization and QT interval.
- QT interval is used as a surrogate marker of arrhythmias; however, its relationship to the arrhythmic events has been seriously questioned in the recent clinical studies.
- It is assumed, but has not been proved, that even a small drug-induced increase in QT interval indicates some risk of arrhythmias.

Given these limitations it is clear that in order to adequately address pro-arrhythmic risk of drugs it is necessary to look beyond the drug-induced changes of QT interval. Other drug-induced ECG changes, associated pro-arrhythmic risks, and threshold of magnitude of changes should be considered as a cause for concern. Therefore, novel advanced ECG technologies should be develop do better define drug-induced arrhythmogenesis.

8. References

[1] Myerburg RJ, Kessler KM, Castellanos A. Sudden cardiac death: epidemiology, transient risk, and intervention assessment. Ann Intern Med 1993; 119: 1187–97.

[2] Myerburg RJ, Castellanos A. Emerging paradigms of the epidemiology and demographics of sudden cardiac arrest. Heart Rhythm 2006; 3: 235–9.
[3] Priori SG, Aliot E, Blomstrom-Lundqvist C, Bossaert L, Breithardt G, Brugada P, Camm AJ, Cappato R, Cobbe SM, Di Mario C, Maron BJ, McKenna WJ, Pedersen AK, Ravens U, Schwartz PJ, Trusz-Gluza M, Vardas P, Wellens HJ, Zipes DP. Task Force on Sudden Cardiac Death of the European Society of Cardiology. Eur Heart J 2001; 22: 1374–450.
[4] M, Wellens HJ. Implantable defibrillators and sudden cardiac death. Circulation 2004; 109: 2685–91
[5] Hurst W. Naming of the waves in the EKG, with a brief account of their genesis. Circulation 1998; 98:1937-42.
[6] Dudel J. Information transfer by electrical excitation. In: Schmidt RF, Thews G , eds. Human physiology.Berlin: Springer-Verlag; 1989: 19-42.
[7] Yan GX, Antzelevitch C. Cellular basis for the normal T wave and the electrocardiographic manifestations of the long-QT syndrome. Circulation 1998;98:1928–36.
[8] Williams EMV. QT and action potential duration. Br Heart J 1982; 47: 513-4.
[9] Antzelevitch C, Shimizu W. Cellular mechanisms underlying the long QT s yndrome. Curr Opin Cardiol 2002;17:43–51. [PubMed]
[10] Magnano AR, Holleran S, Ramakrishnan R, Reiffel JA, Bloomfield DM. Autonomic nervous system influences on QT interval in normal subjects. J Am Coll Cardiol 2002; 39:1820–6.
[11] Malik M, Färbom P, Batchvarov V, Hnatkova K, Camm AJ. Relation between QT and RR intervals is highly individual among healthy subjects: implications for heart rate correction of the QT interval. Heart. 2002;87(3):220-8.
[12] Schwartz PJ. The idiopathic long QT syndrome: progress and questions. Am Heart J 1985; 109: 399–411.
[13] Curran ME, Splawski I, Timothy KW, et al.: A molecular basis for cardiac arrhythmia: HERG mutations cause long QT syndrome. Cell 1995;80:795–803.
[14] Wang Q, Curran ME, Splawski I, et al. Positional cloning of a novel potassium channel gene: KVLQT1 mutations cause cardiac arrhythmias. Nat Genet 1996;12: 17–23.
[15] Bednar MM, Harrigan EP, Anziano RJ, et al. The QT interval. Prog Cardiovasc Dis 2001;43:1–45.
[16] Tomaselli GF, Marban E: Electrophysiological remodeling in hypertrophy and heart failure. Cardiovasc Res 1999;42:270–283.
[17] Vrtovec B, Delgado R, Zewail A, Thomas CD, Richartz BM, Radovancevic B. Prolonged QTc interval and high B-type natriuretic peptide levels together predict mortality in patients with advanced heart failure. Circulation. 2003;107(13):1764-9.
[18. Priori SG, Napolitano C, Schwartz PJ, Grillo M, Bloise R, Ronchetti E, Moncalvo C, Tulipani C, Veia A, Bottelli G, Nastoli J: Association of long QT syndrome loci and cardiac events among patients treated with beta-blockers. *JAMA* 2004, 292:1341-1344.
[19] Schwartz PJ, Priori SG, Cerrone M, Spazzolini C, Odero A, Napolitano C, Bloise R, De Ferrari GM, Klersy C, Moss AJ, Zareba W, Robinson JL, Hall WJ, Brink PA, Toivonen L, Epstein AE, Li C, Hu D: Left cardiac sympathetic denervation in the

management of high-risk patients affected by the long QT-syndrome. *Circulation* 2004, 109:1826-1833.
[20] Crotti L, Celano G, Dagradi F, Schwartz PJ. Congenital long QT syndrome. Orphanet J Rare Dis. 2008 Jul 7;3:18.
[21] Poglajen G, Fister M, Radovancevic B, Vrtovec B. Short QT interval and atrial fibrillation in patients without structural heart disease. J Am Coll Cardiol. 2006 May 2;47(9):1905-7.
[22] Schimpf R, Borggrefe M, Wolpert C. Clinical and molecular genetics of the short QT syndrome. Curr Opin Cardiol. 2008;23(3):192-8.
[23] Boriani G, Biffi M, Valzania C, Bronzetti G, Martignani C. Short QT syndrome and arrhythmogenic cardiac diseases in the young: the challenge of implantable cardioverter-defibrillator therapy for children. Eur Heart J. 2006; 27(20):2382-4.
[24] Gaita F, Giustetto C, Bianchi F, Schimpf R, Haissaguerre M, Calo L. Short QT syndrome: pharmacological treatment. J Am Coll Cardiol 2004;43:1494– 9.
[25] Schimpf R, Bauersfeld U, Gaita F, Borggrefe M, Wolpert C. Short QT syndrome: successful prevention of sudden cardiac death in an adolescent by implantable cardioverter defibrillator treatment for primary prophylaxis. Heart Rhythm 2005;2:416–7.
[26] Wolpert C, Schimpf R, Giustetto C, Antzelevitch C, Cordeiro J, Dumaine R, et al. Further insights into the effect of quinidine in short QT syndrome caused by a mutation in HERG. J Cardiovasc Electrophysiol 2005;16:54–8.
[27] Antzelevitch C, Fish J. Electrical heterogeneity within the ventricular wall. Basic Res Cardiol 2001;96:517–527.
[28] Berger RD, Kasper EK, Baughman KL et al. Beat-to-beat QT interval variability. Novel evidence for repolarization lability in ischemic and nonischemic dilated cardiomyopathy. Circulation 1997;96:1557-65.
[29] Starc V, Schlegel TT. Real-time multichannel system for beat-to-beat QT interval variability. J Electrocardiol. 2006;39(4):358-67.
[30] Saksena S, Epstein AE, Lazzara R, Maloney JD, Zipes DP, Benditt DG, Camm AJ,Domanski MJ, Fisher JD, Gersh BJ, et al. NASPE/ACC/AHA/ESC medical/scientific statement special report--clinical investigation of antiarrhythmic devices: astatement for healthcare professionals from a Joint Task Force of the North American Society of Pacing and Electrophysiology, the American College ofCardiology, the American Heart Association, and the Working Groups on Arrhythmias and Cardiac Pacing of the European Society of Cardiology. Pacing Clin Electrophysiol. 1995;18(4 Pt 1):637-54.
[31] Murabayashi T, Fetics B, Kass D, Nevo E, Gramatikov B, Berger RD. Beat-to-beat QT interval variability associated with acute myocardial ischemia. J Electrocardiol 2002;35:19–25.)
[32] Atiga L, Fananapazir L, McAreavey D, Calkins H, Berger RD. Temporal repolarization lability in hypertrophic cardiomyopathy caused by beta-myosin heavy-chain gene mutations. Circulation 2000;101:1237–1242.
[33] Haigney MC, Zareba W, Gentlesk PJ et al. QT interval variability and spontaneous ventricular tachycardia or fibrillation in the Multicenter Automatic Defibrillator Implantation Trial (MADIT) II patients. J Am Coll Cardiol 2004;44:1481–1487.

[34] Piccirillo R, Magri L, Matera S et al. QT variability strongly predicts sudden cardiac death in asymptomatic subjects with mild or moderate left ventricular systolic dysfunction: a prospective study. Eur Heart J 2007;28:1344–1350.
[35] Darpo B.The thorough QT/QTc study 4 years after the implementation of the ICH E14 guidance. Br J Pharmacol. 2010;159(1):49-57.
[36] Roden DM. Drug-induced prolongation of the QT interval. N Engl J Med. 2004; 350(10):1013-22.
[37] Valentin JP. Reducing QT liability and proarrhythmic risk in drug discovery and development. Br J Pharmacol. 2010;159(1):5-11

7

A Novel Technique for ECG Morphology Interpretation and Arrhythmia Detection Based on Time Series Signal Extracted from Scanned ECG Record

Srinivasan Jayaraman, Prashanth Swamy,
Vani Damodaran and N. Venkatesh
Innovation Labs, Tata Consultancy Services, Bangalore
India

1. Introduction

Cardiovascular disease (CVD) is the one of the biggest health problem in Indian and around the world as well. Electrocardiogram is a traditional method used for the diagnosis of heart diseases for about a century. Maintaining and retrieving patient history during a course of treatment is a essential but a laborious process. More particularly, over a decade ago thermal ECG records were stored physically, off late, due to advancement in technology; it has been stored as scanned ECG images. Storing the scanned ECG trace images requires considerable storage space. This necessitated the development of an automated solution capable of storing the ECG digitally, retrieving it quickly and detecting cardiac arrhythmia automatically.

Majority of the ECG's clinical information is said to be found in the intervals and amplitudes defined by its features (characteristic wave peaks and time durations).According to author's knowledge, very few researchers [Lawson et al., 1995, Silva et al., Wang et al., 2009, Chebil et.al., 2008, Kao et al.,2001] have approached the extraction of ECG digital time series signal from scanned ECG trace images. Lawson et al., chose a scanning resolution of 200 dpi and used global thresholds to separate the ECG trace from the background grid lines. The low resolution results in loss of data accuracy and global thresholds results in missing pixels which are replenished by linear interpolation. Fabio Badilini et al., 2005 developed an application for extraction of the ECG trace from the image. But the method requires the user to fix anchor points for missing peaks and thus the accuracy comes down. Shen et al., separated the ECG trace from the background grids using the histogram. The missing pixels are replenished by checking the value of the pixel in the original image. This is a tedious process. Kao et al., employed a color filter to remove the background gridlines in the color image. There was a problem of missing pixels in the process which was replenished by linear interpolation. Jalel Chebil et al., performed a comparative study of the extracted trace accuracy by scanning the image at various resolutions. Global thresholds and median filtering were employed to remove background grids. The threshold to separate the trace from the background should be selected based on the nature of the image to avoid any missing pixels. All conventional techniques use morphological operations such as erosion, dilation, thinning etc [Rafael C. Gonzalez and Richard E.Woods 2008] to extract the ECG trace from the background. However, all the above work addresses the issue of one-dimensional time series signal alone.

In this work, we propose an improved methodology to extract the digitized ECG time series dignal from scanned ECG records. As a novelty, we are using the Radon transform for de-skewing the scanned images. Even though the conventional morphological techniques are adapted, they are applied in an iterative fashion on the binarized de-skewed images. This results in more accurate extraction of the time series trace. Further, a simple and useful way of axis identification is proposed. In addition to ECG digitization, we have extended this work to ECG morphological extraction and report generation. As a novelty, we have applied slope method for morphological extraction that eliminates the pre-processing of noise and baseline wandering technique. This method reduces the retrieval and computational time and improves the accuracy of ECG image.

This chapter is divided into three subtopics: Converting thermal ECG trace to Digital ECG signal, Report generation from ECG morphology and automated arrhythmia detection. This chapter explains various techniques, adapted to extract the digital time series signal from scanned thermal ECG records. This process of digitally converting ECG trace reduces the storage space and retrieval time with increased viewing accuracy. The challenges here are as follows. Firstly, the analysis algorithms requires the ECG signal to be digital. Therefore, the conversion of scanned ECG records to digital time series is a pre requisite. The algorithms are also capable of handling data from the digital ECG device that provide a digital signal as an output. Secondly, the digital signal from scanned ECG requires standardization, i.e. based on the ECG records, the ECG digital signal must be re-sampled and voltage levels adjusted automatically. In addition to digital signal conversion, this chapter explains the technique used to interpret ECG morphology and generate reports based on the interpretation. A challenge in report generation is estimation of time and amplitude level from pixel information and ECG morphological interpretation techniques. After ECG morphology analysis, automatic cardiac arrhythmia classification is performed for diagnosis. In this automated cardiac arrhythmia detection we would discuss about various classification technique and there efficiency.

2. Methodology

The following sections explains in detail the various stages involved in capturing the ECG trace, its storage and retrieval, signal extraction and digital signal generation, report generation and finally abnormality classification.

2.1 Data acquisition and image processing

Figure 1 gives an overview of the image processing techniques involved in the signal extraction process.

12 lead ECG signals were recorded at a paper speed of 25mm/sec and printed in thermal paper. These stored paper ECG trace is scanned at resolution of 600 dpi (dots per inch) black and white images and stored in jpeg format. Radon transform is applied on these images to detect and correct the skewness, which is incurred during the scanning process. The de-skewed image is adaptively binarized by choosing local thresholds. To limit the area to be binarized, the image is iteratively filtered by morphological filters. Each time the

image retained is a cropped version of the original image. An envelope detection operation has been performed on the resultant binary ECG image to yield the upper and lower boundaries. The pixel values are then averaged to obtain the Digital ECG signal. The digital signal is windowed and re-sampled in accordance with the ECG record as shown in Figure. 1.

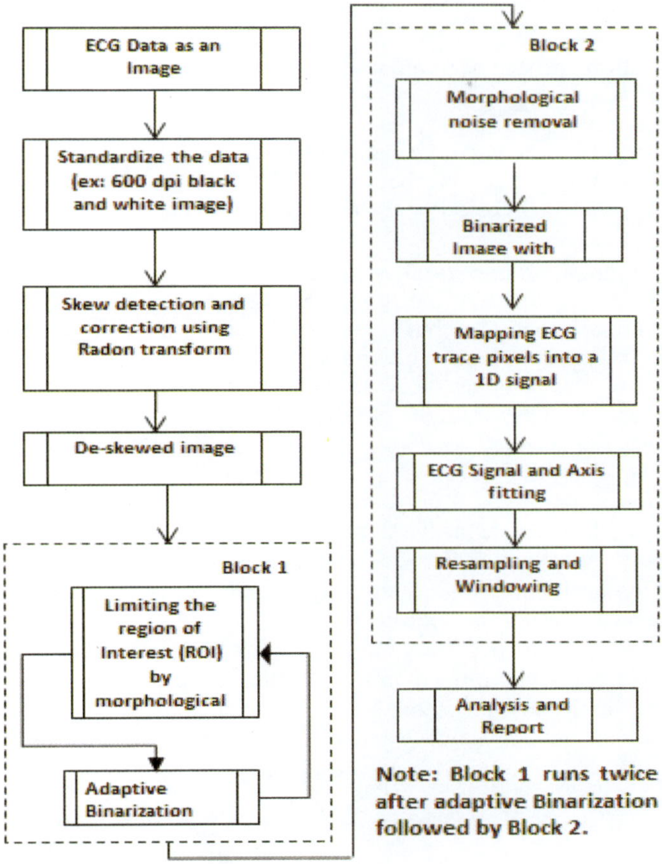

Fig. 1. Overview of the Digitization Process

2.1.1 Scanning and standardization

Table 1, lists out various scanning resolution and formats that that can be handled by the algorithm proposed. Based on the resolution of scanning and paper speed the pixel is defined in terms of time and amplitude units. For example, a resolution of 600 dpi implies 600 pixels in an inch (25.4 mm). Thus the number of pixels per mm can be calculated. Paper speed of 25 mm/sec i.e. 1 sec = 25 mm and calibration mark of 1mV amplitude = 10 mm is used to evaluate the value of each pixel in the time scale and amplitude scale. Pixel value in time scale is found to be 1.693 ms and amplitude scale to be 4.233 mV. These values are used during the digital time series signal generation.

Scanning Resolution in dpi	Type/Color	Image Format
200	True Color	Jpeg/Tiff/Bmp/Png
300	Gray Scale	Jpeg/Tiff/Bmp/Png
600	True Color/Gray Scale/B&W	Jpeg/Tiff/Bmp/Png

Table 1. Various scanning resolution

2.1.2 Skew detection and correction using radon transform

Scanning process of paper ECG may results in skewness in scanned images either due to human error or faulty scanners. In order to extract faithfully the ECG signal from images, the skewness has to be eliminated. To remove the skew we have applied Radon transform [Lins R. D. and Ávila B. T., 2004, Prashanth et al., 2010] to find the angle of skewness. The skew angle has been selected, based on the maximum variance.

2.1.3 Adaptive binarization and iterative morphological operations

Our next objective is to binarize the image. Extracting the ECG signal from the image depends on the accuracy with which it is separated from the rest of the attributes present in the image like grid lines, textual characters etc. From elaborate experimentation, it is observed that, using various image processing filters and tweaking the thresholds, could not eliminate the noise completely from the ECG signal.

In this work Otsu's algorithm [Otsu N., 1979] has been performed for image adaptive binarization. Adaptive threshold technique for image binarization yields better results compared to global thresholds. This process of adaptive binarization ensures that the threshold is selected based on an active signal region using morphological operation and not on the entire image. Morphological operations include dilation and erosion as shown in the figure 2 (c). Erosion operation on the binary image results in the loss of ECG signal as shown in Figure 2c. However, during this process of erosion, we record the upper and lower limit in the Cartesian coordinate. The boundary limit values are assigned as threshold and the image clipping operation has been performed on the ECG trace. The clipped image is again fed back to the adaptive binarization algorithm and the whole process is repeated again. This methodology reduces the original image to the requisite binarized image containing the useful information. Further this has been achieved through reduced processing time.

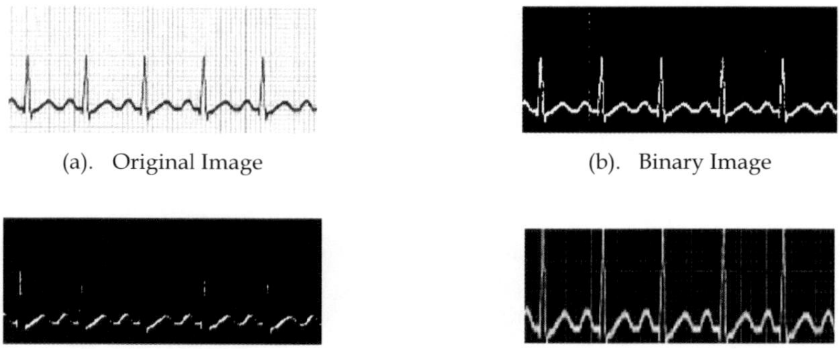

(a). Original Image (b). Binary Image

(c). Dilated Image (d). Clipped Image

Fig. 2. Iterative Morphological operations

2.2 Signal extraction and report generation

Once the ECG waveform in the image is separated from the gridlines, it must be converted to a digital format. Data logged as X-Y coordinates represent the signal. The binarized imaged is subjected to envelope detection to obtain a complete digital signal.

2.2.1 Envelope detection and axis identification

The result as shown in figure 2 (b), contains only the binary ECG trace whose thickness is more than a single pixel. An envelope detector is applied in order to obtain a time series. In an envelope detector, the image is scanned column wise, at each column the uppermost and lowermost non zero values are recorded. Plotting all the upper and lower bound values, we obtain upper and lower envelopes of the ECG signal respectively. Figure 3 (a) shows a original gray scale ECG trace. Figure 3 (b) shows its corresponding envelopes.
The mean of ECG signal is represented as

$$X = [Xub + Xlb]/2 \tag{1}$$

Where, X is the mean ECG signal, Xub and Xlb is upper and lower envelope of ECG signal respectively

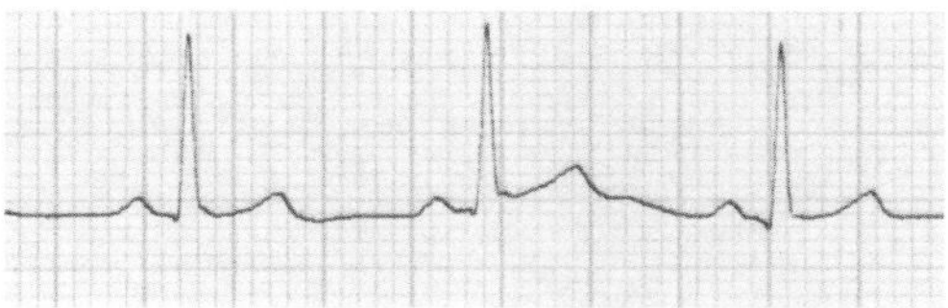

(a) Binary Image of the scanned ECG

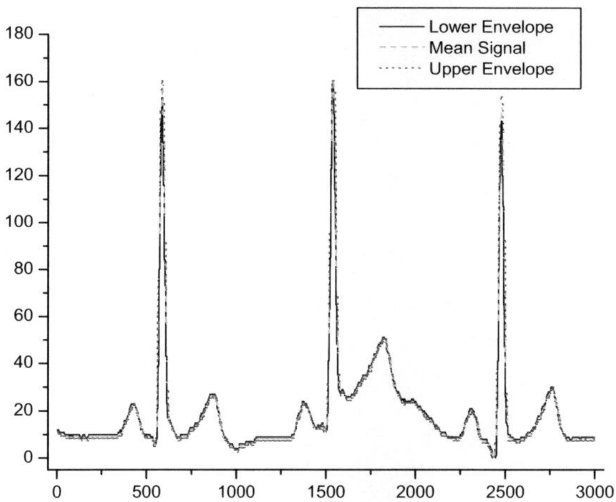

(b) Digital Signal

Fig. 3. (a) shows original paper ECG image of size 3000x250 pixels and (b) shows its corresponding digital ECG signal.

Axis identification plays a vital role in further diagnosis and automatic report generation of the ECG records. The test square pulse present in the starting of any ECG trace is used as reference for the axis. However, in most practical scanning procedures and data capture, square pulses are often absent due to the sheer length of the ECG paper. In order to overcome this, a novel and simple technique to identify the axis is proposed in this paper. The obtained signal X can be represented as $X = [x_1, x_2, x_3 \ldots x_n]$, where the values of each element in the vector correspond to an ECG signal pixel location. By observation, it was found that the most significant and recurring pixels usually represent the axis of the signal along the horizontal. As the signal obtained can be treated as a vector, the axis is obtained by calculating the mode of the vector. Hence, we can represent it as:

$$\text{ECG Axis} = \text{Mode}(X) \tag{2}$$

In most cases, the axis will be non-zero; therefore there is a need to offset the axis to the horizontal zero in order to standardize the signal. Equation 2 describes the offset process.

$$\text{ECG zero axis} = \text{Offset}(\text{Mode}(X)) \tag{3}$$

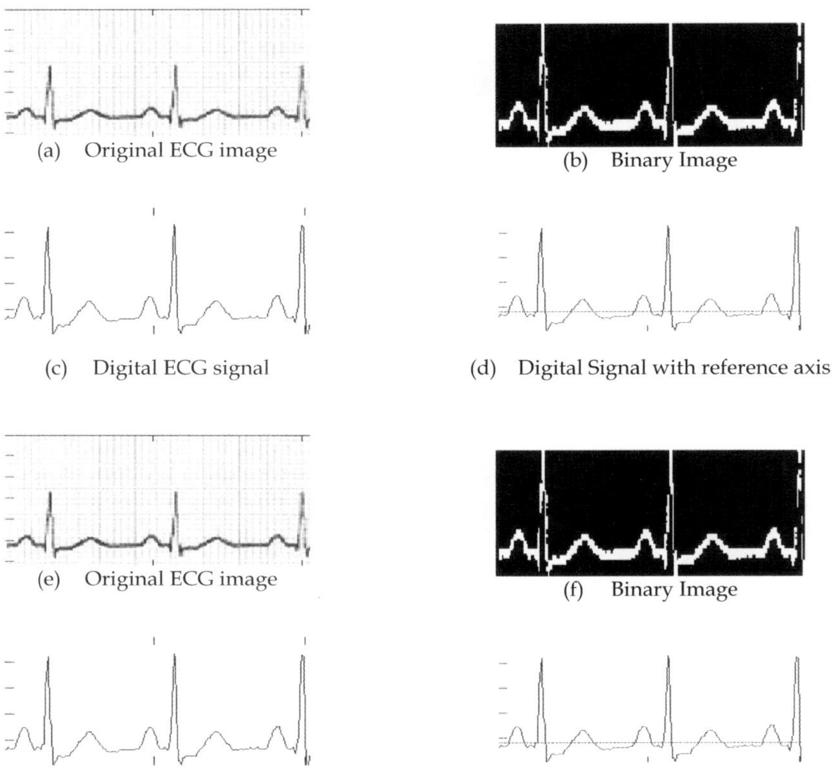

(a) Original ECG image
(b) Binary Image
(c) Digital ECG signal
(d) Digital Signal with reference axis
(e) Original ECG image
(f) Binary Image
(g) Digital ECG signal
(h) Digital Signal with reference axis

Fig. 4. A typical ECG extraction process is as shown in figure 4 (a – c). (d) represents the signal with the reference axis plotted as a dotted horizontal line

2.2.2 Normalising and R-peak detection

The R-peaks which have maximum amplitude in an ECG signal which is extracted by differentiating the ECG signal. Taking the first derivative of the ECG signal and discarding the negative values provides the location of the R-peaks. Subsequently, the number of peaks is used to calculate the heart rate.

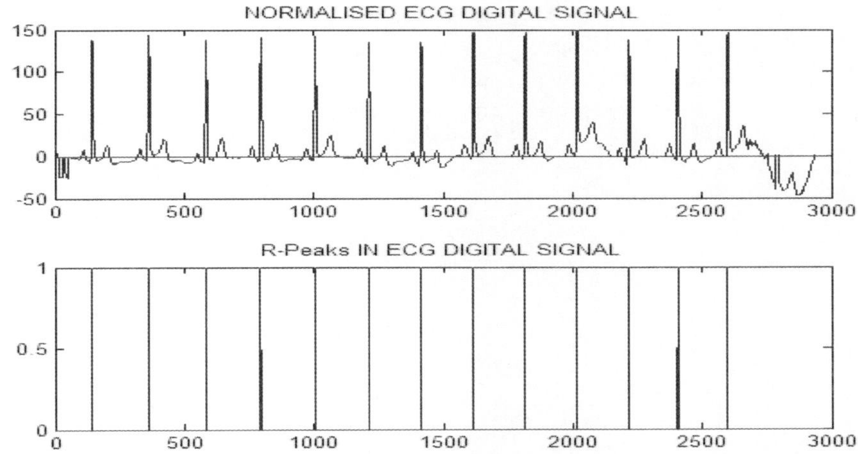

Fig. 5. Normalized ECG signal with reference axis and location of the corresponding R-Peaks. Normalized signal with reference axis is used to extract the r-peaks. All peak locations are represented as 1's in the x-axis ranging between – to 3000.

2.3 ECG morphological feature extraction

A database of 25 patients paper ECG were recorded from 12 lead ECG machine is created and the digital signals are generated. The obtained ECG signals are processed to extract morphological features. The morphological feature extraction is carried out by two methods: time based method and slope based method. The morphological features extracted are P wave duration, QRS complex duration, T duration, PR interval, QT interval and ST intervals and P, R and T amplitudes.

2.3.1 Time based feature extraction

In this method, the digital ECG was filtered using a bandpass filter designed for a frequency range of 0.05 to 30 Hz. Obtained digital ECG signal is differentiated and the R peaks were identified. Heart Rate is calculated by mean of calculating the distance between two peaks. Heart rate is calculated using the formula

$$\text{Heart Rate} = \frac{60}{\text{RR Interval}} \tag{4}$$

In this method, morphological features are extracted by traversing the windowing function on either side of the R peak, based on the ascending and descending nature of the waveform the various peaks and onset and offset of each peak is identified. The window size for Q and

S is 120 ms and for P and T is 150 ms. The Q and S peaks are found by traversing on the left and right side of the R peak within the specified window and locating the minimum or negative peak values. From the Q peak, by traversing on its left side, the maximum value is found to be the P peak. Similarly, by traversing to the right side of the S peak, the maximum value is found to be the T peak.

The P_on and P_off points are identified by traversing the window function on either side of the P peak until they descend and reach the baseline. Similarly, T_on and T_off points are detected with respect to T peak. Using these data point various morphological features such as the duration of P, QRS and T waves, intervals such as PR, QT and ST and the amplitude of P, R and T waves were identified and marked on the digital signal plot as shown in Figure. 6.

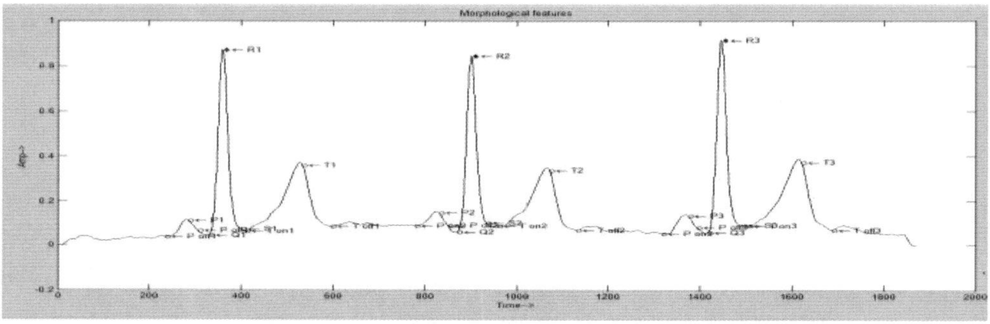

Fig. 6. Time based morphological feature extraction

The accuracy of 94.9% had been obtained for this method for a database of 25 patient's digial ECG records

2.3.2 Slope based feature extraction

In this method, slope of the ECG signal [Damodaran, et al., 2011]within a window size of 'n' number of samples is evaluated to extract the morphological details. The slope of the signal has both positive and negative values due to Increasing and decreasing peaks in an ECG waveform. Slope of the signal is calculated using Equation 5.

$$S_{slope}(i) = \tan^{-1}\left(S(i+n) - S(i)\right) / n \tag{5}$$

where i =1, 2...N-n,

S(t) = Extracted ECG Signal with samples 1 to N and n=Window size

$S_{slope}(t)$ = Slope signal

The window size depends on the number of samples between the Q peak and R peak in the ECG signal. For finding the window size, the R peak is found by differentiating the ECG signal and the Q wave is detected as the negative peak immediately prior to the detected R peak. The window is placed at the 1st sample and the slope between the 1st and the (n+1)th sample is found and stored. The window is then placed on the 2nd sample and the slope between the 2nd and (n+2)th is found. The window is placed at all samples till the (N-n)th sample and the slope values found is stored as the S_{slope} signal.

A standard range of values is defined for the inclination angle of the P wave, QRS complex and T wave for both normal and abnormal ECG. Thus from the defined range of slope values for the ECG waveform, the slope values between the minimum positive slope value and the maximum negative slope values are removed to eliminate any noise.
For finding the window size, the R peak is found by differentiating the ECG signal and the Q wave is detected as the negative peak immediately prior to the detected R peak. The slope of the signal within this window is found for the entire signal is shown in Figure. 7.

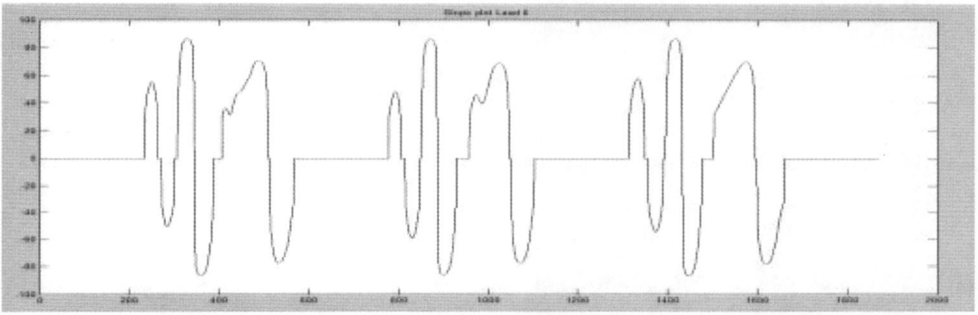

Fig. 7. Slope plot for the digital ECG extracted form the paper ECG. Plotting of the slope values result in three peaks, each one for P, QRS and T waves respectively

The first positive peak is the P_on, the first negative peak is P and the following zero crossing is P_off. Similar procedure is followed to identify the Q, R and S peaks and T wave. The features extracted using slope method is marked on the signal plot as shown in Figure. 8. Accuracy of 97.09% had been obtained for this method for a database of 25 patient's digital ECG records

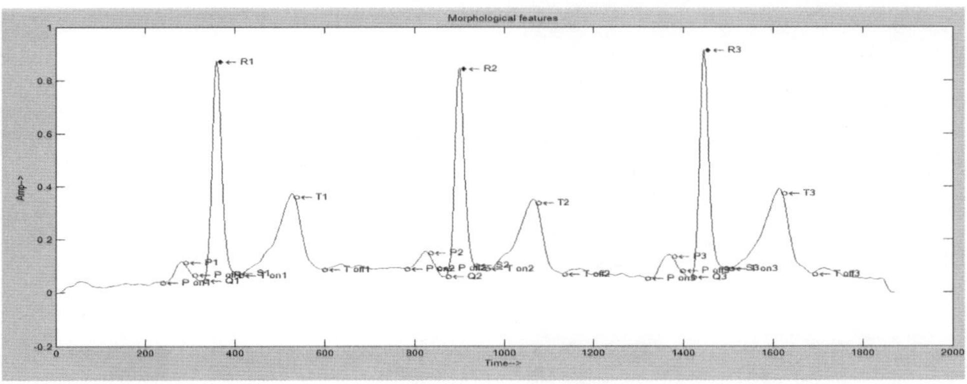

Fig. 8. Slope based morphological feature extraction

As an extension, we have also performed a comparitive study between the slope method and the time base method as shown in table 2.

MORPHOLOGY	MANUAL	TIME BASED	SLOPE BASED
HR	66	65	66
P Duration	0.12	0.13	0.1222
QRS Duration	0.11	0.12	0.115
T Duration	0.24	0.25	0.24
PR Interval	0.16	0.15	0.16
QT Interval	0.42	0.44	0.42
ST Interval	0.3	0.31	0.3
P Amplitude	0.1	0.09	0.11
R Amplitude	0.86	0.82	0.85
T Amplitude	0.3	0.33	0.3

Table 1. Comparison of the time based method and slope method for a single patient ECG patient record

2.4 Automated arrhythmia detection

The morphological features extracted were used to detect the arrhythmias. In this study we have considered three different abnormalities, namely, Sinus Bradycardia, Sinus Tachycardia and PVC. Feature parameter chosen were P wave duration, QRS complex durations, T wave duration, PR intervals, QT intervals and ST intervals. Two classifiers are used to detect arrhythmias, namely Dynamic time warping (DTW) and Adaboost and their performance were compared.

2.4.1 Dynamic Time Warping (DTW)

The DTW classifier [Niranjan et.al., 2004, Venkatesh N and Srinivasan J.,2011] is based on the ranking of the prototypes by the distance to the query.

Let, F = (f1.....fn) and G = (g1.....gm) be two time series of length n and m, respectively. To align the two sequences using DTW, we construct an n-by-m matrix whose (i,j)th element is the Euclidean distance d(i,j) between two points fi and gj. The (i,j)th matrix element corresponds to the alignment between the points fi and gj. A warping path, R is a contiguous sets of matrix elements that defines a mapping between F and G and is written as R={r1.....rS} where, max(m, n) < S < m + n - 1. To limit the warping path, several constraints such as boundary conditions, continuity, monotonicity, and windowing [Bishop, 2006] are used. The DTW algorithm finds the point-to-point correspondence between the curves, which satisfies the above constraints and yields the minimum sum of the costs associated with the matching of the data points. There are exponentially many warping paths that satisfy the above conditions. The path that minimizes the warping cost is,

$$D(F,G) = \min \sum_{s=0}^{S} r_s \tag{6}$$

The warping path can be found efficiently using dynamic programming to evaluate a recurrence relation, which defines the cumulative distance $\gamma(i,j)$ up to the element (i, j) as the sum of d(i, j), the cost of dissimilarity between the ith and the jth points of the two sequences and the minimum of the cumulative distances up to the adjacent elements:

$$\gamma(i,j) = d(i,j) + \min\{\gamma(i-1,j), \gamma(i,j-1), \gamma(i-1,j-1)\} \quad (7)$$

The classification procedure based on DTW yielded the following results.

Types	Total No. Of Records	Classified	Misclassified
Normal	25	24	1
Sinus Tachycardia	8	8	0
Sinus Bradycardia	7	7	0
Pvc	5	5	0

Table 2. DTW classification results

2.4.2 Adaboost classifier

In this study, multiclass adaboost has been used to identifying the arrhythmias detection. Adaboost classifier increases the accuracy of weak classifier by reinforcing training on misclassified samples and assigns appropriate weights to each weak classifier. The final classification is given by

$$h(x)\begin{cases} 1, & if \sum_{i=1}^{t} \alpha_t h_t \geq threshold \\ & 0, otherwise \end{cases} \quad (8)$$

where, 1 indicates the sample has been correctly classified. In this experiment, stumps are used as a weak classifier. For reassigning the weights to the weak classifier 5000 iterations were performed and this was experimentally found to yield better results.

Because it may have potential advantages such as higher classification performance, more rapid recognition process time and extension of recognition features, Adaboost was applied for the detection of cardiac arrhythmia. Each class of ECG type i.e. normal or arrhythmic, a label +1 or -1 is assigned to it. A large number of weak classifiers around 5000 are chosen. Decision stumps are chosen for classification. Decision stumps make prediction based on the value of just a single input feature. The input value if greater than the prediction value then the feature vector belongs to one class else it belongs to another class. Initially a set of training vectors are fed for classification. Labels are assigned for each input. A set of testing vectors are given as inputs for classification. Based on the labels assigned to each of the testing vector, the classification or misclassification is decided.

Types	Total No. Of Records	Classified	Misclassified
Normal	25	24	1
Sinus Tachycardia	8	8	0
Sinus Bradycardia	7	7	0
Pvc	5	5	0

Table 3. Adaboost classification results

The Adaboost classifier is implemented and the classification results are as shown in Table 4. The sensitivity of the classifier is evaluated and the average sensitivity is found to be 99%. Table 5 presents the performance of the classification system for different arrhythmias. The performance of an arrhythmias detection is measured based on the confusion matrix with parameters false rejection (FR), false acceptance (FA), false acceptance rate (FAR) and false rejection rate (FRR) for different cases. In case-1, normal is made one class with PVC, Sinus Bradycardia and Sinus Tachycardia together is made into another class. Similarly in case-2, Sinus Bradycardia is one class, in case-3 Sinus Tachycardia is one class and in case-4 PVC is one class with the other three types together is the second class respectively.

	Precision (%)	Sensitivity (%)	Specificity (%)	Accuracy (%)
Case1	100	96	100	97.78
Case2	87.5	100	97.37	97.78
Case3	88.89	100	97.29	97.78
Case4	83.33	100	97.5	97.78

Table 4. Classification of ECG for different arrhythmias, Case -1 is normal, Case-2 is sinus Bradycardia, Case –3 sinus Tachycardia, and Case –4 is PVC.

2.5 Report generation

Based on the various morphological features extracted using the proposed method and the arrhythmia detection using classifiers, a report is generated for each patient record. This ECG Report consists of Heart Rate, Morphological features duration and arrhythmias will be listed as a report.

3. Conclusion

The conversion of the scanned ECG record to a digital time series signal has been performed by an improved method of binarisation accurately. The digital time series data obtained is scaled in terms of amplitude and time. The digital signal is further processed for ECG morphological extraction procedure, by two methods namely, time based and slope based methodology. The accuracy of both the methods is evaluated by comparing the obtained results with manually read data from the paper record. Slope method is more accurate than other methods, in addition, this method eliminate the base line correction issues, noise removal issues with ECG signals. Further, this work has been extended to classification of ECG using DTW and Adaboost classifier for arrhythmia detection. The paper ECG converted will be provided as report with consists of Heart Rate, Morphological features duration and arrhythmias. This could be an aid tool to physician and electronic medical record maintains. This can function as a second option tool for initial screening producer for ECG.

4. Acknowledgment

The authors wish to thank Mr.Balamuralidhar.P, Head, Innovation Lab, TCS, for his continuous support.

5. References

Bishop M. C., "Pattern Recognition and Machine Learning", Springer (2006).

Chouhan, V.S., and Mehta, S.S., "Detection of QRS complexes in 12-lead ECG using adaptive quantized threshold", International Journal of Computer Science and Network Security, Vol.8, No.1, pp.155-163, January 2008.

Chouhan V.S. and Mehta S.S., "Threshold-based Detection of P and T-wave in ECG using New Feature Signal", International Journal of Computer Science and Network Security, Vol.8, No.2, February 2008.

Congi, M., Poli, S., Calcagnini, G., Censi, F., Bartolini, P., Damiani, S. and Barbaro, V., "An Automated Measure of P-Wave Duration from Surface ECG Maps", Proceedings of the 25th Annual International Conference of the IEEE EMBS, Mexico, 2003.

Chebil Jalel, Jamal Al-Nabulsi and Mohammed Al-Maitah, "A Novel Method for Digitizing Standard ECG Papers", Proceedings of the International Conference on Computer and Communication Engineering, Kuala Lumpur, Malaysia, pp.1308-1312, 2008.

Fabio Badilini, Tanju Erdem, Wojciech Zareba and Arthur Moss, J., "ECGScan: a method for conversion of paper electrocardiographic printouts to digital electrocardiographic files", Journal of Electrocardiology, Elsevier, Vol. 38, pp. 310-318, 2005.

Francis Morris, June Edhouse, William J Brady and John Camm, "ABC of Clinical Electrocardiography", BMJ publishers, 2003.

Gomes E Silva, A.R., De Oliveria, H.M., and Lins, R.D., "Converting ECG and other legated biomedical maps into digital signals", XXV Simposio Brasileiro de Telecomunicacoes, Brazil, 2007.

Kao T, Len-Jon Hwang, Yui-Han Lin, Tzong-Huei Lin and Chia-Hung Hsiao, "Computer Analysis of the Electrocardiograms from ECG Paper recordings", Proceedings of the 23rd Annual EMBS International Conference, Istanbul, Turkey, pp. 3232-3234, 2001.

Lawson, WT., Wagner, GS., Startt-Selvester, RS., and Ybarra, GA., "New method for Digitization and Computerized Analysis of Paper Recordings of Standard 12-Lead Electrocardiograms", Computers in Cardiology, IEEE, pp. 41-44, 1995.

Lins R. D., and Ávila, B. T. "A New Algorithm for Skew Detection in Images of Documents," Proceedings of ICIAR 2004, Lecture Notes in Computer Science, vol. 3212, pp. 234-240, Springer Verlag, 2004.

Morales, E., Sevilla, D., Pierluissi, J.H., and Nazeran, H., "Digitization and Synchronization Method for Electrocardiogram Printouts", Proceedings of the 2005 IEEE Engineering in Medicine and Biology 27th Annual Conference, Shangai, China, pp.1588-1591, 2005.

Niranjan J., G Sita, A G Ramakrishnan and M. Sriganesh,. "Tamil handwriting recognition using subspace and DTW based classifiers", Proc. 9th International Workshop on Frontiers in Handwriting Recognition (IWFHR-9), Tokyo, Oct 2004

Otsu N., "A threshold selection method from gray-level histogram,"IEEE Trans. Syst., Man, Cybern., vol. SMC-8, pp. 62–66, 1979.

Peter Chia, Kenneth Ong and Harsangeet Kaur Bhullar, "An Accurate and Automatic System for Extracting Features from ECG Paper Recordings: Its Use in Clinical Studies and Telemedicines", Computers in Cardiology, pp. 469-472, 1996.

Ping-Sung Liao, Tse-Sheng Chen and Pau-Choo Chung, "A Fast Algorithm for Multilevel Thresholding", Journal of Information Science and Engineering, Vol 17, pp. 713-727, 2001.

Prashanth Swamy, J Srinivasan, M.Girish Chandra, "An Improved Method for Digital Time Series Signal Generation from Scanned ECG Records," IEEE Proceeding, Issue April 2010, pp: 400-403

Rafael C. Gonzalez and Richard E.Woods, "Digital Image Processing (3rd Edition)", Prentice Hall, 2008.

Sanroman-Lunquera, M., Mora-Jimenez, I., Everss, E., "Quality Evaluation and Effect of Time Synchronization on the Digital Recovery of Intracardiac Electrograms", Computers in Cardiology, Vol. 36, pp. 801-804, 2009.

Silva Gomes e A. R., H.M. de Oliveira, R.D. Lins., "Converting ECG and other paper legated biomedical maps into digital signals," XXV Simpósio Brasileiro de Telecomunicações, Setembro 3-6, Recife - PE, Brasil.

Shen, TW., and Laio, TF., "Image Processing on ECG Chart for ECG Recovery", Computers in Cardiology, pp. 725-728, 2009.

Tanveer Syeda-Mahmood, David Beymer and Fei Wang, "Shape-based matching of ECG Recordings", IEEE Interational Conference on Engineering in Medice and Biology, 2007.

Vani Damodaran, J Srinivasan and S. Poonguzhali "A Novel Method to Extract ECG Morphology from Scanned ECG Records", ICBPE, Singapore, 2011

Venkatesh N and Srinivasan J., 'Human Electrocardiogram for Biometrics using DTW and FLDA', ICPR 2010

Wang Fei, Tanveer Syeda-Mahmood And David Beymer, "Information Extraction from Multimodal ECG Documents", 10th International Conference on Document Analysis and Recognition, 2009.

8

Medicines and QT Prolongation

Ryuji Kato, Yoshio Ijiri and Kazuhiko Tanaka
Osaka University of Pharmaceutical Sciences
Japan

1. Introduction

Significant QT interval prolongation may induce severe polymorphic ventricular tachycardia called Torsade de Pointes (TdP). TdP is a type of ventricular tachycardia (VT) characterized by a twist of the QRS wave around the baseline. In some cases this leads to fatal ventricular fibrillation (VF), which is why it is of particular importance among cases of arrhythmia.

QT prolongation causes TdP which may then induce fatal VF. Common causes of QT prolongation include idiosyncratic causes such as gene deficiency, drugs, and drug-drug interactions. There are many cases of QT prolongation caused by drugs used to treat non-cardiac related conditions; these cases involve unintended, adverse 'collateral' effects. Consequently, most of the drug-related cases fall outside the scope of the doctor's area of speciality and/or expectations, which makes it difficult to take preventive and therapeutic measures. It is for this reason that it is important to identify drugs that are likely to cause QT prolongation. Here, we outline drug that may cause QT prolongation and drug-drug interaction induced QT prolongation that could cause serious arrhythmia.

2. What is QT prolongation?

QT interval defines the start of the Q wave and the end of the T wave in an electrocardiogram, representing the time between depolarization and repolarization of the ventricles. Its value is a measurement from phase 0 (upstroke), through phase 1 (spike) and phase 2 (plateau) to phase 3 (rapid repolarization) (Fig. 1). Phase 4 is a phase between action potentials. QRS represents the depolarization of the ventricle, reflecting the membrane potential range as the ventricular depolarization wave propagates from subendocardial to subepicardial. The T wave represents the potential differences of ventricular repolarization. Factors that cause QT interval prolongation include the prolongation of cardiac ventricular action potential duration (APD), and an increase in nonuniformity of repolarization.

The QT interval shortens in tachycardia but prolongs in bradycardia. There is no significant difference based on gender, while there is a weak tendency for the QT interval to prolong in females as they age. It is necessary to distinguish between two types of bradycardia: the PP interval prolongation on the one hand, and the QT interval prolongation on the other. When comparing QT intervals under different pulse rates, it is standard practice to use the corrected QT interval using Bazett's formula ($QTc = QT/\sqrt{RR}$). Other formulae include Fredericia's ($QTc = QT/\sqrt[3]{RR}$) and Van de Water's ($QTc = QT-0.087\times(RR-1000)$) (Kato et al., 2009). The Bazett QTc values are smaller than actual QT measurements as the RR

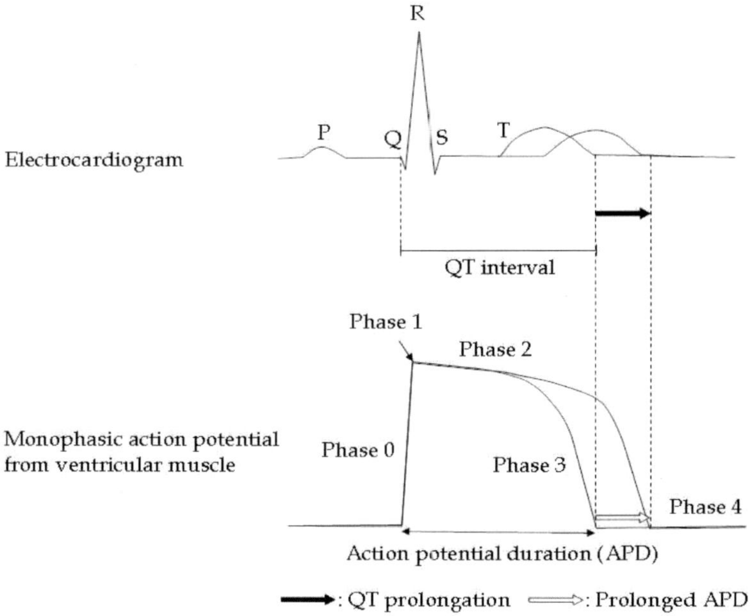

Fig. 1. The relation between electrocardiogram and monophasic action potential from ventricular muscle.

interval prolongs in bradycardia, while in tachycardia they are larger. Here, we adopt the formula among those mentioned above that shows the lowest correlation between the QTc and the RR interval. Normally, QTc values remain constant during both rest and exercise. QT prolongation occurs when QTc values fluctuate to greater than 0.44 sec. When the QTc values are normal (constant), the QT interval should be shortened under exercise compared with resting. QT prolongation occurs when this balance was disrupted. Significant QT interval prolongation may induce a severe polymorphic ventricular tachycardia called Torsade de Pointes (TdP). TdP is a type of ventricular tachycardia (VT) characterized by a twist of the QRS wave around the baseline. The pulse rate can reach 150-300 beats per minute, leading to severe symptoms such as fainting. In some cases this leads to fatal ventricular fibrillation (VF), which is why it is of particular importance amongst cases of arrhythmia. QT prolongation causes TdP that may induce fatal VF, which is why it is important to distinguish PP interval prolongation from QT interval prolongation.

3. What causes QT prolongation?

Long QT syndrome (LQTS) is roughly classified into two types, namely hereditary and acquired LQTS. The former is known to be caused by a disparity between the left and right sympathetic nerve systems stemming from some genetic defect, or by defect in *SCN5A* (the Na^+ channel encoding gene) (Lehnart et al., 2007) or *hERG* (the K^+ channel encoding gene) (Lehnart et al., 2007). Risk factors for the latter include: 1. An electrolyte abnormality such as hypokalemia (outward K^+ current decreases, with APD prolonging) and magnesium deficiency (diuretics can also be a significant cause); 2. Bradycardia; 3. Hypothyroidism; 4. Myocardial infarction with abnormality of K^+ channel; 5. Drugs, and interactions between them.

Next, let us turn now to the electrophysiological mechanism of LQTS. There are a number of different kinds of membrane currents on myocardial cells that are involved with resting potential and action potential formation. Extracellular Na^+ and Ca^{2+} concentration levels are higher than intracellular levels, and the Na^+ current that moves inward (from outside to inside of the cell) forms the depolarization phase (fast channel) while the Ca^{2+} current forms the plateau phase (slow channel). On the other hand, K^+ concentration levels outside the cell are lower than levels inside, and the repolarization phase involves the delayed outward rectifying K^+ current as well as the time-independent inward-rectifying K^+ current. When factors such as drugs are introduced and suppress these K^+ currents, the QT interval prolongs as the prolongation of action potential duration. In the case of TdP accompanying the acquired LQTS, the triggered activity by early afterdepolarization (EAD) or delayed afterdepolarization (DAD) is presumed to play an important role with a possible re-entry involvement.

EAD is an oscillatory potential that occurs in the vulnerable period at the end of the plateau phase when APD prolonged. Triggered activity is generated when EAD reaches the threshold potential and triggers a new action potential. Proposed causes of EAD include: 1. K^+ conductance reduction (K^+ channel blocking); 2. Na^+ conductance increases (aconite poisoning, familial LQTS); 3. Ca^{2+} conductance increases (sympathetic nervous system excitation, catecholamine administered). DAD, on the other hand, is an oscillation in the membrane potential immediately after the myocardinal action potential, or oscillatory after potential. The DAD oscillation can get big enough to constitute triggered activity. One way to grasp the effects on EAD and DAD is to measure the monophasic action potential (MAP) of the myocardium. The MAP measurement makes it possible to examine the Na^+, Ca^{2+} and K^+ currents. MAP_{30} (MAP duration at 30% of repolarization) indicates the Ca^{2+}-ion inward current. MAP_{90} (MAP duration at 90% of repolarization) indicates the K^+-ion outward current. MAP triangulation (MAP_{90-30}) indicates if Ca^{2+} channels or IKr channels are involved (Kato et al., 2009).

In the case of arrhythmia from digitalis, Na^+/ K^+-ATPase inhibition increases intracellular Na^+ which activates the Na^+/ Ca^{2+} exchange mechanism. This in turn increases the intracellular Ca^{2+} concentration level, generating an inward current which makes the sarcoplasmic reticulum unstable. Ca^{2+} may then be released from the sarcoplasmic reticulum during phase 4 in the action potential, again causing depolarization leading to DAD. However, DAD from digitalis should follow a relatively mild development, as it is caused by the pumping function of Na^+/K^+-ATPase; it is unlikely to induce TdP that leads to VF.

4. TdP's clinical manifestations, outcome and treatment

While a number of TdP cases go unnoticed with no recognizable clinical symptoms, there are also cases with clear manifestations. Initial symptoms include increased dizziness, palpitation, pain in the chest, and discomfort in the epigastric region and in the chest. These are attributable to the elimination of the P wave by VT; blood ejection from the heart is suspended and no palpable pulse is detected, although the heart is still beating. At this stage, it is possible to manage the situation by discontinuing or reducing medication if there is any suspected drugs. Symptoms may worsen to include anacatesthesia, fainting, and convulsion before proceeding to VF that causes sudden death. It is necessary at this stage to discontinue medication immediately (if any) and arrange for an AED as well as for an ambulance. The patient needs to be admitted to an ICU or CCU for treatments such as electrolyte correction, defibrillation, lidocaine administration, and temporary pacing.

5. Drugs that may cause QT prolongation

Drugs that may cause QT prolongation include anti-arrhythmics, psychotropics, and antibiotics among others (Table 1).

5.1 Anti-arrhythmic drugs

The drugs that fall under Ia in the Vaughan Williams classification reduce action potential slew rate (dP/dt max), and prolong APD by Na^+ channel inhibition (depolarization phase). It follows then that reducing dP/dt max prolongs APD, but there is a limitation on the overloading of Ca^{2+} from sustained depolarization. Abnormal Na^+ channel activities are unlikely to cause TdP unless there is a deficiency of *SCN5A*. TdP tends to occur in K^+ currents where the K^+ channel is inhibited, which delays repolarization time, with the result that APD is prolonged; K^+ channel inhibition can prolong ADP indefinitely. Under Ic, propafenone is also thought to be a factor because of its β-blockade function that causes bradycardia.

Under III, amiodarone, sotalol and bretyrium can prolong APD mainly by inhibiting outward K^+ current (depolarization phase). They also share β-blocking properties that lead to bradycardia and hence to TdP.

Under IV, bepridil, which is classified as Ca antagonist, is thought to inhibit Na^+ channel and outward K^+ current, which causes APD prolongation and TdP.

5.2 Psychotropic drugs

QT prolongation and TdP can be caused by antipsychotic drugs (chlorpromazine, phenothiazine; haloperidol, butyrophenone), tricyclic antidepressants (amitriptyline) and tetracyclic antidepressants (maprotiline). The mechanism appears to involve a quinidine-like effect, while a range of factors are also cited such as electrolyte imbalance, myocardial membrane enzyme disorder, myocardial tissue degeneration, and effects on autonomic nervous system, among others (Hunt et al., 1995).

5.3 Peripheral anti-histamine drugs

Antiallergic drugs with antihistaminic properties such as terfenadine and astemizole fall under this group. Terfenadine and astemizole are prodrugs whose metabolites have antihistaminic properties. Their parent compounds significantly inhibit K^+ currents. There have been fatal cases involving astemizole overdose as well as terfenadine administration where ventricular arrhythmia accompanied QT prolongation. In the five years after going on sale, seven severe side-effect cases of arrhythmia involving terfenadine were recognized. In 1995, a 'warning' section was added and the instructions for use were revised. However, in the two years following that, ten potentially fatal side-effect cases surfaced that involved QT prolongation and ventricular arrhythmia. In 1997, 'Urgent Safety Information' was submitted to call for extra care for the use of the drug before its sale was suspended in 2001.

The sale of astemizole was suspended in 1999. The mechanism of QT prolongation by terfenadine is thought to involve prolongation of myocardial repolarization time via delayed outward K^+ current inhibition; it appears that antihistaminic metabolites do not significantly inhibit the K^+ channel (Valenzuela et al., 1997). QT prolongation or TdP caused by these drugs is due not to antihistaminic properties but to K^+ current inhibition. At present, there have been no reports of QT prolongation involving ebastine though it has been known to block delayed rectifier K^+ current, albeit to a significantly lesser degree when compared to terfenadine (Valenzuela et al., 1997; Ko et al., 1997). It is in this context that fexofenadine, a metabolite of terfenadine, was developed. Fexofenadine is presumed to be safe, but its structural similarity to terfenadine suggests a possible parallel effect. Ebastine and fexofenadine need further careful study.

5.4 Gastrointestinal prokinetic agents

Cisapride was withdrawn from the market after the claim was made that it caused diabetic QT prolongation. Cisapride causes APD prolongation in extracted myocardial cells of laboratory animals, and dose-dependent prolongation of monophasic action potential duration (MAPD) in anesthetized animals, leading to QT prolongation and TdP (Carlsson et al., 2007). Mosapride is another gastrointestinal prokinetic agent with a similar chemical structure to that of cisapride. Animal testing has shown that it does not affect APD or MAPD, and it does not induce abnormal ECG such as QT prolongation or TdP (Carlsson et al., 2007).

It appears then that QT prolongation caused by this group of drugs is based not on the serotonin agonist property, which is the drug's main effect, but rather on its inhibition of the K^+ channel.

5.5 Macrolide anti-biotics

Erythromycin causes QT prolongation by inhibiting the delayed rectifier K^+ current (Rubart et al., 1993; Daleau et al., 1995). When combined with terfenadine or cisapride (discussed above), erythromycin enhances QT prolongation by blocking drug-metabolizing enzymes.

5.6 Anthracycline anti-cancer drugs

Among anthracycline anti-cancer drugs, doxorubicin is known to cause myocardial damage. It appears to enhance the sensitivity of depolarization in phase 4 (Mitrius et al., 1990).

5.7 Azole anti-fungal drugs

Azole anti-fungal drugs such as fluconazole and voriconazole are also known to cause QT prolongation. They are metabolized by the drug-metabolizing enzyme CYP3A4 while simultaneously inhibiting it. QT prolongation is caused either by the increasing serum concentration of the drug itself, or by increasing the serum concentration of some other drug that would otherwise be metabolized by CYP3A4; the latter case may involve a drug such as erythromycin. This calls for extra care for combinatory use of these drugs.

5.8 Sulfonylureas (SUs) and Glinides as Oral Anti-diabetic Drugs

SU and glinide agents are known to inhibit ATP-dependent K^+ channels. The similarity in mechanism is also increasingly evident between Class Ia anti-arrhythmic drugs and the hypoglycemic function of SUs and glinides (Kakei et al., 1993; Hayashi et al., 2004). SUs and glinides can potentially induce QT prolongation when they affect the heart's ATP-dependent K^+ channels.

5.9 Sulfa drugs

Like SUs, a pentamidine and ST mixture may cause QT prolongation and hypoglycemia. Considering that SUs are modified sulfa drugs, they belong to the same strain that may affect ATP-dependent K^+ channels.

5.10 New quinolones

There have been cases of TdP from QT prolongation caused by sparfloxacin and moxifloxacin, both new quinolones. The mechanism appears to involve K^+ channel inhibition.

5.11 Molecular targeted cancer drugs

There have been cases of QT prolongation or myocardial damage from sunitinib, bortezomib, sorafenib, lapatinib, and nilotinib, among others.

5.12 Others

A study has been done on probucol induced QT prolongation as a result of a change in catecholamine sensitivity, as well as K^+ current inhibition (Hayashi et al., 2004). Further study and consideration is needed. Meanwhile, QT prolongation is also known to be caused by diuretics that cause hypokalemia and magnesium deficiency, by cimetidine the histamine H_2 receptor antagonist, or even by contrast media.

Anti-arrhythmic Drugs	Class Ia : quinidine, procainamide, disopyramide, cibenzoline
	Class Ic : propafenone
	Class III: amiodarone, sotalol
	Class IV: bepridil
Psychotropic Drugs	phenothiazine: chlorpromazine
	butyrophenone: haloperidol
	tricyclic: amitriptyline, imipramine, nortriptyline
	tetracyclic: maprotiline
Peripheral Anti-histamine Drug	terfenadine*, astemizole*, ebastine
Gastrointestinal prokinetic Agents	cisapride*
Macrolide Anti-biotics	erythromycin, clarithromycin
Anthracycline Anti-cancer Drugs	doxorubicin
Azole Anti-fungal Drugs	fluconazole, voriconazole
Sulfonylureas (SUs) and Glinides	SUs: glimepiride, glibenclamide
	glinides: mitiglinide**, nateglinide
Sulfa Drugs	pentamidine, ST mixture
New Quinolones	sparfloxacin, moxifloxacin
Molecular Targeted Cancer Drugs	sunitinib、bortezomib、sorafenib、lapatinib、nilotinib
Others	probucol

*The drugs were withdrawn from the market in Japan.
**Mitiglinide is marketed only in Japan and China.

Table 1. Drugs that may cause QT prolongation.

6. Drug-drug interaction induced QT prolongation

Drug interaction is an important factor for QT prolongation. Drug-drug interaction is divided into pharmacodynamic interaction and pharmacokinetic interaction.

6.1 Pharmacodynamic Interaction

Drugs that are likely to cause QT prolongation are shown in Table 1. Combining two or more reinforces medicinal action additively; doses should be reduced or avoided altogether.

6.2 Pharmacokinetic Interaction

This involves cases where drug metabolism inhibition increases serum concentration, resulting in QT prolongation. Erythromycin, azole anti-fungal drugs, and molecular targeted cancer drugs are metabolized by CYP3A4, a microsomic drug metabolizing enzyme (that does exist outside the liver). When the above mentioned drugs were combined with a drug metabolized by enzymes of the same molecular kind or with a CYP3A4 blocking drug, the serum concentration to increase compared with a single dose of the drug (Table 2). The former is known as competitive antagonism, the latter as non-competitive antagonism; it is the latter that causes a sharper increase in serum concentration.

An abnormal terfenadine-induced ECG is thought to be the result of increasing serum concentrations of an parent compound, produced by the combined use of terfenadine and a CYP3A4-blocking drug from Table 2. Drug-drug interactions like that just described are why the drugs shown under Table 2 were contraindicated for combined use. An active carboxylic acid metabolite of terfenadine called fexofenadine went on the market. It is claimed that fexofenadine does not have the same cardiac related side effects that tefenadine has, however the structural similarity between the two is enough to warrant some caution. Ebastine metabolism is thought to involve CYP3A4, a microsomic enzyme, as well a another metabolizing enzyme. In theory, ebastine should be less likely to lead to TdP than terfenadine, though extra care must be taken when extrapolating data from clinical and non-clinical testing.

Grapefruit juice is known to inhibit CYP3A4, which means it can cause QT prolongation by increasing the serum concentration of erythromycin, azole anti-fungal drugs, and molecular targeted cancer drugs.

1. CYP3A4-blocking drug (competitive inhibition)	
HIV protease inhibitor:	indinavir, saquinavir, ritonavir, nelfinavir
2. CYP3A4-blocking drug (noncompetitive inhibition)	
Azole Anti-fungal Drugs:	itraconazole, ketoconazole, miconazole, fluconazole, voriconazole
Macrolide Anti-biotics:	erythromycin, clarithromycin

Table 2. Drugs that are likely to cause QT prolongation by CYP3A4-blocking.

7. QT prolongation - what measures to take

In the case of drug-induced QT prolongation, the crucial clinical concern is not the QT prolongation itself, but TdP or VF that may follow. It is important then to determine whether QT prolongation is just a simple case of bradycardia (PP interval prolongation), or bradycardia caused by the QT prolongation. The main and intended effect of anti-arrhythmic drugs classified under Ia is QT prolongation. However, drugs intended for other parts of the body can also cause the same QT prolongation in the heart; this is their collateral effect. Under these circumstances it has been extremely difficult for doctors to recognize early symptoms, largely because it falls outside the physician's area of specialty when the case involves drugs other than those described under section 5-1 ('Anti-arrhythmic Drugs'). There was a case of antipruritic (anti-histamine agent) that caused a totally unexpected fatal arrhythmia. Cisapride disappeared from the market, leaving the new term 'Diabetic QT Prolongation'. Furthermore, it is intriguing to note the similarity in mechanism between SUs and cibenzoline, an anti-arrhythmic drug classified under Ia of the Vaughan-Williams classification. Far too many QT prolongation cases that could have been predicted have gone unnoticed. The intended effect of the drug was the focus of attention, while the obvious 'collateral effect' was unobserved.

In order to detect early symptoms of the collateral effect, attention must be paid to: 1. What drugs can cause a collateral effect; 2. Factors on the part of the patient (e.g. certain conditions obtained when sick); 3. Drug-drug interaction. When encountered with early symptoms of TdP such as increased dizziness, palpitation, pain in the chest, and discomfort in the epigastric region and in the chest, medication should be discontinued and immediate medical attention should be sought.

8. Conclusion

Side effects are classified into toxic (dose-dependent) and allergic. The former is a simple extension of the main effect: serum concentration increases dose-dependently in a predictable fashion. The latter is hard to predict because it increases dose-independently in an idiosyncratic fashion. The QT prolongation under discussion belongs to the former and is indeed predictable. When QT prolongation is an extension of the main drug effect (anti-arrhythmic effect) and is confirmed by a specialist as such, preventive or therapeutic measures can be taken before it is too late. However, when QT prolongation is caused by the drugs discussed under sections 5-2 through 5-12 (psychotropics, anti-histamines, gastrointestinal prokinetic agents, anti-biotics, anti-cancer agents, etc.), it is difficult to take preventive or therapeutic measures against these 'collateral' effects because most of these cases are simply beyond the scope of the doctor in charge. This has indeed resulted in a number of cases where QT prolongation was not diagnosed, with unfortunate results. It is essential to learn from these past experiences and develop proactive treatments.

A new guideline (ICH S7B) providing provisions for a QT prolongation screening test for new drug development was issued by ICH, the International conference on Harmonization of Technical Requirements for Registration of Pharmaceuticals for Human Use (http://www.ich.org/products/guidelines/safety/article/safety-guidelines.html). Aside from the provided guidelines, it is important to look for substances that do not block K^+ channels when developing drugs; one can make use of *hERG* or a screening method using MAP (Kato et al., 2009) .

9. References

Carlsson, L., Amos, G.J., Andersson, B., Drews, L., Duker, G. and Wadstedt, G. (1997). Electrophysiological characterization of the prokinetic agents cisapride and mosapride in vivo and in vitro: Imprications for proarrythmic potential? *Journal of Pharmacology and Experimental Therapeutics.* Vol.282, No.1, pp.220-227.

Daleau, P., Lessard, E., Groleau, M.F. & Turgeon, J. (1995). Erythromycin blocks the rapid component of the delayed rectifier potassium current and lengthens repolarization of guinea pig ventricular myocytes. *Circulation.* Vol.91, No.12, pp.3010-3016.

Hayashi, K., Shimizu, M., Ino, H., Yamaguchi, M., Terai, H., Hoshi, N., Higashida, H., Terashima, N., Uno, Y., Kanaya, H. & Mabuchi, H. (2004). Probucol aggravates long QT syndrome associated with a novel missense mutation M124T in the N-terminus of HERG. Clinical Science. Vol.107, No.2, pp.175-182.

Horie, M., Hayashi, S., Yuzuki, Y. & Sasayama, S. (1992). Comparative studies of ATP sensitive potassium channels in heart and pancreatic beta cells using Vaughan-Williams class Ia antiarrhythmics. *Cardiovascular Research.* Vol.26, No.11, pp.1087-1094.

Hunt, N. & Stern, T.A. (1995). The association between intravenous haloperidol and Torsades de Pointes. Three cases and a literature review. *Psychosomatics.* vol.36, No.6, pp.541-549.

Kakei, M., Nakazaki, M., Kamisaki, T., Nagayama, I., Fukamachi, Y. & Tanaka, H. (1993). Inhibition of the ATP-sensitive potassium channel by class I antiarrhythmic agent, cibenzoline, in rat pancreatic beta-cells. *British Journal of Pharmacology.* Vol.109, No.4, pp.1226-1231.

Kato, R., Watanabe, R., Miki, H., Ijiri, Y., Hayashi, T. & Tanaka K. (2009). Does the sedative agent, JM-1232(-) cause QT prolongation with subsequent torsades de pointes? *Life Sciences,* Vol.85, No.21-22, pp. 737-741.

Ko, C.M., Ducic, I., Fan, J., Shuba, Y.M. & Morad, M. (1997). Suppretion of mammalian K+ channel family by ebastine. *Journal of Pharmacology and Experimental Therapeutics.* Vol.281, No.1, pp.233-244.

Lehnart, S.E., Ackerman, M.J., Benson, D.W. Jr., Brugada, R., Clancy, C.E., Donahue, J.K., George, A.L. Jr., Grant, A.O., Groft, S.C., January, C.T., Lathrop, D.A., Lederer, W.J., Makielski, J.C., Mohler, P.J., Moss, A., Nerbonne, J.M., Olson, T.M., Przywara, D.A., Towbin, J.A., Wang, L.H. & Marks, A.R. (2007). Inherited arrhythmias: a National Heart, Lung, and Blood Institute and Office of Rare Diseases workshop consensus report about the diagnosis, phenotyping, molecular mechanisms, and therapeutic approaches for primary cardiomyopathies of gene mutations affecting ion channel function. *Circulation.* Vol.116, No.20, pp.2325-2345.

Mitrius, J.C. & Vogel, S.M. (1990). Doxorubicin-induced automaticity in cultured chick heart cell aggregates. *Cancer Research.* Vol.50, No.14, pp.4209-4215.

Rubart, M., Pressler, M.L., Pride, H.P. & Zipes, D.P. (1993). Electrophysiological mechanisms in a canine model of erythromycin associated long QT syndrome. *Circuration.* Vol.88, pp.1832-1844.

Valenzuela, C., Delpón, E., Franqueza, L., Gay, P., Vicente, J. & Tamargo, J. (1997). Comparative effects of nonsedating histamine H1 receptor antagonists, ebastine and terfenadine, on human Kv1.5 channels. *European Journal of Pharmacology*. 1997; Vol.326, No.2-3, pp.257-263.

9

The Electrocardiogram – Waves and Intervals

James E. Skinner, Daniel N. Weiss and Edward F. Lundy
Vicor Technologies, Inc,
USA

1. Introduction

To understand the Electrocardiogram, one must understand *both* the origin of the waves (PQRST) and intervals between them (PQRST to PQRST or R-R). The waves are intrinsically generated within the heart, with some regulation by the cardiac nerves, but the intervals are extrinsically controlled primarily by the brain, through projections to both the auricular pacemakers and the ventricular tissues. That is, the intervals are regulated by the brain, as mediated through the *autonomic effectors*. To understand the R-R interval variations, one must understand the neural mechanism(s) that underlie changes in the T to P segments, which are lengthened and shortened in time to create the R-R variation.

The Society for Neuroscience does not pay substantive attention to Cardiology, and the various societies of Cardiology do not pay much attention to Neuroscience. This two-way neglect has forced the formation of a new society devoted to both fields of inquiry. The Society for Heart-Brain Medicine was formed in 2007, and the plenary talks that established the field on its own foundation included two by the current authors (Skinner, 2007a; 2007b).

A paradigm is a way of thinking, and a new one is a way of "thinking outside the box." Two new paradigms were presented by us at the first SHBM Meeting and each was based on pivotal new discoveries. First, we showed that only nonlinear algorithms are appropriate for analysis of physiological data, because the data themselves are nonlinear--- a nonlinear algorithm is thus a more sensitive measure of the heartbeat dynamics (e.g., of R-R variability) than all previous stochastic measures, such as the, mean, standard deviation, power spectrum, and so on. Secondly, small proteins and peptides are known to regulate physiology in parallel with the nervous system--- that is, the "state" (behavioral / neural) determines the outputs of these two types of physiological effectors. Hibernation, for example, in which the cold eventually shuts off the nervous system, continues to be regulated by neuroendocrine molecules, some of which were indicated in a similar state (REM sleep) to have salutary effects on the ischemic heart (suppression of arrhythmogenesis in the electrocardiogram). This analogy between the similar states enabled conventional proteomics to be used in the other state (e.g., in hibernation) and thus formed the basis for a new way to discover drugs, "state-dependent proteomics." With the method a new (anti-infarction) drug candidate was actually discovered (Skinner, 2007a).

The realization that the heartbeat intervals in the electrocardiogram are primarily regulated by the brain provides us with an entirely new way to look at the electrocardiogram - the intervals are not intrinsically regulated by currents and pacemakers within the heart, as are the waves, but rather are under extrinsic control by the brain, mediated of course through the autonomic nervous system. The time between P-waves, which, in turn, affects the time between QRS's, is mediated by the slow inward pacemaker current present in the sinus node and other atrial and ventricular tissues, called I_f or the "funny current", a mixed Na and K slowly depolarizing inward current. In order for the cardiac-projecting nerves to alter the RR-interval it must be via this current. Also, the intra-QRS complex intervals (PR, QRS, QT) are certainly regulated by all of the currents, which are under external and intrinsic cardiac nervous system influences.

Since the brain is so highly involved in regulating the RR-intervals, the initial studies of the electrocardiogram, mostly carried out in the anesthetized dog, must be carried out anew, but in the unanesthetized animal in a controlled behavioral state. The pig is the animal of choice, as it has endocardial distributions of the arteries and nerves that are homologous to humans, and furthermore the animal is born and raised in a standardize manner and has not been a pet or a mongrel, either of which would of course make their behavioral control less certain. The neurophysiology of the brain (electrophysiology and neurochemistry) of defined behavioral states and their impact on the electrocardiogram of the ischemic heart (in both animals and humans) are the topics of this manuscript.

2. Background - Role of the brain in the regulation of the waves and intervals in the electrocardiogram

As background we now present important results, mostly from our own previous studies in a conscious pig-model of myocardial ischemia / heart attack, out of which emerged the nonlinear and state-dependent paradigms. The rationale for the nonlinear regulation of the heartbeats came naturally out of our previous studies of the brain regulatory centers, which were found to have nonlinear activities. We also present here the physiological data in this conscious pig-model that led to the rationale for the discovery of the state-dependent proteomics (i.e., that specific molecules are released during a specific state or its equivalent, such as for example hibernation and its physiological equivalent REM sleep). The individual results from the pig-model are summarized in Figure 1, and the two in red were pivotal for our later development of the two new paradigms.

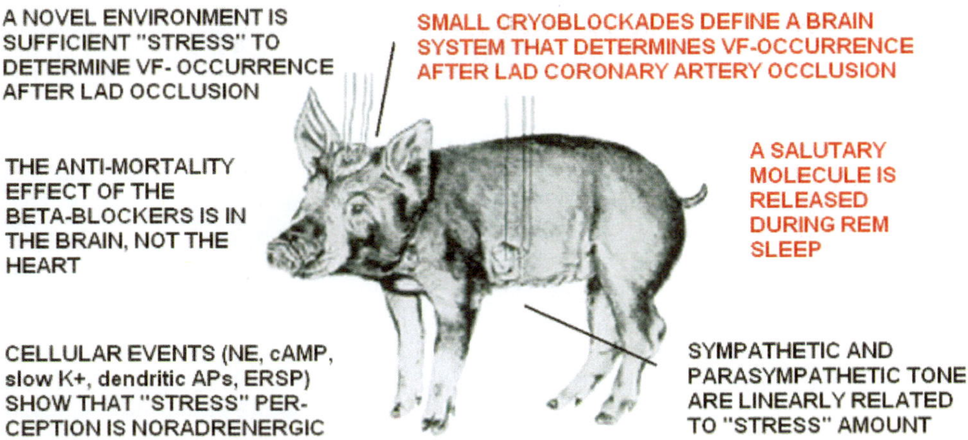

Fig. 1. What we learned from the conscious pig-model of heart attack. These composite results are from several papers and are reviewed in Skinner (2007b).

At the beginning of the conscious animal studies, we were guided by Walter Cannon's theory of a "Cerebral Defense System." He postulated in his 1932 book, "The Wisdom of the Body," that the focus for natural selection that led to the higher evolution of the brain was a cerebral "orchestrator" that simultaneously regulated the sensory input channels (e.g., of attended objects) and the autonomic output channels (e.g., for increasing the heart rate) in a moment of crisis. We already knew from our previous neurophysiological studies that the frontal cortex was the likely site of this hypothesized orchestrator, for we had found that it regulated the sensory input by a mechanism of selective neural inhibition at the thalamic level (Skinner, 1982). We then later stereotaxically implanted cryoneedles along a pathway that extends from the frontal cortex, through the hypothalamus, through the Fields of Forel, through the medulla, and then onward to the motor neurons that give rise to the cardiac nerves. Collateral branches are given off to the various nuclei all along this descending pathway. We found that cryoblockade anywhere within this anatomically interconnected system would prevent the lethal consequence of total occlusion of the left anterior descending (LAD) coronary artery (Skinner and Reed, 1981). A similar effect was reported after surgically cutting the cardiac nerves (Ebert et al, 1970).

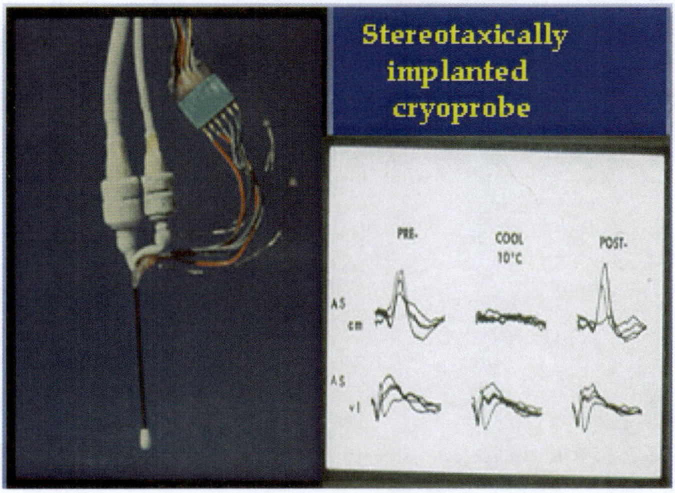

Fig. 2. Reversible cryoblockade in the brain of a conscious animal. From Skinner & Lindsley, 1968. See Skinner (1970) for a simple method.

The cryogenic method illustrated in Figure 2 is actually very easy to master (Skinner & Lindsley, 1968; Skinner, 1970) and enables the conscious animal to serve as its own control. Specific blockades in the brain (i.e., stereotaxic implantation followed by postmortem reconstruction) were found to prevent lethal arrhythmogenesis up to the maximum 25-min period of reversible myocardial ischemia. After recovery from the cryoblockade and reversal of the ischemia, the same animal (pig) could then be used again for the control procedure. The results of this within-subjects as well as between-subjects experimental design is demonstrated in Figure 3 (Skinner & Reed, 1981).

Figure 3 shows the composite results of the various cryoblockades made in the conscious pig-model of heart attack. The cryoprobe tips (always implanted bilaterally) are shown reconstructed on four coronal sections of the pig brain. The locations shown in red are for the 2x4 mm cryoprobe tips that, when cooled (but not when at brain temperature), prevented VF after LAD coronary artery occlusion (i.e., in unadapted or laboratory "stressed" subjects). Also shown (blue) are the locations of control tip-sites that, when cooled bilaterally, had no effect on VF after coronary occlusion. The collected red loci mark the trajectory along a pathway that interconnects the known cardiac regulatory nuclei each of which receive and send information between one another.

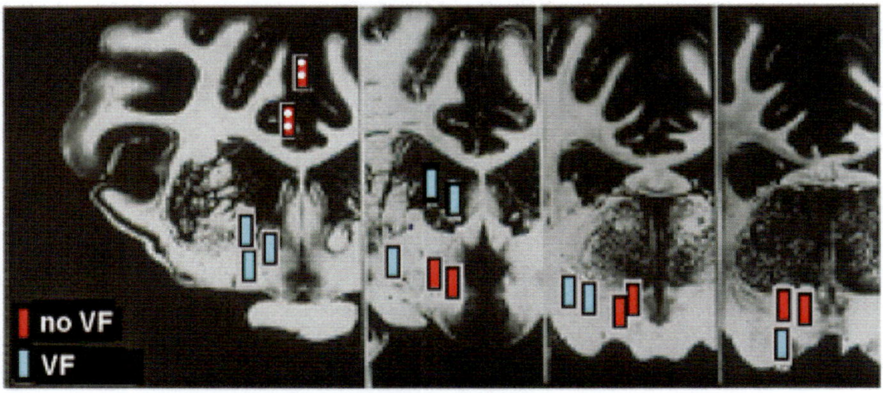

Fig. 3. Composite cryoblockade loci that either prevented VF after LAD occlusion (red) or did not (blue). From Skinner & Reed, 1981; Skinner, 1985.

This neurocardiac system is located between the frontomesial (Figure 3, red with white dots) and orbital cortex at one end and the motor nuclei that project to the heart on the other. Electric stimulations were done in the frontomesial cortex (Figure 4) by our laboratory and these produced cardiac arrhythmias, proving their participation in the system that regulates cardiac vulnerability to arrhythmias. The arrhythmogenic effect of the electric stimulation of each of the other structures in this neuro-cardiac system has been reported by others (reviewed in Skinner, 1985). Thus, a single brain system composed of hierarchically-interconnected telencephalic-, diencephalic-, mesencephalic-, and myelencephalic-loci terminates in the autonomic effectors already shown to control the vulnerability of the heart to lethal VF during an experimental heart attack (i.e., in the mildly-stressed pig).

Once having a conscious animal model, we turned to study the behavioral regulation of this newly discovered neurophysiological system. We found that gradual systematic reduction of laboratory "stress," through learned adaptation to the unfamiliar surroundings, ultimately had the same salutary effect as denervation--- i.e., no VF after LAD occlusion (Skinner, Lie, Entman, 1975). We then showed that the same systematic reduction of stress linearly decreased sympathetic drive on the myocardium, i.e., as measured precisely by phosphorylase activation, using yield-independent cryosamples obtained through a throacic window (Skinner, et al, 1983). This sympathetic effect must have been accompanied by a simultaneous reduction in parasympathetic tone, because the resting heart rate and blood pressure remained the same. The point to be underscored is that behavioral stress-reduction leads to a *loss of autonomic drive.*

We next studied the neuronal responses in the frontal cortex to defined stressors (e.g., novel stimuli, aversive conditioned stimuli, mild noxious stimuli) and found that they all produced the same electrochemical effects: norepinephrine was released from presynaptic terminals, postsynaptic cyclic AMP was activated (as the second messenger) that then controlled a slow outward potassium current, leading to increased excitability in the dendrites of the neurons and the generation of an extracellular event-related slow potential. Each of these data types is learning-dependent and, therefore, is nonlinear in time. So the Cannon-controller of the heartbeats is itself *nonlinear*. This feature is also supported independently by noting that the biophysics of the neuronal action potentials is nonlinear, as modeled by the Hodgkin-Huxley (nonlinear) equations.

These collected cellular responses of the cerebral neurons to transient stressor-events suggested to us that an intracerebral beta-blocker may dampen these mediating neurons and thus have an anti-VF effect in the conscious pig-model similar to that of the cryoblockades. We showed that, indeed, this noradrenergic cerebral system was the site of action for the anti-mortality effect of the beta-blocker drugs, and *not* the noradrenergic cardiac receptors. *Intracerebral* injections of levo-propranolol prevented VF after LAD occlusion, whereas intravenous injections did not (Skinner, 1985; Parker et al, 1993). This interpretation of a cerebral anti-mortality mechanism is supported by clinical studies reported by Aoke Hjalmarson (2000), who showed that the anti-mortality efficacy of the various beta-blocker drugs was related to their lipophilicity. The lipophilic drugs get into the brain at a higher level and thus may explain their greater efficacy in preventing arrhythmic death in post-MI patients.

As shown In Figure 4, electric stimulation (2 sec, 30 Hz) of the mesial frontal cortex (inset, filled, but not unfilled sites) will increase heart rate, reverse the R-waves (as occurs in ischemia), and result in premature beats (arrhythmias) that eventually end in VF if the stimulus is strong and long enough. In contrast to the cryoblockade, the direct electrical stimulation of the frontocortical-brainstem system will evoke malignant cardiac arrhythmias *in a normal heart*. The same effects seen for the mesofrontal cortical stimulation have been shown for stimulation of the other subcortical loci of the structured system indicated in Figure 3 by the red sites (Skinner, 1985). The blockade and stimulation studies *together* suggest a *necessary and sufficient* (i.e., causal) role for this cerebral system to play in VF occurrence. The same cannot be said of the heart as the system, for after cardiac denervation LAD occlusion will not lead to VF (Ebert et al, 1970).

Natural regulation of the brain by REM sleep (Figure 4, lower traces) has a salutary effect on ectopic arrhythmias that result from a previous myocardial infarction. The seconds-long latency between REM onset and the salutary effect (double-headed arrow) suggests mediation by a neurohumoral molecule. Hibernation appears to be a good steady-state model for REM sleep, as both states have the same uncommon features: 1) complete muscle atonia, 2) complete turn-off of both sympathetic and parasympathetic tone (Baust and Bonnert, 1969; Skinner et al, 1975), and 3) multiple endocrine secretions. Using the state of hibernation in which it is easier to collect molecules from fluids, we were able to isolate, identify, synthesize and then inject (IV) a molecule that would prevent tissue damage after 45 minutes of coronary artery occlusion (heart attack) or 1 hour of cerebral artery occlusion (stroke). This anti-infarction effect is illustrated for the stroke model in Figure 5. More details of the state-dependent proteomics methods are provided in Skinner (2007a).

Where the salutary molecule is released is not yet known, but it appears to be from the brain because of the seconds-long latency between the time it is released and the time it is effective in the heart (Figure 4, two-way arrow). A neuroendocrine system is all that is left to

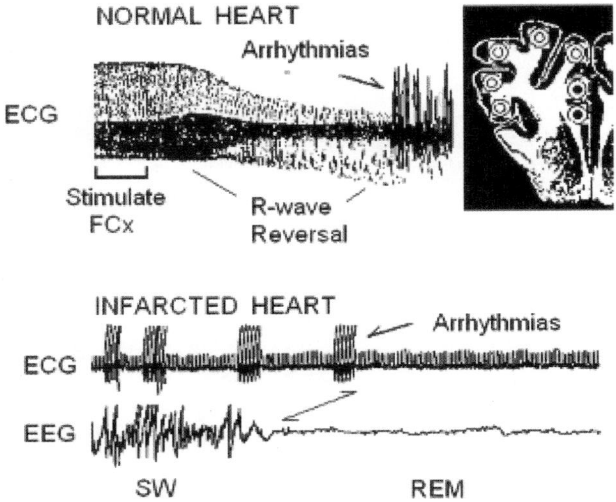

Fig. 4. Effect on the heartbeats produced by a brief electric stimulus to the mesofrontal cortex (upper trace and inset), and an effect of REM sleep on the suppression of arrhythmias in an infarcted heart. From Skinner (1985; 2007a,b).

operate the life-support physiologies during hibernation, because the nervous system is gradually turned off by the cold. Such dual regulation between neuroendocrine and neurophysiological systems is also apparent during other behavioral states, such as the cerebral defensive state (e.g., neural increase in heart rate followed by adrenal gland secretions to increase heart rate). This same dual parallel regulation may also apply to the state of "learned adaptation to stressors," in which state lethal arrhythmogenesis is prevented--- that is, the newly discovered anti-infarction molecule released during REM sleep may be involved in equivalent waking states as well.

Figure 5 shows the mouse model of middle cerebral artery occlusion followed by reflow. The middle cerebral artery is completely occluded, as documented by laser-Doppler flow in the parietal cortex. After 1-hr, the occlusion is then reversed (i.e., a model of thrombolysis in a modern hospital procedure). Immediately after reflow is established, either the control molecule (Figure 5, left) or the synthesized anti-infarction molecule based on a naturally occurring neuropeptide (Figure 5, right) is injected in the tail vein. 24-hrs later the animal's behavior is observed for limb paralysis and its brain is extracted, sliced, and incubated with Tri-Tetrazolium Chloride (TTC), a stain for viable tissue (it binds to functioning mitochorndria). The anti-infarction molecule was found to result in 100% tissue savings in many of the model cases, with no tissue saving effect ever occurring in the controls. The controls manifested hemiplegia associated with the usual lack of TTC staining in the infarcted tissue (Figure 5, left, white). It was concluded from this study that the parallel physiological actions by the neurons and the neuroendocrine secretions exerted during the natural state of REM sleep would then be found to be the same as those exerted during an equivalent model state (hibernation). The important technical discovery was that the neurosecretory molecules collected more easily during the hibernation model could then be found to operate in the more natural state with the same effect--that is, the salutary action on the ischemic heart that occurs during REM sleep (Skinner, 2007a). Who knew that the new "state-dependent proteomics" paradigm would lead to such a powerful molecule as the anti-infarction drug candidate so compellingly presented in Figure 5?

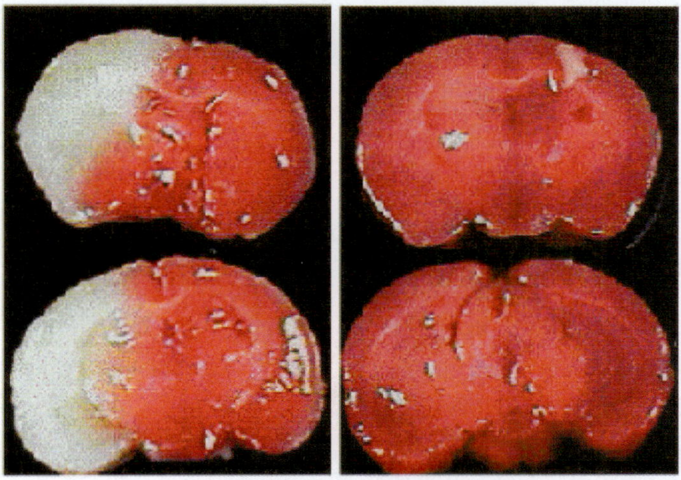

Fig. 5. Mouse model of 1-hr occlusion of the middle cerebral artery, followed by recirculation and IV injection of control (left) or synthesized anti-infarction molecules (right). From Skinner 2007a.

3. Some leading questions about heart rate variability

The following five questions and their simple answers will be further explained by the text, tables, and figures in the sections below. These particular Q & A's are intended to cover some of the common ones raised by physicians and researchers concerning the medical assessment of the heart by studying its rate variability (HRV).

1. **Q.** Why should brain physiology tell you anything about cardiac vulnerability to VF, as assessed by HRV? **A.** Both HRV and VF-initiation involve the *exact same brain structures;* that is, the frontocortical-brainstem system simultaneously controls heart rate and vulnerability to VF.
2. **Q.** The use of measures of HRV is an old warn-out area in cardiology--- they sort of work, but have a lot of false negative and false positive predictions; so, why should a new measure be expected to be any better? **A.** The PD2i uses nonlinear analysis of the heartbeats and is, therefore, better able to extract information from the signal, with the result that it accurately predicts arrhythmic death in chest-pain patients with unprecedented Sensitivity and Specificity compared to the other algorithms.
3. **Q.** What is the nonlinear PD2i algorithm and how is it calculated? **A.** This computerized algorithm uses simple pair-wise comparisons of multi-dimensional vectors made from brief RR-intervals sampled throughout the data, and it reveals how many independent variables (degrees of freedom) are responsible for the heartbeat regulation at that one moment in time; when PD2i indicates reduced degrees of freedom (as measured in dimensions), it means a lot of physiological *cooperation* is going on among the independent brain regulators (neural centers) that control the heartbeats and VF-vulnerability.

4. **Q.** How does PD2i compare to all of the other HRV algorithms out there? **A.** It is superior in both its *discriminability* between experimental and control groups (p<0.0006) and its *ability to analyze noisy, non-stationary data* (see Figure 11 below)
5. **Q.** T-wave Alternans (TWA) was once the hot new heartbeat technology in cardiology that recently fell from grace (Cleland et al, 2008); why would PD2i be any different? **A.** The PD2i measures what is *going on in the brain* (i.e., neural regulation of the heartbeat intervals) and TWA measures what is going *on in the heart* (i.e., recovery from refractoriness, which tends to oscillate if the myocardium is ischemic), and as the new field of heart-brain medicine attests, Sudden Cardiac Death is now considered a brain physiological problem, not an intrinsic heart problem. Although TWA is responsive to neural signals (e.g., the heart reacts to cerebreal defensive neural input), its etiology is derived from the physiology of the heart--- i.e., the refractory cycle of the cardiac cells.

4. The degrees of freedom in the heartbeat intervals

The diagram of the Brain-Heart system in Figure 6 indicates the lower (1) to higher (6) cerebral hierarchy of the structures that regulate the heartbeats. The sensory and motor neurons of the lowest component (1) actually lie within the heart itself, and are capable of performing the same chemo- and stretch- reflexes characteristic of the higher centers above it. The fronto-cortical to brainstem system that controls vulnerability to VF (Figure 3) is isomorphic with these well known sensory-motor loops that control the heartbeats, including the intrinsic afferent-interneuron-efferent loop (Skinner et al, 1996) and the vago-frontocortical-brainstem loop (Chase et al, 1966). This isomorphism led to the rationale for examination of the various measures of heartbeat dynamics in the conscious pig-model that might predict vulnerability to VF. The heartbeats are well known to be regulated by the six afferent-efferent neural loops shown in Figure 6, each of which competes with the others to

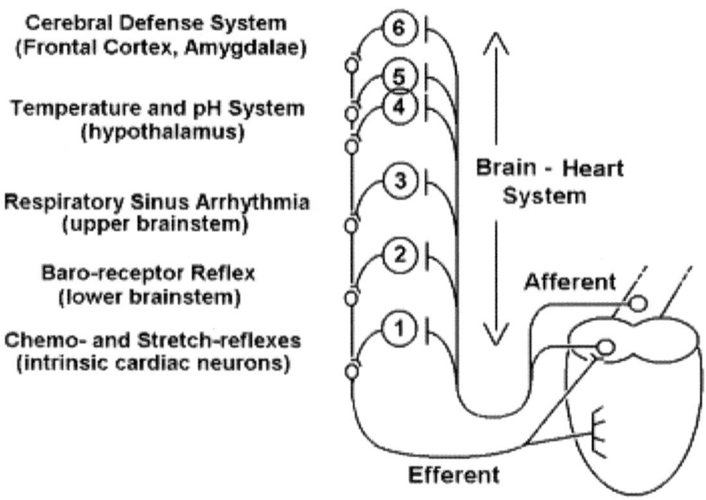

Fig. 6. Brain – heart system thought to simultaneously regulate heart rate and vulnerability to VF. From Skinner (2007b).

control the heartbeat intervals. The close examination of the anatomical structure of each loop shows them all to be highly interconnected, either by sensory collateral branches, bifurcating interneurons, or descending efferent fibers.
There really are six independent regulators of the heartbeats during the resting state. A way was discovered to count them using a nonlinear measure of the degrees of freedom in the heartbeat series. During quiet wakefulness, each of the loops in Figure 6 makes an independent contribution to the regulation of the RR-intervals and this results in a rather "jittery" RR-interval series from which the degrees of freedom can then be calculated. This concept of degrees of freedom and its variation is simply illustrated in Figure 7.

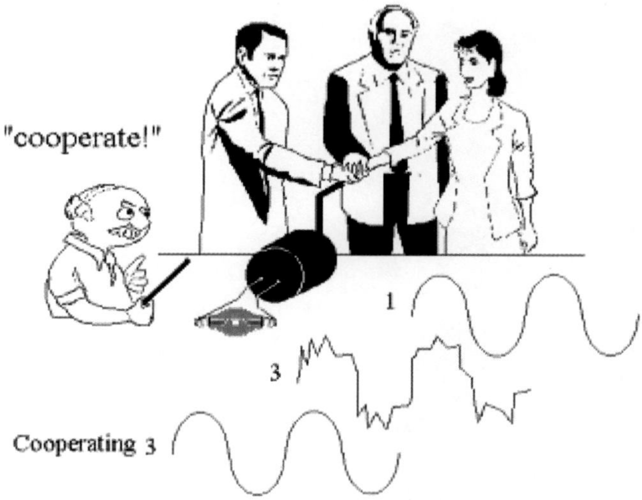

Fig. 7. Illustration of degrees of freedom in a data time series.

Figure 7 illustrates an example of persons turning the crank of an AC generator to light a bulb. A single person turning the crank makes a smooth sinusoid at the output, as shown in the upper trace. In this case the measured degrees of freedom are 1. When three persons attempt to turn the crank, they make a more "jittery" sinusoid (middle trace). The nonlinear measure correctly shows that his output trace has precisely 3 degrees of freedom. If, however, an orchestrator comes by and instructs the crankers to cooperate with his baton, then they *can*, momentarily, make a smooth sinusoid with the degrees of freedom dropping back to 1 (bottom trace; still 3 crankers, but they are cooperating). So the "degree of cooperation" as well as the maximum "number" of independent generators together determine the amount of time-dependent "jitter" in the data series. The next figure shows how this nonlinear algorithm actually works.
In Figure 8, part A., a "jittery" data series is shown. Part B. illustrates a step in making the calculation of the degrees of freedom for the Point Correlation Dimension (PD2i), by gathering two "i" and "j" samples of the data (e.g., R to R heartbeat intervals) and then comparing them by their multi-dimensional vectors (in the illustrated case, m = 3) and then finding the vector difference lengths (VDLs) for all VDLij. The "i" and "j" represent values that are incremented throughout the data series and the VDLs are repetitively calculated

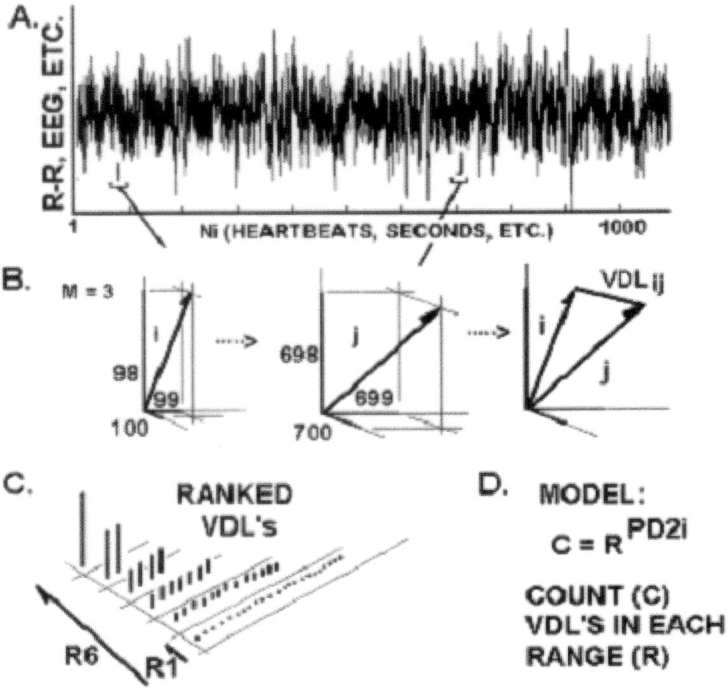

Fig. 8. Making the vector difference lengths to calculate the Point Correlation Dimension (PD2i).

until the end of the data stream is reached for both i and j. Values where i = j are omitted, as they will always be equal to zero; the end of the data stream is not N (number of data points), but N minus the number of data points needed to make the last of the vectors, where m is the number of dimensions of the vectors (m is called the "embedding dimension"). Part C. shows that once the VDLij values are made and collected together for each fixed value of i compared and all j, they are then rank ordered. Imagine that all of the ranked VDLij for a fixed value of i are soldiers ranked by height, with those of the same height being placed behind the one at the front. Now a general takes a series of small to large steps, R1 through R6, with each step starting at the same place just before the small soldier column. With each first step, small to large, the general counts the total number of soldiers in all of the rank columns that are crossed in that step. That is, the general counts (C) the VDL's that increase in number as he systematically increases the range (R) of his step size, and steps across all ranks. Shown in Part D., there will be a new exponent value for each point ("P") in the data series; the "i" in "PD2i" is added to emphasize that PD2i is time-dependent, and the "D2" means that the PD2 approaches the correlation dimension (D2) as N goes to infinity.

As shown at the top of Figure 9, PD2i is the slope of the log-log plot of C vs R. For large data length (Ni approaches infinity) there will be a first long linear scaling region (1) followed by a shorter one (2) that eventually disappears as Ni gets very large. For Ni = 10^{PD2i} there will

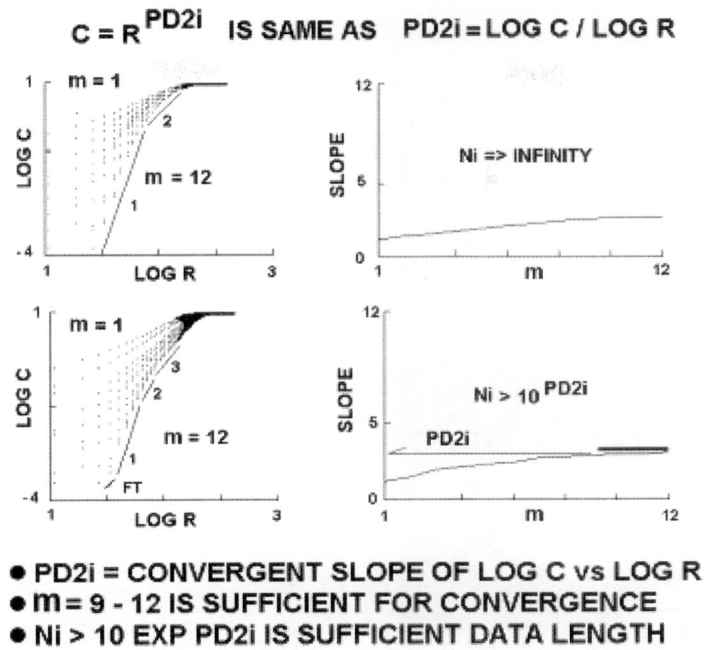

Fig. 9. Log-log plot of C vs R (also called the correlation integral) for each value of m.

be more scaling regions (1-3) because of the finite data length. The minimum Ni-value is experimentally determined according to Kostilich and Swinney (1989), and is required to capture all of the lobes of a physical attractor. This criterion for Ni should be adopted for physiological data, too, as with this data-length there is clear convergence of slope vs m by the 9th embedding dimension (bar above lower right curve for m = 9 to m = 12).

In summary, PD2i is measured as a function of its location in the data series (i), which means that for each i-sample of data it is compared to all possible j-samples. Then position-i is incremented and again compared to all j-samples for the next PD2i. In the left panels of Figure 9 are shown for a given i-sample the log-log plots for embedding dimensions m = 1 (top most data points) through m = 12 (bottom); remember, the embedding dimension is related to the number of selected data points (e.g., RR-intervals) used as coordinates to make the pairwise vectors. Note that slope increases with m, as shown in the upper right plot of Figure 9. After 9 embedding dimensions, the slope (PD2i) is no longer increased with each new embedding dimension and stays the same value; this is the point at which the slope "converges" with embedding dimension. After convergence, m does not have to be increased any more.

The first part of this slope, or scaling region, will contain very few contributions of VDL's made from j-vectors located in non-stationary data with respect to that of the i-vector (i.e., the VDLs will be large), and that is why the scaling region for the PD2i algorithm is restricted--- it makes the PD2i calculation insensitive to the data non-stationarities. In data of smaller total length (Figure 9, bottom two panels), but following the rule that Ni must be greater than 10 to the PD2i power, a "floppy tail" (FT, left) appears. The FT is caused by the finite digitization rate for the data. The use of a "linearity" criterion in conjunction with the "plot length" criterion results in the detection of a stable slope just above the FT.

Figure 10 (middle trace) shows empirically that the running mean PD2i stays within 4% of its known value (D2) when used to analyze non-stationary data made from linking sub-epochs with known degrees of freedom (red). The D2i algorithm, the only other time-dependent algorithm that measures degrees of freedom, shows spurious values, mainly because it requires data stationarity. Its slope length is NOT restricted to lie between the FT and up to 15% of the total plot length. Other investigators are only now just beginning to realize the problem of non-stationary data in the nonlinear analysis of heartbeats. Their methods, however, eliminate data, whereas the PD2i algorithm does not--- it tracks the dimension of the data non-stationarities!

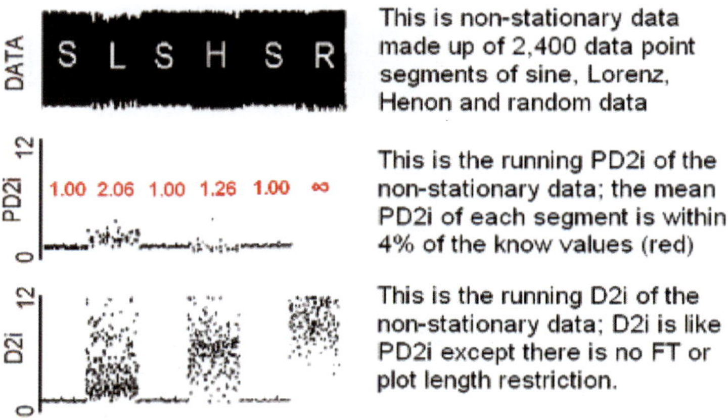

Fig. 10. PD2i of non-stationary data (sine, Lorenz, Henon, random) of known degrees of freedom. From Skinner, Molnar & Tomberg, 1994.

Note that the D2i, which is also known as the "Pointwise Correlation Dimension" according to the nomenclature presented in our 1994 paper in Physiological Reviews (Elbert et al, 1994), is not insensitive to the data non-stationarities. This is because the D2i slope (i.e., linear scaling slope, logC/logR) is not selected the same way. It does not define a "floppy tail" and then find the restricted slope length that lies just above, for a convergent embedding dimension.

5. Early results showing how a PD2i-reduction is related to cardiac events

PD2i tracks changes over time in noisy non-stationary data. The upper left panel of Figure 11 shows the RR-intervals and the lower left panel shows the corresponding accepted PD2i (i.e., accepted for linearity of scaling and for convergence of slope vs m) calculated over the course of blunt chest trauma followed by hemorrhagic shock (i.e., to mimic a traumatic explosion or crash). The experiment was carried out in a lightly anesthetized and ventilated pig and passed Institutional Review Board criteria. Artifacts are produced during anesthesia and intubation and then finally VT and lethal ventricular fibrillation (VF) occur. In the published study in the same pig preparation (Batchinsky et al., 2010), MSE3 (Multiscale

Entropy) and PD2i were compared along with other algorithms. Continuous 200-beat samples of clean and relatively stationary data were used, as MSE3 requires such selection of clean data to be accurate in short files. It is impossible to have such clean noise-free data when recording ECGs in the field, for they resemble the artifact-riddled ECGs observed during intubation. Note that accepted PD2i *could* be recorded during this intubation period.

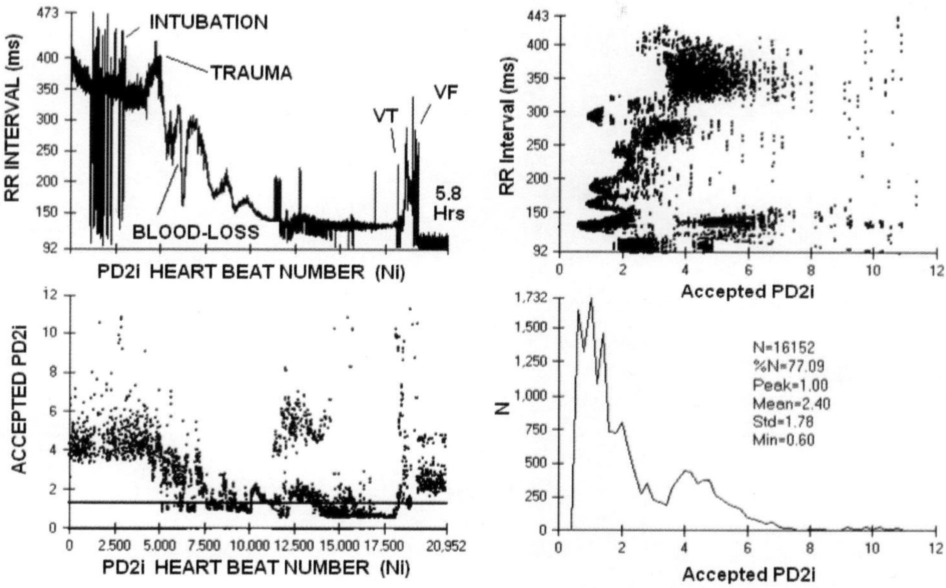

Fig. 11. Effects of trauma (chest thumper) and blood-loss on the RR-intervals (upper left) and corresponding accepted PD2i (lower left) in the anesthized pig. RRi vs PD2i is shown at the upper right and the PD2i histogram is shown at the lower right, along with the accepted PD2i statistics.

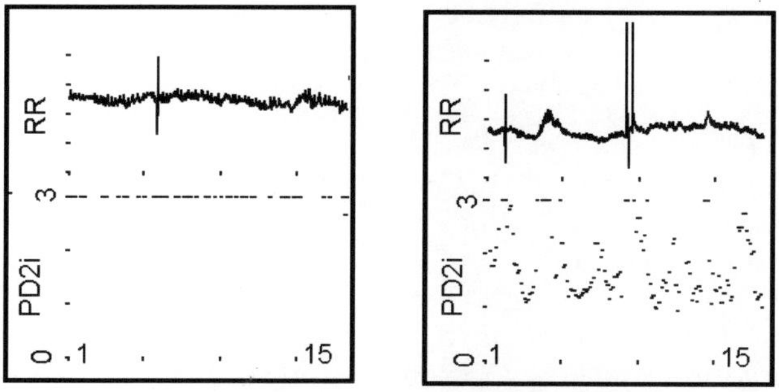

Fig. 12. The PD2i of the RR intervals of two Emergency Department patients presenting with chest pain. The patient with the PD2i between 0 and 3 (right) died of VF within a few days, and the other (left), with similar SDNN and power spectra, lived for at least one year of follow up. The RR interval scale is 600 to 1000 msec.

Figure 12 shows RRi and PD2i data for two typical patients presenting in the Emergency Room with chest pain. Figures 13 and 14 show the same RRi and PD2i results for larger numbers of patients. Table 1 shows the comparison of various HRV algorithms used on the same RRi intervals to predict risk of arrhythmic death. Only the PD2i algorithm is statistically significant for all patient subgroups. These multi-centered studies (Skinner et al, 2008; 2009) were carried out in a total of 918 Emergency Department patients and the results were highly statistically significant for all subgroups, unlike the results for the other comparison algorithms.

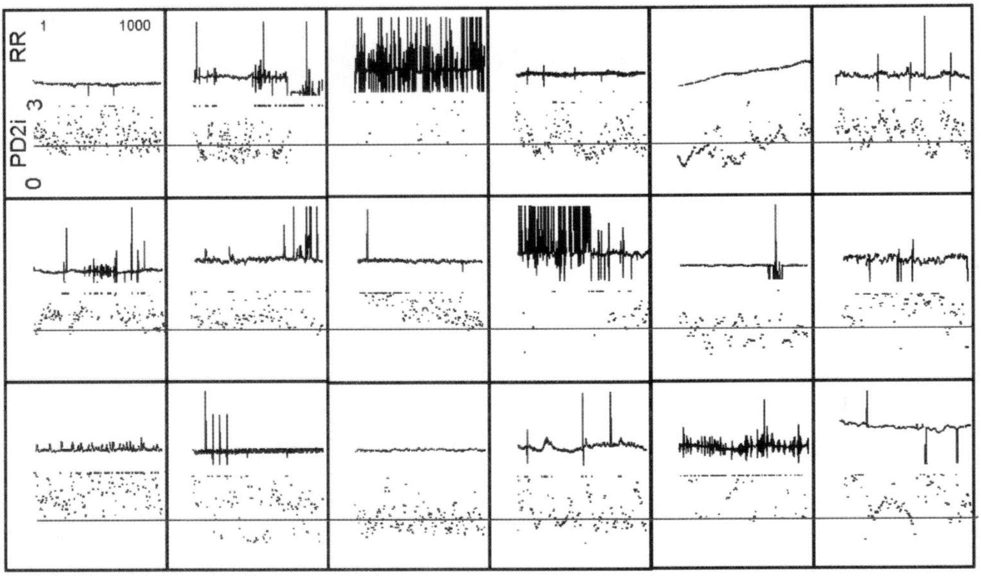

Fig. 13. The PD2i of the RR intervals of 18 consecutive Emergency Department patients presenting with chest pain, who manifested VF within the 1-year of follow-up. The red line is the criterion cut-point of 1.4 indicated by previous studies (Skinner et al,1991; 1993; Vybiral & Skinner, 1993) to separate subjects that would later manifest VF from those that would not. From Skinner et al, 2008a.

T-wave alternans (TWA or Microvolt TWA) was once a popular algorithm for predicting risk of sudden death. Medicare's CMS Committee even approved its use to stratify risk in patients who would receive an ICD (implantable cardiac defibrillator). Unfortunately the MASTER Trial did not show microvolt TWA to identify patients at increased risk of life-threatening ventricular arrhythmias (Cleland et al, 2008). Shown in Figure 15, panels A-C , are the heartbeat intervals (RRi), degrees of freedom (PD2i) and T-wave lability (L; very similar to TWA) for three patients who manifested AD at different times after their ECG was recorded. The T-wave lability is indicated by the range of variation of the T-waves when 5 successive heartbeats are superimposed by alignment of the PQ-intervals. The ECG samples were obtained at the three different times indicated by the numbers above the PD2i trace (1-3). There is an apparent lability (L) in the T-waves in those patients who manifested AD,

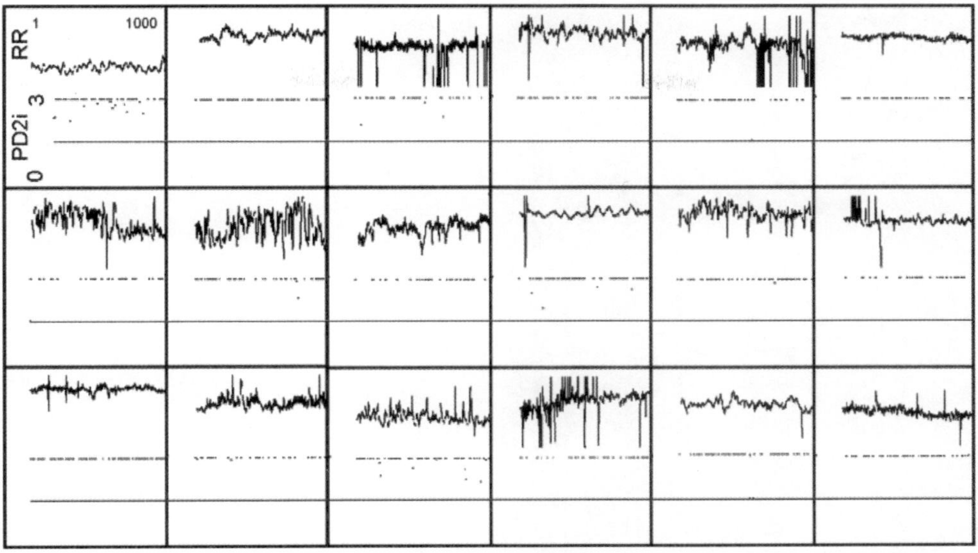

Fig. 14. The PD2i of the RR intervals of 18 Emergency Department patients presenting with chest pain, who were matched to the clinical data of the 18 patients in the previous figure, who did not manifest VF within the 1-year of follow-up. From Skinner et al, 2008a.

either immediately or within a few days (A. and B.). In the patient in B., the lability of the T-waves did not begin until the PD2i temporally descended to the vicinity of 1.4 (horizontal line), a finding which indicates some relationship between PD2i and the lability of refractoriness in this subject. In part C. the patient showed *no T-wave lability*, yet there still was a minimum PD2i (min PD2i) ≤ 1.4 that predicted the later AD.

	AMI	non-AMI	post-MI	non-post-MI
PD2i	>7.39**	>12.17**	>4.51**	>16.85**
DFA	0.70	0.44	0.63	0.48
1/f Slope	1.67	0.56	0.87	0.90
ApEn	0.50	1.44	0.00	0.72
SDNN	0.68	1.75	0.83	1.34
MNN	1.94	>20.82**	3.00	>3.61*
LF/HF	1.08	0.66	2.52	0.61
LF (ln)	1.08	>5.13*	0.73	2.09

The Relative Risk statistic is shown in all cells for the same ED patients (** means $p \leq 0.01$; * means $p \leq 0.05$). Subgroups: AMI = acute myocardial infarction; non-AMI = no acute MI; post-MI is greater than 6 months post MI; non-post-MI = no post MI. Algorithms: PD2i = Point D2; DFA = detrended fluctuation analysis; 1/f Slope = 1/f power spectrum; ApEn = Approximate Entropy; SDNN = standard deviation of normal to normal R-R intervals; MNN = mean of normal to normal R-R intervals; LF/HF = low frequency/high frequency power spectra; LF (ln) = normalized by natural log of low frequency data. From Skinner et al, 2007a; 2009.

Table 1. Comparison of PD2i with other HRV algorithms in various sub-groups

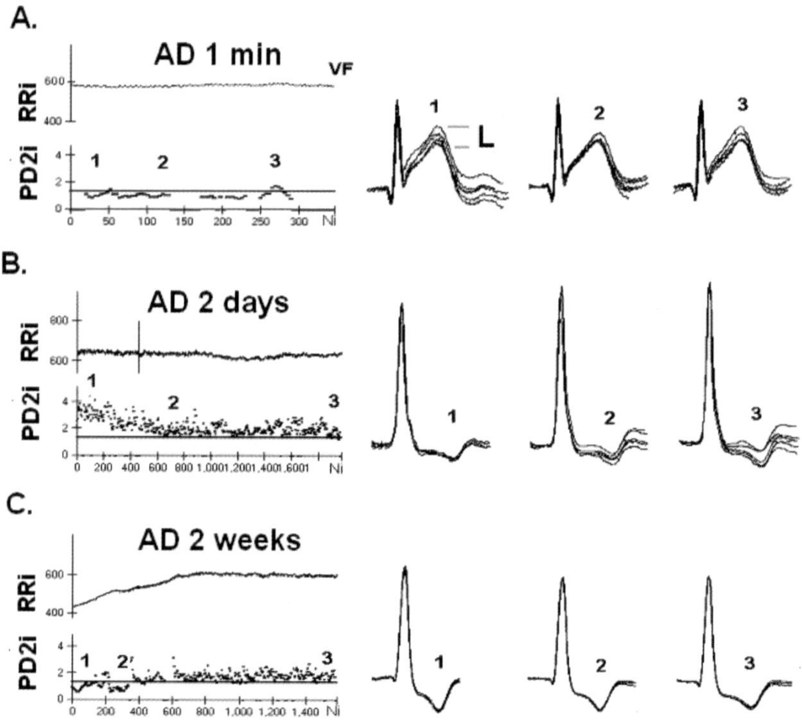

Fig. 15. Comparison of TWL (T-wave lability, similar to TWA) with PD2i of RRi in chest pain patients who manifested arrhythmic death (AD) at different times after the ECG recording. Five successive QRST complexes, sampled at the times shown in the left panels, were superimposed after alignment of the P to Q intervals; the lability of the T-wave is seen as the range of the trace ends at the right. From Skinner (2007a).

It would seem, however, that PD2i *predicts AD at a time when TWA does not* (Figure 15, part C). This might be because TWA is a measure of a "bad heart" (i.e., lability of refractoriness due to myocardial ischemia) and PD2i is a measure of a "bad brain" (i.e., autonomic cooperativity). As we have seen in the pig-model of heart attack, any T-wave lability produced by myocardial ischemia (complete coronary artery occlusion) is *not sufficient* to lead to a VF outcome. It takes a "bad brain," i.e., the cooperativity projected out of the autonomic nervous system, to generate the physiological dynamics suitable to underlie the initiation of VF--- *ischemia alone will not do it!* From the studies listed in Figure 1, it would appear that this cooperation among the heartbeat controllers occurs at a time when sympathetic (and reflexive parasympathetic) tone is high. As will be seen in the next section on the electrogenesis of the waves in the electrocardiogram, these cerebral effects must somehow cause alterations in the wavefront and refractory period and bend the wavefront until it forms a rotating spiral wave (rotor), the immediate cause of VF. The rotor is self-sustaining, splits into other rotating spiral waves and thus becomes VF. The rotor itself seems to result, in nearly all physiological cases of VF ever observed, from a sequellae of arrhythmic events: first a premature beat, followed by ventricular tachycardia and then by VF.

6. Electrogenesis of the waves and intervals in the electrocardiogram

In the previous section we showed that reduction in the degrees of freedom in the variations of the brain-controlled heartbeat intervals is associated with later lethal arrhythmogenesis in Emergency Room patients presenting with chest pain. The rather flat part of the electrocardiogram is where the RR-interval is lengthened or shortened by the brain projections to the heart. The "funny" current (I_f, Brown et al, 1979) controls sodium and potassium channels during the diastolic depolarization phase of each heartbeat, shortening it to increase heart rate and lengthening it to decrease heart rate. The intrinsic pacemaker potential is generally thought to initiate the heartbeat, but I_f determines when that will occur.

Nerve fibers project not only to the pacemaker and Purkinje cells to evoke I_f, and thus control heart rate, but there are also projections to the cardiac arteries and to large interstitial spaces in the ventricular tissues. These latter fibers have terminals that release molecules that can evoke severe vasoconstriction (ischemia) and alter local conduction, propagation and refractoriness so as to produce the various types of ECG anomalies and arrhythmias seen in Figure 4 that result from direct electrical stimulation of the brain. The neural effects of the nerves can no longer be considered to be simple cholinergic and noradrenergic effects that speed up or slow down the oscillatory pacemaker cells.

The P-wave (Figure 16B) is produced during the contractions of the atria that load blood into the ventricles. The contractions of the ventricles force blood through the lungs (right ventricle) and then into the aorta (left ventricle) to pressurize the circulation of the blood. The atrial contractions are initiated at the atrial pacemaker sites. Propagation leads to the spread of excitation to the ventricular surface via the sub-surface and high-speed conduction medium of the Purkinje fibers. The Purkinje fibers end in and first activate the apex (point) of the heart. This initial point of ventricular excitation and contraction then further spreads throughout the heart causing an efficient squeeze that forces blood to move smoothly through the lungs and out into the aorta. The initial apical surface wavefront and its spread throughout the heart produces the QRST-waves.

The electrical properties of the cellular membrane potentials that underlie the excitation, propagation and refractoriness mechanisms were each worked out in the 1950's, in the giant squid axon, by the classical papers of Hodgkin & Huxley (1952). These propagation properties interact with the "funny" current (I_f, Brown et al, 1979), injected primarily into the atrial pacemaker cells to regulate heart rate. But other nerve terminals project directly into the ventricular tissues and release broadly various molecules that can control propagation velocity and direction in the excitable medium. The overall neural effects not only control heart rate at the pacemakers, but also the propagation of wavefronts in the ventricles. These latter controls can bend the wavefronts into curves, that can ultimately lead to rotating waves that can catch their own tails and become self-sustaining "rotors."

Figure 16 shows how the complex of waves is generated during the propagation of an electric wavefront through excitable tissue, such as the wall of a cardiac atrium, cardiac ventricle, cardiac Purkinje-fiber, or a giant squid axon. The atrial tissues containing the sinoatrial and atrioventricular nodes (pacemaker tissues) are innervated by the autonomic nerves and through a complex mechanism cause the P-wave. The wavefront of depolarization of the nerve cells causes a similar action on the atrial pacemaker tissue. A few milliseconds later the R-wave is initiated at the point of the heart (apex) by the Purkinje fibers that rapidly conduct excitation from the AV node to the apex, but in a subsurface route so they do not show in the ECG. The excitation from the apex then spreads throughout the rest of the ventricular tissues until it reaches the base, a line just under the ventricles, and then the excitation stops, the whole heart becomes momentarily refractory and waits for the next heartbeat to begin at the apex. This waiting period is determined by the output of the nerves and I_f and is where the heart beat variation in time is determined. It is the control of the heartbeat rhythm by the brain and its nerves that has been the important subject matter to this point, but its waiting interval (T to P) also should be considered an integral part of the PQRSTP complex of waves known as the electrocardiogram. Nerves project directly into the ventricular tissues and can vary the waiting period independently of the pacemaker initiators.

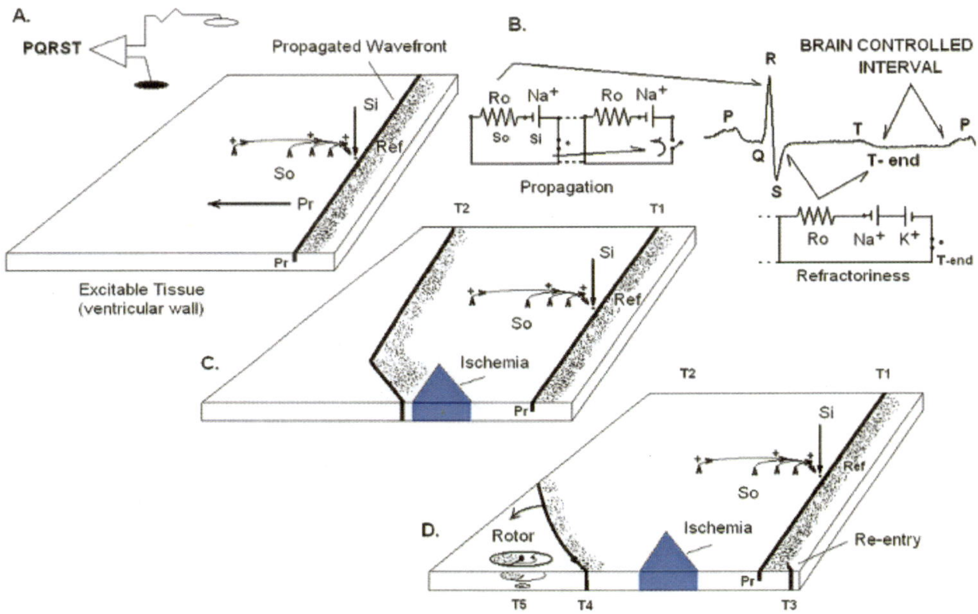

Fig. 16. Electrogenesis of the ECG waves. **A.** Propagation in a three dimensional slab of excitable tissue, showing source currents (So), and sink currents (Si), direction of propagation (Pr arrow) and a band of refractoriness (shaded, Ref) following behind the propagated wavefront. **B.** Electrical schematics of Hodgkin-Huxley model showing how propagation and refractoriness produce the PQRST complex. **C.** Effect of ischemia in slowing segment of propagated wavefront. **D.** Re-entry and Rotor formation.

Propagation of electric activity (Figure 16 A) is akin to that of a fire-front in a prairie grass fire--- the burning grass in the fire-front (excitation) causes the unburned grass next to it to catch on fire (propagation). It can only burn new grass on one side, as it has just burned the grass on the other and it is refractory (i.e., until new grass grows). Thus, the front spreads in a straight line, as does the wavefront in cardiac tissue. The wavefront in the heart is an electric current caused by the depolarization of the cells underneath it. In the schematic diagram in Figure 16B, it is the current flowing through the switch in one membrane compartment (where one sodium channel is switched on, left Na^+) that then turns on the switch in the next compartment (adjacent Na^+ at right). This cascade of switching is due to the voltage-gated conductances of the sodium channels that are packed closely together throughout the cellular membrane (and throughout the whole excitable tissue, by a syncytium of electrically interconnected cells).

Refractoriness is produced by exhaustion of energy (burnt grass), but also is produced more rapidly by another set of batteries (potassium channels, K^+) connected across the membrane in the *opposite* polarity to the sodium channels; these are also voltage-gated, but stay on longer and reduce the effective voltage produced by the Na^+ battery; the K^+ channel being on makes the cell refractory. The K^+ channels being on also causes the long interval out to the T-wave; the interval starts just after the R-wave and lasts until the potassium-switch is off (T-end). Both the Na^+ and K^+ switches automatically turn themselves off, but the K^+ switch stays on longer to create the refractoriness required for propagation in a straight line (i.e., the metaphorical "fire" cannot be started when the K^+ battery is on, so the propagation goes only into the "fresh" grass). There are other channels and batteries in the cardiac membrane, but the main two required for propagation are the sodium and potassium channels.

The sink-current (Si) is at the location of the excitation of the wavefront itself, and draws the source-currents (So) to complete the circuit shown in Figure 16B. As it draws the So it first causes the small Q-wave, and then as the wavefront propagates throughout the heart the R-wave is generated. The S-waves is generated as the R-wave ends. The T-wave is generated by the K^+ battery being turned on and off. The large R-wave produces a large upward deflection in the ECG trace only if it is propagated (travelling) toward the recording electrode (filled electrode in 16A) with respect to the indifferent electrode (unfilled, placed far away so that the source currents at this point are very small). The magnitude of the R-wave deflection is proportional to the current that travels between the electrodes in the resistance of the extracellular spaces (Ro); that is, the recorded potential is the voltage-drop across the resistance of the exracellular space where the source currents flow. The source currents are driven by the plus to minus poles of the batteries, batteries that lie across the membrane and are only on when the membrane compartment switches are on; but these currents travel through the electrically coupled cell's cytoplasm, then back across the high resistance of the membrane and through the low resistance of the extracellular spaces to return to the other pole of the battery located on the outside of the membrane.

Notice that the density of the source currents observed at right angles to the wavefront (16A) are smaller the farther they are away from the battery (i.e., the density of current lines is smaller). But because the membrane resistance is 100 times larger than that of Ro, the extracellular currents produced are by a constant-current generator that pushes the So current density farther away from the battery poles; that is why the currents flow out into, say, the patient's arms. But still, if you want to maximize the size of the R-wave deflection, you want the recording electrode (filled electrode) to be as close to the heart as possible. In the precordial recordings of a 12-lead ECG, some electrodes will be below the apex and some above the base, so to maximize the deflection of the R-wave you want to record a bipolar lead between an electrode toward which the wavefront is traveling (lead-1 or -2) and one from which the wavefront is traveling away (lead-4 or -5). This bipolar recording will eliminate the in-phase 60-cycle artifacts while maximizing the amplitude of the PQRSTP waves.

As shown in Figure 16 C., time T2, myocardial ischemia will slow down the propagation of the wavefront; this delay is caused by many tortuous pathways of conduction through the ischemic zone and/or by the circulatory loss of high energy phosphates which energize the polarization process (i.e., make the batteries work). The delay may have other causes (e.g., neurally-induced ischemia and conduction losses), and the refractory period in and around the ischemic zone can become quite complex. In part D, T3, the delay causes the next wavefront to occur in the excitable tissue just behind the refractory period; thus a beat is created that is either shorter or longer than that of the previous beat depending on exactally where it occurs. A shorter beat leads to a reflexive compensatory pause in its next beat (i.e., seen in the ECG as a two-beat, premature, ventricular complex, PVC). The ischemic zone may cause more severe delays (Figure 16, D., T4), and can lead to the severe bending of the wavefront and the development of a rotating spiral wave (rotor) spinning around a pivot point in which the rotating wavefront constantly re-enters marginally recovered tissue; this spinning rotor is observed in the standard-lead electrocardiogram as ventricular tachycardia (VT). The pivot point meanders randomly, like that of a spinning top, and the rotor will eventually enter an area with a non-conductive piece of tissue, such as a coronary artery or infarcted tissue, and then split into two rotors; these rotors split, and so on, until the electrocardiogram manifests ventricular fibrillation (VF). A sequellae of waveforms in the ECG occurs in most cases of VF--- first PVCs, then VT, then VF.

Arthur Winfree (1987) has seen these rotors in a three dimensional computer model that uses the Hodgkin-Huxley (nonlinear) equations. Instead of a delay in conduction that leads to a re-entrant beat, he simply injects the re-entrant wavefront current near the T-wave. But injection of current on top of a T-wave, or its equivalent through an ischemia-caused delay in propagation, are not the only ways to cause VF, for as was shown in Figure 4 (top ECG), electric stimulation in the brain can also cause VF in a normal heart. How this happens is not known, but the same sequellae of arrhythmias occur--- PVCs, VT and VF, so the underlying patterns of excitation and refractoriness must be equivalent to those associated with ischemia. Note that in Figure 6, the diagrammed efferent nerve fibers project not only to the pacemaker sites, but also directly into the ventricles where they can influence excitation, propagation, and refractoriness in the cardiac tissue.

If one is interested in saving the life of a patient, then the rhythm of the heart should be the focus. That is not to say that the PQRST waves of the electrocardiogram are not important, but they are more directly related to the intrinsic properties of excitation, propagation and refractoriness dictated by the heart cells, properties which cannot explain the onset of lethal arrhythmias. We will now show that the consideration of the extrinsic properties of the nonlinear rhythm of the heartbeats imposed on the heart by the brain is best able to accurately predict risk of VF onset in a variety of clinical patient groups.

7. Clinical results of PD2i tests

Table 2 presents results of 3 independent studies of the heartbeat intervals (Skinner et al, 1993; 2008a; 2008b) showing that one or more PD2i ≤ 1.4 is a statistically significant ($p \leq 0.001$) predictor of lethal arrhythmias (VF) in hospitalized patients: 1) in patients admitted to the Cardiology floor having episodes of non-sustained ventricular tachycardia; 2) in patients presenting in the Emergency Room with chest pain; 3) in patients with various types of arrhythmias placed in the public Physiobank website. The Sensitivity and Specificity of prediction in each study were about the same, and the few cases of rejection-from-study were mostly due to high arrhythmia rates (>10% of beats), of either sinus or ventricular origin. High arrhythmia rates tend to randomize the remainder of RR-intervals and make their PD2i infinite. These 3 studies listed below are confirmed by an independent one in 24 patients with anterior wall infarctions compared to normal controls (Nashishoni et al, 2004a)

In Table 2 Sensitivity = TP/(TP+FN), Specificity = TN/(TN+FP); Negative Predictive Value = TN/(TN+FN); Positive Predictive Value = TP/(TP+FP); Relative Risk = TP/FN x (TP+FN)/(FN+FP). Relative Risk is the more important contingency table statistic, as it is most sensitive to the highly undesireable FNs (i.e., cases where the physician tells the patient "you are OK" and then the patient goes home from the hospital and dies). Each of the statistics in Table 2 is highly statistically significant ($p < 0.001$) by the Fisher Exact Test for contingency tables. Relative Risk may be even higher because the number of FN's approaches zero.

1. Skinner, Pratt, Vybiral (1993) *American Heart Journal*, 125:731-743.
   37 Total Enrolled, 7 Rejections, 30 Completed Study.

True Positive (7)	**False Positive (4)**
False Negative (0)	**True Negative (19)**
Sensitivity = 100%	**Specificity = 83%**

2. Skinner, et. al, (Emergency Room, 5 Tertiary Care Hospitals, Philadelphia, Newark, Camden, Detroit, Allentown). *TCRM*, August 2008
   918 Total Enrolled, 173 Rejections, 745 Completed Study.

True Positive (23)	**False Positive (104)**
False Negative (1)	**True Negative (617)**
Sensitivity = 96%	**Specificity = 86%**

3. Skinner, et. al., (MIT-BI PhysioBank Study). *TCRM*, August 2008
   44 Total , 11 Rejections, 33 Analyzed.

True Positive (17)	**False Positive (3)**
False Negative (0)	**True Negative (13)**
Sensitivity = 100%	**Specificity = 81%**

Table 2. Sensitivity and Specificity of PD2i prediction of VF in cardiac patients with non-sustained ventricular tachycardia (1), presentation with chest pain (2), or having various types of arrhythmias (3).

The majority of deaths in patients with diabetes mellitus (DM) is arrhythmic death. The minimum PD2i at rest in young type-1 DM patients having no signs of neuropathy is statistically significantly lower than that in their age-matched controls ($p \leq 0.001$). Table 3 shows the contingency table for the first study, and Table 4 shows the same effects in another type-1 DM study, but one including recovery from exercise with and without atropine.

	DM (+)	DM (-)	Total
PD2i (+)	16	5	21
PD2i (-)	1	12	13
Total	17	17	

Sensitivity = TP/(TP+FN) = 94%**
Specificity = TN/(TN+FP) = 71%**
Negative Predictive Value = TN/(TN+FN) = 92%**
Positive Predictive Value = TP/(TP+FP) = 76%**
Relative Risk = TP/FN x (TP+FN)/(FN+FP) = 16**

** Statistically significant ($p < 0.001$) by the Fisher Exact Test

Table 3. PD2i < 2.0 identifies type-1 Diabetes Mellitus (DM) patients without signs of neuropathy mixed together with age-matched normal controls (From Skinner et al, 2011).

Groups	PD2i min Rest	PD2i min Recovery
DM *mean*	1.822	1.446
Std Dev	0.713	0.608
Control *mean*	2.566	1.984
Std Dev	0.754	0.715
DM atropine* *mean*	1.878	0.645
Std Dev	0.927	0.228
Control atropine* *mean*	2.525	0.938
Std Dev	0.542	0.648
*(atropine given during exercise)		

Group 1	Group 2	P-value
DM rest	Control rest	0.00521
DM rest	DM recovery	0.05553
Control rest	Control recovery	0.02001
DM recovery	DM atrop recovery	0.00002
Control recovery	Cont atrop recovery	0.00001

Table 4. Min PD2i of Heartbeats in type-1 diabetic patients (DM) and Controls after recovery from exercise.

It is well known that immediately after recovery from exercise, the remaining increase in HR due to sympathetic drive is strongly countered by a rise in vagal (parasympathetic) tone to restore the HR to pre-exercise levels. This fast recovery effect can be blocked by atropine, leaving HR increased well into recovery. This same atropine effect is observed in the type-1 DM patients with respect to minimum PD2i, and suggests an association with sympathetic drive. Sympathetic stimulation or parasympathetic blockade lowers PD2i, whereas parasympathetic stimulation or sympathetic blockade raises PD2i. This study (Vicor, in progress) already has around 50 subjects, so the alpha-statistics shown in the lower panel of Table 3 also have high beta-power.

Hemorrhage causes an immediate reduction in PD2i from baseline in the lightly anesthetized animal (Skinner, Nester, Dalsey, 2000). When bleeding is started after blunt chest trauma, to mimic an explosion, it immediately causes a larger and more extreme reduction in PD2i (Figure 11; Batchinsky et al, 2010).

Table 5 shows that a small loss of blood (1 pint), after voluntary donation at a blood bank, causes a significant PD2i reduction (p = 0.0011; Jett et al, 2010). It is noted that more than half of the subjects, however, may have had a low resting min PD2i score; that is, they were all lower than the mean of the normal controls seen in Table 4 or of most of the values seen for the hospitalized controls in Figure 14.

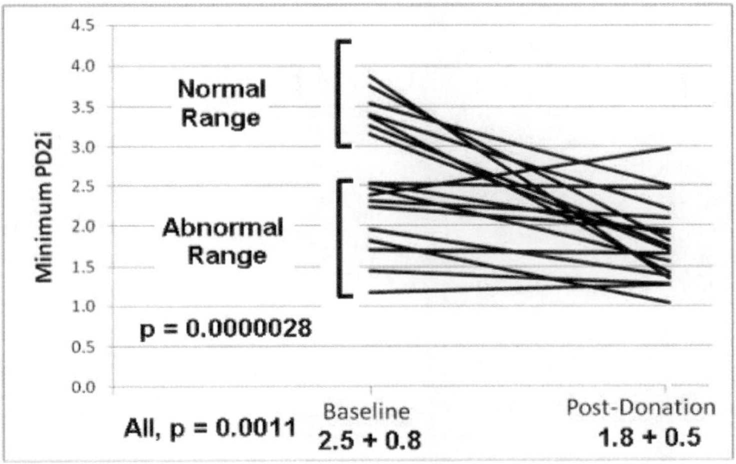

Table 5. Reduction of the min PD2i in normal subjects after donation of 1 pint of blood.

Variable	Sensitivity	Specificity	PPV	NPV
pPD2 <3.90	100	100	100	100
HR >88 bpm[a]	73	73	73	73
HR >100 bpm[b]	36	100	100	61
SBP <122 mm Hg[a]	55	64	60	58
SBP <110 mm Hg[b]	9	91	50	50
DBP <68 mm Hg[a]	46	36	42	40
DBP <60 mm Hg[b]	0	73	0	42

Entries are percentages. All variables refer to baseline (prespinal) measurements.

PPV = positive predictive value; NPV = negative predictive value; pPD2 = peak point correlation dimension measure of heart rate variability; HR = heart rate; SBP = systolic blood pressure; DBP = diastolic blood pressure.

[a] Selection of the discriminant was based on the median value of the entire cohort of 22 patients.

[b] Arbitrary selection of the discriminant was based on common clinical judgment. Note: no patient had SBP <100 mm Hg or DBP <50 mm Hg, making selection of these discriminants specious.

Table 6. Comparison of Baseline Hemodynamic Variables to Predict Postspinal Hypotension.

It would appear then that the rather novel environment of "hypodermic needles and hanging bags of blood" may have had a sympathomimetic effect on the heart similar to that of, say, the "unfamiliar laboratory" in the pig, in which case the sympathetic tone was measured quantitatively (Skinner, Lie, Entman, 1975; Skinner, Beder, Entman, 1983). In normal humans performing simple psychological "stress" tasks, Shubert et al (2009) showed that the heartbeat PD2i is statistically significantly reduced from baseline. They also found the same stress-related reduction in PD2i for chronic-stress subjects compared to non-stressed subjects, where stress was assessed by a chronic stress scale.
Spinal anesthesia often results in a hypotensive crisis ended clinically by injection of catecholamines. In women about to give birth at term, it is desirable to know in advance whether or not they are likely to manifest the hypotensive crisis so that prophylactic measures can be taken to prevent any untoward affects on the mother or fetus. It seems that the peak PD2i of the heartbeats observed prior to the spinal injection is able to predict the hypotensive crisis (Chamchad et al, 2004). Table 6 shows that if *peak* PD2i (pPD2i) at rest lies below 3.90, then the manifestation of a hypotensive crisis is highly likely following the spinal injection. Neither blood pressure nor heart rate has any predictive value, whereas the sensitivity and specificity of peak PD2i < 3.9 are both 100% ($p = 0.001$). Again a "novel environment" stress-effect may be differentially causing the reduction of the baseline PD2i scores in the women at risk. But in this case, it is the maximum value of the resting range that is lower, not the minimum value.

Algorithm	**Non LSI**	**LSI**
ApEn	1.14 ± 0.03	0.99 ± 0.09
SampEn	1.19 ± 0.04	0.99 ± 0.11
MSE (3)†	3.41 ± 0.17	1.84 ± 0.41***
PD2i	1.31 ± 0.10	0.82 ± 0.11**
pNN30	14.89 ± 2.4	4.60 ± 2.13*
HF	167.17 ± 30.53	36.17 ± 18.73**

† = post hoc selection of 3; requires clean data
* p = 0.05
** p = 0.01
*** p = 0.001

Table 7. Comparison of algorithms used on the heartbeats of wounded soldiers (N=70) to predict a prehospital life-saving intervention (LSI). (Vicor, unpublished data). (Cancio & Skinner, unpublished).

Comparison of PD2i with other nonlinear "complexity" algorithms has recently been done by the Army in a cohort of wounded soldiers, as shown in Table 7. Several measures reached statistical significance. Notable, though, was the fact that the data set of 70 patients was culled from a larger set of 132 patients. Whereas all 132 could be analyzed by PD2i, only these current 70 could be analyzed by the other methods, due to their more restrictive ECG length requirements and their intolerance of extrasystoles and noise. The performance of PD2i when applied to the entire 132 patient data set was similar to that shown here, while the other measures tended to lose their predictability (Cancio and Skinner, 2011).

For Multi Scale Entropy (MSE), the scale of 1 to 4 is selected after the analyses to determine which one is the most discriminating. This type of *post hoc* selection is not really allowed when making a statistical inference. Computationally this selection of scale is like selecting the embedding dimension (m = 1 to 4) for the PD2i. MSE with a scale of 1 is the same as Sample Entropy (SampEn), which is not a statistically significant discriminator.

Very recently, PD2i analysis has been used in a large cohort of 651 chronic heart failure (CHF) patients (Zareba et al., 2011). The study population was observed for 44 months on average with total mortality as primary endpoint and cardiac mortality, sudden cardiac death, and heart failure death as secondary endpoints. The PD2i was computed based on 20-minute supine high-resolution Holter recording and was categorized as positive (PD2i≤1.4) or negative (PD2i>1.4) based on prespecified criteria. Among the 651 chronic heart failure patients, 537 had successful PD2i analyses resulting in 144 (27%) patients showing positive results and 393 (73%) negative results. The multivariate results are shown below.

	Hazards Ratio	95% CI	p value
Univariate Analysis			
PD2i	1.73	1.18-2.53	0.005
Multivariate Analysis			
Age >65 years	1.56	1.07-2.29	0.022
Prior myocardial infarction	1.63	1.13-2.37	0.010
EF ≤35%	2.24	1.50-3.35	<0.001
Beta-blocker use	0.60	0.41-0.88	0.009
PD2i	1.55	1.05-2.29	0.026

* After adjustment for the same clinical covariates as in the main model.
There were no other interactions between PD2i: p value for interaction with age was 0.223, with Age >65 0.861, and with beta-blocker use 0.608.

Table 8. Prognostic significance of PD2i for predicting total mortality in heart failure patients.

Table 8 shows that after adjustment for clinical covariates (Zareba et al, 2011) PD2i, was found predictive for total mortality by the Hazards Ratio (HR=1.55; p=0.026). Predictive value of PD2i was observed in heart failure patients with left ventricular ejection fraction ≤35% (HR=1.95; p=0.004), whereas not in patients with >35% (HR=0.87; p=0.716). Further analyses revealed that among patients with ejection fraction ≤35%, PD2i was also predictive for cardiac death and for heart failure death. The conclusion was that the PD2i is predictive for total mortality, cardiac death and heart failure death in heart failure patients with left ventricular ejection fraction ≤35%.

PD2i has also recently been applied to all patients presenting to *the intensive care unit* (ICU) to stratify the risk of mortality at 30 days (Vicor, ongoing study). A min PD2i ≤ 1.4 was found to have a relative risk of death of 8.9 (p = 0.003) at ICU discharge and 11.1 at 30 days (p < 0.001). Thus the PD2i of the heartbeats has been found useful in another defined cohort.

A low PD2i of the heartbeats has also been shown to detect cardiac allograft transplant rejection (Izrailtyn et al., 2000). The partially intact nervous system apparently can continue to distinguish between a new muscular pump that is good and one that is failing.

Interestingly, a low PD2i of the heartbeats has also been found in major depression in human subjects (Nahshoni, Aravot, et al., 2004b). These same authors showed in an animal model that the neuronal spike-intervals thought to give rise to depressive behavior also show a reduction in PD2i compared to controls (Dremencov, Nahshoni et al, 2004; Friedman, Deri et al, 2007). The fact that there is an elevated rate of adverse cardiac events in patients with major depression (Glassman, Bigger, Gafney, 2009) leads to the intriguing speculation that it is due to autonomic derangements, which are detected by the low PD2i of the heartbeats. The PD2i of the heartbeats may provide psychiatrists with a physiological end-point for use in evaluating therapies.

8. Discussion

It has long been known that mostly the hyper "type A" personalities are the ones who die from heart attacks (Friedman and Rosenman, 1974). Death of a spouse dramatically increases the risk of death of the surviving partner (Rees and Lutkins, 1967). We have all heard the statement that he/she died of a broken heart or of marital strife or job insecurity (Rahe et al, 1973). A salient characteristic of people who live to 100 years of age is a positive and optimistic view of life (Rozanski and Kubzansky, 2005). Despite the examples being all around us, this obvious connection between the conscious mind and the heart/body has been underappreciated and poorly studied by the medical community. One of the major reasons for scientific based western medicine's failure to understand, study and appreciated this connection is that, up until now, it has been difficult to objectively *identify and quantify the underlying physiology*. The PD2i has changed all that by giving physicians and scientists an easily administered, reproducible, quantifiable, and sensitive test of how this conscious state exerts it influence on the body.

The connection of the conscious mind to the body is primarily mediated through the autonomic nervous system. It is becoming apparent that the status of and the relative balance of the sympathetic and parasympathetic nervous systems' input to all of the organs has a profound impact on outcomes in a multitude of diseases and pathological conditions. Heart rate variability has served for almost 40 years as a window to the autonomic nervous system, but no real advances were made because the measurements were too inaccurate. Heart rate variability is determined not only by the balance of the sympathetic and parasympathetic components of the autonomic nervous system, which may be caused by unconscious compensatory actions, but also by the nonlinear phase relationships between and within the two types of effectors (i.e., the "cooperativity" among the brain centers that controls the degrees of freedom in the autonomic output). Using an advanced algorithm (PD2i) that detects the nonlinear information lost by the conventional measures used over the past decades, biologists can now accurately quantify the autonomic output in a more meaningful way. The influence of the attentive and conscious Cerebral Defense System combined with the unconscious respiratory, blood-pressure, and temperature controllers is now subject to a composite integrated measure of the output of the nerves to one of its target organs.

Trauma, blood loss and heart failure are states in which the sympathetic nervous system increases its activity in an attempt to maintain homeostasis. But there is something more than sympathetic tone that needs to be considered. For example, in the two patients shown in Figure 12, the heart rates are about the same (same sympathetic drive), but the PD2i is much lower in the one who later died (more autonomic "cooperation" occurring). As would be expected, it has been found in trauma patients, critically ill ICU patients, patients who have lost blood, and heart failure patients, that a low PD2i score--- indicating a higher level of compensatory output--- identifies the "more stressed patient," the one who is sicker, losing more blood, or is more traumatized and trying harder to compensate and, thus, more likely to die or require a life saving intervention.

In certain chronic disease processes, such as diabetes, it is not the reaction of the autonomic nervous system to the acute or chronic disease that affects the heart rate variability signal but, rather, damage to the autonomic nervous system itself, which may, in turn, prove to be a major cause of the end-organ damage. A multitude of studies have found that if autonomic dysfunction is present the outcomes of patients with diabetes and renal disease are far worse; for example, the adverse cardiac event rate is doubled in diabetic patients with autonomic dysfunction (Vinjk et al, 2003). The contribution of autonomic nervous dysfunction to metabolic syndrome and sleep apnea are only now being considered, but the driving hypotheses are quite rational in view of recent discoveries.

The clinical and research implications of being able to easily measure and quantify the nonlinear status of the autonomic nervous system are far reaching and profound. To be able to identify patients with "high sympathetic tone" and/or high autonomic "cooperativity," which correlate with a "more stressed and sicker patient," would obviously be very helpful in anesthesia monitoring during surgery, monitoring of critically ill patients in the ICU, and in the triage and monitoring of trauma patients. At present, identifying occult class I blood loss (<15%) is a diagnostic dilemma. The PD2i's ability to noninvasively identify such low level blood loss would thus be helpful in a multitude of medical situations. Being able to predict and identify which patient will have a more malignant course from their chronic illnesses of heart failure, diabetes and renal disease would clearly also be very helpful to the physicians, the health care providers, and the health care systems who care for them. Finally having a more sensitive and specific "test" of the autonomic nervous system will facilitate research on the contributions of the underlying systems to a wide range of medical conditions. In the years to come the PD2i will help expand our understanding of the autonomic nervous system and its profound contribution to a variety of disease processes and medical conditions.

9. Summary and conclusions

The same loci of cerebral centers that control vulnerability of the ischemic heart to lethal arrhythmogenesis overlaps precisely with the quantified six loci of cerebral centers known to control resting heart rate, thus providing the rational for the hypothesis that patterns in the heartbeat series may be related to the physiological conditions that enable ventricular fibrillation to occur. This hypothesis has been tested and shown to be true in a number of studies in animals and in human patients. The PD2i is a nonlinear measure well suited to extracting signals from any physiological data series (RRi, ECG, EEG, etc.), because all such physiological data are themselves nonlinear. With this new metric it is possible to extract information, even in non-stationary data, that has been hidden to measurement by conventional algorithms that are based on a linear stochastic model—e.g., the mean, standard deviation, power spectra, and so on.

With rather spectacular sensitivity, the PD2i, compared to the other linear and nonlinear algorithms, has been shown to outperform them all in the prediction of future risk of lethal arrhythmias (Table 1). The prediction comes with sufficient sensitivity, specificity, relative risk and low p-values so as to be medically useful in a variety of medical situations. Peer-reviewed and recently published studies illustrating this medical utility are presented in Tables 1 to 8 for various well-defined cohorts with various medical disorders: multiple hospitalized cardiac cohorts (ER-, Cardiology-floor, Physiobank- archive, and ICU); young diabetics without neuropathy; blood-donors and bleeders with or without chest trauma; pre-hospital wounded-soldiers requiring life-saving intervention; patients with chronic (congestive) heart failure.

In cerebral states of short-term stress (public speaking), long-term stress (anxiety scales), or major depressive disorder, the PD2i of the heartbeats is significantly reduced compared to controls, and these negative affective states are also known to be related to an increased incidence of death in both animal models and patients. In contrast, salutary brains states, such as occur in animals during REM sleep, or after adaptation to an unfamiliar environment, appear to be related to neuroendocrine secretions operating in parallel with neural activations. Through the new paradigm of equivalent state-dependent proteomics, new drugs candidates can be isolated, identified, synthesized and tested in biological models. One such candidate is a neuroendocrine molecule that has a potent anti-infarction effect in a model of stroke or heart attack (Figure 5).

The neglected part of the electrocardiogram, the flat and uninteresting T to P interval, appears to be controlled in time by the brain. Modern cardiologists and physicians must take notice of the new extrinsic underpinnings of the electrocardiogram, for there is a wealth of new medical utility and discovery to be unfolded.

10. Acknowledgements

The first author, James E. Skinner, would like to acknowledge Donald B. Lindsley, his mentor during graduate training in Neuroscience at the Brain Research Institute, and Michael E. DeBakey, the Chancellor of Baylor College of Medicine, who first hired him as an Assistant Professor, built him a magnificent laboratory, and supported him throughout his 25-year career research into the Role of the Brain in Cardiovascular Disorders. It was Dr. DeBakey who challenged Skinner "to get his science to the bedside," which meant founding Vicor Technologies, Inc., in 2000, to commercialize his collected science. Skinner would also like to acknowledge the high clinical expertise of his co-authors, Drs Daniel N Weiss (Electrocardiologist) and Edward F Lundy (Thoracic Surgeon), who each have a keen interest in innovative medicine. Skinner would finally like to thank the National Institutes of Health for the many millions of dollars of NS RO1 and PO1 research grants that supported his career work and the SBIR Fast Track grant that help him get Vicor started. The authors disclose that they are employees of Vicor and shareholders.

11. References

Batchinsky AI, Skinner JE, Necsoiu C, Jordan BS, Weiss D, Cancio LC. New measures of heart-rate complexity: effect of chest trauma and hemorrhage. J Trauma. 68:1178-85, 2010.

Baust W and Bonnert B. Regulation of heart rate during sleep. Exp Brain Res 7:169-180, 1969.

Brown HF, DiFrancesco D, Noble SJ. How does adrenaline accelerate the heart? Nature, 280:235-236, 1979.

Cancio L and Skinner JE. PD2i of 200 heartbeats predicts life saving interventions in wounded soldiers. (unpublished data of Vicor Technologies, Inc and the Army Institute of Surgical Research) 2011.

Cannon WB. The Wisdom of the Body. Norton, New York, 1932.

Chamchad D, Arkoosh VA, Horrow JC, Buxbaum JL, Izrailtyan I, Nakhamchik L, Hoyer D, Kresh JY. Using heart rate variability to stratify risk of obstetric patients undergoing spinal anesthesia. Anesth Analg. 99:1818-21, 2004.

Chase MH, Sterman MB, Clemente CD. Cortical and subcortical patterns of response to afferent vagal stimulation. Exp Neurol; 16;36-49, 1966.

Cleland JG, Coletta AP, Abdellah AT, Cullington D, Clark AL, Rigby AS. Clinical trials update from the American Heart Association 2007: CORONA, RethinQ, MASCOT, AF-CHF, HART, MASTER, POISE and stem cell therapy. Eur J Heart Fail. 10:102-8, 2008.

Dremencov E, Nahshoni E, Levy D, Mintz M, Overstreet DH, Weizman A, Yadid G, Dimensional complexity of the neuronal activity in a rat model of depression NeuroReport, Vol 15 No 12, 2004.

Ebert PA, Vanderbeek RB, Allgood RJ, Sabiston DC Jr. Effect of chronic cardiac denervation on arrhythmias after coronary artery ligation. Cardiovasc Res. 4:141-7, 1970.

Elbert, T., Ray, W.J., Kowalik, Z.J., Skinner, J.E., Graf, K.E., and Birbaumer, N. Chaos and Physiology: deterministic chaos in excitable cell assemblies. Physiological Reviews 74:1-47, 1994.

Friedman M and Rosenmen RH. Type A Behavior and Your Heart. Knopf, NY, 1974

Friedman A, Deri I, Friedman Y, Dremencov E, Goutkin S, Kravchinsky E, Mintz M, Levi D, Overstreet DH, Yadid G. Decoding of dopaminergic mesolimbic activity and depressive behavior. J Mol Neurosci, 32:72-9. 2007.

Glassman AH, Bigger JT Jr, Gaffney M. Psychiatric characteristics associated with long-term mortality among 361 patients having an acute coronary syndrome and major depression: seven-year follow-up of SADHART participants. Arch Gen Psychiatry; 66:1022-9, 2009.

Hjalmarson A. Cardioprotection with beta-adrenoceptor blockers:Does lipophilicity matter? Basic Res Cardiol; 95:I41–I45, 2000.

Hodgkin AL and Huxley AF. A quantitative description of ion currents and its applications to conduction and excitation in nerve membranes. *J. Physiol. (Lond.)*, 117:500-544, 1952.

Izrailtyan I, Kresh JY, Morris RJ, Brozena SC, Kutalek SP, Wechsler AS, Early detection of acute allograft rejection by linear and nonlinear analysis of heart rate variability. J Thorac Cardiovasc Surg; 120:737-745, 2000.

Jett PL, Skinner JE, Anchin JM, Weiss DN, Parsell DE, Hughes JJ. Blood donation results in observable changes in heart rate variability pattern. Abstract AABB, 2010.

Kostelich EJ, Swinney HL. Practical considerations in estimating dimension from time series data. Physica Scripta. 40: 436–441, 1989.

Nahshoni E, Strasberg B, Adler E, Shula Imbar S, Sulkes J, Weizman A. Complexity of the dynamic QT variability and RR variability in patients with acute anterior wall myocardial infarction: a novel technique using a non-linear method. J Electrocardiology; 37:173-179, 2004a.

Nahshoni E, Aravot D, Aizenberg D, Sigler M, Zalsman G, Strasberg B, Imbar S, Adler E, Weizman A. Heart rate variability in patients with major depression. psychosomatics; 45:129-134, 2004b.

Parker GW, Michael LH, Hartley CJ, Skinner JE and Entman ML. Central beta-adrenergic mechanisms may modulate ischemic ventricular fibrillation in pigs. Circ Res, 66:259-270, 1990.

Rahe RH, Bennett L, Romo M, Seltanen P, Arthur RS. Subject's recent life changes and coronary heart disease in Finland. Am J Psychiat, 130:1222, 1973.

Rees WD, Lutkins SG, Mortality of bereavement Br Med J 4:13, 1967

Rozanski A, Kubzansky LD. Psychologic functioning and physical health: a paradigm of flexibility. Psychosom Med. 67 Suppl 1:S47-53, 2005.

Schubert C, Lambertz M, Nelesen RA, Bardwell W, Choi JB, Dimsdale JE. Effects of stress on heart rate complexity-a comparision between short-term and chronic stress. Biol Psychol 80:325-332, 2009.

Skinner, J. E. A cryoprobe and cryoplate for reversible functional blockade in the brains of chronic animal preparations. Electroencephalogr Clin Neurophysiol, 29: 204-205, 1970.

Skinner, J.E. The role of the brain in ventricular fibrillation and hypertension: from animal models to early human studies. Clev Clin J Med. 74:S73-S78, 2007a.

Skinner, J.E. New paradigms in heart-brain medicine: nonlinear physiology and state-dependent proteomics. Clev Clinc J Med. 74:S79-S85, 2007b.

Skinner, J. E. Regulation of cardiac vulnerability by the cerebral defense system. In: Electrophysiological Mechanisms Underlying Sudden Cardiac Death, edited by B. E. Sobel, J. V. Dingell, and M. B. Mock. New York: Futura Publishing Company; p. 131-146, 1982.

Skinner JE and Lindsley DB. Reversible cryogenic blockade of neural function in the brain of unrestrained animals. Science, 161: 595-597, 1968.

Skinner JE, Mohr DN, and Kellaway P. Sleep-stage regulation of ventricular arrhythmias in the unanesthetized pig. Circ. Res., 37: 342- 349, 1975.

Skinner JE, Lie JT, and Entman ML. Modification of ventricular fibrillation latency following coronary artery occlusion in the conscious pig: the effects of psychological stress and beta- adrenergic blockade. Circulation, 51: 656-667, 1975.

Skinner JE and Reed JC. Blockade of a frontocortical- brainstem pathway prevents ventricular fibrillation of the ischemic heart in pigs. Am J Physiol, 240: H156-H163, 1981.

Skinner JE, Beder SD, and Entman ML. Psychologic stress activates phosphorylase in the heart of the conscious pig without increasing heart rate and blood pressure. Proc Nat Acad Sci, 80: 4513-4517, 1983.

Skinner JE The regulation of cardiac vulnerability by the cerebral defense system. J Amer Coll Cardiol, 5:88B-94B, 1985.

Skinner JE, Pratt CM, Vybiral TA. Reduction in the correlation dimension of heart beat intervals precedes imminent ventricular fibrillation in human subjects. Am Heart J, 125:731-743, 1993.

Skinner JE, Molnar M, and Tomberg C. The Point Correlation Dimension: Performance with non-stationary surrogate data and noise. Integr Physiol Behav Sci, 29:217-234, 1994.

Skinner JE, Wolf SG, Kresh JY, Izrailtyn I, Armour JA, Huang M-He. Application of chaos theory to a model biological system: evidence of self-organization in the Intrinsic Cardiac Nervous System. Integ Physiol Behav Sci, 31:122-146, 1996

Skinner JE, Nester BA, Dalsey WC. Nonlinear dynamics of heart rate variability during experimental hemorrhage in ketamine-anesthetized rats. Am J Physiol: Heart Circ Physiol. 279:H1669-78, 2000.

Skinner JE, Meyer M, Dalsey WC, Nester, BA, Ramalanjaona G, O'Neil, BJ, Mangione A, Terregino C, Moreyra A, Weiss DN, Anchin JM, Geary U, Taggart P. Risk stratification for arrhythmic death in an emergency department cohort: a new method of nonlinear analysis of RR-intervals. Therap and Clin Risk Manag, 4:1-9, 2008a.

Skinner, J.E., Anchin, J. M., Weiss, D. Nonlinear analysis of the heartbeats in public patient ECGs using an automated PD2i algorithm for risk stratification of arrhythmic death. Therap and Clin Risk Manag, 4:549-557, 2008b.

Skinner JE, Meyer M, Nester BA, Geary U, Taggart P, Mangione A, Ramalanjaona G, Terregino C, Dalsey WC. Comparison of linear-stochastic and nonlinear-deterministic algorithms in the analysis of 15-minute clinical ECGs to predict risk of arrhythmic death. Therap and Clin Risk Manag 5:671-82; 2009.

Skinner JE, Weiss DN, Anchin JM, Turianikova Z, Tonhajzerova I, Javorkova J, Javorka K, Baumert M, Javorka M. Nonlinear PD2i heart rate complexity algorithm detects autonomic neuropathy in patients with type 1 diabetes mellitus. Clin Neurophysiol. Jan 20, [Epub ahead of print], 2011.

Vinik AI, Maser RE, Mitchell BD, Freeman R: Diabetic autonomic neuropathy (Technical Review). Diabetes Care 26:1553–1579, 2003.

Vybiral, T., Skinner, J.E. The Point Correlation Dimension of R-R intervals predicts Sudden Cardiac Death among high risk Patients. Computers in Cardiology, 257-260, 1993.

Winfree A T. When Time Breaks Down: The Three-Dimensional Dynamics of Electrochemical Waves and Cardiac Arrhythmias. Princeton University Press. ISBN 0-691-02402-2, 1987.

Zareba W, Cygankiewicz I, McNitt S, Bayes de Luna A. Prognostic significance of PD2i, novel risk marker in heart failure patients. Abstract: 11-A-8315-ACC, J Amer Colleg Cardiol. 2011.

10

Quantification of Ventricular Repolarization Dispersion Using Digital Processing of the Surface ECG

Ana Cecilia Vinzio Maggio[1], María Paula Bonomini[2], Eric Laciar Leber[3] and Pedro David Arini[1,2]
[1]*Instituto Argentino de Matemática 'A. Calderón', CONICET, Buenos Aires*
[2]*Instituto de Ingeniería Biomédica, Universidad de Buenos Aires, Buenos Aires*
[3]*Gabinete de Tecnología Médica, Universidad Nacional de San Juan, San Juan*
Argentina

1. Introduction

Digital processing of electrocardiographic records was one of the first applications of signal processing on medicine (Taback et al., 1959). There are many ways to analyze and study electrical cardiac activity using the surface electrocardiogram (ECG) and nowadays a good clinical diagnostic and prevention of cardiac risk are the principal goal to be achieved (Sörnmo & Laguna, 2005).

One aim of digital processing of ECG signals has been quantification of ventricular repolarization dispersion (VRD), phenomenon which is mainly determined by heterogeneity of action potential durations (APD) in different myocardial regions (Amlie, 2000). The APD differs not only between myocytes of apex and the base of both ventricles, but those of endocardial and epicardial surfaces (transmural dispersion) and between both ventricles. Also, it was demonstrated the existence of several electrophysiologically and functionally different myocardial cells, like epicardial, endocardial and mid-myocardial M cells (Antzelevitch et al., 1999). The APD inequalities develop global and/or local voltage gradients that play an important role in the inscription of ECG T-wave morphology. In this way, we can assume that T-wave is a direct expression of ventricular repolarization (VR) inhomogeneities on surface ECG.

Experimental and clinical studies have demonstrated a relationship between VRD and severe ventricular arrhythmias (Kuo et al., 1983) (Surawicz, 1997). In addition, patients having increased VRD values have a higher risk of developing reentrant arrhythmias (Shimizu & Antzelevitch, 1998). Frequently the cardiac answer to several pathological states produces an increase of VRD; this phenomenon may develop into malignant ventricular arrhythmia (MVA) and/or sudden cardiac death (SCD). Moreover, it has been shown that the underlying mechanisms in MVA and/or SCD are cardiac re-entry, increased automation, influence of autonomic nervous system and arrhythmogenic substrates linked with cardiac pathologies. These cardiac alterations could be present in ischemia (Janse et al., 1985), hypothermia (Eagle, 1994), electrolyte imbalance (Weinberg et al., 1995), long QT syndrome (LQTS) (Priori et al., 1994), autonomic system effects (Shusterman et al., 1998) and others.

Digital processing of ECG has been proved to be useful for cardiac risk assessment, with additional advantages like its non invasive nature and direct applicability to the general population (Sörnmo & Laguna, 2005). Also, with the aim to identify high cardiac risk patients, the researchers have tried to quantify the VRD with different parameters obtained from mathematic-computational processing of the surface ECG. These parameters are based on detecting changes of T-wave intervals and T-wave morphology during cardiac pathologies, linking these changes with VRD.

Figure 1 illustrates a temporal segment of an ECG acquired in a healthy subject, which includes the representation of different waves, intervals and segments of the cardiac signal. The P-wave reflects the sequential depolarization of the right and left atria, the QRS complex (consisting of Q, R and S waves) reveals the depolarization of both ventricles, and the T-wave displays the VR. The RR interval represents the duration of a cardiac cycle. The QT interval corresponds to the time from the onset of ventricular depolarization to the offset of VR.

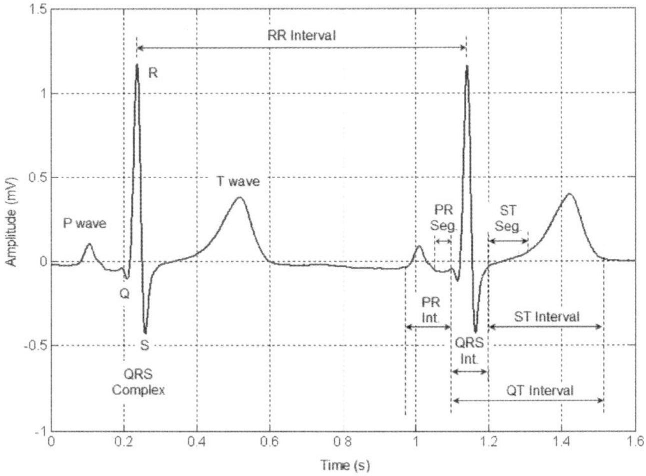

Fig. 1. Schematic representation of ECG waves, intervals and segments for a healthy subject.

In this chapter, we present a review of VRD indexes based on digital processing of ECG signals to quantify cardiac risk. The chapter is organized as follows: Section 2 explains ECG preprocessing and delineation of fiducial points. In Section 3, indexes of VRD quantification, such as: QT interval dispersion, QT interval variability and T-wave duration, are described. In Section 4, different repolarization indexes related to T-wave morphology and energy are examined, including complexity of repolarization, T-wave residuum, angle between the depolarization and repolarization dominant vectors, T-wave morphology dispersion, micro T-wave alternans, T-wave area and amplitude and T-wave spectral variability. Finally, in Section 5 conclusions are presented.

1.1 Most used abbreviations

APD (action potential duration), **C_D** (Dipolar Components), **C_{ND}** (non-dipolar components), **C_R** (complexity of repolarization), **DWT** (dyadic wavelet transform), **ECG** (electrocardiogram), **EMG** (electromyogram), **HR** (heart rate), **HRV** (heart rate variability), **HS** (healthy subject), **IL**

(isoelectric line) **MAPs** (monophasic action potentials), **PVS** (premature ventricular stimulation), **QT_C** (QT interval corrected), **QT_D** (QT interval dispersion), **QT_V** (QT interval variability), **SCD** (sudden cardiac death), **SVD** (singular value decomposition), **T_{CRT}** (total cosine R-to-T), **T_L** (T-wave loop), **T_{MD}** (T-wave morphology dispersion), **T_{PE}** (T-wave peak-to-end), **T_W** (T-wave width), **T_{WR}** (T-wave residuum), **T_{WRa}** (absolute T-wave residuum), **T_{WRr}** (relative T-wave residuum), **T_{WSV}** (T-wave spectral variance), **μT_{WA}** (micro T-wave alternans), **VF** (ventricular fibrillation), **VR** (ventricular repolarization) and **VRD** (ventricular repolarization dispersion).

2. ECG preprocessing

The objectives of ECG preprocessing consist on the application of several digital signal processing techniques in order to: a) attenuate the noise components present in the ECG signal, b) detect all heartbeats in the recording and, c) identify characteristics points of the ECG waves. In order to accomplish these objectives the following signal processing algorithms are used: ECG filtering, QRS complex detection and ECG delineation.

2.1 ECG filtering

Unfortunately, all ECG recordings are contaminated by different types of noise and artifacts sources (Sörnmo & Laguna, 2006) as it is illustrated in Figure 2. These noise sources are:

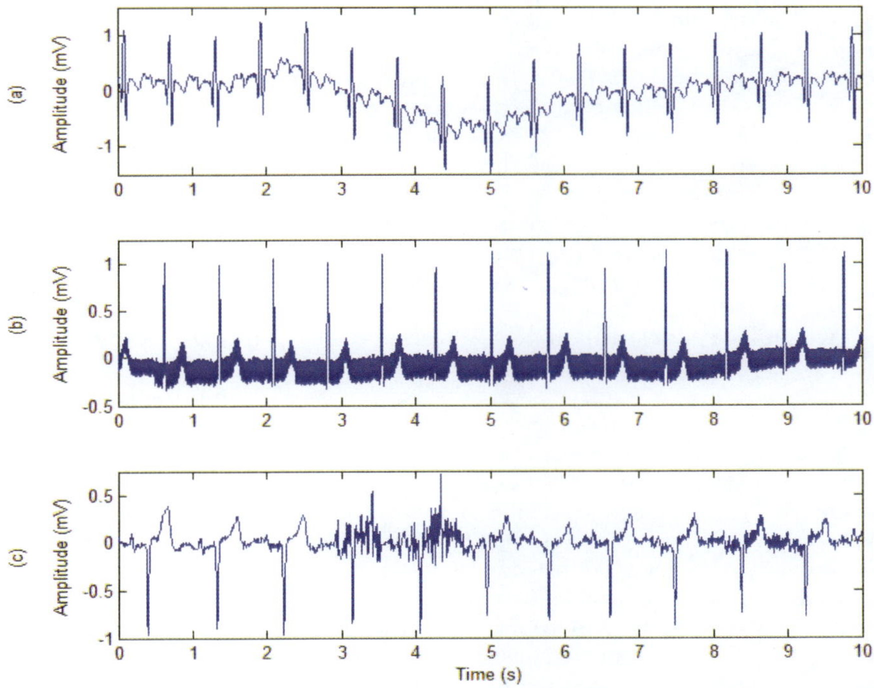

Fig. 2. Common types of noise in ECG recordings. (a) Baseline wander, (b) 50 Hz power line interference, and (c) Electromyographic noise.

a) Baseline wander is a low-frequency component in the ECG (*see Fig. 2.a*) caused by a variety of noise sources including respiration, body movements, and poor electrode contact. Its spectral content is usually confined to frequencies below 0.5 Hz. The magnitude of the baseline wander may exceed the amplitude of QRS complex by several times and it can significantly affect ECG analysis algorithms.

Different filtering techniques are employed for the removal of this low frequency noise, mainly, linear filters and polynomial fitting (Sörnmo & Laguna, 2005). In the first category, linear, time-invariant, highpass filters are used. The cut-off frequency (f_c) and phase response characteristic should be chosen to preserve the morphology of ECG signal. The value of f_c must be lower than the minimum frequency of the ECG; a choice of f_c = 0.5 Hz provides generally good results. A linear filter with time-variable cut-off frequency has been proposed for these ECG acquired during stress test (Sörnmo, 1993). Also, linear phase filters are recommended to prevent phase distortions in the ECG signal and avoid possible errors in the estimation of the wave durations and cardiac intervals. The second approach is to fit a polynomial to representative samples ("knots") of the ECG followed by the subtraction of the resultant polynomial curve. One knot must be defined for each beat, usually in the isoelectric line (IL) of PQ interval. In contrast to linear filtering, this approach requires that QRS complexes first be detected and PQ intervals are determined. After knots are located in the ECG signal, a third-order polynomial is fitted to these points (Sörnmo & Laguna, 2005).

b) Powerline interference is a common noise source in ECG recordings caused by electromagnetic fields of devices coupled to electric power system. It is characterized by a 50 or 60 Hz sinusoidal interference (*see Fig. 2.b*), which can be accompanied by its harmonics. Such narrowband noise makes difficult the further analysis of ECG record, and may affect the performance of the ECG delineation algorithms (Huhta & Webster, 1973). Various precautions may be taken during the acquisition of the ECG recording in order to minimize the level of the interference, such as shielding the leads, grounding property of the ECG system and lowering the skin-electrode impedance (Webster, 1992).

However, it may be still necessary to apply some signal processing to remove the residual powerline interference on the ECG recordings. For this purpose, simple techniques can be used such as straightforward linear bandstop or nonlinear filtering (Sörnmo & Laguna, 2005). A more advanced technique includes the amplitude and phase estimation of the interfering sinusoid in an isoelectric segment, followed by substraction of the estimated sinusoid within the entire heartbeat (Ider & Köymnen, 1995). This last technique requires a correct delineation of PQ interval.

c) Electromyographic noise is due to the electrical activity of skeletal muscles during periods of contraction. It is particularly important in ECGs recorders during ambulatory monitoring or stress tests. It can be either intermittent, e.g. due to a sudden body movement (*see Fig. 2.c*), or have more stationary noise properties, e.g during relaxation or sleep. The frequency components of electromyogram (EMG) noise considerably overlap those of the QRS complexes, making difficult their detection (Sörnmo & Laguna, 2005).

Due to the overlap spectra of both signals, EMG noise filtering is a complicated task which in several cases introduces considerable distortion in the ECG. Since the ECG is a repetitive signal, ensemble averaging is a commonly technique used for EMG noise reduction. However this technique is restricted to signal-averaged ECG analysis and can require much beats to be averaged particularly in ECG records corrupted with high levels of EMG noise (Laciar & Jané, 2001). Other different approach consists on the use of adaptive Gaussian filtering. This technique produces a time-varying lowpass filter with a variable frequency response so that smooth segments on the ECG are subjected to considerable lowpass filtering whereas the QRS interval remains unfiltered (Talmon et al., 1986). The adaptation of the f_c of a linear lowpass filter with the slopes of the ECG has been proposed by Pinto (Pinto, 1991). Although others techniques have been proposed for EMG noise reduction, no single method has gained wide acceptance for use in clinical routine, so the muscle noise problem remains unsolved in ECG signal processing (Sörnmo & Laguna, 2005).

2.2 QRS complex detection

The following step in the ECG signal processing consists on the detection of all heartbeats in the ECG recording. Due to the QRS complex has generally greater amplitude and higher signal to noise ratio than P and T waves (*see Fig. 1*), the heartbeats identification is usually carried out with a QRS detector. Moreover, the QRS complex has a higher frequency content which can be distinguish from low frequency of P and T waves (Thakor et al., 1984). The QRS detector must be able to detect a large number of different QRS morphologies in order to be clinically useful and able to follow sudden or gradual changes of the cardiac rhythm. Consequently, the performance of any ECG automatic analysis system depends on a correct detection of all QRS complexes in the ECG record.

In the literature, it has been proposed several QRS detectors. Köhler et al., produced a rather comprehensive review of the main QRS detecting algorithms (Köhler et al., 2002). One of them, widely used, was proposed by Pan & Tompkins (Pan & Tompkins, 1985). Its implementation is simple reaching high levels of sensitivity and predictivity (both > 99.5%). Bandwidth, slope and pulse duration are the three criteria used by the algorithm. A bandpass filter keeps the spectral portion where most of the QRS energy concentrates, attenuating the P and T waves low frequency components, removing baseline slow changes or drifts and reducing 50/60 Hz line interference and EMG high frequency noise. A differentiator picks out the steep QRS edges, obviously much different that the other components smoother edges. Thereafter, the mean quadratic value of each signal sample is computed by a non-linear unit to obtain only positive values and to emphasize the QRS high frequency components. A moving window integrator adds up the areas under the quadratic signal to produce pulses and to remove short duration artifacts. Such output goes to the decision unit where each pulse is compared to the preestablished threshold singling it out or not and locating it in its proper relative temporal place. The overall output is composed of the temporal marks or spikes, each corresponding to the detected QRS complex.

2.3 ECG delineation

Since important diagnostic information is contained in the wave amplitudes and time durations of a heartbeat (*see Fig. 1*), wave delineation represents an important step in ECG processing (Sörnmo & Laguna, 2005). Basically, ECG delineation consist on the automatic determination of peaks and time limits of the cardiac waves (QRS complex, P and T-waves). Delineation algorithms usually depart from a previous QRS location and define temporal search windows before and after the QRS fiducial point to seek for the other waves. Once the search window is defined, some technique is applied to enhance the characteristic features of each wave (e.g., its frequency band) in order to find the wave peaks.

The localization of ECG wave onsets and offset is a more difficult task, as the signal amplitude is low at the wave boundaries and the noise level can be higher than the signal itself (Martinez et al., 2004). The classical definition of a wave boundary is the time instant at which the wave crosses a certain amplitude threshold. Unfortunately, this definition is not adequate for cardiac waves delineation, particularly in ECG records corrupted with baseline wander, so it is not used in practice (Sörnmo & Laguna, 2005).

In order to solve this problem, many delineation algorithms examine the change in the slope of ECG signal to detect the wave limits. Hence, the first derivate of the signal is computed and analyzed with respect to zero crossing and extreme values. This delineation scheme is particularly appropriate to find QRS onset and offset points, due to the steep changes in the slopes of these waves (de Chazal & Celler, 1996, Daskalov & Christov, 1999).

ECG delineation is especially problematic with the estimation of T-wave end boundary, which is often characterized by a very gradual transition to the IL. The delineation of T-wave end is problematic even among cardiologists, which can exhibits differences up to 100 ms (Sörnmo & Laguna, 2005). A correct determination of this endpoint is extremely important for an accurate estimation of QT interval (*see Fig. 1*). Different algorithms have been proposed for the automatic detection of T-wave end. Xue & Reddy in 1998 compare the performance of five T-wave delineation algorithms based on: (a) the point at which the T-wave intersects the IL plus a threshold, (b) the point at which the first derivate of T-wave intersects a threshold above IL, (c) the intersection of the maximum slope of T-wave and IL, (d) the intersection of the line fitted by least squares to the maximum slope of T-wave and IL (LSI), and (e) the point at which the T-wave area reaches 90% of its total value. They conclude that LSI method has the best reproducibility (Xue & Reddy, 1998). Other ECG delineation algorithm, based on a multiresolution analysis of ECG signal using dyadic wavelet transform (DWT), has proven to be particularly adequate for a correct estimation of T-wave boundaries (Li et al., 1995, Martínez et al., 2004). This wavelet approach can be viewed as a filter bank of lowpass differentiators with varying cut-off frequencies. The wave boundaries are then found through the different decomposition levels of DWT.

3. Indexes of repolarization dispersion based on ECG durations

In this section, we present different VRD indexes obtained from ECG durations. Some of them can measure spatial heterogeneity of repolarization, such as QT dispersion, T-wave width and T-wave peak-to-end duration. Other index, like QT variability can be used to evaluate the dynamic heterogeneity of VR. Also, other spatial heterogeneity indexes, such as, T-wave amplitude, T-wave symmetry and the relationship between T-wave areas, are shortly commented.

3.1 QT interval dispersion

QT dispersion (QT_D) is defined as the arithmetic difference between the maximum and the minimum QT interval (*see Fig. 1*) or as QT interval standard deviation between all ECG-leads. QT_D was first defined on multilead recordings system (Sylven et al., 1984) and then on the standard 12-lead ECG (Cowan et al., 1988), intended to reflect the duration of the monophasic action potentials (MAPs). Thus, the QT_D measured on the 12-lead ECG aims to be a non-invasive index of VRD. The main concept proposed by Day et al., which supports the QT_D as a VRD marker, is the fact that every ECG lead picks up local activity from different heart areas and therefore differences among them directly translate into differences in APD (Day et al., 1990). In consequence QT_D quickly became popular for its non-invasive nature and calculus simplicity.

In the repolarization analysis, many studies focussed on finding a universal formula that corrected QT (QTc) for heart rate (HR) in every patient (Hodges, 1997). However, Malik et al. showed that the QTc must not be universally applied but individually (Malik, 2002). In this way, animal studies have shown that VRD does not change with HR and need not be corrected for it (Zabel et al., 1997). Also, QT_D correction in humans can be misleading since changes in this index at different HR may shows or reflects modifications in cycle length and not changes in VRD (Subramanian et al., 1999).

Later on, QT_D was studied by Day et al. in 1992 (*see Table 1*) under sinus rhythm and controlled ectopic stimulus leading to the conclusion that QT_D reflected regional variations of the cellular recovery time (Day et al., 1992).

Higham et al. (Higham et al., 1992), found a high correlation between VRD measured on MAPs basis and QT_D on both sinus rhythm and ventricular pacing. Also Zabel et al., observed that QT_D was highly correlated to ventricular recovery times and duration of MAPs in isolated rabbit hearts (Zabel et al., 1995). Later on, results were confirmed in humans, comparing QT_D from ECG 24 hs after MAPs recording, increasing accordingly QT_D and endocardic MAPs (Zabel et al., 1998b).

Zabel et al., in 32-months follow-up a prospective study including myocardial infarction (MI) patients, failed to find in QT_D a predictive value of mortality (Zabel et al., 1998a). On the other hand, Mänttäri et al., with a 6.5 years follow-up study, did find QT_D measured to T-wave peak as a predictor of SCD but not of fatal MI (Mänttäri et al., 1997).

Using a modified Langendorff-perfused rabbit heart model, Arini et al. compared QT_D measure from multilead system against the values found when the 12 standard ECG-leads were used. The obtained results supported the importance of multiple recording systems for the evaluation of QT_D and helped to understand the discrepancies found in clinical applications (Arini et al., 2000). Later, Arini et al., using an animal heart model with multiple electrode recording system, showed a differential behavior in the modulation of VRD depending on whether premature ventricular stimulation (PVS) were elicited at the right or left ventricle. They concluded that different ventricles anisotropic properties, dissimilar wall thickness and fiber orientation partially contribute to the explanation of results (Arini et al., 2001).

More controversial issues came up with Lee et al. (*see Table 1*), and Macfarlane et al. who simultaneously showed that QT_D calculated from 12-ECG leads derived from the orthogonal XYZ leads (without any regional information) was similar to that obtained from the standard ECG. Also, Kors et al. (*see Table 1*), found a high correlation between QT_D and the parameters of the T-wave loop (T_L) in the vectocardiogram, concluding that the QT_D would be more a feature of the T_L in 3D more than a local VRD phenomenon. If all the repolarization information is contained in the T_L, then the QT_D would be a result from the projection effect (Lee et al., 1998; Macfarlane et al. 1998; Kors et al., 1999).

Many technical limitations make QT_D not reliable. Great efforts have been addressed to define different ways of measurement (Hnatkova et al., 1994a) as well as to analyze their reproducibility (Macfarlane et al., 1998). Kautzner et al. tested that the greater QT intervals in leads displaying greater T-wave amplitudes. They also found a 27-33% interobserver variability for QT_D whilst a much smaller interobserver variability (2-4%) was found for QT intervals (Kautzner et al., 1994). Lead selection also affects QT_D. Hnatkova et al. analyzed in a systematic way the measurement errors derived from imperfect sets of leads. Due to the great variability found, they concluded that QT_D should be compared with a constant and standard set of leads basis (Hnatkova et al., 1994b). On the other hand, Kors & Van Herpen, postulated a valuable criterion for lead selection based on the frontal leads dependence (Kors & var Herpen, 1998). Another technical problem concerning QT_D measurement is T-wave end delineation which was before mentioned in Section 2.3. Figure 3 shows QT_D calculated between two hypothetical ECG leads where it can be seen the difficultities to distinguish between the dispersion generated by estimation error and the real dispersion.

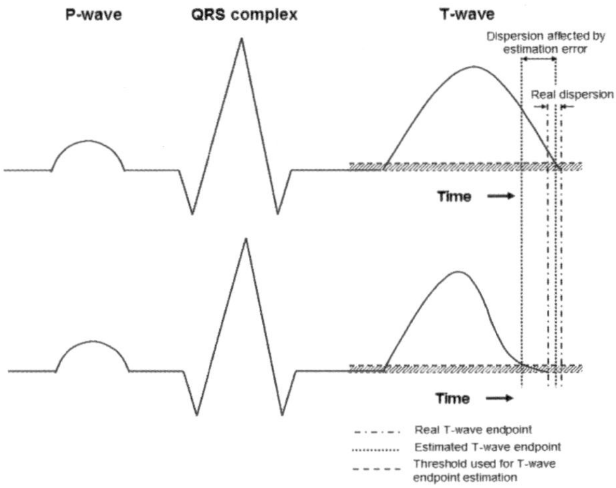

Fig. 3. Both T-waves of the same amplitude have different ends, this results in 'real dispersion' of QT intervals (vertical dashdot lines). Also, from below the threshold level (horizontal dashed lines) defined by an automatic algorithm, there are different proportions of T-waves end (vertical dot lines), this results are called 'Dispersion affected by estimation error' which is different from the 'Real dispersion'.

In spite of the technical limitations and controversies, QT_D is used in a growing number of medical applications. Examples of this are the assessment of cardiac toxicity in anesthesia (Cafiero et al., 2010) or the search of cardiac indexes in malnourished adults (Hanci et al., 2010).

3.2 QT interval variability

In order to separate the heart rate variability (HRV) from the QT variability (QT_V), the QT_V index is redefined as: $QT_{VI}=QT_V/HRV$, being this ratio related to arrhythmic events, SCD and heart failure (Berger et al., 1997, Yeragani et al., 2004). QT_{VI} reflects beat-to-beat changes of the recovery times and such variations in the refractory times can lead to reentrant arrhythmias.

In a prospective study recruiting patients referred to electrophysiological studies, the greater QT_V belonged to those who presented SCD or ventricular fibrillation (VF) (Atiga et al., 1998). Healthy subjects presented low QT_{VI} and considerable HRV, with a low average HR and a high average QT, while patients with dilated cardiopathy presented a high QT_{VI} with low QT average and low HRV with an high HR average.

In 1999, trying to get rid of the T-wave end detection, Courdec analyzed the QT abnormal components in the time-space domain by means of wavelet transform (Couderc et al., 1999) where they found LQTS patients with higher QT_V than the control patients. Burattini and

<table>
<tr><th>Author and year of publication</th><th>Short description</th><th colspan="2">Indexes</th><th colspan="12">Conditions for the evaluation of methodologies</th></tr>
<tr><td rowspan="3">Day et al. (1992)</td><td rowspan="3">9 patients under electrophysiological study of palpitation</td><td rowspan="2" colspan="2"></td><td colspan="6">CI= 300 (ms)</td><td colspan="6">CI= 500 (ms)</td></tr>
<tr><td colspan="2">PSC</td><td colspan="2">VE</td><td colspan="2">FSC</td><td colspan="2">PSC</td><td colspan="2">VES</td><td colspan="2">FSC</td></tr>
<tr><td colspan="2">AQT_D (ms)</td><td colspan="2">22 ±2</td><td colspan="2">80±4</td><td colspan="2">23±6</td><td colspan="2">18±2</td><td colspan="2">87±6</td><td colspan="2">18±2</td></tr>
<tr><td>Lee et al. (1998)</td><td>Conventional and derived ECGs obtain from 129 HS</td><td colspan="2">QT_D (ms)</td><td colspan="6">40 ±20
(12 leads from XYZ)</td><td colspan="6">41±18
(from 12 leads)</td></tr>
<tr><td rowspan="2">Kors et al. (1999)</td><td rowspan="2">1220 standard simultaneous 12 ECG leads.</td><td rowspan="2" colspan="2">QT_D (ms)</td><td colspan="12">54.2±27.1 for narrow and large T-wave loop</td></tr>
<tr><td colspan="12">69.5±33.5 for wide and small T-wave loop</td></tr>
<tr><td rowspan="3">Fuller et al. (2000)</td><td rowspan="3">Correlation coefficients of VRD versus T-wave width (T_W) and QT_D for each lead set</td><td colspan="2"></td><td colspan="3">Ep</td><td colspan="3">BS</td><td colspan="3">Pc</td><td colspan="3">Op</td></tr>
<tr><td colspan="2">T_W</td><td colspan="3">0.91</td><td colspan="3">0.84</td><td colspan="3">0.72</td><td colspan="3">0.81</td></tr>
<tr><td colspan="2">QT_D</td><td colspan="3">0.46</td><td colspan="3">0.47</td><td colspan="3">0.17</td><td colspan="3">0.11</td></tr>
<tr><td rowspan="4">Arini et al. (2001)</td><td rowspan="4">Dispersion Variables (DV) was evaluated as a function of CI and site of stimulation in 12 in vitro rabbit hearts. *p<0.05 vs. 400ms</td><td rowspan="2" colspan="2"></td><td colspan="6">CI for Stimulus RV (ms)</td><td colspan="6">CI for Stimulus LV (ms)</td></tr>
<tr><td colspan="2">400</td><td colspan="2">250</td><td colspan="2">ERP +5</td><td colspan="2">400</td><td colspan="2">250</td><td colspan="2">ERP +5</td></tr>
<tr><td rowspan="2">DV (ms)</td><td>SDJTp</td><td colspan="2">9.6± 0.88</td><td colspan="2">10.2± 0.84</td><td colspan="2">14.9± 0.73*</td><td colspan="2">7.7± 0.55</td><td colspan="2">6.2± 0.55*</td><td colspan="2">11± 1.16*</td></tr>
<tr><td>SDJTe</td><td colspan="2">7.6± 0.55</td><td colspan="2">8.1± 0.7</td><td colspan="2">11± 0.83*</td><td colspan="2">7.1± 0.52</td><td colspan="2">4.6± 0.72*</td><td colspan="2">11± 0.86*</td></tr>
</table>

AQT_D (Adjusted QT_D)= ($max QT_D - min QT_D$)/$\sqrt{}$ nº of leads; *CI (Coupling interval);* PSC (Preceding Sinus Complex); VE (Ventricular Extrasystole); FSC (Following Sinus Complex); Ep (Epicardial); BS (Body Surface); Pc (Precordial); Op (optimal); SD (Standard Deviation); JTp (J point to T-wave peak); JTe (J point to T-wave end) RV (Right Ventricle); LV (Left Ventricle); ERP (Effective Refractory Period). HS (healthy subjects)

Table 1. Some of the principal results of ECG duration indexes explained in Section 3.

Zareba, on the other hand, proposed a temporal method to measure beat-to-beat QT_V consisting on correlating T-waves with a pattern (Burattini & Zareba, 1999). This index was validated with ischemic myocardiopathy who presented a higher index than control patients. Nevertheless, no correlation with left ventricular ejection fraction (LVEF), HR, HRV and QTc were found.

Almeida et al. in 2006 postulated a parametric linear model to explore interactions between QT_V and HRV. The method was applied to simulated series and artificial ECG signals, but validated on real ECG data from healthy subjects, where it was found a 40% of QT fraction not correlated with HRV, suggesting that an important part of QT_V is not linearly driven by HRV and may contain complementary information (Almeida et al., 2006).

Recently, it was shown the relationship between QT_{VI} and cardiac sympathetic activity in hypertensive patients (Baumert et al., 2011).

3.3 T-wave duration

Fuller et al., in 2000 used isolated-perfuse canine hearts (*see Table 1*) to measure QT_D and T-wave width (T_W) from the root-mean-square (RMS) curve obtained from: the available epicardial electrograms, ECG body surface leads, standard precordial ECG leads, and optimal lead set. They induced myocardial VRD by three different ways: changing temperature, modifying the cycle length and changing activation sequence. The VRD, which was measured directly using epicardium recovery times, was compared to T_W and QT_D. VRD was strongly correlated with T_W computed from the RMS series, but not with QT_D (Fuller et al., 2000).

Arini et al., proposed that T-wave widening can result from a result of combined dispersion between apex-base and transmural APD heterogeneities. They used the addition of anthyarritmic drugs and PVS to induce increase VRD in an In Vitro rabbit heart model (*see Table 1*), concluding that VR is reflected in the ECG as a T_W widening, while index QT_D failed as risk stratification (Arini et al., 2008a).

Other studies have shown T-wave peak-to-end (T_{PE}) interval as a measure of transmural dispersion (Zareba et al., 2000), although it is difficult to associate this concept with the ECG standard, since the concept of T_{PE} is mainly associated to the ECG derived from the Wedge preparation (Antzelevitch et al., 1999). In addition, the T_{PE} can replace the T_W to measure dispersion during ischemia, since the measurement of T-wave onset is very unstable during ST-segment modifications (Arini et al., 2008b).

4. Indexes of repolarization dispersion associated to ECG-morphology

In this section, we present VRD indexes obtained from ECG morphology changes. These indexes are based on the hypothesis that morphological changes on the T-wave will appear when VRD is increased. The indexes complexity of repolarization, T-wave residuum, the total cosine R-to-T, the T-wave morphology dispersion, T-wave area and T-wave amplitude, can measure spatial heterogeneity of repolarization. Other indexes from beat-to-beat, such as micro T-wave alternans and T-wave spectral variance can measure dynamic heterogeneity of VR.

4.1 Evaluation of T-Wave morphology employing Singular Value Decomposition

The main technique used to evaluate morphological or energy changes of T-wave during increased VRD is the Singular Value Decomposition (SVD). SVD is a mathematical transformation based on the correlation between signals. In this case, SVD is applied to the eight mutually independent leads (I, II, V1-V6) and then the information is reconstructed in an optimal orthogonal space of eight pseudo-leads (S1-S8) (*see Fig. 4*). In the new space, S1 will have the maximal energy or eigenvalue ($\lambda 1$) in this direction, S2 will contain the maximal energy ($\lambda 2$) perpendicular to S1, S3 will have the maximal $\lambda 3$ perpendicular to the two first pseudo-leads and so on. S1, S2 and S3 have the 98% of total ECG energy approximately, and are named dipolar components (C_D) ($\lambda 1$, $\lambda 2$, $\lambda 3$), whereas S4-S8 have the 2% residual and are called non-dipolar components (C_{ND}). The C_D is the ECG energy represented in 3D, and shows the normal activity, but for C_D are not enough to represent pathological activity adequately, being necessaries the C_{ND}.

The Complexity of Repolarization (C_R) index is represented by the ratios between eigenvalues (Priori et al. 1997). In normality conditions, the T_L can be represented like a 3D vector with eigenvalues λ1 λ2 λ3 relative to the principal axes S_1 S_2 S_3. In general, T_L is concentrated in the λ1 and λ2 values denominated preferential plane and it can be quantified by C_R like a narrow or a rounded loop in this plane. Furthermore, the planarity can be calculated, because in a loop totally plane λ3 is equal to zero.
The ventricular gradient is the resulting vector of all the instantaneous vectors of depolarization and repolarization. Expanding this concept, it can be estimated the wavefront direction descriptor, named Total cosine R-to-R (T_{CRT}). This index was defined like the cosine of the angle formed between the dominant vectors of the VR and depolarization, measured in a 3D loop of SVD space (Acar et al., 1999). Also, the T-wave morphology dispersion (T_{MD}) index measures dissimilarities of the T-wave shapes between different leads and reconstruction vectors of the individual ECG leads and it is calculated as the average of angles among pairs of reconstruction vectors (Zabel & Malik, 2004). Finally, the T-wave residuum (T_{WR}) index was proposed by Malik et al., and estimates the non-dipolar components relative energy. The T_{WR} can be absolute (T_{WRa}) defined like C_{ND} and relative (T_{WRr}), the T_{WRa} normalized by total energy (Malik et al, 2000).

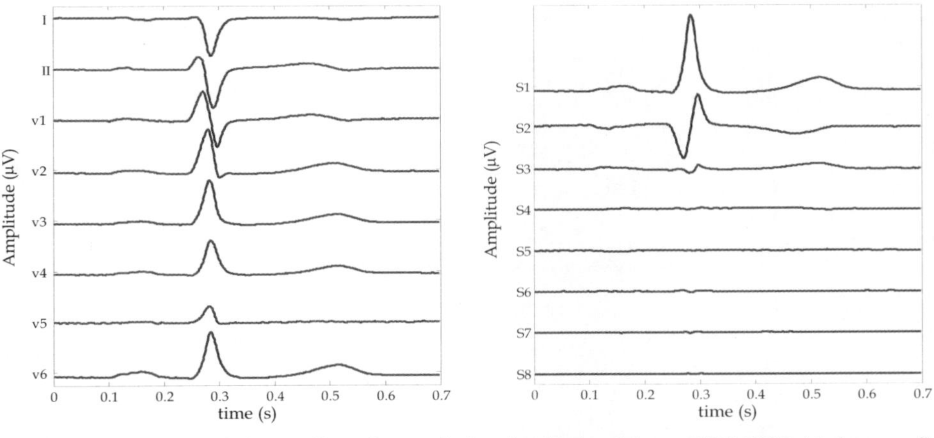

Fig. 4. Standard ECG (left panel) and pseudo-leads obtained from ECG SVD (right panel).

Badilini et al. applied the relationship between 3D T_L morphology and scalar QT_D. This analysis was applied to the XYZ ECG obtaining the normalized eigenvalues with the aim to estimate one loop narrowness parameter and two planarity parameters. They evaluated the parameters in healthy subjects (HS) and post MI and LQTS patients. The scalar measurements were significantly larger in patients with MI and LQTS than in HS but only in 3D analysis was observed a loss of planarity and an increased roundness of the T_L, differentiating MI from LQTS patients. They concluded that the spatial nature of T_L was associated to scalar interlead variability (Badilini et al., 1997).
Almost simultaneously, Priori et al. applied eigenvalues relationship to 12-lead Holter recordings (*see Table 2.*) to estimate the C_R, and compared their results against other methods that characterize QT interval. They found that the ratio of the λ2 to λ1 was more representative of C_R, being C_{R24h} the average of C_R in 24 hs. They observed that CR_{24h} was

significantly higher in LQTS than in HS. They concluded that eigenvalues relationship can be used to quantify the C_R in a non invasive way (Priori et al., 1997).
In addition to those indexes previously described, Acar et al. developed another indexes linked to T_L. They employed ECG records with HS and hypertrophic cardiomyopathy (HCM) (*see Table 2*) to calculate the conventional measures of VR and the ratios among eigenvalues. They concluded that new descriptors were more reproducible than the conventional QT interval descriptors and T_{MD} and T_{CRT} indexes were the best indexes for discrimination between groups (Acar et al., 1999).

Author and year of publication	**Short description**	**Indexes**	**Conditions for the evaluations of methodologies**			
Priori et al., (1997)	Were studied 36 LQTS patients and 40 control subjects.		*Normal*	*LQTS*	*Sen %*	
		QTc (ms)	414±18	514±59	88	
		QT_{DC} (ms)	38±9	82±37	69	
		C_{R24h}	13±3	34±12	88	
Acar et al., (1999)	Were employed 76 normal subjects and 63 patients with HCM. p-value of separation between normal and HCM for each index evaluated		*Normal*	*HCM*	*p- value*	
		T_{MD}	10.72±4.784	41.1±26.85	$2.818x10^{-18}$	
		T_{CRT}	0.522±0.274	-0.351±0.522	$3.548x10^{-19}$	
		λ_2/λ_1	15.56±6.162	23.56±10.85	$9.886x10^{-7}$	
		λ_3/λ_1	4.826±2.373	7.765±4.235	$6.603x10^{-9}$	
Malik et al., (2000)	The study was realized with a group of 78 HS, 68 HCM, 72 DCM and 81 acute MI patients.		*Normals*	*HCM*	*DCM*	*acute MI*
		QT_D (ms)	33.6±18.3	47±19.3	37.8±21.2	57.5±25.3
			Normals vs DCM: NS, other p<0.009			
		T_{WR} (%)	0.029 ±0.031	0.067 ±0.067	0.112 ±0.154	0.186 ±0.308
			HCM vs DCM: NS, other p<0.006			
		QT_D and T_{WRr} correlation	-0.0446	0.2805	-0.1531	0.0771
			p=0.03 for HCM , other NS			
Arini et al., (2008a)	The experiments were carried out in 20 isolated rabbit hearts during PE and after DS		*Control*	*PVS*	*Control*	*DS*
		T_W (ms)	78±10.3	118.5 ±15.7	78±10.3	95.2±7.9
		SDQT (ms)	7.6±2.2	13±3.4	6.5±1.4	11.6±1.9
		θ_{PT} (°)	137±65	129±61	35±51	117±49

NS (non significant); QT_{DC} (QT dispersion corrected); SD (Standard Deviation).

Table 2. Some relevant results from ECG SVD and the comparison with another indexes

A research in which QT_D and T_{WRr} was calculated in 12-lead resting supine ECGs records corresponding to HS, HCM patients, dilated cardiomyopathy patients (DCM) and survivors of acute MI (*see Table 2.*) was carried out by Malik et al. They concluded that C_{ND} differ in clinically well-defined groups, and that QT_D is unrelated to them, so, QT_D is not a direct measure of local VRD (Malik et al., 2000).

Zabel et al., during a prospective study for risk stratification in post-MI patients evaluated C_R, T_L dispersion (T_{LD}), T_L area, T_{CRT} and T_{MD}, and where correlated with QT_D and clinical data. Zabel et al. found that T_{CRT} and T_{LD} is suitable for risk discrimination. They realized a multivariate analysis including other predictive risk stratifiers. They concluded that T-wave morphology analysis can be used in the post-MI risk estimation and in combination with other risk markers enhanced the final results (Zabel et al., 2000). Later, Zabel et al. presented a study to assess the prognostic value of the same parameters evaluated in 2000, adding the T_{WRa}, T_{WRr} and QT interval in long term survivals in US veterans with cardiovascular disease and the patients were follow up 10.4 ± 3.8 years. They showed that T_{WR} presents a significant long-term prognostic power in the population studied (Zabel et al., 2001).

The C_D and C_{ND} were analyzed by Biagetti et al., in isolated rabbit hearts model. The aim was to analyze the role of both components in the determination of T_{WR} observing that both increased significantly during PVS and after D-sotalol (DS) exposure. Despite the increase of T_{WRa}, the T_{WRr} decreased during PVS and did not change after DS. They concluded that due to the fact that C_D and C_{ND} can change simultaneously, T_{WRr} may not reflect regional heterogeneity of VR with accuracy and that C_{ND} of the 2nd half of the T-wave can be related to transmural VRD (Biagetti et al., 2004).

A study that analyzed Principal Component Analysis (PCA) parameters in relation to conduction disturbances in patients with chest pain and ECG nondiagnostic of acute MI was developed by Kesek et al. in 2004. They calculated C_R, T_{WRa} and T_{WRr} which were assessed against clinical and ECG parameters, discharge diagnosis and total mortality during 35-months follow up. They found that a T_{WRr} increased with conduction disturbances, which were associated with augmented VR inhomogeneity (Kesek et al., 2004).

Malik et al. in 2004 carried out a research in which stratified risk of arrhythmic events by mean of LVEF and HR, HRV, the slope of HR turbulence and T_{CRT} in patients who might benefit from prophylactic antiarrhytmic intervention. It was evaluated individual risk characteristics and the combinations of them. They concluded that T_{CRT} was a strongest risk stratifier that compared very favorably to LVEF and was also strongest in combination with other stratifiers like LVEF (Malik et al., 2004).

Arini et al., evaluated indexes that quantify the VRD for cardiac risk. The study was carried out in multilead ECG records from animal heart model (*see Table 2*); employing DS and PVS achieved to increment VRD. They calculated indexes from the absolute ECG summation signal (T-wave amplitude, area and width) and from the SVD of the ECG: θ_{PT} (angle between the 1st SVD axis and the VR axis), T_{WR}, T_{MD}, unnormalized T_{MD}, and T_{CRT}. They compared the results with the classical indexes based on QT and concluded that the globally increased VRD can be reflected by T_W (Arini et al., 2008a).

T-wave morphology parameters were studied in LQTS patients by Anttonen et al. in 2009. They wanted to determine if these parameters presented abnormal value in these patients and whether can be used to diagnose LQTS. They measured T_{CRT}, T_{LD} among others and concluded that patients with short QT interval and with a history of arrhythmic events presented abnormal values of T-wave morphology parameters (Anttonen et al., 2009).

4.2 Other T-wave morphology indexes

T-wave amplitude, T-wave symmetry and the relationship between T-wave areas were proposed as markers of cardiac arrhythmogenic. In ischemia, symmetry and amplitude of T-wave changes (Hartikainen, 2004) agreed with a computer model (Di Bernardo et al., 2001) in which this disease was simulated. Studies have found differences in amplitude, area and symmetry of the T-wave stress test (Langley et al., 2002), antiarrhythmic and PVS with respect to control (Arini et al., 2005).

The beat-to-beat variability of VR using QT interval (Section 3.2) approach is largely influenced by criteria used to detect T-wave end point, as was mentioned in Section 2.3. In order to solve this problem, Steinbigler et al. developed the technique of T-wave Spectral Variance (T_{WSV}) using the two dimensional Fast Fourier transform. This technique can detect dynamic changes in VR pattern either in amplitude or duration independently of the exact delineation of T-wave end (see Fig. 3). Steinbigler et al. tested T_{WSV} capacities to detect inhomogeneities of VR in retrospective way of post-MI patients with and without a history of arrhythmias (Steinbigler et al., 1998). Later on, Valverde et al., using an animal model of myocardial infarction, verified the presence of dynamic VR heterogeneity associated with chronic MI and further contributes to identify the infarcted animals (Valverde et al., 2002).

4.3 Micro T-wave alternans

The electrical T-wave alternans is defined as a variation in VR morphology on an alternate beat basis (Murda'H et al., 1997) and can be distinguished in macro and micro alternans.

Macro T-wave alternans refers to a systematic or beat to beat alteration in amplitude, width, and/or shape which can be visualized easily in surface ECG. Micro T-wave alternans (μT_{WA}) is a microscopic alteration of ST-T complex or T-wave, which are revealed through the digital processing of ECG signal (Lux & Brockmeir, 2004) showing dynamic heterogeneity of VR. Experimental and clinical evidence shows that μT_{WA} are linked to abnormal electrophysiological functions and are cardiac risk markers in patient with coronary artery disease (Ikeda et al., 2002; Nearing et al., 1991; Pires 2002; Rosenbaum et al., 1996 as cited in Lux & Brockmeir, 2004) dilated cardiomyopathy (Adachi et al., 1999 as cited in Lux & Brockmeir, 2004), myocardial hypertrophy (Kon-No et al., 2001, as cited in Lux & Brockmeir, 2004) and hypertension (Hennersdorf et al., 2001, as cited in Lux & Brockmeir, 2004). Pastore et al. measured cellular APD employing optical mapping techniques in the epicardial surfaces of guinea pigs revealing more details about μT_{WA} mechanism. They demonstrated that when HR is incremented to critical values, spatial gradients of VR can be developed by neighboring cells membrane repolarization alternating with the opposite phase. This behavior can be detected in surface ECG at microvolt levels and the heterogeneities produced are the cause of regional VRD. Also, these gradients have enough magnitude to induce unidirectional block and reentrant VF (Pastore et al., 1999).

The principal technique used to detect μT_{WA} is spectral analysis and their presence is defined by a magnitude of 1.9 μV or greater, the relationship between μT_{WA} and HR and alternans ratio (Bloomfield et al., 2002).

The spectrum depicts the frequencies at which beat-to-beat fluctuations in the amplitude of the T-wave occur. The μT_{WA} is present with a periods generally of two beats (2:1 relationship) and this appears in the spectrum at a frequency of 0.5 cycles per beat (cpb), hence, the magnitude of the peak at this frequency is a direct measure of electrical alternans allowing differentiate it from another signals occurring at other frequencies like noise or the breathing signal (Murda'H et al., 1997).

The measurement of μT_{WA} is highly dependent on HR, appearing when the HR increases above 90 beats per minutes (Bloomfield et al., 2002). The μT_{WA} measurement can be done in a non invasive way during exercise stress testing or in an invasive way during atrial stimulation with the final objective of keeping HR invariant (Constantini, 2004).
Another important feature of spectral analysis is the alternans ratio (AR), whose value represents the number of standard deviation for which the alternans magnitude exceeded the noise level (Bloomfield et al., 2002).
The significant finding was done by Adam et al. between 1981 and 1984 quantifying from a non-invasive way in dogs (*see Table 3*) μT_{WA} to determine the existence of relation between temporal variability of VR and susceptibility to VF, measured with an index called VF Threshold (VFT). The VFT was reduced inducing hypothermia, tachycardia and by coronary artery ligation (CAL). They found that when VFT was reduced, a μTWA pattern was developed. They made an index, T-wave Alternans Index (TWAI), defined as the square root of the amplitude of the power spectrum minus the noise (Adam et al., 1984) and it was called spectral method (SM).
Smith et al., in 1988 quantified the degree and statistical significance of waveform alternation present in the magnitude of the three orthogonal-lead ECG. Smith et al. reported the relationship between electrical alternans and electrical stability that was found in experimental models with dogs and clinical studies (*see Table 3*). The electrical alternans was measured with an index called Alternating Electrocardiographic Morphology Index (AEMI) and electrical stability in dog preparations was assessed via VFT measurement and in the clinical studies via programmed stimulation (Smith et al., 1988).
Nearing et al. in 1991 implemented the Complex Demodulation Method (CDM) which detected the oscillatory nature of ECG signal during μT_{WA}, modeling it like a sinusoidal signal of 0.5 cpb with phase and amplitude variable. The amplitude was estimated demodulating the 0.5 cpb signal components. They revealed that μT_{WA} is concentrated during the first half of the T-wave coinciding with the vulnerable period of cardiac cycle, linking μT_{WA} with vulnerability of VF (Nearing & Verrier, 1991).
Rosembaum et al. in 1994 tested the Smith et al. hypothesis in humans by mean of electrophysiologic studies (*see table 3*). The μT_{WA} was expressed by two indexes Cumulative Alternans Voltage (CAV) defined as the square root of the alternans peak minus the noise mean and the alternants ratio is defined like the ratio between the alternans peak minus the noise mean and the noise standard deviation. The electrophysiologic test was considered positive if sustained Ventricular Tachycardia (VT) or VF was induced after applied extra stimuli. They concluded that μT_{WA} was a significant predictor of inducible arrhythmias on electrophysiologic testing (Rosembaum et al., 1994).
The method proposed by Laguna et al. consists on applying the Karhunen-Loeve Transform (KLT) to each element of an ST-T vector. Then they calculated the Power Spectral Density (PSD) of the KLi series by the FFT during fixed periods of time. Finally the power band is estimated in those bands around the frequency where alternans appear (0.5 and 0.25cpb). The μTWA is detected when a threshold is exceed. This robust method was validated using simulated and real ECG recordings (Laguna et al., 1996).
Burattini et al. in 1997 performed a time domain Correlation Method (CM) for μT_{WA} detection and compared it with the SM using simulation data. They analyzed the ability of these methods to detect non-stationary μT_{WA} and μT_{WA} under different factors which affect

<table>
<tr><th>Author and year of publication</th><th>Short description</th><th>Index or indication of μT_{WA}</th><th colspan="6">Conditions for the evaluations of methodologies</th></tr>
<tr><td rowspan="3">Adam et al. (1984)</td><td rowspan="3">The experiments were performed in 20 dogs</td><td rowspan="3">TWAI</td><td colspan="2">Hypothermia</td><td colspan="2">Tachycardia</td><td colspan="2">CAL</td></tr>
<tr><td colspan="2" rowspan="2">(7e.)
7/7 VFT↓
p<0.03
6/7 TWAI↑
p< 0.03</td><td colspan="2">Epicardial ECG (6 e.)
6/6 TWAI↑
p< 0.02</td><td colspan="2">Epicardial ECG (11 e.)
11/11 TWAI↑
p< 0.001</td></tr>
<tr><td colspan="2">Surface ECG (10 e.)
07/10 TWAI↑
p< 0.09</td><td colspan="2">Surface ECG (10 e.)
07/10 TWAI↑
p< 0.08</td></tr>
<tr><td rowspan="3">Smith et al. (1988)</td><td rowspan="2">The experiments were performed in 10 dogs</td><td rowspan="2">AEMI (ST-T)</td><td colspan="3">Hypothermia</td><td colspan="3">Transient occlusion of the LAD</td></tr>
<tr><td colspan="3">(10 e.)
10/10 AEMI↑
p<0.0001</td><td colspan="3">(10 e., 24 m)
17/24 AEMI↑
p<0.002</td></tr>
<tr><td>23 studies to predict inducibility of VT or VF</td><td>Presence or absence of alternation</td><td colspan="6">Alternation identify the inducible population with Sen.: 92 % and Spec.: 50%
p< 0.05</td></tr>
<tr><td rowspan="3">Rosembaum (1994)</td><td rowspan="3">83 patients examined to evaluate if levels of μT_{WA} predicted vulnerability to arrhytmia. 66 patients were follows up for 20 months</td><td></td><td colspan="3">General analysis</td><td colspan="3">Patients follow up</td></tr>
<tr><td>AR>2.5</td><td colspan="3">Sen.: 81 %, Spec.: 84%
p< 0.001</td><td colspan="3" rowspan="2">μT_{WA} and inducibility of ventricular arrhythmias, significant predictors of survival without arrhythmia p<0.001</td></tr>
<tr><td>CAV>10 (μV)</td><td colspan="3">Sen: 80 %, Spec: 79%
p< 0.003</td></tr>
<tr><td rowspan="2">Nearing & Verrier (2002)</td><td rowspan="2">Simulated ECG and studies in 13 dogs with CAL to assess vulnerability to VF</td><td rowspan="2">Not specified</td><td colspan="3">Simulation Studies</td><td colspan="3">Experimental Studies</td></tr>
<tr><td colspan="3">The tests present a ρ= 0,999 indicating precision in μT_{WA} detection</td><td colspan="3">Revealed vulnerability to MI-induced VF Sen.: 100 %,Spec.:100 %</td></tr>
</table>

The expression x/z means x experiments (e) or measures (m) achieve a result from z experiments or measures made in total. Abbreviations employed in the table: Sen(Sensibility), Spec (Specificity), ρ (correlation coefficient), isch. (ischemic), CAL (Coronary Artery Ligation), LAD (left anterior descendent)

Table 3. Some relevant results for TWA

real ECG records. The study proved that SM is not adequate for detecting non- stationary μT_{WA}, and while both methods are suitable to detect μT_{WA} in noise presence, with CM were obtained better results (Burattini et al., 1997). In 1999 CM was applied to ECG Holter records from LQTS patients and healthy subjects (Burattini et al., 1999).

Martínez et al. in 2000 evaluated the CDM and CM before mentioned and proposed two alternative methods, one of them was a variation of CDM called Capon Filtering Method (CFM) and the other one based on the KLT. CFM consisted on the replacement of the deterministic filter by a data dependent Capon filter. In addition, Martinez et al. proposed transform the ST- T complex by means of KLT and then apply the CFM. The evaluation of the different detectors was carried out using simulated and real data. This study concluded that CM performed worse than the other methods, which showed a similar performance, having the method that employ KLT and CFM higher computational complexity (Martinez et al., 2000).

In 2002 was proposed a new method to analyze μT_{WA} called Modified Moving Average (MMA) (*see Table 3*). This one consists on dividing the beats in even beats (A) and odd beats (B) and making a moving average for A and another for B. The μT_{WA} is determined like the maximum absolute difference between A and B MMA within the ST segment and T-wave region. They concluded that MMA is better than CDM because the MMA signal processing features are superior to CDM which can be affected by artifacts (Nearing &Verrier, 2002).

A work published in 2002 by Martínez & Olmos showed that the SM and CDM can be interpreted like a Generalized Likelihood Ratio Test (GLRT) for detection of μT_{WA} and tried to prove that Laplacian distribution is more appropriate to model the noise in μT_{WA} than Gaussian. For this they developed a Laplacian Likelihood Ratio (LLR) method which looked for estimate μT_{WA} with the maximum likelihood estimator (MLE) and detect them employing a GLRT. LLR for Laplacian noise was tested with simulated data and founding that LLR is more robust than SM and CDM but the results obtained were not as significant as was expected (Martínez & Olmos, 2002). In 2003 they employed this model with nonstationary noise obtaining similar results (Martínez & Olmos, 2003).

Monasterio & Martínez in 2009 developed a multilead scheme (MS) in which combined LLR with PCA comparing it with a single- lead (SLS) approach in which detected μT_{WA} lead by lead using Laplacian GLRT and alternans estimation is achieved with MLE (Martínez & Olmos, 2002). The MS consists on finding the eigenvectors matrix applying PCA to the output of a detrending filter which input was a data matrix, obtaining the transform leads and μT_{WA} detection is achieved applying Laplacian GLRT to them. The MS was tested with simulated data and showing better results with a lower SNR than the SLS. Moreover both methods were applied on stress ECG records in healthy and ischemic patients. With MS better results were obtained (Monasterio et al., 2009). In 2010 they presented a MS based on periodic component analysis (πCA) concluding that the new πCA MS detect most efficiently than the MS detector based on PCA, and the SLS approach (Monasterio & Martinez, 2010)

5. Conclusions

It has been proposed in the literature several indexes to quantify hetereogeneity of VR using surface ECG. These indexes could be divided into two groups: those based on ECG duration and those founded on ECG morphology. Also, in general, these indexes can be used to evaluate: a) In an individual beat simultaneously recorded leads (spatial heterogeneity) which can be calculated as: QT_D, T_W, T_{PE}, C_R, T_{CRT}, T_{MD}, T_{WR}, T-wave area and

T-wave amplitude or b) in a sequence of beats (dynamic heterogeneity) which can be calculated as: QT_V, T_{WSV}, and μ_{TWA}.
The nature of the relationship between QT_D and VRD is controversial, as was showed in Fig. 3. First, due to technical issues, involving the determination of the T-wave end, the existence of U-wave and notched T-waves, as was showed in Fig. 3. Second, the problems with determining increased heterogeneity of VR using QT_D are the effects generated by the projections of T_L that have different shapes and different angles onto the axis of each ECG lead, which results in T-waves that have different amplitudes and morphologies. That is how to emerge the necessity to find indexes that allow study another aspects of VR and caracterize their anormalities, solving at the same time the problems with measures in the time-domain transforming the ECG signals to another domain obtained by SVD (*see Fig. 4*).
C_R has been evaluated in different cardiac pathologies. This index was employed using 12 standard ECG-lead and, although certain commercial equipment include it, its role in diagnostic is not well defined. In general, the T-wave morphology indexes, such as, T_{CRT}, T_{MD}, T_{WR}, T_{WSV}, have detected medium and high cardiac risk, however, the association between pathological mechanisms and these indexes still need further study.
In another sense, the T_W evaluated from RMS curve or absolute ECG summation signal, could measure apex-base or transmural VRD or both simultaneously, but it is necessary to study these parameters in different cardiac conditions. Although, T_{PE} was measured in a few clinical studies, the results are controversial. While T-wave symmetry and the relationship between T-wave areas has been proposed like cardiac risk markers (Zareba et al., 2000), its use is not widespread.
The μT_{WA} index have shown as a promising risk stratification index of SCD in some clinical populations, and as an important marker of cardiac electrical instability linking μT_{WA} with VRD and ventricular arrhythmias. Despite this, there are still technical limitations in the determination of μT_{WA} and controversy about its clinical validity under certain circumstances. On the other hand, there are a lot of techniques which detect and measure μT_{WA}, but have not been standardized the optimal times, conditions and methods for the measurement of μT_{WA}. Also , μTWA has not been evaluated in combination with other markers of SCD risk. All these aspects not covered yet, can be explored in future studies.
In conclusion, some indexes presented and evaluated in this chapter have restricted capacity to predict cardiac risk, and others have shown potential but still need to validate in medical practice. Also most of them have been evaluated in small patient populations and some of them only in animal models. Hence, in general, it should be carried out more tests for their implementation in the clinical practices. Finally, it would be important an expert consensus to unify criteria for assessment of the parameters to evaluate VRD in the same way that was done for another ECG computational techniques like late potentials in high-resolution ECG (Breithardt et al., 1991) or heart rate variability, (Heart rate variability-Standard, 1996) for which have been developed several standard documents by specialized committees.

6. Acknowledgements

This work has been supported by Consejo Nacional de Investigaciones Científicas y Técnicas (PIP 538) and Agencia Nacional de Promoción Científica y Tecnológica (PICT 2108), both institutions from Argentina.

7. References

Acar, B., Yi, G., Hnatkova K. & Malik M. (1999). Spatial, temporal and wavefront direction characteristics of 12-lead T-wave morphology. *Medical & Biological Engineering & Computing*, Vol.37, pp. 574- 584, ISSN 0140-0118

Adam D., Smith J., Akselrod S., Nyberg S., Powell A. & Cohen R.(1984). Fluctuations in T-Wave Morphology and susceptibility to ventricular fibrillation. *Journal of Electrocardiology*, Vol.17, pp. 209- 218, ISSN 0022-0736

Almeida R., Gouveia S., Rocha A., Pueyo E., Martinez J. & Laguna (2006). QT Variability and HRV interactions in ECG: quantification and reliability. *IEEE Transactions on Biomedical Engineering*, Vol. 53, No. 7, pp 1317-1329, ISSN 0018-9294.

Amlie J. (2000). Increased dispersion of repolarization: A major mechanism behind the genesis of malignant ventricular arrhythmias in cardiac diseases. In: *Dispersion of ventricular repolarization: State of the art*, Olsson S., Amlie J., Yuan S. (Editors), pp. 143-163, Futura Publishing Company, Inc., ISBN 0-87993-458, Armonk, New York

Anttonen O., Junttila J., Giustetto C., Gaita F., Linna E., Karsikas M., Seppänen T., Perkiömäki J., Mäkikallio T., Brugada R. & Huikuri H. (2009). T-Wave morphology in short QT syndrome. *Annals of Noninvasive Electrocardiology*, Vol. 14, No. 3, pp. 262-267, ISSN 1082-720X

Antzelevitch C., Shimizu W., Yan G., Sicouri S., Nesterenko W., Burashnikov A. ,Di Diego J., Saffitz J., & Thomas G. (1999). The M cell: Its contribution to ECG and to normal and abnormal electrical function of the heart. *Journal of Cardiovascular Electrophysiology*, Vol. 10, pp. 1124–1152, ISSN 1045-3873

Arini P., Bertrán G., Valverde E. & Laguna P. (2008a). T-wave width as an index for quantification of ventricular repolarization dispersion: Evaluation in an isolated rabbit heart model. *Biomedical Signal Processing and Control*, Vol. 3, pp. 67-77, ISSN 1746- 8094

Arini P., Baglivo F, Martinez J. & Laguna P. (2008b). Ventricular repolarization dispersion during ischemia course measured by temporal and spatial electrocardiographic parameters. *Computers in Cardiology*, Vol. 35, pp. 323-326, ISSN: 0276-6574

Arini P., Quinteiro R., Valverde E., Bertrán G. & Biagetti M. (2000). Evaluation of QT interval dispersion in a multiple electrodes recording system vs. 12-leads standard ECG in an In Vitro model. *Annals of Noninvasive Electrocardiology*, Vol. 5, No. 2, pp. 125-132, ISSN 1082-720X

Arini P., Valverde E., Quinteiro R., Bertrán G. & Biagetti M. (2001). Differential modulation on ECG indexes of dispersion of ventricular repolarization depending on the site of pacing during premature Stimulation. *Journal of Cardiovascular Electrophysiology*, Vol. 12, No. 1, pp. 36-42, ISSN 1045-3873

Arini P., Valverde E., Bertrán G. & Laguna P (2005). Geometrical and temporal ECG features for quantification of increased ventricular repolarization dispersion in an experimental heart rabbit model. *Computers in Cardiology*, Vol. 32, pp. 89-92, ISSN 0276-6574

Atiga W.L., Calkins H., Lawrence J., Tomaselli G, Smith J & Berger R (1998). Beat-to-beat repolarization lability identifies patients at risk for sudden cardiac death. *Journal of Cardiovascular Electrophysiology*, Vol. 9, No. 9. pp. 899-908, ISSN 1045-3873

Badilini F., Fayn J., Maison-Blanche P., Leenhardt A., Forlini M., Denjoy I., Coumel P. & Rubel P. (1997). Quantitative aspects of ventricular repolarization: relationship between three-dimensional T-wave loop morphology and scalar QT dispersion. *Annals of Noninvasive Electrocardiology*, Vol. 2, No. 2, pp. 146-157, ISSN 1082-720X

Baumert M., Schlaich M, Nalivaiko E., Lambert E., Ika Sari C., Kaye D.M., Esler M., Sanders P. & Lambert G. (2011). Relation between QT interval variability and cardiac sympathetic activity in hypertension. *Amerincan Journal of Physiology – Heart and Circulation Physiology*, Vol. 300, No. 4, pp. 1412-1417, ISSN 0363-6135

Berger R., Kasper E., Baughman K., Marban E., Calkins H. & Tomaselli G. (1997). Beat-to-beat QT interval variability: novel evidence for repolarization lability in ischemic and nonischemic dilated cardiomyopathy. *Circulation*, Vol. 96, No.5, pp. 1557-1565, ISSN 0009-7322

Bexton R., Vallin H. & Camm A.J. (1986). Diurnal variation of the QT interval-influence of the autonomic nervous system. *British Heart Journal*, Vol. 55, pp. 253-258, ISSN 0007 0769

Biagetti M., Arini P., Valverde E., Bertrán G & Quinteiro R. (2004). Role of dipolar and nondipolar components of the T wave in determining the T wave residuum in an isolated rabbit heart model. *Journal of Cardiovascular Electrophysiology*, Vol. 15, pp. 356- 363, ISSN 1045-3873

Bloomfield D., Hohnloser S. & Cohen R. (2002). Interpretation and classification of microvolt T wave alternans test. *Journal of Cardiovascular Electrophysiology*, Vol.13, No.5, pp. 502-512, ISSN 1045-3873

Breithardt G., Cain M., el-Sherif N., Flowers N, Hombach V., Janse M., Simson M. & Steinbeck G. (1991). Standards for analysis of ventricular late potentials using high-resolution or signal-averaged electrocardiography: a statement by a task force committee of the European Society of Cardiology, the American Heart Association, and the American College of Cardiology. *Journal of the American College of Cardiology* 1991, Vol. 17, pp. 999-1006, ISSN 0735-1097

Burattini L., Zareba W. & Moss A. (1999). Correlation method for detection of transient T-wave alternans in digital Holter ECG recordings. *Annals of Noninvasive Electrocardiology*, Vol. 4, No. 4, pp. 416-424, ISSN 1082-720X

Burattini L., Zareba W., Courdec J., Titlebaum E. & Moss A. (1997). Computer detection of non- stationary T wave alternans using a new correlation method. *Computers in Cardiology*, Vol. 24, pp. 657-660, ISSN 0276-6574

Burattini L. & Zareba W. (1999). Time-domain analysis of beat-to-beat variability of repolarization morphology in patients with ischemic cardiomyopathy. *Journal of Electrocardiology*, Vol.32, pp. 166-172, ISSN 0022-0736

Cafiero T., Di Minno, R. & Di Iorio, C. (2010). QT interval and QT dispersion during the induction of anesthesia and tracheal intubation: a comparison of remifentanil and fentanyl. *Minerva Anestesiologica*, Vol. 77, No. 2, pp. 160-165, ISSN 0375 9393

Costantini O. (2004). Microscopic T wave Alternans, In: *Dynamic Electrocardiography*, Malik M. & Camm J., pp. 439 – 447, Blackwell Futura, ISBN 0-4051-1960-8, USA

Couderc J., Zareba W., Burattini L. & Moss A. (1998). New method for the quantification of beat-to-beat T wave temporal variablility based on interscale changes in wavelet transform of the ECG: Application to simulated ECG signals. *Proceeding of the*

IASTED international conference on Signal processing and communications, ISBN 0-88986-580-9, Nevada, USA, October, 1998

Cowan J., Yusoff K., Moore M., Amos P., Gold A., Bourke J., Tansuphaswadikul S. & Campbell R. (1988). Importance of lead selection in QT interval measurement. *American Journal of Cardiology* Vol. 61, No. 1, pp. 83-87, ISSN 0002- 9141

Daskalov I. & Christov I. (1999). Electrocardiogram signal preprocessing for automatic detection of QRS boundaries. *Medical engineering & physics,* Vol. *21,* pp. 37-44, ISSN: 1350-4533

Day C., McComb J. & Campbell R. (1990). QT dispersion: an indication of arrhythmia risk in patients with long QT intervals. *British Heart Journal,* Vol. 63, No. 6, pp. 342-344., ISSN 0007 0769

Day C., McComb J. & Campbell R. (1992). QT dispersion in sinus beats and ventricular extrasystoles in normal hearts. *British Heart Journal,* Vol. 67, No. 1, pp. 39-41, ISSN 0007 0769

de Chazal, P. & Celler B. (1996). Automatic measurement of the QRS onset and offset in individual ECG leads. *Proceedings of the 18th Annual International Conference of the IEEE Engineering in Medicine and Biology Society,* ISBN 0-7803-3811-1, Amsterdam, The Netherlands, October, 1996

Di Bernardo D. & Murray A. (2001). T wave shape in clinical research. *Circulation*; pp.104:e80

Eagle K. (1994). Images in clinical medicine. Osborn wave of hypothermia. *New England Journal of Physiology,* Vol. 10, pp. 680, ISSN 0028-4793

Fuller M., Sándor G., Punske B., Taccardi B., MacLeod R., Ershler P., Green L., & Lux R. (2000). Estimation of repolarization dispersion from electrocardiographic measurements. *Circulation,* Vol. 102, pp. 685–691, ISSN 0009 7322

Hanci V., Ayoglu H., Yurtlu S., Yildirim N., Okyay R., Erdogan G., Sayin E. & Turan I. (2010). An evaluation of P wave dispersion, QT, corrected QT and corrected QT dispersion intervals on the electrocardiograms of malnourished adults. *Anesthesia and Intensive Care,* Vol. 38, No. 1, pp. 122-127, ISSN 0310- 057X

Hartikainen J. (2004). T wave and QT interval changes related to myocardial ischaemia, In: *Dynamic Electrocardiography,* Malik M., Camm J., (Editors). pp. 380 – 389, Blackwell Futura, ISBN 0-4051-1960-8, USA

Heart rate variability. Standards of measurement, physiological interpretation, and clinical use. Task Force of the European Society of Cardiology and the North American Society of Pacing and Electrophysiology (1996). *Circulation,*Vol. 93, pp. 1043-1095, ISSN 0009-7322

Higham P., Hilton C., Aitcheson J., Furniss S., Bourke J. & Campbell, R. (1992). Does QT dispersion reflect dispersion of ventricular recovery? *Circulation,* Vol. 86(Suppl.), pp. 392-392, ISSN 0009-7322

Hnatkova K., Kulakowski P., Staunton A., Keeling P., Yi G., Camm A. & Malik M. (1994a). Influence of filtering techniques on the time-domain analysis, diagnosis, and clinical use of signal-averaged electrocardiogram. *Pacing Clinical Electrophysiology,* Vol. 17, No.6, pp. 1107-1117, ISSN 0147 8389

Hnatkova K., Malik M., Kautzner J., Yi G. & Camm J. (1994b). Adjustment of QT dispersion assessed from 12 lead electrocardiograms for different numbers of analyzed electrocardiographic leads: comparison of stability of different methods. *British Heart Journal,* Vol. 72, No.4, pp. 390-396, ISSN 0007 0769

Hodges M. (1997). Rate correction of the QT interval. *Cardiac Electrophysiology Review*, Vol. 3, pp. 360-363, ISSN 1385 2264

Huhta J. & Webster J. (1973). 60-Hz interference in electrocardiography. *IEEE Transactions on Biomedical Engineering*, Vol. 20, No. 2, pp. 91-101, ISSN 0018-9294

Ider Y. & Köymen H. (1995). Removal of power line interference monitoring and reduction in biopotential amplifiers, *IEEE Transactions on Biomedical Engendering*, Vol. 37, pp. 731-735, ISSN 0018-9294

Janse M., Capucci A., Coronel R. & Fabius M. (1985).Variability of recovery of excitability in the normal and ischaemic porcine heart. *European Heart Journal*, Vol. 6 (suppl), pp. 41-52, ISSN 0195-668x

Kautzner J., Yi G., Camm J. & Malik M. (1994). Short- and long-term reproducibility of QT, QTc, and QT dispersion measurement in healthy subjects. *Pacing clinical Electrophysiology*, Vol. 17, pp. 928-937, ISSN 0147 8389

Kawataki M., Kashima T., Toda H. & Tanaka H. (1984). Relation between QT interval and heart rate. Applications and limitations of Bazett's formula. *Journal of Electrocardiology*, Vol. 17, pp. 371-375, ISSN 0022-0736

Kesek M., Jernberg T., Lindahl B., Xue J. & Englund A. (2004). Principal component analysis of the T wave in patients with chest pain and conduction disturbance. *Pacing and Clinical Electrophysiology*, Vol. 27, pp. 1378-1387, ISSN 0147-8389

Kligfield P., Lax K. & Okin P. (1996). The QT interval-heart rate relationship during exercise in normal men and women: definition by linear regression analysis. *Journal of the American College of Cardiology* Vol. 28, pp. 1547-1555, ISSN 0735-1097

Köhler B., Hennig C. & Orglmeister R. (2002). The principles of software QRS detection, *IEEE Engineering in Medicine and Biology Magazine*, Vol. 21, No. 1, pp. 42:57, ISSN 0739-5175

Koponen H., Alaraisanen A., Saari K., Pelkonen O., Huikuri H., Raatikainen M., Savolainen M. & Isohanni M. (2008). Schizophrenia and sudden cardiac death: a review. *Nordic Journal of Psychiatry*, Vol. 62, No.5, pp. 342-345, ISSN 0803-9488

Kors J., van Herpen G. & van Bemmel J. (1999). QT dispersion as an attribute of T-loop morphology. *Circulation*, Vol. 99, No.11, pp. 1458-1463, ISSN 0009-7322

Kors J. & van Herpen G. (1998). Measurement error as a source of QT dispersion: A computerized analysis. *Heart*, Vol. 80, pp. 453-458, ISSN 1355-6037

Kuo C., Munakata K., Reddy P. & Surawicz B. (1983). Characteristics and possible mechanism of ventricular arrhythmia dependent on the dispersion of action potential. *Circulation*, Vol. 67, pp. 1356–1367, ISSN 0009 7322

Laciar E. & Jané R. (2001). An improved weighted signal averaging method for high-resolution ECG signals. *Computers in Cardiology*, Vol. 28, pp. 69-72, ISSN: 0276-6574

Laguna P., Ruiz M., Moody G. & Mark R. (1996). Repolarizacion alternance detection using the KL transform and the beatquency spectrum. *Computers in Cardiology*, Vol.23, pp. 673-676, ISSN 0276-6574

Langley P., Bernardo D. & Murray A. (2002). Quantification of T wave shape changes following exercise *Pacing and Clinical Electrophysiology*, Vol. 25, pp. 1230-1234, ISSN 0147-8389

Lee K., Kligfield P., Okin P. & Dower G. (1998). Determinants of precordial QT dispersion in normal subjects. *Journal of Electrocardiology*, Vol. 31 Suppl, pp. 128-133, ISSN 0022-0736

Li C., Zheng C. & Tai C. (1995). Detection of ECG characteristics points using wavelet transforms. *IEEE Trans Biomed Eng.*, Vol. 42, pp. 21-28.

Lux R. & Brockmeier K. (2004). Macro T wave alternans, In: *Dynamic Electrocardiography*, Malik M. & Camm J. (Editors), pp. 433 – 438, Blackwell Futura, ISBN 0-4051-1960-8, USA

Macfarlane P., McLaughlin S. & Rodger, J. (1998). Influence of lead selection and population on automated measurement of QT dispersion. *Circulation*, Vol. 98, No. 20, pp. 2160-2167, ISSN 0009- 7322

Malik M., Acar B., Gang Y., Yap G., Hnatkova K. & Camm J. (2000). QT dispersion does not represent electrocariographic interlead heterogeneity of ventricular repolarization. *Journal of Cardiovascular Electrophysiology*, Vol. 11, pp. 835-843, ISSN 1045- 3873

Malik M., Hnatkova K. & Batchvarov V. (2004). Post infarction risk stratification using the 3-D angle between QRS complex and T-wave vectors. *Journal of Electrocardiology*, Vol. 37, pp. 201-208, ISSN 0022-0736

Malik, M. (2002). The imprecision of heart rate correction may lead to artificial observations of drug-induced QT interval changes. *Pacing and Clinical Electrophysiology*, Vol. 25, pp. 209-216, ISSN 0147-8389

Mänttäri M, Oikarinen L., Manninen V., & Viitasalo M. (1997). QT dispersion as a risk factor for sudden death and fatal myocardial infarction in a coronary risk population. *Heart*, Vol. 78, pp. 268-272, ISSN 1355-6037

Martínez J. & Olmos (2003). Detection of T wave alternans in non- stationary noise: a GLRT approach. *Computers in Cardiology*, Vol. 30, pp. 161-164, ISSN 0276- 6574

Martínez J. & Olmos. (2002). A robust T wave alternans detector based on the GLRT for Laplacian noise distribution. *Computers in Cardiology*, Vol. 29, pp. 677- 680, ISSN 0276- 6574

Martínez J., Olmos S. & Laguna P. (2000). Simulation study and performance evaluation of T- wave alternans detector. *Proceedings of the 22nd Annual EMBS International Conference*, ISSN 0-7803-6465, Chicago IL.,USA, July 23-28, 2000.

Martínez J., Borges de Almeida R., Olmos S., Rocha A. & Laguna P. (2004). A wavelet-based ECG delineator: Evaluation on standard databases. *IEEE Transactions on Biomedical Engineering*, Vol. 51, No. 4, pp. 570-581

Monasterio V., Clifford G., Laguna P. & Martínez J. (2010). A multilead scheme based on periodic component analysis for T- wave alternans analysis in the ECG. *Annals of Biomedical Engineering*, Vol. 38, No 8, pp. 2532- 2541, ISSN 0009 6964

Monasterio V., Laguna P. & Martínez J. (2009). Multilead analysis of T- wave alternans in the ECG using principal component analysis. *IEEE Transactions on Biomedical Engineering*, Vol. 56, No 7, pp. 1880- 1890, ISSN 0018-929

Murda'H M., Mckenna W. & Camm J. (1997). Repolarization alternans: techniques, mechanisms and cardiac vulnerability. *Pacing and Clinical Electrophysiology*, Vol.20, pp. 2641- 2669, ISSN 01478389

Nearing B. & Verrier R. (2002). Modified moving average analysis of T- wave alternans to predict ventricular fibrillation with high accuracy. *Journal of Applied Physiology*, Vol. 92, No. 2, pp. 541- 549, ISSN 8750-7587

Nearing B., Huang A. & Verrier R. (1991). Dynamic tracking of cardiac vulnerability by complex demodulation of the T wave. *Science*, Vol. 252, pp. 437-440, ISSN 0036 8075

Pan J. & Tompkins W. (1985). A real-time QRS detection algorithm. *IEEE Transactions on Biomedical Engineering*, Vol. 32, pp 230-236, ISSN 0018-9294.

Pastore J., Girouard S., Laurita K., Akar F. & Rosembaum D. (1999). Mechanism linking T wave alternans to the genesis of cardiac fibrillation. *Circulation*, Vol. 99, pp. 1385-1394, ISSN 0009-7322

Pinto V. (1991). Filters for the reduction of baseline wander and muscle artifact in the ECG, *Journal of Electrocardiology*, Vol. 25 (Suppl.), pp. 40-48, ISSN 0022-0736

Priori S., Napolitano C., Diehl L. & Schwartz P. (1994). Dispersion of the QT interval. A marker of therapeutic efficacy in the idiopathic long-QT Syndrome. *Circulation*, Vol. 89, pp. 1681-1689, ISSN 0009-7322

Priori S., Mortara D., Napolitano C., Diehl L., Paganini V., Cantù F., Cantù G. & Schwartz P. (1997). Evaluation of the spatial aspects of T-wave complexity in the long- QT syndrome. *Circulation*, Vol. 96, No.9, pp. 3006-3012, ISSN 0009-7322

Rosembaum D., Jackson L., Smith J., Garan H., Ruskin J. & Cohen R. (1994). Electrical alternans and vulnerability to ventricular arrhythmias. *The New England Journal of Medicine*, Vol.330, No.4, pp. 235- 241, ISSN 0028-4793

Shimizu W. & Antzelevitch C. (1998). Cellular basis for the ECG features of the LQT1 form of the long QT syndrome. Effects of β- adrenergic agonist and antagonist and sodium channel blockers on transmural dispersion of repolarization and torsades de pointes. *Circulation*, Vol. 98, pp. 2314–2322.

Shusterman V, Aysin B & Gottipaty V. (1998). Autonomic nervous system activity and the spontaneous initiation of ventricular tachycardia. *Journal of American College of Cardiology*; Vol. 32, pp. 1891-1899, ISSN 0363 6135

Smith J., Clancy E., Valeri R., Ruskin J. & Cohen R. (1988). Electrical alternans and cardiac electrical inestability. *Circulation*, Vol. 77, No. 1, pp. 110-121, ISSN 0009-7322

Sörnmo L. & Laguna P. (2005). *Bioelectrical Signal Processing in Cardiac and Neurological Applications, Elsevier Academic Press,* ISBN 0-12-437552-9, Amsterdam, The Netherlands.

Sörnmo L. & Laguna P. (2006). Electrocardiogram (ECG) Signal Processing. In: *Wiley Encyclopedia of Biomedical Engineering*, Metin Akay (Editor), John Wiley & Sons, Inc, Vol. 2, pp. 1298-1313, ISBN 0-471-24967-X.

Sörnmo L. (1993). Time-variable digital filtering of ECG baseline wander, *Medical & Biological Engeniering & Computing*., Vol. 31, No. 5, pp. 503-508, ISSN 0140-0118.

Steinbigler P., Haberl R. & Steinbeck G. (1998). T wave spectral variance. A new method to determine inhomogeneous repolarization by T wave beat-to-beat variability in patients prone to ventricular arrhytmias, *Journal of Electrocardiology*, Vol. 30, suppl., pp. 137-144.

Subramanian R., Shalaby A. Campbell R. & Sager P. (1999). Is QT dispersion altered by changes in heart rate? *Journal of American College of Cardiology*, Vol. 33, pp. 113A-114A, ISSN 0735-1097

Surawicz B. (1997). Ventricular fibrillation and dispersion of repolarization. *Journal of Cardiovascular Electrophysiology* , Vol. 8, pp. 1009–1012, ISSN 1045-3873

Sylven J., Horacek B., Spencer C., Klassen G., Campbell, R. & Montague T. (1984). QT interval variability on the body surface. *Journal of Electrocardiology*, Vol. 17, No.2, pp. 179-188, ISSN 0022-0736

Taback L., Marden E., Mason H.L. & Pipberger H.V. (1959). Digital recording of electrocardiographic data for analysis by digital computer. *IRE Trans Med Electron*, Vol. 6, pp. 167-171, ISSN 0097-1049

Talmon J., Kors J. & van Bemmel J. (1986). Adaptive Gaussian filtering in routine ECG/VCG analysis, *IEEE Transactions in Acoustic, Speech and Signal Processing* Vol. 34, pp. 527-534, ISSN 0096-3518

Thakor N., Webster J. & Tompkins W. (1984). Estimation of QRS complex power spectrum for design of a QRS filter, *IEEE Transactions on Biomedical Engineering.*, Vol. 31, No. 11, pp. 702-706, ISSN 0018-9294

Valverde E., Quinteiro R., Arini P., Bertrán G. and Biagetti M. (2002). Beat-to-beat repolarization variability measured by T wave spectral variance index in chronic infarcted animals. *Annals of Noninvasive Electrocardiol*, Vol.7, nro. 4, pp. 319-325.

Webster J. (1992). *Medical Instrumentation. Application and Design*, J. Webster (Editor), 2nd Edition, Houghton Mifflin Co., ISBN 0-395-59492-8, Boston, USA.

Weinberg G. (1995). Mechanism of cardiac arrhytmias, In: *Design of cardiac pacemaker*, Webster J (Editor), pp. 35-63, IEEE Press, ISBN 0-7803-1134-5, Piscataway

Xue Q. & Reddy S. (1998). Algorithms for computerized QT analysis. *Journal of Electrocardiology*. Vol. 30, Suppl 1., pp. 181-186.

Yeragani, V., Adiga S., Desai N. & Berger R. (2004) Beat-to-beat QT interval variability in atrial fibrillation with and without congestive cardiac failure. *Ann Noninvasive Electrocardiol*ogy, Vol. 9, pp. 304-305, ISSN 0009- 6964

Zabel M. & Malik M. (2004). Morphological assessment of T wave patterns, In: *Dynamic Electrocardiography*, Malik M. & Camm J., pp. 351 – 357, Blackwell Futura, ISBN 0-4051-1960-8, USA

Zabel M., Acar B., Klingenheben T., Franz M., Hohnloser S. & Malik M. (2000). Analysis of 12- Lead T- Wave Morphology for Risk Stratification After Myocardial Infarction. *Circulation*, Vol. 102, (April, 2000), pp. 1252-1257, ISSN 0009-7322

Zabel M., Malik M., Hnatkova K., Papademetriou V., Pittaras A., Fletcher R. & Franz M. (2001). Analysis of T-wave morphology from the 12- leads electrocardiogram for prediction of long- term prognosis in male US veterans. *Circulation*, Vol. 105, (February, 2002), pp. 1066-1070, ISSN 0009-7322

Zabel M., Kligenheben T., Franz M.R. & Hohnloser S.H. (1998a). Assesment of QT dispersion for prediction of mortality or arrhythmic events after myocardial infarction. Results of a prospective, long-term follow-up study. *Circulation*, Vol. 97, pp. 2543-2550, ISSN 0009-7322

Zabel, M., Lichtlen, P.R., Haverich, A. & Franz, M.R. (1998b). Comparison of ECG variables of dispersion of ventricular repolarization with direct myocardial repolarization measurements in the human heart. *Journal of Cardiovascular Electrophysiology*, Vol. 9, No.12, pp. 1279-1284, ISSN 1045-3873

Zabel M., Portnoy S. & Franz M. (1995). Electrocardiographic indexes of dispersion of ventricular repolarization: an isolated heart validation study. *Journal of American College of Cardiology*, Vol. 25, No. 3, pp. 746-752, ISSN 07351097

Zabel M., Woosley R. & Franz M.R. (1997). Is dispersion of ventricular repolarization rate dependent? *Pacing and Clinical Electrophysiology*, Vol. 20, pp. 2405-2411, ISSN 0147-8389

Zareba W., Couderc J. & Mos, A. (2000). Automatic detection of spatial and temporal heterogeneity of repolarization. In: *Dispersion of ventricular repolarization*, Olsson S., Amlie J. & Yuan S. (Editors), pp. 85–107. Futura Publishing Company, Inc., ISBN 0-87993-458, Armonk, New York

11

Recognition of Cardiac Arrhythmia by Means of Beat Clustering on ECG-Holter Recordings

J.L. Rodríguez-Sotelo[1], G. Castellanos-Domínguez[2] and C.D. Acosta-Medina[3]

[1]*Grupo de Automática, Facultad de Ingeniería, Universidad Autónoma de Manizales,*
[2]*Grupo de Procesamiento y Reconocimiento de Señales, Universidad Nacional de Colombia*
[3]*Grupo de Computación Científica y Modelamiento Matemático, Universidad Nacional de Colombia*
Colombia

1. Introduction

The development of bio-signal analysis systems, mostly, has become a major research field due to technological progress in signal processing. Electrocardiography (ECG) had been amongst the most studied type of bio-signals for several decades. Research on this type of signals has become an important tool for the diagnosis of cardiac disorders. Because of its simplicity, low cost and a non-invasive nature it is still widely used despite newer available techniques.

This chapter deal with the problem of long-term recording analysis corresponding to ECG signals of Holter recordings. The motivation for studying this issue focuses on the development of methods for cardiac arrhythmia analysis to identify particular events occurring at specific periods of time. Such events are associated to cardiac disorders that may become potentially harmful to the patient. The developed methods are aimed at further building up of specialized equipment that will provide clinical monitoring for both the patient and the specialist, as well as the support for real time diagnosis.The above mentioned will decrease mortality rates regarding heart problems specially for people living in rural areas. This technology will benefit them to have access to a quicker and efficient specialized medical diagnostics.

This chapter focuses on analyzing two major aspects of Holter recordings: The first one corresponds to the large amount of data stored in such recordings, reaching up to 100.000 heartbeats for its evaluation, which becomes a hard task for the specialist to assess the information and to decide what heartbeats are important for a determined analysis. There are cases where only a few beats allow to identify a certain pathology or to prevent deadly diseases. Therefore, a detailed analysis of the complete record is needed. The second aspect corresponds to the intrinsic characteristics of the signal, such as heart rate variability, morphological variety, among others. They may result from problems in the cardiac system or the patient's physical and physiological characteristics. In addition, the electrical nature of ECG signals and its transmission to electronical devices increase the noise sensitivity, which can completely alter the diagnostic information contained in the signal, changing the training processes in the identification of cardiac pathologies.

Consequently, both aspects have been strongly considered in the automatic ECG processing and analysis procedures to detect, classify, and cluster heartbeats. Thus, several methods have been reported in the scientific literature to carry out those classification–related tasks, using either supervised Ceylan & Özbay (2007); De-Chazal et al. (2004); Wen et al. (2007); Özbay et al. (2006) or unsupervised Cuesta et al. (2007); Lagerholm et al. (2000); Rodríguez-Sotelo et al. (2009) approaches. Due to a large variability in ECG heartbeat morphology; the former methods tuned for a specific ECG dataset may decrease performances in other datasets. In addition, these techniques require a considerable amount of known and labeled heartbeats which are not feasible when having long–term ECG monitoring.

Regarding unsupervised methods, even though their performance does not usually overperform supervised training, they can be applied to a broader set of ECG recordings because they can dynamically adapt to new signal features. However, additional factors must be taken into account in the unsupervised analysis, such as highly unbalanced classes, uncertainty of the number of classes, signal variability, artifacts, etc. This type of analysis is more convenient for Holter monitoring.

There are still some open issues when implementing unsupervised analyses, such as computational cost, unbalanced clusters, unknown number of clusters and initial partition. They are also described in this chapter ending up in an unsupervised analysis methodology that can be implemented in oriented devices for analysis in real time. The considered methodology does not require prior training or heartbeat labeling by the specialist and can be applied to ECG signals that have great variability in time and morphology, identifying the main arrhythmias set by the AAMI standard.

Objective

To describe a non-supervised methodology for analysing ECG signals of Holter recordings including preprocessing, feature estimation, relevance analysis and clustering stages, in order to identify cardiac arrhythmias, according to ANSI/AAMI EC57:1998 standards, and to provide a proper trade-off between computational cost and performance.

Abbreviations and operators

ECG	Electrocardiogram
QRS	Complex of three graphical deflections seen on a typical ECG
AAMI	Association for the Advancement of Medical Instrumentation
HRV	Heart Rate Variability
PCA	Principal Component Analysis
WPCA	Weighted Principal Componente Analysis
MSE	Mean Square Error
GEMC	Gaussian Expectation Max-minimization-based Clustering
MSSC	Minimum Sum of Squares-based Clustering
DTW ($\mathrm{dtw}(\cdot,\cdot)$)	Dynamic Time Warping
$\langle\cdot,\cdot\rangle$	Inner product
$\langle\cdot,\cdot\rangle_{\boldsymbol{A}}$	M-inner product regarding matrix $\boldsymbol{A}$
$\mathcal{E}\{\cdot\}$	Expectation operator

2. Cardiac arrhythmias

In general, the pathologies observed using the ECG are divided into three categories:

1. Heart rhythm disturbances, or arrhythmias.
2. Dysfunctions of blood perfusion in the myocardium or cardiac ischemia.
3. Chronic disorders of mechanical structure of the heart, such as left ventricular hypertrophy.

We will describe the characterization and identification of the first type of pathologies above mentioned. The methods are developed over the entire *QRS* complexes that are associated with ventricular electrical activity. They contain clinic important information, for example their morphology has significant changes in abnormal ventricular heartbeats. *QRS* complexes are also present in most of the heartbeats and their signal to noise ratio is the highest among all waves present in the signal.

2.1 Not imminently life-threatening cardiac arrhythmias

Broadly speaking, arrhythmias can be divided into two groups: The first group includes ventricular fibrillation and tachycardia, which are life-threatening disorders and require immediate therapy with a defibrillator. Identification of these arrhythmias and successful detectors have been developed with high sensitivity and specificity degree. However, this study just analyzes the second group, which includes arrhythmias that are not imminently life-threatening but may require therapy to prevent further problems.
According to the AAMI standard (ANSI/AAMI EC57:1998/(R)2003) as is described in De-Chazal et al. (2004), the following arrhythmia groups shown in Table 1 are of interest to be examined: Normal–labeled heartbeat recordings (termed *N*), Supraventricular ectopic beat (*Sv*), Ventricular ectopic beat (*V*), Fusion beat (*F*), as well as unknown beat class (*Q*) are taken into consideration. One or more classes of such arrhythmias can be present during Holter analysis.
The MIT/BIH arrhythmia database Moody & Mark (1982) is one of the most representatives, at a scientific level, to evaluate the design of algorithms regarding the analysis of cardiac arrythmias. The database contains several types of beats within each group of arrhythmias recommended by the AAMI, for example, in the Normal group we can find the following arrhythmia types: Left bundle Branch Block (*LBBB*), Right Bundle Branch Block (*RBBB*), Atrial Escape (*AE*) and junctional Nodal Escape (*NE*). The Table 1 shows a classification of arrhythmias previously mentioned.

2.1.1 Group of arrhythmias *N*

It corresponds to any beat that does not belong to *Sv*, *V*, *F* or *Q* classes (Table 1), as shown in Figure 1. Bundle Branch Block (BBB) is a disorder in the conduction of electrical impulses to the ventricles Braunwald (1993). The electrical impulse conduction to the ventricles is carried out via the *His* bundle and its divisions: right and left bundle branch. When one of these branches is altered, the electrical impulse spreads throughout the ventricular muscle itself rather than spreading in the Purkinje system. This reduces the conduction velocity. In case there is blockage in one of the branches, the complex will take more time than normal Guyton & Hall (n.d.). Branch blocks also originate morphological changes (*R*-prime) within the *QRS* complex.
In the *LBBB*, cardiac depolarization spreads much faster in the right ventricle compared to the left ventricle. Therefore, the left ventricle remains polarized longer than the right one. This is

AAMI heartbeat	Description	MIT/BIH heartbeat types
N	Any beat not in the *Sv*,*V*,*F* or *Q* classes	Normal (*N*), Left Bundle Branch Block (*LBBB*), Right Bundle Branch Block (*RBBB*), Atrial Escape (*AE*), Nodal (junctional) escape beat(*NE*)
Sv	Supraventricular ectopic beat	Atrial Premature (*AP*), Aberrated Atrial Premature (*aAP*), Nodal (junctional) Premature (*NP*), Supraventricular Premature (*SP*),
V	Ventricular ectopic beat	Premature Ventricular Contraction (*PVC*), Ventricular escape (*VE*)
F	Fusion beat	Fusion of ventricular and normal (*fVN*), Fusion of paced and normal beat (*fPN*)
Q	Unknown beat	Paced (*P*), Unclassified (*Q*)

Table 1. Set of analyzed arrhythmias according to the AAMI standard.

observed in left precordial leads (V_5 and V_6) through an extension and a morphological change (RR') of the *QRS*. Besides, in the *RBBB*, the impulse conduction through the right ventricle is delayed regarding the left one, in this way, the *QRS* is prolonged and generates a morphology known as *rsR* observed in the right precordial leads (V_1 and V_2).
The *BBB* does not necessarily mean heart disease, since it can occur also in healthy patients. It may have a good prognosis and may not progress to a higher degree block Micó & Ibor (2004). However, in some studies Brugada et al. (1998); ginsburg et al. (2006); Pabón (2001) it was found that the presence of *RBBB* is correlated with arterial hypertension, heart failure, coronary disease, pulmonary embolism, and increased mortality and the presence of *LBBB* increases the risk of coronary heart disease, mortality and ventricular myocardial infarction Balaguer (n.d.), Li et al. (n.d.). Thus, it is necessary to detect such arrhythmias because of the prognostic value they have.
The *AE* are characterized by occasionally appearing and interrupt the pace of the rate base. The most common are those identified ahead of that cadence or extrasistoles and those delayed or escape heartbeats. Depending on the morphology of the waves,it will be possible to know the origin of the heartbeats (atrial, nodal or ventricular) and the type of the existing AtrioVentricular (*AV*) conduction.

2.1.2 Group of arrhythmias type *Sv*

It includes both, atrial and supraventricular premature beats as well as their variants. An example is illustrated in Figure 2. An Atrial Premature Beat (APB) is also called Atrial Ectopic Beat (AEB) or Premature Atrial Contraction (PAC). It is an extra heartbeat caused by electrical activation of the atrium from an abnormal site before a normal heartbeat happens. Generally, APBs occur in healthy people that rarely have symptoms. It is common among people who have lung problems, specially in adults instead of young people. Recent studies on risk factors for stroke have shown that frequent APB heartbeats are an independent risk factor for suffering a stroke Rodríguez-Sotelo et al. (2009).

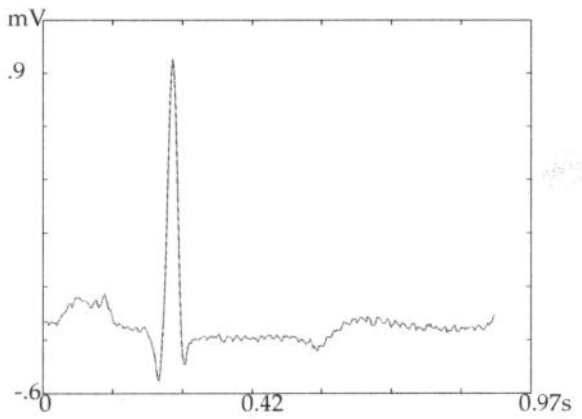

(a) Normal heartbeat

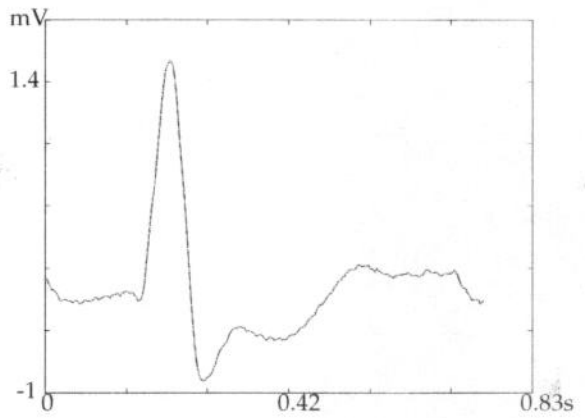

(b) LBBB beat

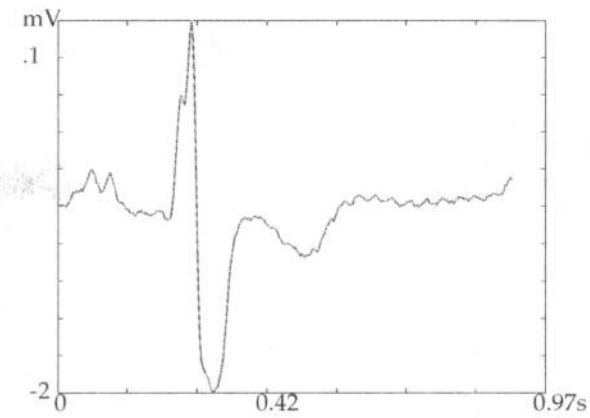

(c) RBBB beat

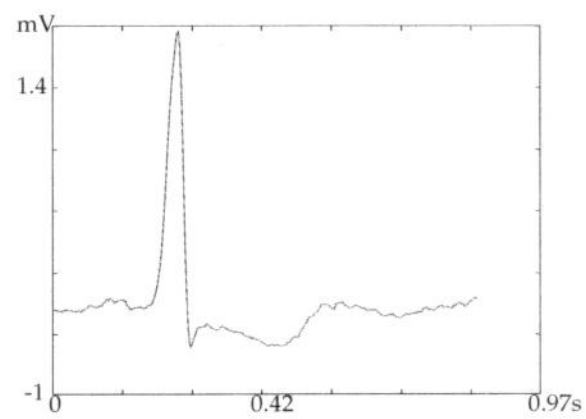

(d) Atrial Escape beat

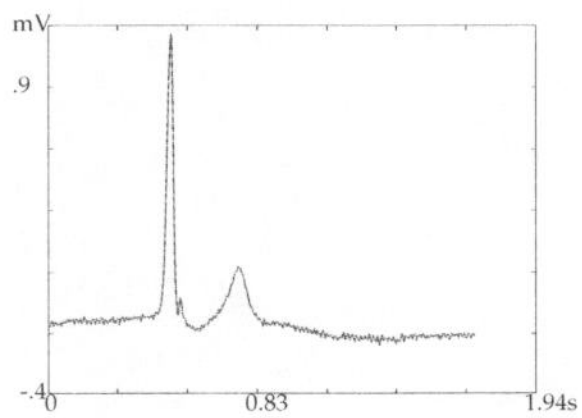

(e) Nodal escape beat

Fig. 1. Heartbeats of *N* group, extracted from MIT/BIH database.

Although, APBs are often considered a benign disorder, it has been shown in clinical practice that frequent APBs could be an early symptom of heart failure and may precede atrial fibrillation.

Frequent APBs can be an indicator for other risk factors, such as severe hypertension, asymptomatic atherosclerosis, structural abnormalities causing stroke, calcified mitral valve or enlargement of the left atrium. These risk factors might increase in the formation of thromboembolism Engström et al. (2000).

Experts have usually analysed Holter recordings for detecting APB beats due to their frequency and they have found that detecting them is troublesome because of their nature. They have shown similar morphological characteristics in contrast to normal heartbeats which accounts for the majority. Particularly, ventricular depolarization and repolarization have displayed similar morphology between *QRS* complexes and *T* waves. Atrial depolarization has also been used for identifying such beats, it means analysing *PR* intervals and *P* waves. Nevertheless, there may exist beats that do not have *P* waves, since beats overlap with a previous *T* wave which results in a slight increase of its amplitude. Heart rate variability (HRV) is another more effective technique used to detect APB heartbeats.

From a physiological point of view, before there is a completion of ventricular repolarization, there is a premature excitement in the atrial area different from the sinus node. This fact results in a premature beat. Besides, there will be a delay in the activation of the sinus node for the next cardiac cycle, triggering both an increase and a later decrease of the heart rate. The HRV's drawback is that if there is continuous premature beats, the pattern just described disappears. In some cases this is interpreted as normal pace beats reducing possibilities to succeed in the detection of APB beats through this technique.

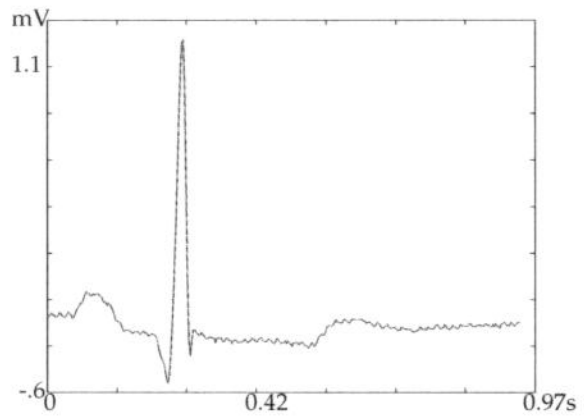

(a) Atrial Premature Beat (APB)

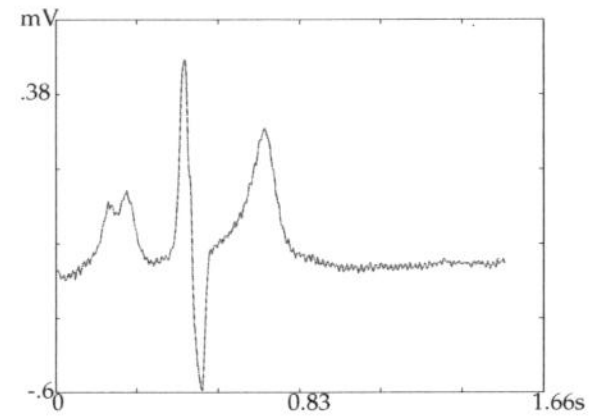

(b) Aberrated APB

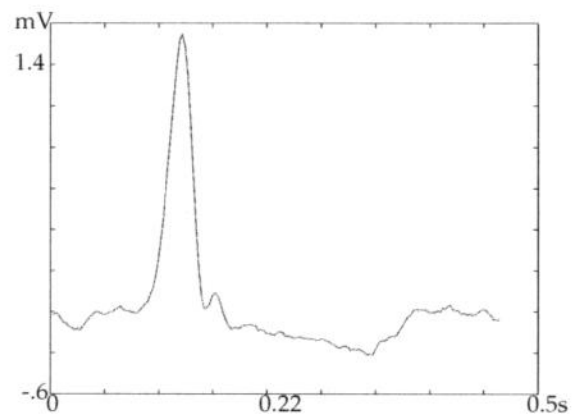

(c) Nodal Premature Beat

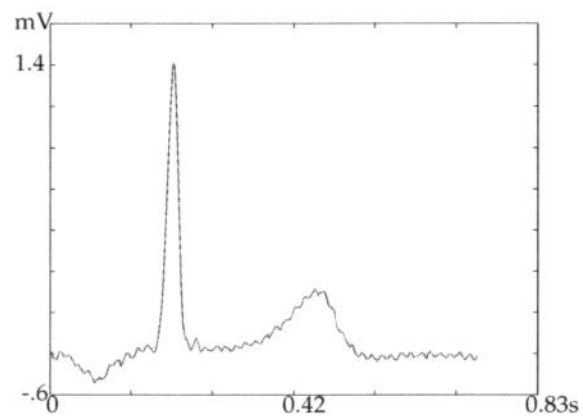

(d) Supraventricular Premature Beat

Fig. 2. Heartbeats of *Sv* group, extracted from MIT/BIH database.

2.1.3 Group of arrhythmias type *V*

A ventricular premature beat (ventricular ectopic beat, premature ventricular contraction) is an extra heartbeat resulting from abnormal electrical activation originated in the ventricles before a normal heartbeat occurs. See Figure 3. The main symptom is a perception of a skipped heartbeat. ECG is used to diagnose such condition. In some avoiding stress, caffeine, and alcohol may be usually enough to treat this condition. Ventricular premature beats are more common in adults. This arrhythmia may also be caused by physical or emotional stress, intake of caffeine (in beverages and foods) or alcohol, or use of cold or fever remedies containing drugs that stimulate the heart, like pseudoephedrine. Other causes include coronary artery disease (especially during or shortly after a heart attack) and disorders that cause ventricles to enlarge, like heart failure and heart valve disorders.

VE beats are hardly found in ECG of 12-leads, therefore Holter recordings are used for their detection Holter (n.d.). VEs can be identified following certain criteria of morphological features of the ECG Dave et al. (2005); Friedman (1989):

- *QRS* duration: It is higher than the average *QRS* dominant. It is due to an abnormal activation of the ventricle.
- Different morphologies in the *QRS* complexes are present: There are not preceding *P* waves prematurely. *T* wave is often found in the opposite direction of *R* wave. If heartbeats originated from a single focus, all the VPC would have the same morphology, although different from the normal one.
- RR intervals: They are shorter than RR average and later a complete compensatory pause can be observed in the heartbeat.

- VEs originated from the left ventricle normally produce heartbeat patterns of RBBB and the ones originated from the right ventricle normally produce heartbeat patterns associated with LBBB.

A ventricular escape beat is another type of ventricular extrasystole. It is a self-generated electrical discharge initiated by the ventricles that causes their contraction. It has been stated that the heart rhythm begins in the atria of the heart and is subsequently transmitted to the ventricles. The ventricular escape beat is followed after a long pause in ventricular rhythm to prevent from a possible cardiac arrest. It indicates a failure of the electrical conduction system of the heart to stimulate the ventricles (This would lead to the absence of heartbeats, unless ventricular escape beats occur).
Ventricular escape beats happen when the rate of electrical discharge reaches the ventricles and they in turn alter the base rate. An escape beat usually occurs around 23s after an electrical impulse has failed to reach the ventricles.

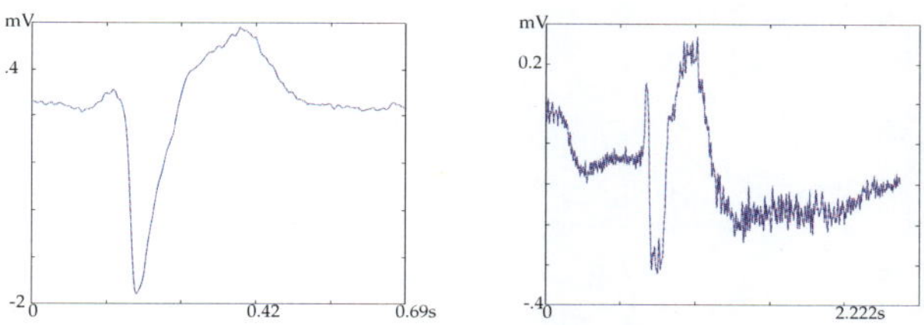

(a) Premature Ventricular Contraction (PVC) (b) Ventricular escape beat

Fig. 3. Heartbeats of *V* group, extracted from MIT/BIH database.

2.1.4 Group of arrhythmias type *F*

Fusion heartbeats develop when either the atria or the ventricles are activated by two simultaneously invading impulses and they can be assessed in *P* wave or *QRS* complex of the ECG. An atrial fusion beat results when: the sinus beat coincides with an atrial ectopic beat, two atrial ectopic beats coincide, or an atrial or sinus beat coincide with retrograde conduction from a junctional focus. A ventricular fusion beat results when: a ventricular beat coincides with either a sinus beat, a ventricular ectopic beat, or a junctional beat. A couple of examples are shown in Figure 4.

2.1.5 Group of arrhythmias type *Q*

Unclassified heartbeats (heartbeats *Q*) correspond to heartbeats that do not contain relevant medical information, mainly due to some external conditions as artifacts, electrode disconnection, saturation of acquisition system, or heartbeats by pacemakers. In some systems, it is necessary to isolate this kind of heartbeats from the training space in order to give an adequate diagnosis. Normally, These heartbeats are considered as outliers because of their low importance in the diagnosis. Figure 5 shows two types of *Q* heartbeats: Paced beat and Unclassified beat.

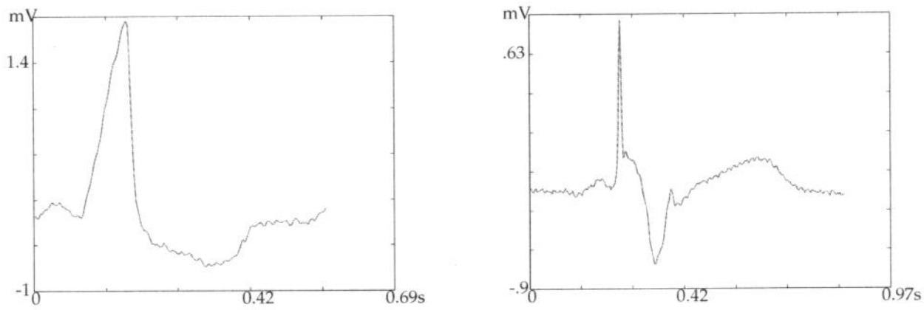

(a) Fusion of ventricular and normal beat (b) Fusion of paced and normal beat

Fig. 4. Heartbeats of *F* group, extracted from MIT/BIH database.

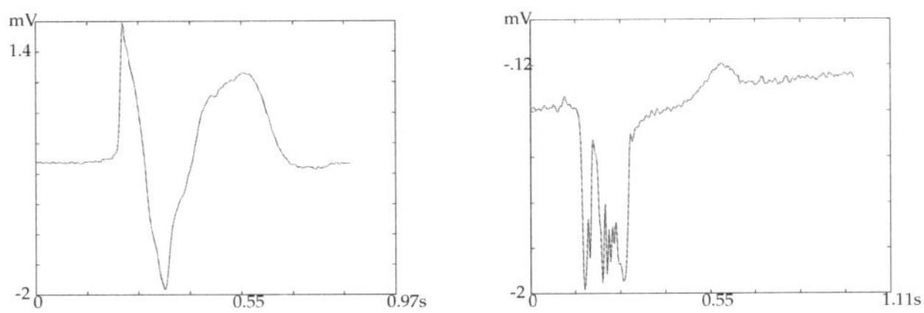

(a) Paced beat (b) Unclassified beats

Fig. 5. Heartbeats of *Q* group, extracted from MIT/BIH database.

3. Ambulatory electrocardiography

During the last two decades, acquisition systems for physiological signals have been developed and improved. It has been stated that they are lighter, smaller and capable of recording multiple signals up to 48 hours. These systems also called ambulatory record systems are used in ECG analysis to detect infrequent arrhythmias or transient abnormalities in heart function often associated to everyday life stress, besides transient ischemic events or silent myocardial ischemia. This type of disorders cannot be detected in short-time ECG or 12 leads ECG recordings. Holter recorders have been used to detect this type of abnormalities. Nowdays, signals are recorded in flash-type semiconductor memories, which can be transferred to a workstation for further analysis J. Segura-Juárez et al. (2004).

On the other hand, the increase of health costs makes an urgent need to develop ambulatory systems to reduce the number of patients going to hospitals. Therefore, it is necessary the design of a portable, low cost, high performance and simple system that allows an automated analysis and diagnosis. Such system has to fulfill certain requirements such as integrate various data analysis techniques, for instance: signal processing, pattern recognition, decision making and human-machine interaction. The existing portable devices have improved in size and performance due to technological reasons, the need to record the signal over a specific period of time, which is constrained by the storage capacity of the devices. For example, a typical signal of 24 hours consists of approximately 100.000 heartbeats that can be morphologically grouped (*clustered*) into a much smaller number of classes. Most of the classes where the heartbeats have a typical pattern, it is enough to know the number of heartbeats and a representative template of the morphology for grouping them, but in the time span where cardiac activity presents anomalies or symptoms of illness, the whole recording is needed.

This is only possible if the portable device for analysis is able to do both record the signal, and process it.
Some technical issues with regard to the ECG processing have been discussed, such as the problem of the wide variability into signal morphology, not only among patients, but also due to patients movements, electrical conduction changes, body characteristics, among others. In addition, the ECG signal is contaminated by several noise sources, both external sources (interference of the power line, movement of the electrodes) and biological sources (muscle movement causing high-frequency interference and breathing causing baseline displacement). Because of this, it is not possible to have a general training set that takes into account all cases of interest. That is the reason why, this kind of analysis requires special care to choose appropriate techniques for signal conditioning (pre-processing), since the quality of input signal for further classification has a direct impact on its performance.

4. A novel methodology for analysis of cardiac arrhythmias

Figure 6 depicts the methodology proposed for Holter arrhythmia analysis that considers the following stages: a) Preprocessing, b) Feature extraction, c) Analysis of relevance, and c) Clustering. As input data, Holter recordings are initially preprocessed to reduce the influence of interferences and artifacts. Next, recordings are segmented based on estimation of fiducial point of *QRS* complexes. Heartbeat features extracted using variability, prematurity, morphology and representation measurements of the heart rate variability, are calculated by weighted linear projection. After that, projected data is grouped by soft clustering algorithm. The restrictions for reducing computational load lead to framing along the time axis the input data into a equal number (N_s in Figure 6) of successive divisions of the Holter recordings, where each frame is separately processed. Therefore, according to the assumed criterium of homogeneity between two given consecutive frame divisions, resulting clusters can be either merged or split. Finally, such clusters, which represent different types of arrhythmia present in the recording, are analyzed by the specialists, and serve them as a supporting tool for the medical diagnosis.

4.1 Preprocessing and segmentation

The heartbeat set from recorded Holter ECG signals is to be processed. Let $s(t)$, that is subject to discrete time transformation, $\boldsymbol{s} = \{s_k\}$; where $s_k \triangleq s[kT_s]$, being $k \in \mathbb{N}$, and T_s the sampling period. At the beginning, recordings are normalized by the z–scores approach to prevent biasing, i.e., $\boldsymbol{s}^0 = (\boldsymbol{s} - \boldsymbol{\mathcal{E}}\{\boldsymbol{s}\})/(|\max\{\boldsymbol{s}\}|)$, where the notation $\boldsymbol{\mathcal{E}}\{\cdot\}$ stands for the expectance operator. Then, unbiased vector $\boldsymbol{s}^0$ is filtered to reduce signal disturbances and artifacts. Specifically, power line interference is reduced using an algorithm based on adaptive sinusoidal interference canceller that provides significant signal–to–noise ratio improvement Martens et al. (2006). Also, the baseline wandering is cancelled out by the method described in Roddy (1991) that is based on a two–pole, phase–compensated filter, developed for real–time processing of long ECG segments. Although, the signal is also partially filtered, this preprocessing is supposed not to affect the separability among the underlying heartbeat groups.
R–peak locations are previously estimated accordingly to the procedure given in Laguna & Sörnmo (2005), since the analysis of arrhythmias under consideration is supported on fixed changes of both *QRS* complex, as well as the *HRV*. The following sequential procedures are included: band–pass filtering, *R* peak enhancement and adaptive thresholding. Furthermore, their segmentation is carried out for a fixed window length

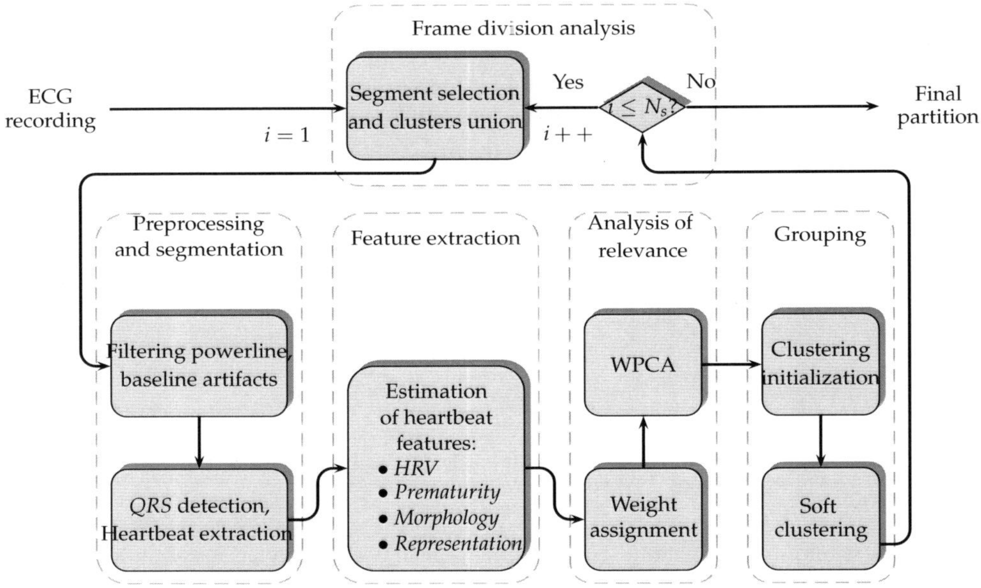

Fig. 6. Block diagram of proposed unsupervised methodology for Holter monitoring of cardiac arrhythmias.

to avoid analysis over *QRS* complexes of different length, that is, each j–th complex $\boldsymbol{d}_j$ is accomplished as follows: $\boldsymbol{d}_j = \{s_k^0\}; \forall k \in [l_j - aF_s, l_j + bF_s]$, where l_j is the R–peak time location of the j-th heartbeat and $F_s = 1/T_s$ is the sampling frequency. Nonetheless, it must be quoted that some morphologies such as VE, might exhibit S–waves lasting exceptionally more than usual, and therefore, they can be missed if using such a short processing window. *QRS* width is fixed to be of 200 ms length, i.e., $a = b = 0.1$.

4.2 Feature extraction

Heartbeat characterization is achieved by taking into consideration the wide set of features previously proposed for arrhythmia analysis over Holter ECG recordings Cuesta et al. (2007); Cvetkovic et al. (2008); Lagerholm et al. (2000); Rodríguez-Sotelo et al. (2009). The whole set of studied features can be divided into the following groups, as shown in table 2:

4.2.1 Prematurity and variability based features

When considering *Sv* labelled arrhythmias, their morphology is highly similar to the normal heartbeat shape. Therefore, the following set of features, which are extracted from variability of cardiac rhythm, are mainly considered Rodríguez-Sotelo et al. (2009):

– *HRV–derived features* (x_1, x_2, x_3): Interval parameters providing information about sequences of heartbeats with unusual timing, namely De-Chazal et al. (2004):

$$\begin{aligned} x_1 &= l_j - l_{j-1}, \quad (RR \text{ interval}) \\ x_2 &= l_{j-1} - l_{j-2}, \; (pre - RR \text{ interval}) \\ x_3 &= l_{j+1} - l_j, \quad (post - RR \text{ interval}) \end{aligned}$$

Index	Type	Description
x_1	HRV and Prematurity	• RR interval
x_2		• pre-RR interval
x_3		• post-RR interval
x_4		• Difference between RR and pre–RR intervals, $x_4 = x_1 - x_2$
x_5		• Difference between post–RR and RR intervals, $x_5 = x_3 - x_1$
x_6		• Continuous APB^* heartbeat type, (eq. 1)
x_7	Morphology and representation	• QRS matching by Dynamic time warping
x_8		• Polarity of QRS complex
x_9		• Energy of QRS complex
$x_{10}, \ldots, x_{19}$		• First 10 Hermite–based coefficients
$x_{20}, \ldots, x_{90}$		• Db2 (A4: $20-25$, D4: $26-31$, D3: $32-41$, D2: $43-58$, D1: $59-90$)
$x_{91}, \ldots, x_{100}$		• $\text{var}\{\text{A4}, \text{D4}, \text{D3}, \text{D2}, \text{D1}\}$, $\max\{A4, D4, D3, D2, D1\}$

The notation APB^* stands for Atrial Premature Beat, being a sort of S heartbeats.

Table 2. Feature set considered for Holter monitoring of cardiac arrhythmias.

It should be noted that atrial (S) and ventricular (V) ectopic beats manifest abrupt changes on fiducial point intervals, which in turn, affect the respective values of heartbeat interval features.

– *Prematurity features* (x_4, x_5, x_6): Defined parameters, $x_4 = x_1 - x_2$ and $x_5 = x_3 - x_1$, are assumed to be relevant, since they make possible the identification of S type arrhythmia, when reflecting the increase or decrease of heart rate. Besides, if any heartbeat occurs after another S–labeled event, it is regarded as normal, and the above mentioned features will change of sign. Feature x_6 accounts for the number of consecutive S that is also sensitive to an increase of the heart rate, exceeding the normal range set for x_4. The parameter x_6 is expressed as follows:

$$x_6 = \left(\frac{x_3}{x_1}\right)^2 + \left(\frac{x_2}{x_1}\right)^2 - \left(\frac{1}{3}\sum_{i=1}^{3} x_i^2 \log(x_i)^2\right). \tag{1}$$

The first and second squared terms in Eq. (1) are sensitive to abrupt changes of heart rate, whereas, the last addend is inferred as unnormalized Shannon entropy, which increases the value of x_6 whenever heart rate is steadily increasing.

4.2.2 Morphological and spectral features ($x_7, \ldots, x_{100}$).

Since most analyzed arrhythmias change the shape of QRS complexes, their characterization can be achieved by commonly used time and spectral–based techniques Cuesta et al. (2003). Therefore, regarding the former techniques, the following features are worth to be considered: A couple of features that are sensitive to abnormal QRS complexes: x_7, It computes a morphological dissimilarity by means of Dynamic Time Warping (DTW) approach between current QRS complex and linearly averaged QRS complex of the last n heartbeats Cuesta et al. (2003).

$x_8 = \left|\max\{\boldsymbol{d}_j\}/\min\{\boldsymbol{d}_j\}\right|$, being $\boldsymbol{d}_j$ the current QRS complex. This feature is sensitive to ventricular arrhythmias that exhibit abnormal QRS complexes such as ventricular extrasystoles or branch blocks Cuesta et al. (2007). Because of the noticeable morphological characteristic of branch block heartbeats, the QRS energy, which is a straightforward feature to detect previously described type of heartbeats, is estimated as $x_9 = \sum_{i=1}^{L_d} d_j[i]^2$, where L_d is the processing length of the j-th QRS complex.

On the other hand, spectral–based representation features used in the field of signal compression are also taken into account, since only a few coefficients are needed to reconstruct the signal Lagerholm et al. (2000). In this line of analysis, the Hermite coefficient h_i related to i-th order base is used and calculated as follows:

$$h_i = \frac{1}{F_s} \langle \boldsymbol{d}_j, \phi_i^{\sigma} \rangle, \quad \phi_i^{\sigma}(t) = \frac{e^{-t^2/2\sigma^2}}{\sqrt{2^i i! \sqrt{\pi}}} H_i(t/\sigma) \tag{2}$$

where $\langle \cdot, \cdot \rangle$ is the inner product, H_i is a Hermite polynomial of degree i and σ a parameter determining the window length.

Wavelet decomposition coefficients are also studied. Specifically, 4–level coefficients of Daubechies–2 class (*dB2*) are computed. They have been proved to describe properly different heartbeat morphologies, as discussed in Cvetkovic et al. (2008). The following statistical descriptors are extracted from decomposition coefficients: mean value, variance, and maximum values are estimated.

As a result, given an i-th observation heartbeat, the respective feature vector $\{\boldsymbol{x}_i \in \mathbb{R}^p : i = 1, \ldots, n\}$, $p = 100$, is assumed to be the input training space toward arrhythmia classification stage.

4.3 Analysis of relevance

Since there is a huge amount of information stored during Holter monitoring, classification of heartbeats usually becomes quite time–consuming; that is the reason why any automated processing of the recording would be of benefit; particularly, the dimensional reduction procedure can be considered. In this sense, and based on multivariate representation of input data, a direct approach is the use of linear decomposition methods to decrease the dimensionality of the resulting feature space from heartbeat characterization. Among linear decomposition methods, the PCA and its variations have shown to be a good alternative for this aim Perlibakas (2004). Moreover, the non–parametric nature, feasibility of implementation and versatility are some advantages of PCA. Nonetheless, Holter monitoring of cardiac arrhythmias is an application where the conventional PCA might not be recommended because it gives the same importance to all observations, being sensitive to the presence of outliers and noise in the data. In fact, strong asymmetry among class observations requires a properly selection of heartbeat features to provide convenient separability among heartbeat types Cuesta et al. (2007); Sotelo, Frau, Ordónez, Domínguez & Novak (2009). To that end, a weighted version of PCA (termed WPCA) is used, where introduced weights are given depending on variable–wise relevance criteria; this in turn makes possible to assess the relative importance of each feature (variable) immersed on the original data representation by using a kind of weighting factor. The following two linear projection methods to estimate the feature–wise weighting factor, namely, Minimum Square Error (MSE) and M–inner product are described in the next paragraphs.

Given a set of p-dimensional vector data, $\{\boldsymbol{x}_i\}$, being centered, i.e., $\boldsymbol{\mathcal{E}}\{\boldsymbol{x}_i\} = \boldsymbol{0}, \forall i$, where all n observations can be aligned in the input matrix $\boldsymbol{X} = [\boldsymbol{x}_1 \mid \cdots \mid \boldsymbol{x}_n]^{\top} \in \mathbb{R}^{n \times p}$, then the respective linear projection is $\boldsymbol{Y} = \boldsymbol{X}\boldsymbol{V}$, $\boldsymbol{Y} \in \mathbb{R}^{n \times p}$. Generally, the ortonormal projection is performed to a q–dimensional space ($q < p$), being $\boldsymbol{V} \in \mathbb{R}^{p \times p}$ an orthogonal matrix, where the representation quality of $\boldsymbol{X}$ is measured by using a given error function ε between the original data and the truncated orthonormal projection $\widehat{\boldsymbol{V}} \in \mathbb{R}^{p \times q}$. This can be expressed as a distance measure: $\varepsilon = d(\boldsymbol{X}, \widehat{\boldsymbol{X}})$, where $\widehat{\boldsymbol{X}} = \widehat{\boldsymbol{Y}}\widehat{\boldsymbol{V}}^{\top}$, being $\widehat{\boldsymbol{X}} \in \mathbb{R}^{n \times p}$ the truncated input matrix. There exist several alternatives for calculating this distance, such as, the Minkowski distance (L_p metrics), square Euclidean distance, angle–based distance, Mahalanobis, among others, as discussed in Perlibakas (2004). Commonly, analysis of relevance methods aim to minimize ε.

Denoting $\widetilde{\boldsymbol{X}} = \boldsymbol{X}\boldsymbol{W}$ as the weighted data matrix, we can estimate a set of their q most relevant eigenvalues. The weighted relevance (weighting covariance) matrix is introduced as follows Yue & Tomoyasu (2004):

$$\widetilde{\boldsymbol{\Sigma}}_{\boldsymbol{X}} = \widetilde{\boldsymbol{X}}^{\top}\widetilde{\boldsymbol{X}} = \boldsymbol{W}^{\top}\boldsymbol{X}^{\top}\boldsymbol{X}\boldsymbol{W},\ \widetilde{\boldsymbol{\Sigma}}_{\boldsymbol{X}} \in \mathbb{R}^{p\times p} \tag{3}$$

where $\boldsymbol{W} \in \mathbb{R}^{p\times p}$ is a diagonal weighting matrix.

4.3.1 MSE–based approach

The main goal of conventional PCA is to find out the optimum fitting for a given data in terms of least squares. This technique has been considered as the simplest eigenvector–based multivariate analysis, where the linear decomposition of matrix $\boldsymbol{X}$ by singular value decomposition takes place, $\boldsymbol{X} = \boldsymbol{U}\boldsymbol{\Lambda}_{\boldsymbol{X}}\boldsymbol{V}^{\top} = \sum_{i=1}^{p}\mu_i\boldsymbol{u}_i\boldsymbol{v}_i^{\top}$. Matrix $\boldsymbol{\Lambda}_{\boldsymbol{X}} = \operatorname{diag}(\boldsymbol{\mu})$ is the singular values matrix, $\boldsymbol{U} \in \mathbb{R}^{n\times n}$ corresponds to eigenvectors of $\boldsymbol{X}\boldsymbol{X}^{\top}$, and $\boldsymbol{V}$ holds eigenvectors of $\widetilde{\boldsymbol{\Sigma}}_{\boldsymbol{X}}$ when $\boldsymbol{W} = \operatorname{diag}(\mathbf{1}_p)$ and $\mathbf{1}_p$ is a p-dimensional all–ones vector.

Therefore, the minimum square error (MSE) distance is achieved to assess the representation quality, which yields to the following minimization problem:

$$\min_{\widehat{\boldsymbol{V}}^{\top}}\{\varepsilon\} = \boldsymbol{\mathcal{E}}\left\{\min\{(\boldsymbol{X} - \widehat{\boldsymbol{Y}}\widehat{\boldsymbol{V}}^{\top})^{\top}(\boldsymbol{X} - \widehat{\boldsymbol{Y}}\widehat{\boldsymbol{V}}^{\top})\}\right\} \tag{4}$$

Let, $\boldsymbol{x}^{(l)} \in \mathbb{R}^{n\times 1}, l = 1,\ldots,p$, the l-th feature of the input matrix, $\boldsymbol{X}$ that can be approximated by its truncated version in a q-dimensional ortonormal space by the following linear combination:

$$\widehat{\boldsymbol{x}}^{(l)} = \sum_{i=1}^{q} c_i^{(l)}\boldsymbol{u}_i \tag{5}$$

then, the MSE value between the original and the reconstructed features is estimated as,

$$\overline{e^2} = \boldsymbol{\mathcal{E}}\left\{(\boldsymbol{x}^{(l)} - \widehat{\boldsymbol{x}}^{(l)})^{\top}(\boldsymbol{x}^{(l)} - \widehat{\boldsymbol{x}}^{(l)})\right\} = \boldsymbol{\mathcal{E}}\left\{(\sum_{i=q+1}^{p} c_i^{(l)}\boldsymbol{u}_i)^{\top}(\sum_{i=q+1}^{p} c_i^{(l)}\boldsymbol{u}_i)\right\} \tag{6}$$

that can be minimized if maximizing its complement, and therefore the following expression takes place:

$$\boldsymbol{\mathcal{E}}\left\{(\sum_{i=1}^{q} c_i^{(l)}\boldsymbol{u}_i)^{\top}(\sum_{i=1}^{q} c_i^{(l)}\boldsymbol{u}_i)\right\} = \boldsymbol{\mathcal{E}}\left\{\sum_{i=1}^{q} \left(c_i^{(l)}\right)^2\right\} \tag{7}$$

The coefficients of the linear combination in Eq. (5) are given by $c_i^{(l)} = \mu_i v_i^{(l)}$ where $v_i^{(l)}$, estimated for the matrix $\boldsymbol{V}$, is the i-th element of the respective l feature. Replacing $c_i^{(l)}$, the expression (7) is rewritten as follows:

$$\boldsymbol{\mathcal{E}}\left\{\sum_{i=1}^{q} \left(c_i^{(l)}\right)^2\right\} = \boldsymbol{\mathcal{E}}\left\{\sum_{i=1}^{q}(\mu_i)^2(v_i^{(l)})^2\right\} = \boldsymbol{\mathcal{E}}\left\{\sum_{i=1}^{q}\lambda_i(v_i^{(l)})^2\right\} \tag{8}$$

where $\boldsymbol{\lambda} = [\lambda_1, \ldots, \lambda_p]$ is the vector of the eigenvalues of $\widetilde{\boldsymbol{\Sigma}}_{\boldsymbol{X}}$. As a result, generalizing the last expression for the p features, and having the simple average as an estimation of expectance operator, then the relevance measure is assumed as follows:

$$\boldsymbol{\rho} = \frac{1}{q} \sum_{i=1}^{q} \lambda_i \boldsymbol{\nu}_i, \tag{9}$$

where $\boldsymbol{\nu}_i$ is a vector composed by the square of each of $\boldsymbol{v}_i$ elements. It should be remarked that vector $\boldsymbol{\rho}$ yields a relevance index, which measures the accumulated variance of eigenvalues and eigenvectors, and such vector is used as a weighting factor. Then, accordingly to the quadratic form of the generalized covariance matrix (see Eq. (3)), the weighting matrix can be obtained as $\boldsymbol{W} = \operatorname{diag}(\sqrt{\boldsymbol{\rho}})$. Lastly, the commonly known criterion of variance explained is used to find q, which rejects the elements that do not significantly contribute to the accumulated variance of data set. In addition, since the first principal component holds most of explained variance, the particular case $q = 1$ is also analyzed throughout this section.

4.3.2 M-inner product approach

This case considers the M-inner product as an error measure between the original variable and its orthonormal projection. Let $\boldsymbol{U}_p \in \mathbb{R}^{p \times p}$ be an arbitrary orthonormal matrix, and $\widehat{\boldsymbol{x}}^{(l)} = \boldsymbol{u}_p^{(l)\top} \boldsymbol{X}$ the linear combination to estimate the l-th feature. Then, the error measure for each feature is given by:

$$d_{\boldsymbol{A}}(\boldsymbol{x}^{(l)}, \widehat{\boldsymbol{x}}^{(l)}) = \langle \boldsymbol{x}^{(l)}, \widehat{\boldsymbol{x}}^{(l)} \rangle_{\boldsymbol{A}} = \boldsymbol{x}^{(l)\top} \boldsymbol{A} \widehat{\boldsymbol{x}}^{(l)} \tag{10}$$

where $\langle \cdot, \cdot \rangle_{\boldsymbol{A}}$ is the M-inner product regarding a symmetric positive definite matrix $\boldsymbol{A} \in \mathbb{R}^{n \times n}$, which is related to the inner product between observations, i.e., $\boldsymbol{A} = \sum_{i=1}^{p} \boldsymbol{x}_i \boldsymbol{x}_i^\top$. If definition for the l-th estimated feature $\boldsymbol{x}^{(l)}$, given by Eq. (5), is replaced in Eq. (10), the following expression holds:

$$(\boldsymbol{x}^{(l)} - \widehat{\boldsymbol{x}}^{(l)})^\top \boldsymbol{A} (\boldsymbol{x}^{(l)} - \widehat{\boldsymbol{x}}^{(l)}) = \left(\sum_{i=q+1}^{p} c_i^{(l)} \boldsymbol{u}_i \right)^\top \boldsymbol{A} \left(\sum_{i=q+1}^{p} c_i^{(l)} \boldsymbol{u}_i \right) \tag{11}$$

that can be minimized if maximizing its complement, i.e, $\widehat{\boldsymbol{x}}^{(l)\top} \boldsymbol{A} \widehat{\boldsymbol{x}}^{(l)}$. Thus, replacing $\boldsymbol{A}$ and $\widehat{\boldsymbol{x}}^{(l)}$ given in Eq. (5), and generalizing for all variables, the following expression yields the value:

$$\operatorname{tr}(\boldsymbol{X}^\top \boldsymbol{A} \boldsymbol{X}) = \operatorname{tr}(\boldsymbol{X}^\top \boldsymbol{X} \boldsymbol{X}^\top \boldsymbol{X}) = \sum_{i=1}^{q} \lambda_i^2 \tag{12}$$

where λ are the eigenvalues of $\boldsymbol{X}\boldsymbol{X}^\top$.

Furthermore, the eigenvalues of $\widehat{\boldsymbol{X}}^\top \widehat{\boldsymbol{X}}$ matrix are the first p eigenvalues of $\widehat{\boldsymbol{X}} \widehat{\boldsymbol{X}}^\top$, then, maximizing Eq. (12) is equivalent to maximizing the expression:

$$\operatorname{tr}(\boldsymbol{X}\boldsymbol{X}^\top \boldsymbol{X}\boldsymbol{X}^\top) = \operatorname{tr}(\boldsymbol{A}\boldsymbol{A}) = \sum_{i=1}^{q} \lambda_i^2 \tag{13}$$

Next, establishing a weighted relevance matrix, $\boldsymbol{A}_{\boldsymbol{\alpha}} = \boldsymbol{X}\boldsymbol{W}\boldsymbol{W}\boldsymbol{X}^\top$, where $\boldsymbol{W} = \operatorname{diag}(\sqrt{\boldsymbol{\alpha}})$ and $\boldsymbol{\alpha} \in \mathbb{R}^{p \times 1}$ is a weighting vector, and assuming the orthonormal invariance criterion

Algorithm 1 Power-embedded $Q-\alpha$ method Wolf & Shashua (2005)

1. Initialize: $\boldsymbol{M} = \boldsymbol{X}^\top$, chose at random $k \times n$ matrix $\boldsymbol{Q}^{(0)}$ $(\boldsymbol{Q}^{(0)\top}\boldsymbol{Q}^{(0)} = \boldsymbol{I}_n)$, $\boldsymbol{m}_i \leftarrow (\boldsymbol{m}_i - \mu(\boldsymbol{m}_i))/\|\boldsymbol{m}_i\|$.
2. Make $\boldsymbol{G} : g_{ij} = (\boldsymbol{m}_i^\top \boldsymbol{m}_j)\boldsymbol{m}_i^\top \boldsymbol{Q}\boldsymbol{Q}^\top \boldsymbol{m}_j$
3. Compute $\boldsymbol{\alpha}$ as the eigenvector associated with the major eigenvalue of $\boldsymbol{G}$.
4. Compute auxiliar matrix $\boldsymbol{C}_{\boldsymbol{\alpha}} = \boldsymbol{M}^\top \mathrm{diag}(\boldsymbol{\alpha})\boldsymbol{M}$
5. Compute the orthonormal transformation: $\boldsymbol{Z}[r] = \boldsymbol{C}_{\boldsymbol{\alpha}}[r]\boldsymbol{U}[r-1]$
6. Compute QR decomposition: $[\boldsymbol{Q}[r], \boldsymbol{R}] = \mathrm{qr}\ (\boldsymbol{Z}[r])$
7. Make $r \leftarrow r+1$ and return to the step 2

Yu & Shi (2003), the optimization problem can be rewritten as:

$$\max_{\boldsymbol{\alpha}} \ \mathrm{tr}(\boldsymbol{Q}^\top \boldsymbol{A}_\alpha \boldsymbol{A}_\alpha \boldsymbol{Q}) = \sum_{i=1}^{q} \lambda_i^2 \qquad (14)$$
$$\text{s.t.} \qquad \boldsymbol{\alpha}^\top \boldsymbol{\alpha} = 1, \quad \boldsymbol{Q}^\top \boldsymbol{Q} = \boldsymbol{I}$$

being matrix $\boldsymbol{Q} \in \mathbb{R}^{n \times n}$ an arbitrary orthonormal matrix that will be explained in detail further. Besides, the weighting vector is adjusted to be $\sqrt{\boldsymbol{\alpha}}$ to make the optimization problem in hand to be bilinear regarding $\boldsymbol{\alpha}$, thus, $\widetilde{\boldsymbol{X}} = \boldsymbol{X}\mathrm{diag}(\sqrt{\boldsymbol{\alpha}})$. The weighting vector α and the orthonormal matrix $\boldsymbol{Q}$ are determined at the maximal point of the optimization problem. Finally, the objective function can be rewriting as the following quadratic form:

$$\max_{\boldsymbol{\alpha}} \boldsymbol{\alpha}^\top \boldsymbol{G} \boldsymbol{\alpha} \qquad (15)$$
$$\text{s.t.} \qquad \boldsymbol{\alpha}^\top \boldsymbol{\alpha} = 1$$

where $\boldsymbol{G} \in \mathbb{R}^{p \times p}$ is a matrix with $g_{ij} = (\boldsymbol{m}_i^\top \boldsymbol{m}_j)\boldsymbol{m}_i^\top \boldsymbol{Q}\boldsymbol{Q}^\top \boldsymbol{m}_j$, $i, j = 1, \ldots, p$, elements and $\boldsymbol{M} = \boldsymbol{X}^\top$. As a consequence, the previous equation becomes the objective function to be used in the unsupervised $Q-\alpha$ algorithm, as described in Wolf & Shashua (2005).
It must be quoted that the matrix $\boldsymbol{G}$ is obtained from an arbitrary orthonormal transformation, it is necessary to apply an iterative method to tune the matrix $\boldsymbol{Q}$ and the weighting vector $\boldsymbol{\alpha}$. From the optimization problem, described by Eq. (15), it can be observed that vector $\boldsymbol{\alpha}$ points out to the direction of most relevant features, whereas matrix $\boldsymbol{Q}$ means its rotation. Therefore, the adjustment of these parameters should be mutually dependent and must be achieved on an alternating way, as shown in algorithm 1. In steps 5 and 6, it introduces an auxiliar orthonormal projection of $\boldsymbol{C}_{\boldsymbol{\alpha}}$ and QR decomposition, respectively, to refine matrix $\boldsymbol{Q}$ at each iteration. Then, the q most relevant features are those elements of $\boldsymbol{M}$ that satisfy $\sum_{i=1}^{q} \alpha_i^2 \approx \sigma_e/100$, for a given percentage fraction σ_e of explained variance.
Convergence of the algorithm 1 is discussed in detail in Wolf & Shashua (2005) (with $r < 5$ iterations). However, an indicator of the algorithm convergence could be the change of the vector $\boldsymbol{\alpha}$, i.e, the difference between the current and preceding vector: $\|\boldsymbol{\alpha}[r] - \boldsymbol{\alpha}[r-1]\| < \delta$, where $\delta \geq 0$ stands for any needed accurate amount, being $\boldsymbol{\chi}[r]$ the achieved value of $\boldsymbol{\chi}$ at the r-th iteration.
The procedure for computing the weighting vector, $\boldsymbol{\alpha}$, is refined iteratively, and the whole data set is to be used, where the orthonormal matrix is updated per iteration to get the

Algorithm 2 Projection of weighted data.

1. (Initialization): Normalize $\boldsymbol{X}$, $\mu(\boldsymbol{x}_i) = 0$, $\|\boldsymbol{x}_i\| = 1$, $1 \leq i \leq p$
2. Choose a method to find the weighting vector $\boldsymbol{w}$

(a) $\boldsymbol{w} \leftarrow \sqrt{\boldsymbol{\alpha}}$, Eigenvector corresponding to the largest eigenvalue of $\boldsymbol{G}$ (algorithm 1, $r \leftarrow$ last iteration)

(b) $\boldsymbol{w} \leftarrow \sqrt{\widehat{\boldsymbol{\alpha}}}$, Eigenvector corresponding to the largest eigenvalue of $(\boldsymbol{X}^{\mathsf{T}}\boldsymbol{X})^{\cdot 2}$.

(c) $\boldsymbol{w} \leftarrow \sqrt{\boldsymbol{\rho}}$, see Eq. (9), removing eigenvectors $[q+1, \ldots, p]$ that do not significantly contribute to variance.

(d) $\boldsymbol{w} \leftarrow \sqrt{\widehat{\boldsymbol{\rho}}}$, see Eq. (9), $q = 1$.

3. Weight original data $\widetilde{\boldsymbol{X}} = \boldsymbol{X}\mathrm{diag}(\boldsymbol{w})$
4. Compute principal components $\widetilde{\boldsymbol{V}}$ of $\widetilde{\boldsymbol{X}}$
5. Project data $\boldsymbol{Y} = \widetilde{\boldsymbol{X}}\widetilde{\boldsymbol{V}}$

subset of relevant features. As a result, the computational load may increase. Nonetheless, based on variance criterion, it can be inferred that the first q components of $\widehat{\boldsymbol{x}}^{(l)}$ hold the most informative directions of weighting data. Thus, the l $(q+1 \leq l \leq p)$ directions do not contribute significantly to the explained variance. Time calculation when computing the vector $\boldsymbol{\alpha}$ can be diminished just to one iteration with no significant decrease of accuracy Wolf & Shashua (2005). With this in mind, the feature relevance may be preserved optimizing the p original variables or the first q variables. Indeed, maximizing $\mathrm{tr}(\boldsymbol{Q}^{\mathsf{T}}\boldsymbol{A}_{\boldsymbol{\alpha}}\boldsymbol{A}_{\boldsymbol{\alpha}}\boldsymbol{Q})$ is equivalent to maximize $\mathrm{tr}(\boldsymbol{A}_{\boldsymbol{\alpha}}\boldsymbol{A}_{\boldsymbol{\alpha}}) = \mathrm{tr}(\boldsymbol{X}\mathrm{diag}(\boldsymbol{\alpha})\boldsymbol{X}^{\mathsf{T}}\boldsymbol{X}\mathrm{diag}(\boldsymbol{\alpha})\boldsymbol{X}^{\mathsf{T}})$. Since, this expression is bilinear regarding $\boldsymbol{\alpha}$, the objective function can be re-written as $\boldsymbol{\alpha}^T\boldsymbol{H}\boldsymbol{\alpha}$, where $\boldsymbol{H}_{ij} = \mathrm{tr}(\boldsymbol{x}_i^{\mathsf{T}}\boldsymbol{x}_i\boldsymbol{x}_j^{\mathsf{T}}\boldsymbol{x}_j) = \boldsymbol{x}_i\boldsymbol{x}_j^{\mathsf{T}}\,\mathrm{tr}(\boldsymbol{x}_i^{\mathsf{T}}\boldsymbol{x}_j) = (\boldsymbol{x}_i\boldsymbol{x}_j^{\mathsf{T}})^2$. Accordingly, it can be inferred that the approximate vector of relevance $\widehat{\boldsymbol{\alpha}}$ is the eigenvector corresponding to the largest eigenvalue of $(\boldsymbol{X}^{\mathsf{T}}\boldsymbol{X})^{\cdot 2}$ (where notation $(\chi)^{\cdot 2}$ stands for the square of each one of the elements of the involved matrix χ).
In conclusion, the weighting factor is related to either vectors: $\boldsymbol{\alpha}$ (complete case) and $\widehat{\boldsymbol{\alpha}}$ (approximate case). The weighting matrices become $\boldsymbol{W}_{\alpha} = \mathrm{diag}(\sqrt{\alpha})$ and $\boldsymbol{W}_{\widehat{\alpha}} = \mathrm{diag}(\sqrt{\widehat{\alpha}})$, respectively.

4.3.3 Projection of weighted data

As described above, the data are weighted by the diagonal matrix $\boldsymbol{W} = \mathrm{diag}(\boldsymbol{w})$, where $\boldsymbol{w}$ is the weighting vector calculated using either the MSE or the M inner-product-based approaches previously explained. Therefore, weighting data $\widetilde{\boldsymbol{X}} = \boldsymbol{X}\boldsymbol{W}$ is linearly projected, so: $\boldsymbol{Y} = \widetilde{\boldsymbol{X}}\widetilde{\boldsymbol{V}}$, where $\widetilde{\boldsymbol{V}}$ are the principal components of $\widetilde{\boldsymbol{X}}$, $\widetilde{\boldsymbol{V}} = \boldsymbol{V}$, if $\boldsymbol{W} = \mathrm{diag}(\mathbf{1}_p)$. The achieved procedure for relevance analysis and rotation of weighted data based on described methods is described in algorithm 2.

4.4 Clustering of cardiac arrhythmias

The projected weighted data $\boldsymbol{Y}$ are clustered in three stages. Firstly, the estimation of number of groups is carried out by means of spectral analysis of affinity measure, as described in Ng et al. (2001). Secondly, center initialization is achieved based on the *J–H–means* clustering algorithm Hansen & Mladenovic (2001), where objective function corresponds to the Minimum Sum–of–Squares (MSS), as suggested in Rodríguez-Sotelo et al. (2009). To carry out the above process, a random initialization is developed where every point $\boldsymbol{y}_i$ out of a sphere of radius ϵ has a center at $\boldsymbol{\zeta}_j$, $j = 1 : k$ ($\boldsymbol{\zeta}_j$ is the j-th of the k centers)and is considered a center candidate. $\boldsymbol{y}_i$ replaces a current center $\boldsymbol{\zeta}_j$. Once updating and computing the MSS, the process is repeated as long as MSS reaches the optimal value. The process stops whenever there is no further MSS optimization. This initialization is aimed to avoid local minima. Lastly, the third clustering stage computes the final partition based on the Gaussian Expectation Maximization Clustering (GEMC) algorithm Cvetkovic et al. (2008), having as an objective function a linear combination of centered gaussian distributions over each centroid:

$$\theta(\boldsymbol{Y}, \boldsymbol{\zeta}) = -\sum_{i=1}^{n} \log \left(\sum_{j=1}^{k} p(\boldsymbol{y}_i \mid \boldsymbol{\zeta}_j) p(\boldsymbol{\zeta}_j) \right), \tag{16}$$

where $p(\boldsymbol{y}_i \mid \boldsymbol{\zeta}_j)$, assumed as gaussian distribution centered at $\boldsymbol{\zeta}_j$, is the probability of $\boldsymbol{y}_i$, and $p(\boldsymbol{\zeta}_j)$ is the a priori probability of the j-th cluster. For sake of simplicity, the *log* function is used, while the minus sign accounts for minimization. Besides, the GEMC employs a soft member function, $f_m(\cdot)$, assigning a membership level to $\boldsymbol{y}_i$ for every cluster, as described in Hamerly & Elkan (2002).

Further decreasing of computational load can be reached if sectioning the whole input recording into divisions for localized processing. At the beginning, a proper length of frame division to be clustered is estimated. It is assumed that its validity measures provide an equivalent performance compared to the full length processing of input recordings. Selecting proper number of localized clustering segments is constrained by the following restrictions: twice of number of features must exceed the amount of heartbeats per segment, and the minimum computational cost should be reached. At the end of the grouping step, combination of clustered segments is developed based on estimation of the proximities between each chosen cluster and the remaining clusters.

In this regard, DTW algorithm, noted as $\mathrm{dtw}(\cdot,\cdot)$, is used as a dissimilarity measure among heartbeats related to the set of centroids of a given cluster, as detailed in Cuesta et al. (2007). Thus, considering $\boldsymbol{P}^i = \{\boldsymbol{J}_1^i, \ldots, \boldsymbol{J}_{k^i}^i\}$ as the partition estimated for i–th segment, where $\boldsymbol{J}_{j^i}^i$ is the j-th cluster associated to i-th segment and k^i is the number of assumed groups for the same partition, $\{\zeta_1^i, \ldots, \zeta_{k^i}^i\}$ are the centroids of i–cluster, and $\boldsymbol{Y}(\boldsymbol{\zeta})$ stands for the projected data related to $\boldsymbol{\zeta}$ centroid, then, a combination of clusters follows next rule:

$$v(j^i, j^{i-1}) = \mathrm{dtw}\left(\boldsymbol{y}(\zeta_{j^i}^i), \boldsymbol{y}(\zeta_{j^{i-1}}^{i-1})\right) \tag{17}$$

that is, if an estimated measure $v(j^i, j^{i-1})$ lies within assumed proximity interval, then both chosen clusters are to be combined. Otherwise, following comparison of cluster is accomplished. Nonetheless, if there is any cluster not fulfilling the proximity measure during the current i-th iteration, it is no discarded but considered later during the coming next iterations. Therefore, incorrect clustering of minority classes is avoided whereas computational load is decreased.

4.5 Performance measures

clustering index, as a validity measure, is expressed as the relationship between the expected value of the GEMC objective function, given in Eq. (16), and assessed if considering an

ideal partition (θ_2), and the current value estimated for the final partition (θ_1), i.e θ_1/θ_2, as introduced in Sotelo, Peluffo, Frau, Ordónez & Domínguez (2009). Since $\theta_2 \geq \theta_1$, one might infer that index is regarded to a proper clustering if its value lies closer to 1. It must be quoted that the proposed above measure is not sensitive to the assumed number of clusters.
Another cluster validity measure that can be considered is the clustering quality developed by spectral graph partitioning Yu & Shi (2003), when a proper clustering means that tight connection is reached within partitions, there is a loose connection between partitions. Thus, the cluster coherence is computed as follows:

$$\epsilon_{\boldsymbol{B}} = \frac{1}{k}\sum_{l=1}^{k}\frac{\boldsymbol{B}_l^{\mathsf{T}}\boldsymbol{A}\boldsymbol{B}_l}{\boldsymbol{B}_l^{\mathsf{T}}\boldsymbol{D}\boldsymbol{B}_l} \tag{18}$$

where $\boldsymbol{B} = [\boldsymbol{B}_1, \ldots, \boldsymbol{B}_k]$, $\boldsymbol{B} \in \mathbb{R}^{n \times k}$ is a binary matrix comprised by the membership values of all elements to each cluster: $b_{ij} = \lfloor \max \arg_j f_m(\boldsymbol{y}_i/\zeta_j) \rfloor$, $j = 1, \ldots, k$, where $\lfloor \cdot \rfloor$ is 1 if its argument is true and 0 otherwise. $\boldsymbol{A}$ is the affinity matrix and $\boldsymbol{D} \in \mathbb{R}^{n \times n}$ is the degree of matrix $\boldsymbol{A}$.
Due to normalization with respect to the affinity matrix, the maximum value of $\epsilon_{\boldsymbol{B}}$ is 1, resulting in evidencing a good clustering if its value is closer to 1. Clustering is penalized when there is a large set of groups. In addition, supervised measures are accomplished to contrast with another similar references, taking advantage of recording labels, as further described. Particularly, each assembled cluster can be split into two clases: one holding the majority heartbeats regarding to the class of interest (*MC*), and another having the minority beatings being of different classes (*OC*). The following quantitative measures are defined: True Positive (T_P), heartbeats *MC* classified correctly, True negative (T_N), heartbeats *OC*, classified correctly, False positive (F_P), heartbeats *OC* classified as *MC* and False negative (F_N), heartbeats *MC* classified as *OC*.
After computing the above described measures, the following values of sensitivity (Se), specificity (Sp), and clustering performance (CP) are estimated:

$$\begin{aligned} Se &= \frac{T_N}{T_N + F_P} \\ Sp &= \frac{T_P}{T_P + F_N} \\ CP &= \frac{T_N + T_P}{T_N + F_P + T_P + F_N} \end{aligned}$$

Since there is no ideal partition, there are more clusters than classes expected. Therefore, the partition might be penalized when holding a relatively large number of clusters, for instance, by means of a factor as $e^{\eta k_r/k_a}$, where k_r is the number of groups resulting from the clustering, k_a is the admissibility value of groups, and η, $0 < \eta \leq 1$, is an adjusting value. In this way, the measure φ that can be S_e, S_p or C_P is weighted as follows:

$$\varphi = \begin{cases} \varphi e^{\eta k_r/k_a} & k_r > k_a \\ \varphi, & k_r \leq k_a \end{cases} \tag{19}$$

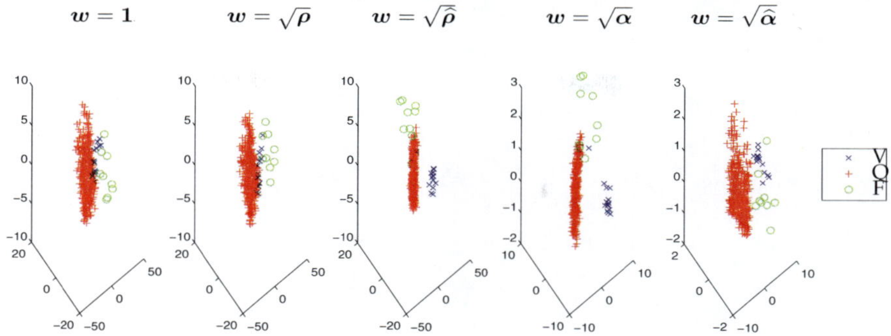

Fig. 7. First 3 principal components after weighting the data matrix for recording 217 with different $\boldsymbol{w}$ (algorithm 2)

5. Relevant experiments and discussion

Training is carried out over a set of ECG MIT-BIH database, which holds different types of arrhythmia, as previously discussed 1. The analysis is carried out over the whole data set for the MIT/BIH arrhythmia database that holds 48 recordings each one being of about 30 minutes long. It is important to note that the recording analysis is performed one by one, and some recordings exhibit strong unbalanced number of observation per class. Namely, it can be found some recordings holding just one–two heartbeats of class *F*, a few of *S* (less than 10), whereas its number of normal heartbeats may be very huge (more than 3000!).

5.1 Analysis of relevance results

Figure 7 shows an example for relevance analysis stage using the proposed scheme, taking into account the last 5 minutes of recording numbered as 217. It can be observed that there is a short separation of first 3 principal components. Remaining subfigures show the transformed data using the methods studied, where a better separability can be noted when using $\boldsymbol{w} = \sqrt{\widehat{\boldsymbol{\rho}}}$ and $\boldsymbol{w} = \sqrt{\boldsymbol{\alpha}}$. Particulary, in case of $\widehat{\boldsymbol{\rho}}$, the ignored eigenvectors (see Eq. (9)) for computing the relevance generate an homogeneous weighting of the analyzed features set, resulting in a lower selectivity, i.e., $\boldsymbol{w} = \sqrt{\boldsymbol{\rho}}$, having similar separability to $\boldsymbol{w} = \mathbf{1}_p$ (i.e. Conventional PCA). The variable weighting using the analyzed methods is shown in Fig. 8. It exhibits a similarity between $\boldsymbol{w} = \sqrt{\boldsymbol{\alpha}}$ and $\boldsymbol{w} = \sqrt{\widehat{\boldsymbol{\rho}}}$. The weighting obtained from iterative $Q - \alpha$ algorithm stands out mainly due to the quadratic nature of the objective function to be maximized, which employs M-inner product as distance measure. Although, it is not possible to generalize the results to all recordings because of ECG signal variability, this behavior is observed in most cases.

Figure 9 shows the dynamic of the calculated relevance of variables according to morphology type of each recording. Three segments of 207-th recording are analyzed. The first segment corresponds to the first 5 minutes of recording, which contains type *L*, *R* and *V* beats. The second one corresponds to a period between 20 minutes and 25 minutes, that only has type *L* and *V* beats. The last one contains type *A* and *E* beats corresponding to the last 5 minutes of recording.

It can be seen that in the first segment, the relevant variables correspond to the WT features (table 2) while in the second one, the Hermite coefficients had higher weight since these coefficients characterize appropriately to the morphology of type *L* and *V* beats. Finally, in

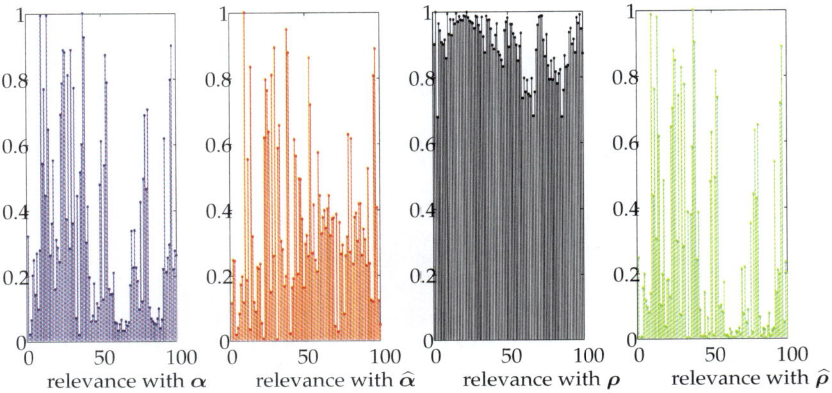

Fig. 8. Relevance of the features (table 2) for the last 5 minutes of recording 217 using all methods to estimate $\boldsymbol{w}$ (algorithm 2)

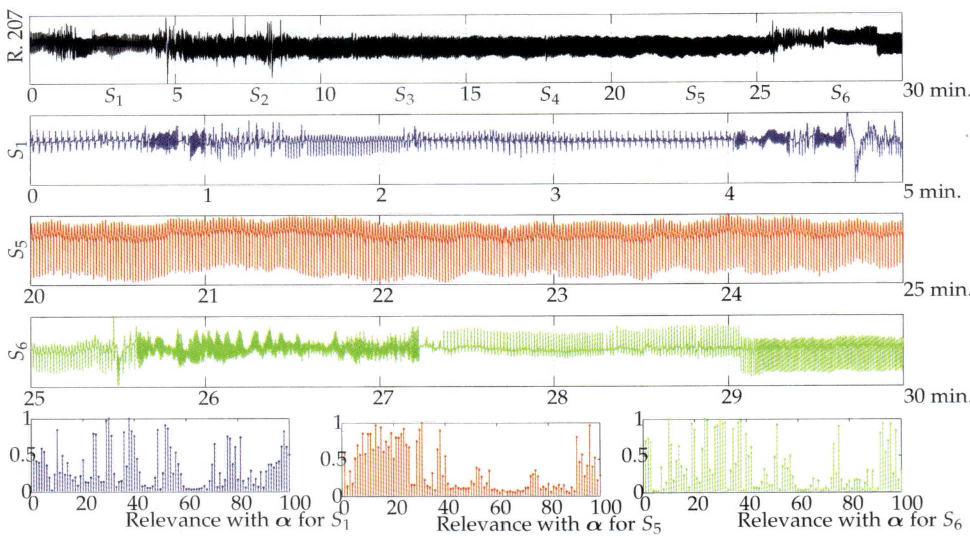

Fig. 9. Results of the relevance of the features with Q-α method, for 3 segments of the recording 207. S_i, corresponds to the i-th segment of the recording 207, which holds 5 minutes of length.

the last analyzed segment the weight for each one of the first 3 variables (*HRV* features) is increased. According to this, it can be concluded that segment analysis allows a local analysis of relevance and achieves good performance after the final partition, as discussed in the following section.

	θ_1/θ_2	$\epsilon_{\boldsymbol{B}}$	k_{end}	q	Time [s]
			$\mu - \sigma^2$		
α	0.95 - 0.08	0.86 - 0.12	9 - 2.43	6 - 0.86	37.20 - 7.65
ρ	0.94 - 0.10	0.82 - 0.14	11 - 2.67	10 - 1.78	38.52 - 7.52
$\widehat{\rho}$	0.94 - 0.10	0.83 - 0.14	11 - 2.66	9 - 1.77	37.47 - 7.66
$\widehat{\alpha}$	0.95 - 0.08	0.84 - 0.12	9 - 2.44	6 - 1.16	36.20 - 7.54

Table 3. Clustering performance using non–supervised indices (θ_1/θ_2, $\epsilon_{\boldsymbol{B}}$), number of resultant groups (k_{end}), number of relevant features (q) and processing time $[s]$.

It can be highlighted the fact that the variability features (*HRV*, table 2) are essential to discriminate between normal heartbeats and supraventricular ectopic beats, both of them having similar morphology. Most important morphological features correspond to those based on WT, which discriminate between type *V* and *Q* heartbeats.

5.2 Computing clustering performance

The results of clustering are accomplished by framing each recording into 6 divisions and the resulting clusters are merged as described in section 4.4. The number of segments is achieved experimentally, improving the trade–off among the number of segments, computational cost and quality of partition. Thus, the segment analysis enhances the performance if compared to the whole data clustering. In fact, it reduces the probability that a minority class heartbeat might be clustered wrongly. Furthermore, in most cases, the sum of processing times over all segments turns out to be considerably shorter than the time of analysis of the whole recording data for one iteration. As a result, the introduced framing approach significantly reduces the computational cost.

Table 3 depicts the whole system performance using the non–supervised indices, as discussed in section 4.4, and parameters for computational cost and the number of resulting groups are displayed, as well. The first column refers to the index θ_1/θ_2, the second one to $\epsilon_{\boldsymbol{B}}$, the third one corresponds to the resulting clusters (k_{end}) after processing all segments of each recording, the fourth one is the number of selected features before projecting the data, and the last one is the time fixed from filtering to clustering stages. The rows show the methods considered for weighting of variables.

Evaluation of the quality of partition is provided by the index θ_1/θ_2 that has been introduced in Sotelo, Peluffo, Frau, Ordónez & Domínguez (2009), where a maximum index value of $\theta_1/\theta_2 = 0.98$ was achieved over only 14 recordings of the entire MIT/BIH database. In this chapter, the maximum index achieved is close to ($\sim$ 0.96), over the whole recording set if providing framed division analysis; pointing out to have a better generalization ability. If increasing the number of groups k, then index θ_1/θ_2 tends to 1. Nonetheless, a very high number of k leads to a more difficult evaluation by specialists. Specifically, in Lagerholm et al. (2000), the total number of groups representing the entire MIT/BIH database is assumed to be 25, while in Rodríguez-Sotelo et al. (2009), when considering only some recordings from MIT/BIH database, the average number of groups diminishes to 15. In this chapter, for the entire MIT/BIH database the value k ranges within $9 \leq k \leq 11$, still showing a better performance.

As discussed above, the non–supervised measure $\epsilon_{\boldsymbol{B}}$ penalizes the number of groups after the final partition. In fact, if the clustering procedure is carried out for a value less than or equal to the proper value of k, then $\epsilon_{\boldsymbol{B}}$ tends to 1. Otherwise, this value becomes far from 1, as the amount of k is increased, due to the upper bound monotonicity theorem Yu & Shi (2003).

	N	S	V	F	Q
	$\mu-\sigma^2$	$\mu-\sigma^2$	$\mu-\sigma^2$	$\mu-\sigma^2$	$\mu-\sigma^2$
			$\boldsymbol{\alpha}$		
Se	99.25– 2.48	91.11–15.66	96.11– 8.24	70.73–32.05	91.9 –17.83
Sp	95.77– 9.12	99.36– 2.19	99.87– 0.24	99.59– 0.77	99.79– 0.47
CP	99.16– 2.5	96.18– 6.15	98.29– 3.37	93.29–10.62	99.91– 0.21
			$\widehat{\boldsymbol{\alpha}}$		
Se	99.06– 3.5	90.52–16.54	96.31– 7.03	50.59–35.33	87.88–26.77
Sp	95.32– 9.49	99.49– 1.62	99.84– 0.31	99.51– 0.99	99.6 – 0.73
CP	99.25– 2.01	96.24– 6.67	98.13– 3.86	81.64–32.51	99.96– 0.06
			$\widehat{\boldsymbol{\rho}}$		
Se	99.27– 2.55	91.26–15.26	91.5 –21.52	50.57–34.63	79.91–44.67
Sp	92.19–19.06	99.5 – 1.51	99.86– 0.26	99.6 – 0.76	99.85– 0.34
CP	99.14– 2.46	95.68– 7.47	93.71–20.77	81.05–33.04	79.93–44.68
			$\boldsymbol{\rho}$		
Se	99.24– 2.79	90.08–18.57	91.62–21.61	42.44–39.57	87.86–26.75
Sp	92.17–19.37	99.58– 1.22	99.85– 0.28	99.53– 0.92	99.79– 0.47
CP	99.12– 2.58	96.16– 6.07	93.77–20.79	68.87–41.56	99.91– 0.21

Table 4. Clustering results by using supervised measures for all groups of arrhythmias

Concretely, a value of k less than 6 can be taken as an admisible number of groups because 5 classes are considered in the present arrhythmia analysis.
Table 3 shows that the achieved values for $\epsilon_{\mathcal{B}}$ are ranging within interval $0.82 \leq \epsilon_M \leq 0.86$, which can be considered as a realistic outcome to quantify the resultant partition. Still, this measure does not reach the value 1, as if grouping were absolutely correct, because of the effect of penalization regarding the number of groups and also the sensitivity to the affinity matrix. Besides, the average number is shown for the relevant features q before the WPCA projection (see section 4.3) that most of them contribute to the clustering process. As seen, the range of values of q is $6 \leq q \leq 10$, showing admisible values with respect to the total number of features. Additionally, the average computing time needed to process the whole recording is 37 s, being a reasonable time for each considered recording.
Table 4 shows the arithmetic mean (μ) and variance (σ^2) of supervised measures, discussed in section 4.4, over the entire database for each group of arrhythmias, using the proposed weighting methods (see algorithm 2). In Rodríguez-Sotelo et al. (2009), the clustering performance is evaluated only considering three arrhythmia groups, namely, *N*, *S* and *V* (see table 1). Nonetheless, the performance measures are calculated by couples of arrhythmias and, as a consequence, the value of measures tends to increase. The reported results are $Se_S = 93.3\%$ and $Sp_S = 99.5\%$, which can be compared with the second column of table 4, where the maximum values are $Se_S = 91.3\%$ and $Sp_S = 99.5\%$. Although, sensitivity is less than the reported in Rodríguez-Sotelo et al. (2009), it should be noted that among results of this work, all recordings from the database with *S*-type arrhythmias (the class of interest) and the remaining groups as another class are analyzed. Thus, the proposed method provides more robustness when considering other types of arrhythmias.
For some considered arrhythmia groups, the performance results in table 4 became remarkable, e.g. $Se_N = 99.25\%$, $Se_V = 96.5\%$. In other cases, e.g. *F* group, the performance values decreases, $Se_F = 70.7\%$, due to the low number of representative heartbeats of some classes. Still, one can infer that the best performance is provided when the data are weighted by using $\boldsymbol{\alpha}$.
Finally, in Figure 10, an example of clustered heartbeats is presented by using the recording 217 of the MIT/BIH arrhythmia database which contains heartbeats of type: N, V, f and P (in

Figure, the symbol P is represented as /, which corresponds to the original tag for paced beats in the MIT/BIH database).

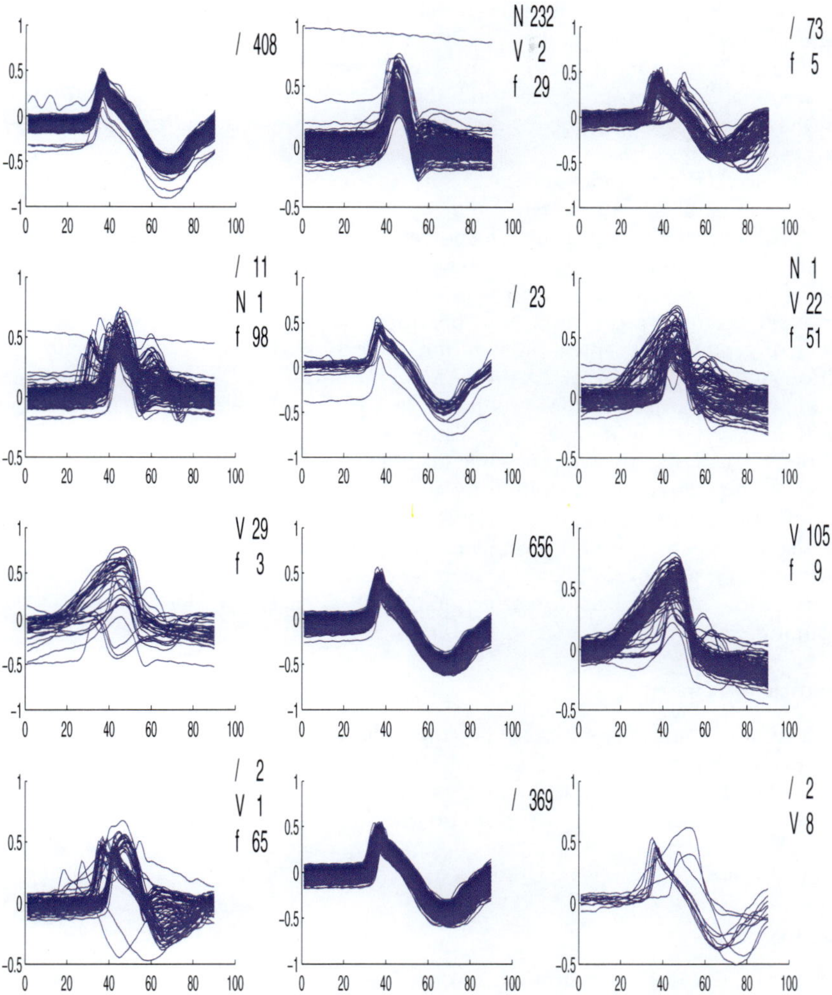

Fig. 10. General methodology applied over recording 217.

6. Conclusions

The proposed methodology for unsupervised Holter monitoring of cardiac arrhythmias that is based on variable–wise relevance analysis leads to an improvement of clustering of those heartbeat types recommended by AAMI. Because of strong asymmetry among class observations, the heartbeat–derived features should be properly selected by their weighting projection. This makes possible to assess the relative importance of each feature immersed on the original data representation. In addition, because of restrictions for reducing computational load, proposed methodology is carried out by successive division analysis along the time, where each recording is separately processed, and thus significantly reduces the processing time.

It must be noted that the relevance analysis provides enough generalization capability, mainly, because of most informative features are weighted and projected. In general, in this work, the M-inner product-based approach showed better performance than MSE-based approach, and although its iterative nature leads to high computational cost, the segment analysis compensates for this effect. This it is possible its implementation for real time applications. Besides, the assuming grouping that includes initial parameters estimation (estimation of number of groups and center initialization), which is based on spectral techniques and soft partitional clustering, generates a proper final partition.

The methodology provides an useful tool to analyze cardiac arrhythmias with suitable quality since it is based on non-supervised training. That is, there is no need for labelling of recordings, which mostly is not feasible for Holter monitoring.

Testing of considered methodology by using introduced cluster validity measures shows a comparable performance in comparison to another referenced works based on either supervised or unsupervised training and carried out for the MIT/BIH database.

As future work, additional spectral clustering stages should be explored with the possibility of unifying the stages of feature selection and clustering, in order to improve accuracy and computational load for the system.

7. Acknowledgment

This study was financially supported by the project "Cálculo Científico Para El Procesamiento Avanzado De Bioseñales", code: 20201006570, Universidad Nacional de Colombia, and was supported by the project "Sistema automatizado para la estimación del tamaño de lesión en el ventrículo izquierdo a causa de infarto de miocardio usando electrocardiografía", code: 249-028, Universidad Autónoma de Manizales. Additionally, The authors thank to the "Language Institute (Translation Center)", Universidad Autónoma de Manizales.

8. References

Balaguer, I. (n.d.). Los estudios longitudinales en la prevención de las enfermedades cardiovasculares, *Revista Española de Salud Pública*. pp. 1135–5727.

Braunwald, E. (1993). *Tratado de Cardiología.*, Vol. 1, 4 edn.

Brugada, J., Brugada, R. & Brugada, P. (1998). Síndrome del bloqueo de rama derecha, elevación del segmento st de v1 a v3 y muerte súbita cardíaca, *Medicina General* .

Ceylan, R. & Özbay, Y. (2007). Comparison of fcm, pca and wt techniques for classification ecg arrhythmias using artificial neural network, *Expert Systems with Applications* 33(2): 286 – 295. URL: *http://www.sciencedirect.com/science/article/B6V03-4K48JG7-1/2/e55c48da65949dc6b8965a7f172c763a*

Cuesta, D., Biagetti, M., Quinteiro, R., Mico-Tormos, P. & Aboy, M. (2007). Unsupervised classification of ventricular extrasystoles using bounded clustering algorithms and morphology matching, *Medical and Biological Engineering and Computing* 45(3): 229–239.

Cuesta, D., Pérez-Cortés, J. & Andreau-García, G. (2003). Clustering of ecg signals in computer-aided holter analysis, *Computer Methods and Programs in Biomedicine* 72: 179–196.

Cvetkovic, D., Übeyli, E. D. & Cosic, I. (2008). Wavelet transform feature extraction from human ppg, ecg, and eeg signal responses to elf pemf exposures: A pilot study, *Digital Signal Processing* 18(5): 861 – 874.
URL: *http://www.sciencedirect.com/science/article/B6WDJ-4NX2NHW-4/2/bcd26d87922d-1691141f30adfbaab88b*

Dave, J., Gandhi, G., Nazeer, S., Jha, S. & Kocheril, A. (2005). Ventricular premature complexes. emedicine, *www.emedicine.com ([Online])* .

De-Chazal, P., O'Dwyer, M. & Reilly, R. (2004). Automatic classification of heartbeats using ecg morphology and heartbeat interval features, *IEEE transaction on biomedical engineering* 51(7): 1196–1206.

Engström, G., Hedblad, B., Juul-Möller, S., Tydén, P. & Janzon, L. (2000). Cardiac arrhythmias and stroke increased risk in men with high frequency of atrial ectopic beats, *Stroke, American Heart Association, Inc.* pp. 2925–2929.

Friedman, H. (1989). *Diagnostic electrocardiography and vectorcardiography*, 3ra edn, Mc. Graw Hill.

ginsburg, G., Sunder, N. & Grace, P. (2006). Acute right bundle branch block as a presenting sign of acute pulmonary embolism, *Anesth Analg* pp. 789 – 791.

Guyton, A. & Hall, J. E. (n.d.). *Tratado de fisiología médica*, 10 edn.

Hamerly, G. & Elkan, C. (2002). Alternatives to the k-means that find better clusterings, *Pattern Recognition* .

Hansen, P. & Mladenovic, N. (2001). J-means: a new local search heuristic for minimum sum of squares clustering, *Pattern Recognition* 34: 405–413.

Holter, N. (n.d.). *New methods for heart studies*, Science.

J. Segura-Juárez, D. C., Samblas-Pena, L. & Aboy, M. (2004). A microcontroller-based portable electrocardiograph recorder, *IEEE transaction on biomedical engineering* 51: 1686–16906.

Lagerholm, M., Peterson, C., Braccini, G., Edenbrandt, L. & Sörnmo, L. (2000). Clustering ecg complexes using hermite functions and self-organising maps, *IEEE trans. on. Biomed.* 48: 838–847.

Laguna, P. & Sörnmo, L. (2005). *Bioelectrical signal processing in cardiac and neurological applications*, Vol. 1.

Li, Z., Devereux, R., Kjeldsen, S., Julius, S., Wachtell, K., Ibsen, H., Nieminen, M., Jern, S., Okin, P. & Dahlof, B. (n.d.). Association of left bundle branch block with cardiovascular morbidity and mortality in hypertensive patients with left ventricle hypertrophy: the life study, *Posters: Clinical Trials* .

Martens, S., Mischi, M., Oei, S. & Bergmans, J. (2006). An improved adaptive power line interference canceller for electrocardiography, *IEEE transactions on Biomedical Engineering* 53(11): 2220 – 2231.

Micó, J. A. & Ibor, P. (2004). Medicina general, *Medicina General* (66): 426.

Moody, G. & Mark, R. (1982). Development and evaluation of a 2-lead ecg analysis program, *in Computers in Cardiology, IEEE Computer Society Press* pp. 39–44.

Ng, A. Y., Jordan, M. I. & Weiss, Y. (2001). On spectral clustering: Analysis and an algorithm, *Advances in Neural Information Processing Systems 14*, MIT Press, pp. 849–856.

Pabón, G. (2001). Indicación de estudio electrofisiológico en pacientes con bloqueo intraventricular crónico, *Primer consenso sobre recomendaciones de estudio electrofisiológico y ablación con energía de radiofrecuencia* .

Perlibakas, V. (2004). Distance measures for pca-based face recognition, *Pattern Recognition Letters* 25(16): 711–724.

Roddy, A. (1991). A filter to suppress ecg baseline wander and preserve st-segment accuracy in a real-time environment, *Journal of Electrocardiology* 24(4): 315–323.

Rodríguez-Sotelo, J., Cuesta-Frau, D. & Castellanos-Domínguez, G. (2009). Unsupervised classification of atrial heartbeats using a prematurity index and wave morphology features, *Medical and Biological Engineering and Computing* 47(7): 731–741.

Sotelo, J. L. R., Frau, D. C., Ordónez, D. P., Domínguez, G. C. & Novak, D. (2009). Unsupervised feature selection in cardiac arrhythmia analysis, *Engineering in medicine and conference. EMBC* .

Sotelo, J. L. R., Peluffo, D., Frau, D. C., Ordónez, D. P. & Domínguez, G. C. (2009). Non-parametric density-based clustering for cardiac arrhythmia analysis, *Computers in cardiology. CINC* .

Wen, C., Yeh, M. & Chang, K. (2007). Ecg beat classification using greyart network, *Signal Processing, IET* 1(1): 19–28.

Wolf, L. & Shashua, A. (2005). Feature selection for unsupervised and supervised inference: The emergence of sparsity in a weight-based approach, *Journal of machine learning* 6: 1855 – 1887.

Yu, S. X. & Shi, J. (2003). Multiclass spectral clustering, *ICCV '03: Proceedings of the Ninth IEEE International Conference on Computer Vision*, IEEE Computer Society, Washington, DC, USA, p. 313.

Yue, H. H. & Tomoyasu, M. (2004). Weighted principal component analysis and its applications to improve fdc performance, *Conference on decision and control*.

Özbay, Y., Ceylan, R. & Karlik, B. (2006). A fuzzy clustering neural network architecture for classification of ecg arrhythnmias, *Computers in Biology and Medicine* 36: 376–388.

12

Concealed Conduction

Hasan Ari and Kübra Doğanay
Bursa Postgraduate Hospital,
Departments of Cardiology,
Bursa,
Turkey

1. Introduction

Concealed conduction is a phenomenon which could be rarely seen on the surface of electrocardiography (ECG). The surface ECG must be evaluated carefully for determination of concealed conduction. Because concealed conduction manifests itself in different shape and level. This evaluation could prevent misdiagnosis and unappropriate treatment. In this chapter we want to contribute to understanding this phenomenon.

2. Historical perspective

Concealed conduction of sinus impulse at the level of the AV node was documented in animal models in 1925 (1). Nearly 20 years after the animal models, concealed conduction was shown in human heart by Langendorf et al (2). Initial animal and human models showed that concealed conduction occurred in the sinus node, around the sinus node, atrium, AV node and Hiss-Purkinje system (3-5). Following years many studies was published about the effect and electrophysiological mechanism of concealed conduction.

3. Concealed conduction mechanism

A number of investigators had since observed similar phenomena but it was not until the studies of Langendorf and Pick that the concept of concealed conduction was firmly established in electrocardiology (6,7). A wide variety of phenomenology has been described as consequences of penetration of impulses that do not emerge from the AV node (8). Some of these: delay of conduction of a succeeding propagated response, block of a succeeding atrial impulse that occurs at a time when the AV node should have been excitable, delay of the expected discharge of an AV nodal pacemaker. When an impulse penetrates the AV node but it does not traverse completely, at one point it becomes subthreshold for cells located distal to the site of block. This subthreshold event may be manifested in the distal cells as an electrotonic depolarization at a distance that depends on the membrane resistance and the degree of electrical coupling among cells.

It was demonstrated initially by Antzelevitch and Liu (9,10) many of the phenomena described in terms of concealed conduction may be a consequence of the inhibitory action of subthreshold electrotonic potentials on subsequent responses in the Purkinje fiber and numerical experiments in models of AV nodal cells. Thus, electrotonic inhibition explain the

clinically observed phenomenon of concealed AV conduction. Subthreshold potentials in the AV node may result in delay of excitation or even failure of responses occurring later in time, that at least some variants of concealed AV conduction may be explained by electrotonically mediated reduction of $I_{Ca.T}$ (10).
Electrotonic inhibition and concealed conduction are widespread in cardiac tissues. However, we have very little knowladge about ionic mechanisms of electrotonic inhibition and concealed conduction. Electrotonic inhibition of excitability has been demonstrated in ventricular myocytes. Indeed, repetitive stimulation in myocytes, with depolarizing current pulses of threshold amplitude may elicit action potentials in a one-to-one manner. Furthermore, subthreshold pulse during a single diastolic interval may lead to a transient decay in excitability and even to complete failure of subsequent excitation.
Liu et al, demonstrated that the specific role of $I_{Ca.T}$ in the dynamic modulation of AV nodal excitability by premature inputs and suggest a plausible ionic mechanism for the regulation of action potential propagation through the AV nodal conducting system (10). Premature depolarization can modulate the amplitude of the transient calcium current, the time course of such modulation is compatible with the diastolic time window during which electrotonic inhibition is permissible. The modulation is directly associated with a decrease in $I_{Ca.T}$ (10). I_F may be responsible for electrotonic inhibition in Purkinje fibers (9). Previous experiments in pig ventricular myocytes have shown that diastolic excitability is modulated by the long time course of deactivation of I_K (11). If conditioning pulse intervals were much longer than expected intervals for complete deactivation of I_K , electrotonic inhibition occurred. Under such conditions, the basis of changes in the kinetics of $I_{Ca.T}$ may easily explain this phenomenon.

4. Concealed conduction

The concealed conduction, is an extra impulse from the heart which penetrate the electrical system of heart on refractory period, regardless the impulse change characteristics of conduction system, it does not cause any contraction. The effect on subsequent events is an important part of the definition of concealed conduction because it differentiates the concept of concealed conduction from other forms of incomplete conduction, such as conduction blocks. It should be recalled that although the ECG reflects the electrophsiological properties of the myocardium, alterations of conduction more often reflect electrophysiological changes in the specialized tissues, the activity of which is not recorded on the surface ECG.
The concept of concealed conduction, was introduced before (6,7), an explanation for the effects of incomplete penetration of an impulse into a portion of the A-V conduction system. The phenomena could observe on the surface ECG, but that was incompletely penetrating impulse and not directly reflected on the surface ECG; hence the term *concealed.*
The manifestations of concealed conduction are numerous, because of variations of the site of impulse formation, the different effects of the anatomical site, the direction of the concealment (e.g., the heart rate, automatic tone, drugs, or electrolyte balance).
The manifestations of concealed conduction include;

a. prolongation of conduction,
b. failure of propagation of an impulse,
c. facilitation of conduction by "peeling back" refractoriness, directly altering refractoriness, and/or summation (12,13), and
d. pauses in the discharge of a spontaneous pacemaker.

The concealed conduction usually occur in AV node and/or His-purkinje system. The conduction of AV node is silent, so that does not occur any deflexion on surface ECG. The conduction of AV node can be determined by measuring duration of PR. Sometimes, an extra impulse is originated from atria or ventricle which incompletly penetrate in AV node because of refractoriness of the AV node. The incomplete penetration of extra impulse to AV node cause prolongation of the PR interval or blockage of AV conduction (figure 1,2,3,4).
A common example may be interpolated premature ventricular contraction (PVC) during normal sinus rhythm; the PVC does not cause an atrial contraction, because the retrograde impulse form the PVC does not completely penetrate the AV node. However this AV node stimulation can cause a delay in subsequent AV conduction by modifying the AV node´s subsequent conduction characteristic. Hence, the PR interval after the PVC is longer than the baseline PR interval. (figure 1,3).

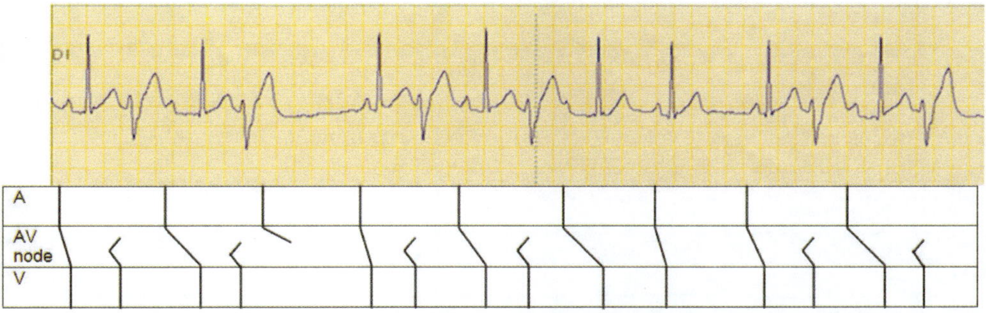

Fig. 1. Sinus rhythm and bigeminal PVC. P waves which follow PVC are blocked, Lewis diagram: A: Atrium, AV: Atrio ventricular, V: Ventricle.

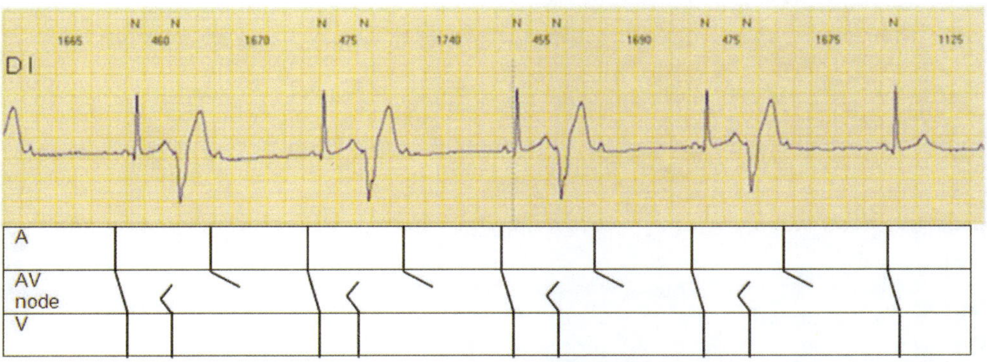

Fig. 2. First and second narrow QRSs are followed by PVCs with progressive prolongation of the PR interval and the blockage of the third sinus beat (Mobitz type I AV block). The third sinus beat is obscured by the T wave. The third and fourth narrow QRSs are also followed by PVCs and PR interval shows progressive prolongation. Since the fifth narrow QRS is not followed by a PVC, this prolongation does not end with the blockage of the next (7th) P wave, which is conducted with a normal PR interval. First, third, fourth, and fifth PVCs are interpolated, Lewis diagram: A: Atrium, AV: Atrio ventricular, V: Ventricle.

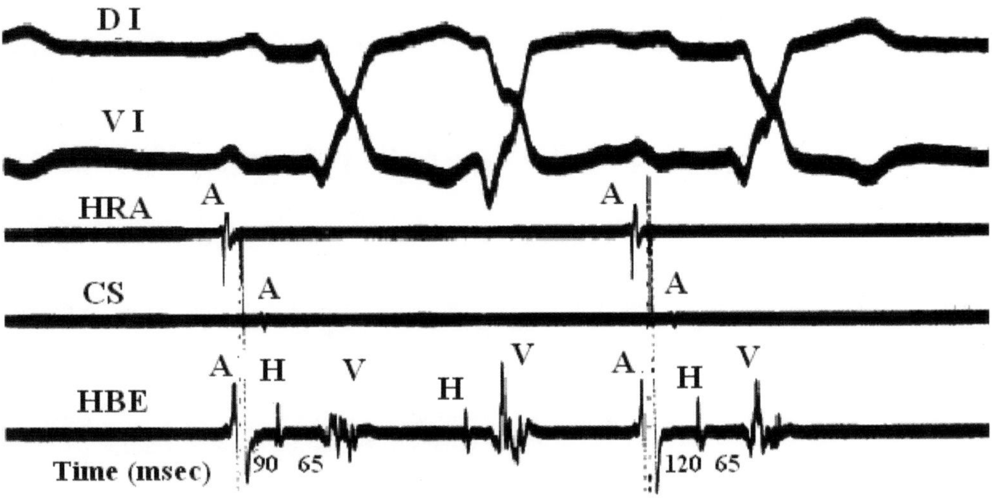

Fig. 3. Because of retrograde concealed conduction by a fascicular extrasystole (second beat) the next sinus impulse A-H interval is longer than before.

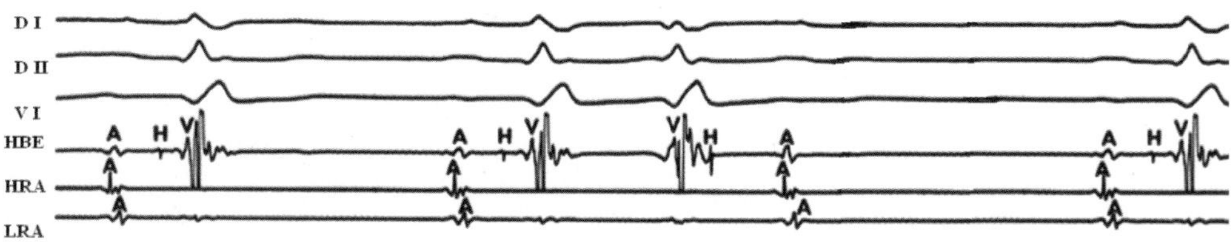

Fig. 4. Concealed conduction by PVC (third beat) the subsequent sinus complex is a block in the A-V node (third atrial beat).

Another example on concealed conduction concept is seen in atrial flutter and fibrillation. Some of the atrial activity fails to get through the AV node in an anterograde direction as a result of the rapid atrial rate. A long RR interval after repeated concealments is usually followed by an AV junctional escape impulse. If the RR is longer than the expected junctional escape interval, a concealed impulse of the junctional pacemaker could be suspected.

In some cases, concealed conduction (extra impulse is orginated from atria or ventricle which has incompletly penetrated in AV node) repair the AV node refractory period and subsequent impulse conduct with normal or short duration of PR. This phenomen is called ''peeling'' or peeling back of the refractory period (figure 5).

Concelaed conduction may be seen in bundle branch system. Functional bundle branch block may be seen as a result of rapid increase of ventricular rate and bundle branch block could continue until ventricular rate return to baseline heart rate. The functional bundle branch block may be explained by transseptal concealed conduction (figure 6). Atrial impulse is conducted to the ventricle via a branch which is in non refractory period and the other branch of conduction system is stimulated via transseptal concealed conduction which is in refractory period during atrioventricular conduction. The next atrial impulse is conducted by the same branch because of ongoing refractory period of the other branch. This stituation causes vicious cycle. This vicious cycle has been continued until heart rate decreases to critical ventriculer rate which elicits refractory period of all branches of cardiac conducting system.

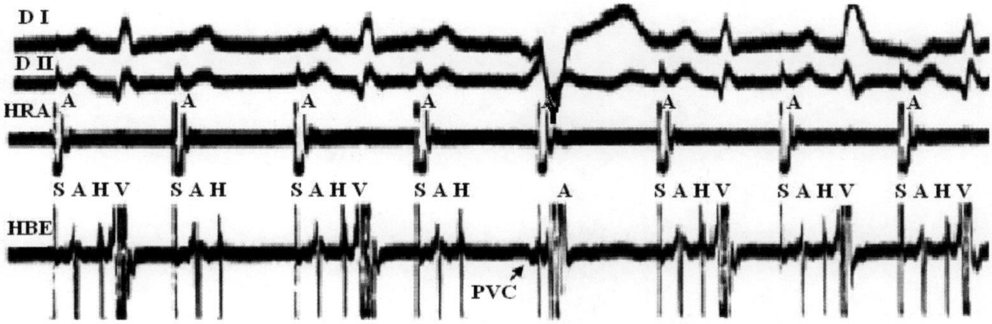

Fig. 5. During atrial pacing at a cycle length of 400 msec, 2:1 block below the His bundle occurs. After a PVC (arrow, the fifth complex), the P wave that block in the 2:1 sequence conducts to ventricle as other conducted complexes. The PVC repair the AV node refractory period and subsequent impulse conduct with normal duration. (S: stimulation, A: atrium, H: His, V: Ventricle).

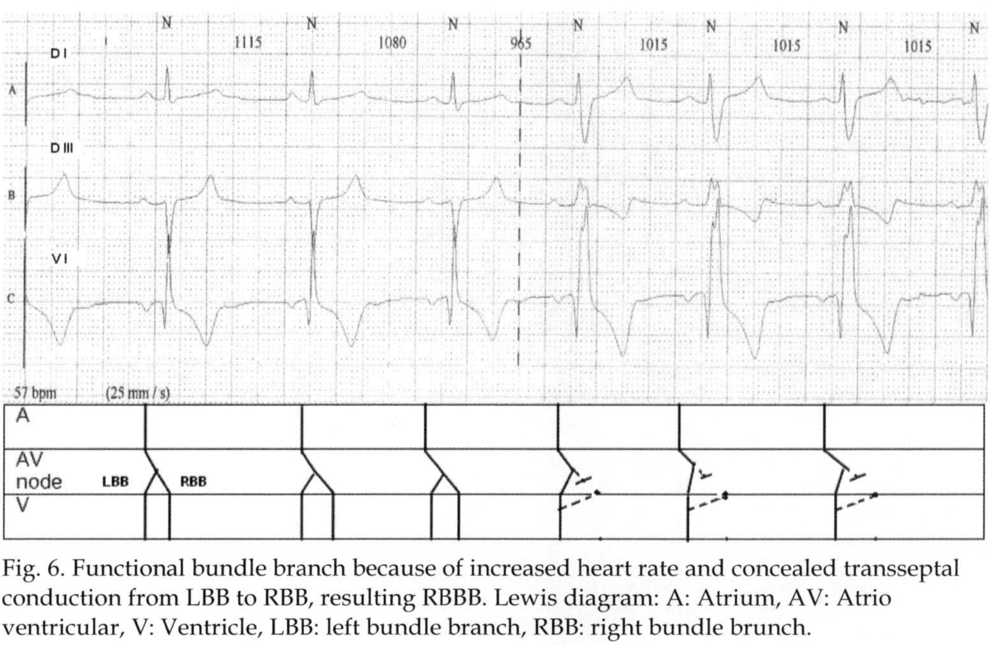

Fig. 6. Functional bundle branch because of increased heart rate and concealed transseptal conduction from LBB to RBB, resulting RBBB. Lewis diagram: A: Atrium, AV: Atrio ventricular, V: Ventricle, LBB: left bundle branch, RBB: right bundle brunch.

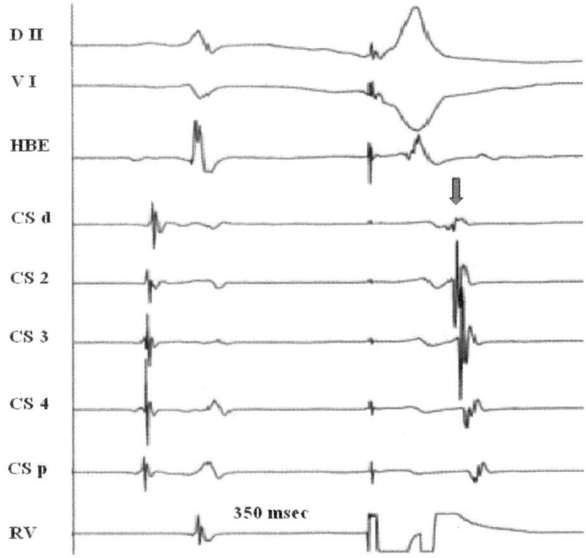

Fig. 7. Right ventricular extrastimulus with 350 msec coupling interval showing retrograde conduction over a left-sided accesory pathway (arrow) (because of short coupling interval the concealed conduction can not arrive to accesory pathway and accesory pathway can be suitable for retrograde conduction).

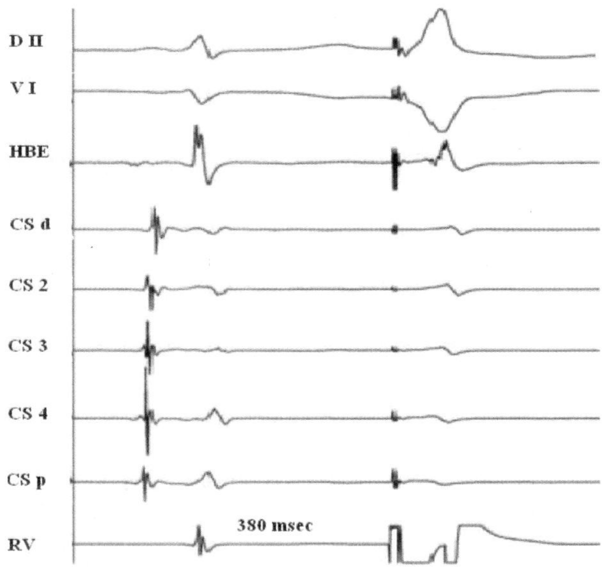

Fig. 8. Right ventricular extrastimulus with 380 msec coupling interval showing no retrograde conduction (the concealed conduction to accesory pathway prevents the retrograde conduction which cause resiprocating tachycardia).

One of circumstance related with concealed conduction is WPW sendrome. Atrial stimulation is conducted to the ventricle by passing AV node and lead to resiprocating tachycardia result of recycling retrograde conduction via accesory pathway (figure 7). However, concealed conduction to accesory pathway causes refractory period of accesory pathway and inhibition of retrograde conduction of accesory pathway, so the concealed conduction to accesory pathway prevents resiprocating tachycardia (figure 8).
The concealed conduction to the sinus node because of an extra atrial impulse (the impulse changes sinus node pacemaker function) lead to delay in the next stimulus of the sinus node. As a result, this event represents itself with a longer duration of PP than the previous duration of PP on surface ECG (figure 9).

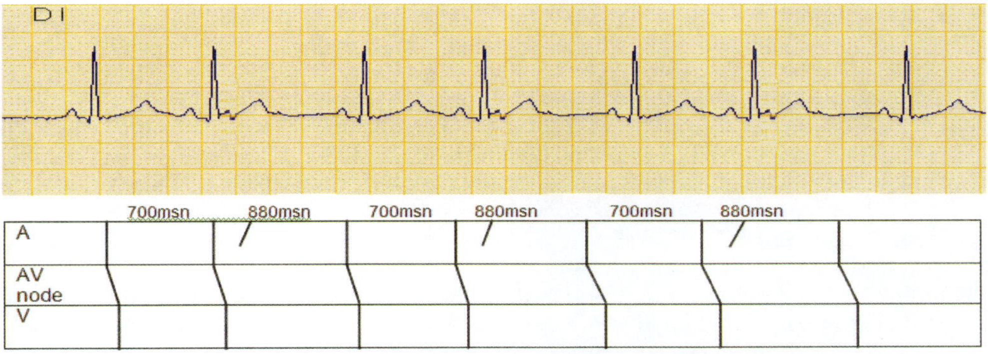

Fig. 9. Lewis diagram: Concealed conduction to sinus node. A: Atrium, AV: Atrio ventricular, V: Ventricle.

5. Summary

Heart conduction system sites and mechanisms of concealed conduction.

- Sinüs node:
  Changing the sinüs node pacemaker function by concealment of an extra atrial impulse; lead to delay the next stimulus.
- AV node:
  1-Anterograde AV node concealment manifest with;
  a. Delay of AV conduction
  b. Block of AV conduction
  c. Block of retrograde VA conduction
  d. Slowing of ventricular rate due to concealment of atrial fibrillatory waves
  e. Peeling back of the AV node refractory period and subsequent impulse conduct with normal or short duration of PR.
  2-Retrograde VA concealment manifest with;
  a. Delay of AV conduction
  b. Block of AV conduction
  c. Peeling back of the AV node refractory period and subsequent impulse conduct with normal or short duration of PR.
- Bundle branch system:

Functional bundle branch block because of rapid ventricular rate and the other branch of conduction system is stimulated via transseptal concealed conduction.

- Accesory pathway:
  Concealed conduction to accesory pathway inhibition the retrograde conduction of accesory pathway. The concealed conduction prevents tachycardia which is related with accesorf pathway.

6. Disclosure

Authors have no relevant conflict of interest to disclose

7. References

[1] Lewis T, Master AM. Observations upon conduction in the mammalian heart. A-V conduction. Heart 1925;12:209 e69.
[2] Langendorf R, Pick A, Edelist A, Katz LN. Experimental Demonstration of Concealed AV Conduction in the Human Heart. Circulation, 1965;32:386.
[3] Langendorf R, Pick A. Concealed intraventricular conduction in the human heart. Recent advences in ventricular conduction. Adv Cardiol 1975, 14:40.
[4] Sung RJ, Myerburg RJ, Castellanos A. Electrophysiological demostration of concealed conduction in the human atrium. Circulation, 1978;58: 940.
[5] Rosen KM, Rahimtoola SH, Gunnar RM. Pseudo AV block secondary to premature nonpropagate His bundle depolatization. Documentation by His bundle electrocardiography. Circulation, 1970;42: 367.
[6] Langendorf R. Concealed AV conduction: the effect of blocked impulses on the formation and conduction of subsequent impulses. Am Heart J 1948; 35:542.
[7] Langendorf R, Pick A. Concealed conduction further evaluation of a fundamental aspect of propagation of the cardiac impulse. Circulation 1956; 13:381-399.
[8] Pick A, Langendorf R. Interpretation of ComplexArrhythmias. Philadelphia, Pa: Lee & Febiger; 1979:471-541.
[9] Antzelevitch C, Moe GK. Electrotonic inhibition and summation of impulse conduction in mammalian Purkinje fibers.Am J Physiol. 1983;245:H42-H53.
[10] Liu Y, Zeng W, Delmar M, Jalife J. Ionic Mechanisms of Electrotonic Inhibition and Concealed Conduction in Rabbit Atrioventricular Nodal Myocytes. *Circulation* 1993;88;1634-1646.
[11] Delmar M, Michaels DC, Jalife J. Slow recovery of excitability and the Wenckebach phenomenon in the single guinea pig ventricular myocyte. Circ Res. 1989;65:761-774.
[12] Moore EN, Knobel SB, Spear JF. Concealed conduction. Am J Cardiol. 1971;28: 406-413.
[13] Zipes DP, Mendez C, Moe GK. Evidence for summation and voltage dependency in rabbit atrioventricular nodal fibers. Circ Res 1973; 32: 170-177.

Part 4

Heart Rate Variability

13

Associations of Metabolic Variables with Electrocardiographic Measures of Sympathovagal Balance in Healthy Young Adults

Richard M. Millis[1], Mark D. Hatcher[1], Rachel E. Austin[1], Vernon Bond[2] and Kim L. Goring[3]
[1]Department of Physiology & Biophysics, Howard University College of Medicine,
[2]Department of Health, Human Performance & Leisure Studies,
Howard University Graduate School of Arts & Sciences,
[3]Department of Medicine, Howard University Hospital
Washington, DC,
USA

1. Introduction

Although obesity affects African-Americans disproportionately to their representation in the U.S. population, few studies have been performed to elucidate the mechanisms of maintaining body fat stores in healthy adolescent or young adult African-Americans with low and high percentages of body fat, before they have developed obesity-related diseases. Research has suggested some explanations, such as distrust and hesitancy about invasive procedures, to account for the sparse representation of African-Americans as subjects in research (Hamilton et al., 2006; Farmer et al., 2007; Braunstein et al., 2008). Indeed, advances in our knowledge of the obese phenotype have been impeded by the lack of noninvasive technologies for measuring the impact of body fat on physiological regulatory mechanisms. However, this impediment has effectively been overcome by the advent of heart rate variability analyses for elucidating autonomic mechanisms (Lucini et al., 2002). Such analyses make it possible to differentiate a wide variety of conditions with common autonomic etiologies (Vanninen et al., 1996; Narkiewicz et al., 1998; Salo et al., 2000; Gutierrez et al., 2002; Pichon et al., 2004).

Previous studies have shown correlations between increments in vagal signaling and high frequency heart rate variability spectral power during controlled (paced) breathing (De Meersman et al., 1995; Sanderson et al., 1996; Badra, 2001). Although the percentage of body fat may be a determinant of heart rate variability spectral power measured at rest (Nagai et al., 2003; Chen et al., 2008), the influence of body fat on heart rate variability measurements was found to be nil when performed at rest and significant only during an autonomic challenge (Matsumoto et al., 1999). We have demonstrated positive correlations of the low frequency/high frequency heart rate variability spectral power ratio with the respiratory quotient before and after feeding (Millis et al., 2009) and negative correlations with the percentage of body fat in healthy young adult/adolescent African-American males after overnight fasting; and the latter only during periods of uncontrolled, and not during periods of paced, breathing (Millis et al., 2010). Other researchers have reported that changes in the percentage of body fat may be correlated with changes in the very low frequency spectral power, a measure of sympathetic thermoregulatory and metabolic energy signaling (Fujibayashi et al., 2009). However, the significances of very low frequency spectral power to measures of body fat stores during trials of uncontrolled and paced breathing associated with different physiological states such as fasting or feeding remain unclear. Therefore, we designed this study to determine the role of sympathetic thermoregulatory and metabolic energy signaling in the same healthy adolescent/young adult African-American male population as previously reported (Millis et al., 2010) during trials of uncontrolled and paced breathing, associated with states of overnight fasting and 3 h post-feeding, the latter associated with the metabolism of foods. We tested the hypothesis that, in healthy resting subjects, the percentage of very low frequency power of heart rate variability, an indicator of sympathetic thermoregulatory and metabolic energy signaling, is significantly correlated with percent body fat, body temperature and energy expenditure.

2. Materials and methods

2.1 Study participants and design

This experimental protocol was approved by the Howard University Human Participants Institutional Review Board, and each subject provided informed consent. The study population of 10 healthy 18-20 year-old African-American male university students was recruited and 8 subjects were included in the experiment. Each subject was studied twice, on separate days at which time they ingested isocaloric (900 Cal) high-carbohydrate and high-fat beverages after overnight fasting. An unsupervised, self reported period of overnight fasting (mean ± SD 12 ± 2 h) was used to limit the potentially confounding effects of diet related differences in autonomic responsiveness that we have described in a previous report (Millis et al., 2009; Millis et al., 2010). Two subjects were excluded because of inadequate fasting as determined by respiratory quotient measurements >0.85. Other criteria for inclusion in the experiment were non-smoking status, absence of alcohol abuse (less than two standard alcohol drinks a day), absence of use of medication that could interfere with autonomic modulation, resting systolic/diastolic blood pressure < 140/90 mm Hg. Table 1 summarizes the relevant characteristics of this study group determined with the subjects at rest after overnight fasting. The respiratory quotient indicates utilization of fatty acids as the main energy substrate and the low frequency/high frequency ratio shows a predominance of vagal modulation of the heart rate.

2.2 Uncontrolled and paced breathing

The subjects were instrumented and instructed as to the experimental procedures. Subjects were instructed to breathe normally while lying recumbent at 45 degrees in a bed of the General Clinical Research Center (GCRC) at Howard University Hospital. Following the normal uncontrolled breathing protocol, subjects were instructed to perform 5 min of paced breathing by following a visual tracking image on a computer monitor for periodic durations of inspirations and expirations set to 12 breaths min^{-1} (0.2 Hz). Each subject practiced paced breathing for a period of 1-3 min and was then instructed to perform the paced breathing for the 5 min paced breathing trial during which time the electrocardiogram signal was recorded using a Biopac MP100 data acquisition system (Biopac Systems, Santa Barbara, CA). The electrocardiogram electrodes were placed on the subject's chest in a standard three-lead position with recordings obtained from standard lead II.

Age (years)	19 ± 1
Weight (kg)	82 ± 25
Height (cm)	174 ± 20
Body mass index (kg · m^{-2})	27 ± 8
Systolic blood pressure (mm Hg)	130 ± 13
Diastolic blood pressure (mm Hg)	70 ± 10
Heart rate (beats · min^{-1})	65 ± 12
Respiratory quotient	0.75 ± 0.05
Energy expenditure (Cal · d^{-1})	1980 ± 369
Body temperature (°F)	97 ± 1

Values in mean ± standard deviation, n = 8

Table 1. Characteristics of study participants

2.3 Heart rate variability analyses

Heart rate was measured in beats · min^{-1}. Fast Fourier transform analysis of the electrocardiogram RR intervals was used to spectrally decompose heart rate variability in the frequency domain. For the frequency domain analysis, vagal modulation was represented by the area under the high frequency power spectrum (HF: 0.15-0.4 Hz), sympathetic cardiovascular modulation by the area under the low frequency power spectrum (LF: 0.04-0.14) and cardiac sympathovagal balance by the ratio LF/HF has been previously reported in this population (Millis et al. 2010). In this study, we analyzed the area under the very low frequency power spectrum (VLF: 0.001-0.04 Hz) expressed as the power in raw ms^2 and in normalized units using specialized autonomic neural software (Nevrokard, Version 6.3, Ljubljana, Slovenia). All time and frequency domain analyses were carried out in accordance with the guidelines put forth by the *Task Force of the European Society of Cardiology and the North American Society of Pacing and Electrophysiology* (1996). The very low frequency band (0.001-0.04 Hz) has been considered by the *Task Force of the European Society of Cardiology and the North American Society of Pacing and Electrophysiology* (1996) guidelines to be too small to be a reliable indicator during short-term recordings. However, recent investigations have challenged this assertion (Nagai et al., 2005; Nagai et al., 2006; Fujibayashi et al., 2009) and we have found that 5-min recordings produced VLF measurements that represented a significant proportion (23%-52%) of the total heart rate spectral power expressed in normalized units. The present study was designed, partly, to test the physiological significance of the very low frequency band as an indicator of sympathetic thermoregulatory and metabolic energy signaling.

2.4 Anthropomorphic, cardiovascular and metabolic measurements

Axillary body temperature was measured after overnight fasting and 3 h after ingesting a 900 Cal beverage. Body weight and height were also measured (Detecto scale) and these values were used to compute body mass index as the quotient kg body weight/m^2 height.

Blood pressure was determined using an automated sphygmomanometer (Criticare Systems Model 506DXNT, Waukesha, WI). To validate the effectiveness of overnight fasting, respiratory quotient and resting energy expenditure were measured by indirect calorimetry using an isolated flow-directed breathing chamber (Deltatrac, SensorMedics, Yorba Linda, CA). The participants were taken to the Howard University Exercise Science Laboratory for an assessment of the body fat percentage measured by dual energy x-ray absorptiometric (DEXA) whole body scanning (LUNAR Model DPX-L DEXA, Madison, WI).

2.5 Statistical analyses

The study design consisted of a comparison and correlation analysis of measurements of body temperature and the area under the very low frequency power spectrum of heart rate variability measured at rest after overnight fasting and 3 h after ingesting a 900 Cal beverage, during trials of uncontrolled and paced breathing with the measurement of body fat percentage (n = 8, 18-20 year-olds). The significance of differences between the post-fasting and post-feeding states and between the uncontrolled and paced breathing trials was evaluated by analysis of variance using a multivariate general linear model with significance set at $P < 0.05$. A correlation analysis between the normalized and percentage units of the very low frequency band of heart rate variability, the low frequency/high frequency power ratio, body temperature, resting energy expenditure and body fat percentage measurements after overnight fasting and 3 h after ingesting a 900 Cal beverage (feeding state) was based on linear regression and Pearson's correlation coefficient during uncontrolled and paced breathing trials with significance at $P < 0.05$. A statistical software package was used for the computations and analyses (SPSS, Chicago, IL).

3. Results

Table 2 compares the body temperature, resting energy expenditure and heart rate variability very low frequency spectral power for the uncontrolled and paced breathing trials after fasting and feeding. Normalized and percentage units of very low frequency spectral power (VLFnu, VLF%) and body temperature for the uncontrolled breathing trials were increased 3 h after feeding; changes for the paced breathing trials were not significant.

Heart rate variability	**Fasting spontaneous breathing condition**	**Fasting paced breathing condition**	**Feeding spontaneous breathing condition**	**Feeding paced breathing condition**
Total power (nu)	122 ± 5	140 ± 19	202 ± 22*	141 ± 7**
Very low frequency (nu)	28 ± 5	43 ± 19	105 ± 22*	45 ± 7**
Very low frequency (%)	23 ± 3	31 ± 5	52 ± 4*	32 ± 3**
LF/HF	0.6 ± .09	0.8 ± .3	1.1 ± 0.2	1.2 ± 0.4

Values in mean ± standard error, nu = normalized units, n = 16
LF/HF = low frequency/high frequency
*Difference between fasting and feeding significant at $P<0.01$.
**Difference between spontaneous and paced breathing significant at $P<0.01$.

Table 2. Heart rate variability measurements after fasting and feeding

Table 3 shows that percent body fat was significantly correlated with body temperature during fasting (r=0.78, P<0.01) but not during feeding (r=0.13, P>0.1). Percent body fat was also significantly correlated with VLFnu and VLF% for the fasting uncontrolled breathing (r=-0.57 and -0.63, P<0.01) but not for the fasting or feeding paced breathing condition or for the feeding uncontrolled breathing condition (P>0.1). Body temperature was correlated with VLFnu and VLF% (r=-0.39, P<0.05 and r=-0.47, respectively, P<0.01) for the uncontrolled breathing trials after fasting but not for the uncontrolled or paced breathing trials after feeding (P>0.1).

Resting energy expenditure, before correction for inter-individual differences in body mass index and percent body fat, was not significantly correlated with VLF% (r=0.04, P>0.1). After correction, the resting energy expenditure/BMI and resting energy expenditure/percent body fat ratios were significantly correlated with VLF% (r=0.50, P<0.01 and r=0.82, P<0.001) for the uncontrolled breathing trials after fasting. The significant correlations between resting energy expenditure and VLFnu were the same as those for VLF%.

Correlate of very low frequency spectral power percentage	Fasting, spontaneous breathing	Fasting, paced breathing
Body fat (%)	-0.63**	-0.31
Body temperature (°F)	0.47**	0.19
Energy expenditure (Cal · d⁻¹)	0.04	-0.13
Energy expenditure/body mass index	0.50**	0.18
Energy expenditure/percent body fat	0.82***	0.23

Values in Pearson's correlation coefficient, n = 16
*Significant at P<.05
**Significant at P<.01
***Significant at P<.001

Table 3. Correlations of very low frequency percentage of total spectral power with percentage of body fat, body temperature and resting energy expenditure after overnight fasting

Correlate of very low frequency spectral power of heart rate variability	Feeding, spontaneous breathing	Feeding, paced breathing
Body fat (%)	-0.41*	-0.15
Body temperature (°F)	0.41*	0.14
Energy expenditure (Cal · d⁻¹)	0.53**	0.19
Energy expenditure/body mass index	0.54**	-0.35
Energy expenditure/percent body fat	0.35	-0.56**

Values in Pearson's correlation coefficient, n = 16
*Significant at P<.05
**Significant at P<.01
***Significant at P<.001

Table 4. Correlations of percentage of very low frequency spectral power with percentage of body fat, body temperature and resting energy expenditure after feeding

Table 4 shows that, after feeding, the direct correlation between VLF% and resting energy expenditure, uncorrected for body mass/fat, was significant for the paced breathing trials. The correlation between VLF% and energy expenditure/percent body fat was also significant for the paced breathing trials; however, the correlation was inverse (negative correlation) to that of the similarly corrected energy expenditure for the uncontrolled breathing trials. The significant correlations between resting energy expenditure and VLFnu were the same as those for VLF%.
Figure 1 depicts the results of linear regression analyses showing that physiological state was a determinant of the significant negative correlation between VLF% and percent body fat for the uncontrolled breathing trials after overnight fasting ($r=-0.63$, $P<0.01$) which was not significant for the uncontrolled breathing trials after feeding ($r=-0.31$, $P>0.1$).
Figure 2 shows the linear regression analyses demonstrating that respiration was a determinant of the significant correlation between VLF% and LF/HF for the uncontrolled breathing trials after fasting ($r=0.61$, $P<0.01$) which was not significant for the paced breathing trials after fasting ($r=0.34$, $P>0.1$). The correlation of VLF% and LF/HF was also significant for the uncontrolled breathing trials after feeding ($r=0.58$, $P<0.01$) and was not significant for the paced breathing trials after feeding ($r=0.14$, $P>0.1$).
Interference of paced breathing with the correlations between VLF% and body temperature after fasting and feeding are shown in Table 3.

4. Discussion

The main findings of this study are significant positive correlations between the very low frequency spectral power of heart rate variability and body temperature and significant negative correlations between percentage of body fat and both body temperature and the very low frequency power. These correlations were significant during trials of uncontrolled breathing after fasting but not during trials of paced breathing or after feeding. These findings suggest that, under steady-state conditions such as overnight fasting and uncontrolled breathing at rest, the very low frequency spectral power may be indicative of autonomic adaptations for maintaining metabolic energy stores which could contribute to the development of obesity-related diseases. The guidelines for standardizing heart rate variability measurements state that the very low frequency spectral power may represent too small a proportion of the total spectral power to be worthy of analysis during short intervals of electrocardiographic recordings (*Task Force of the European Society of Cardiology and the North American Society of Pacing and Electrophysiology* 1996). More recent studies have suggested that the very low frequency power could, under appropriate conditions, be an indicator of sympathetic thermoregulatory and metabolic energy signaling (Nagai et al., 2005; Nagai et al., 2006; Fujibayashi et al., 2009). The significant positive correlation between body temperature and very low frequency power that we found during fasting, but not during paced breathing, corroborates the previous reports of a thermoregulatory and metabolic energy signaling function of the very low frequency band.
In a previous study, we reported the association of a low percentage of body fat with a shift in heart rate variability spectral power toward greater sympathetic modulation and the association of a high percentage of body fat with a shift in spectral power toward greater vagal modulation after overnight fasting (Millis et al., 2010). A shift in sympathovagal balance toward greater vagal modulation is reported during the ingestion of water (Routledge et al., 2002) and, thereby, implies that healthy individuals with high percentages of body fat may exhibit less sympathetic signaling activity during night-time hours than their leaner counterparts.

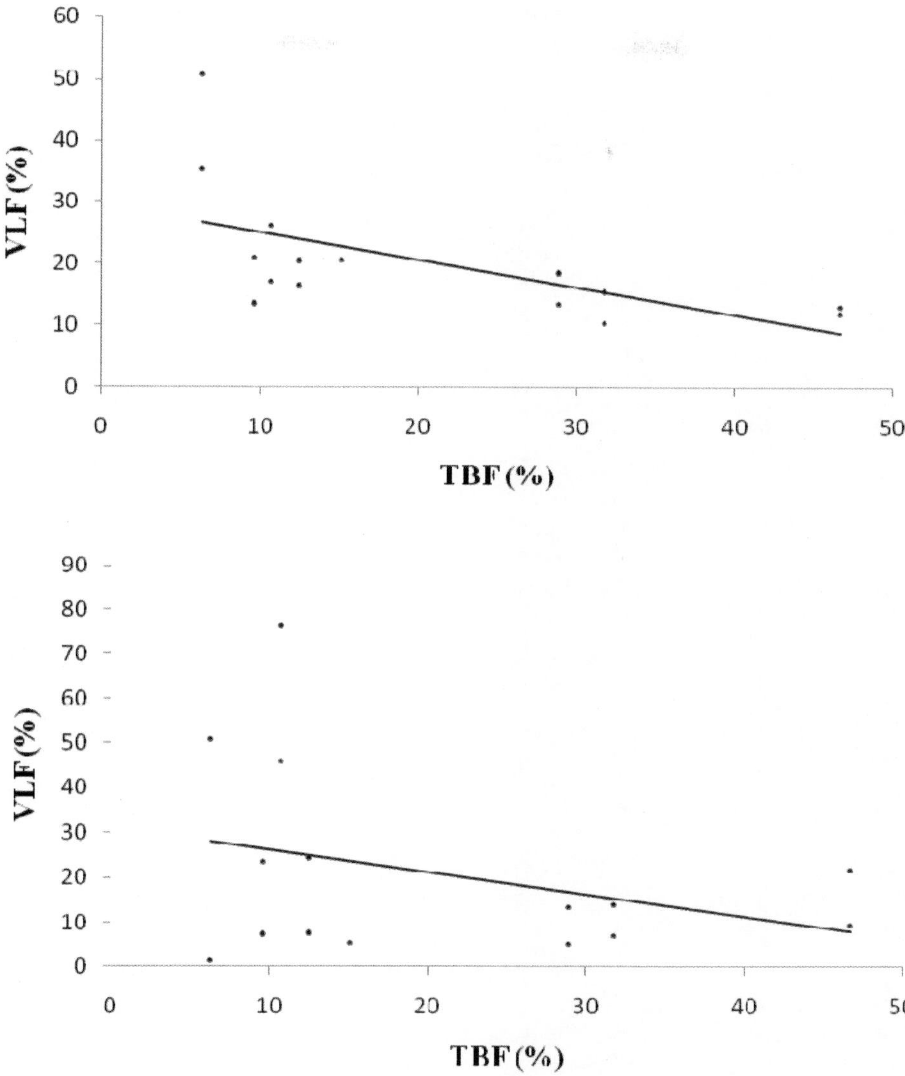

Fig. 1. **Correlation of very low frequency spectral power of heart rate variability with percentage of body fat.** Linear regression for heart rate variability percentage of very low frequency power (VLF) computed from fast Fourier transform analysis of the electrocardiogram RR intervals with percentage of body fat (TBF) measured by dual x-ray absorptiometric, DEXA whole body scanning for eight healthy 18-20 year-old African-American males during uncontrolled (spontaneous) breathing. Top: After overnight fasting, Pearson's correlation coefficient $r=-0.63$, $P<0.01$. Bottom: 3 h after feeding a 900 Cal beverage, Pearson's correlation coefficient $r=-0.31$, $P>0.1$.

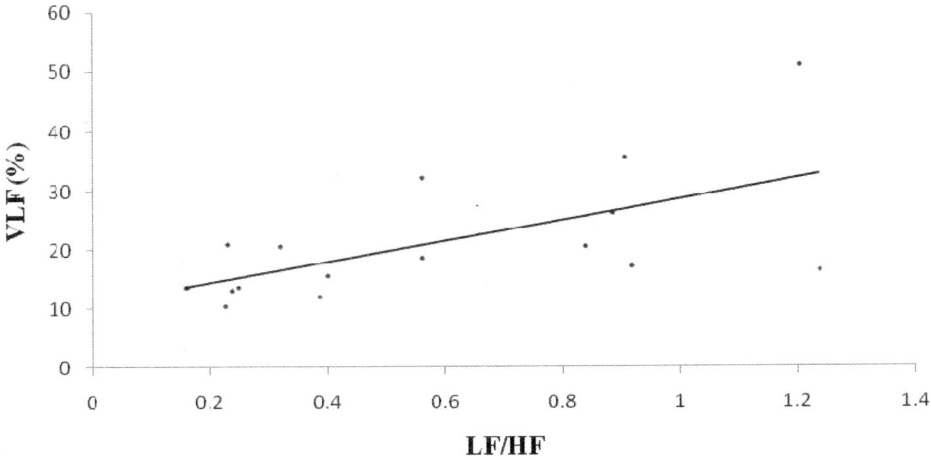

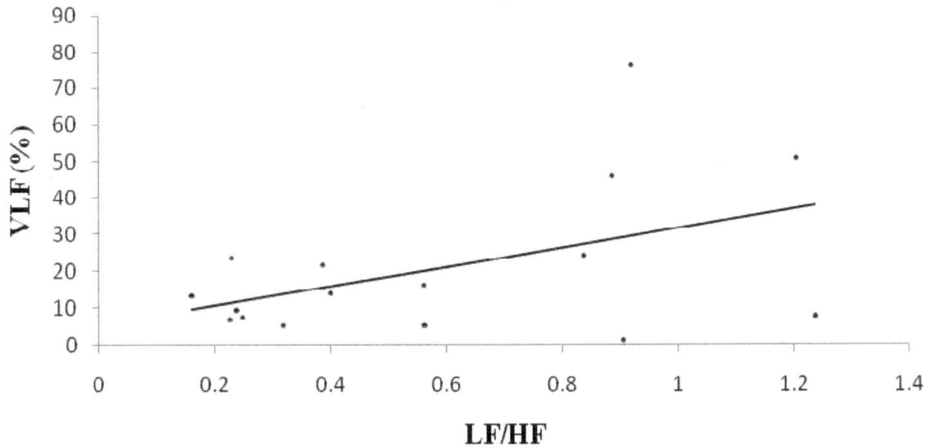

Fig. 2. **Correlation of very low frequency spectral power with low frequency/high frequency spectral power ratio of heart rate variability.** Linear regression for percentage of very low frequency power (VLF) with low frequency/high frequency (LF/HF) power ratio computed from fast Fourier transform analysis of the electrocardiogram RR intervals for eight healthy 18-20 year-old African-American males after overnight fasting. Top: During uncontrolled (spontaneous) breathing, Pearson's correlation coefficient $r=0.61$, $P<0.01$. Bottom: During controlled (paced) breathing at 0.2 Hz, Pearson's correlation coefficient $r=0.34$, $P>0.1$.

The metabolism of food produces a shift in sympathovagal balance toward greater sympathetic modulation, similar to that associated with postural changes (Piccirillo et al. 1998; Paolisso et al. 2000; Martini et al., 2001; Rabbia et al., 2003; Guizar et al., 2005; Kaufman et al., 2007a; Kaufman et al., 2007b; Nagai and Moritani, 2004). Higher body mass index is associated with greater sympathetic responsiveness to postural changes, higher plasma leptin levels (Paolisso et al., 2000) and greater lipolytic activity of adipocytes (Berlan et al., 2002; Tentolouris et al., 2008). These findings suggest that inferences based on heart rate variability measurements of autonomic modulation vary with the physiological state. In the present study, we found significant correlations after overnight fasting but not after feeding. Moreover, we found that the aforementioned correlations were significant only during uncontrolled, and were obscured by paced, breathing. We previously reported that the correlations between percentage of body fat and the low frequency/high frequency spectral power ratio, a measure of cardiorespiratory sympathovagal balance, were masked by paced breathing and were observed only during trials of uncontrolled breathing (Millis et al., 2010).

The requirement for controlling respiratory frequency during measurements of heart rate variability is controversial. Paced breathing is thought, by some researchers, to be necessary for controlling the respiration-related variability (respiratory sinus arrhythmia) of the electrocardiogram inter-beat (RR) intervals on which heart rate variability measurements are based (De Meersman et al., 1995; Sanderson et al., 1996; Badra et al., 2001). Several mechanisms have been attributed to this requirement; e.g., respiratory sinus arrhythmia might be amplified by increased tidal volume (De Meersman et al., 1995). We previously reported no significant difference in low frequency/high frequency ratio during uncontrolled versus paced breathing at 0.2 Hz, (Millis et al., 2010). Respiratory frequency controlled at 0.17 Hz, 0.25 Hz and 0.33 Hz is reported to have no effect on low frequency power and to modulate high frequency power only (Sanderson et al., 1996). Increase in tidal volume is reported to increase high frequency power (Grossman et al., 2004; Pöyhönen et al., 2004) and paced breathing at 0.2 Hz, the respiratory frequency that we used, to increase tidal volume (Pinna et al., 2006). We also previously reported an increase in the low frequency spectral power, a measure of cardiovascular sympathetic modulation, associated with paced breathing at 0.2 Hz (Millis et al., 2010). The subjects were lying recumbent during both the paced and uncontrolled breathing conditions; thereby, ruling out changes in sympathetic modulation associated with changes in posture. However, increased low frequency power has been shown to occur in association with an increased respiratory rate during conditions of mental stress (Bernardi et al. 2000) and could have occurred in the present study because of experimental stress, differences in tidal volumes associated with paced breathing, or differences in respiratory frequency during the uncontrolled breathing trials. The mechanisms responsible for the interferences of paced breathing at 0.2 Hz with the correlation between percent body fat, body temperature and the very low frequency spectral power of heart rate variability are unknown. However, we found the correlations between very low frequency power and low frequency/high frequency power ratio were significant for the uncontrolled, but not for the paced, breathing trials. These findings suggest the possibility that the aforementioned interferences of paced breathing with the correlates of very low frequency power, are likely related to significant interactions between sympathetic thermoregulatory/metabolic signaling indicated by the very low frequency band and the cardiorespiratory sympathovagal signaling indicated by the low frequency/high frequency ratio, which need to be further elucidated. Similar interactions might also be responsible for our findings that, after feeding, the direct correlation between very low frequency power and resting energy expenditure, uncorrected for body mass/fat and the correlation between very low frequency power and the energy expenditure/percent body fat ratio were significant only for the paced breathing trials; however, the latter correlation was inverse (positive changed to negative correlation) to that of the similarly corrected energy expenditure for the uncontrolled breathing trials.

5. Conclusion

In this study, we showed that the very low frequency spectral power of heart rate variability was an autonomic signaling correlate of body temperature, resting energy expenditure and percentage of body fat in healthy adolescent/young adult African-American males. The correlations were significant after fasting and during uncontrolled breathing but not after feeding or paced breathing. We found associations of high body temperature, low resting energy expenditure and low percentage of very low frequency spectral power in individuals with high percentage of body fat during trials of uncontrolled breathing. These findings suggest that the very low frequency band of heart rate variability may be correlated with sympathetic thermoregulation and related to an autonomic adaptation for maintaining metabolic energy stores. A comparison between the healthy young adult/adolescent population that we studied and a young population affected by diabetes mellitus or the metabolic syndrome should further elucidate the role of the very low frequency band of heart rate variability for sympathetic metabolic signaling in populations at high risk for developing an obese phenotype.

6. Acknowledgments

Supported in part by grants from the Cooperative Extension Service of the University of the District of Columbia & United States Department of Agriculture, Center for Diet, Nutrition & Health, from the Mordecai Wyatt Johnson Fund and by the Howard University General Clinical Research Center grant [M01 RR10284]), funded through the National Institutes of Health National Center for Research Resources, and the VIDDA Foundation.

7. References

Badra, L.J., Cooke, W.H., Hoag, J.B., Crossman, A.A., Kuusela, T.A., Tahvanainen, K.U., Eckberg, D.L (2001). Respiratory modulation of human autonomic rhythms. *American Journal of Physiology. Heart and Circulatory Physiology.* 280 (6), H2674-H2688.

Bernardi, L., Wdowczyk-Szulc, J., Valoenti, C., Castoldi, S., Passino, C., Spadacini, G., Sleight, P. (2000). Effects of controlled breathing, mental activity and mental stress with or without verbalization on heart rate variability. *Journal of the American College of Cardiology.* 35 (6), 1462-1469.

Braunstein, J.B., Sherber, N.S., Schulman, S.P., Ding, E.L., Powe, N.R. (2008). Race, medical researcher distrust, perceived harm, and willingness to participate in cardiovascular prevention trials. *Medicine* (Baltimore). 87(1), 1-9.

Chen, G.Y., Hsiao, T.J., Lo, H.M., Kuo, C.D. (2008). Abdominal obesity is associated with autonomic nervous derangement in healthy Asian obese subjects. *Clinical Nutrition.* 27(2), 212-217.

De Meersman, R.E., Reisman, S.S., Daum, M., Zorowitz, R., Leifer, M., Findley, T. (1995). Influence of respiration on metabolic, hemodynamic, psychometric, and R-R interval power spectral parameters. *American Journal of Physiology.* 269 (4Pt2), H1437-H1440.

Farmer, D.F., Jackson, S.A., Camacho, F., Hall, M.A. (2007). Attitudes of African American and low socioeconomic status white women toward medical research. *J Health Care Poor Underserved.* 18(1), 85-99.

Fujibayashi, M., Hamada, T., Matsumoto, T., Kiyohara, N., Tanaka, S., Kotani, K., Egawa, K., Kitagawa, Y., Kiso, Y., Sakane, N., Moritani, T. (2009). Thermoregulatory sympathetic nervous system activity and diet-induced waist-circumference reduction in obese Japanese women. *American Journal of Human Biology*. 21(6), 828-635.

Grossman, P., Wilhelm, F.H., Spoerle, M. (2004). Respiratory sinus arrhythmia, cardiac vagal control, and daily activity. *American Journal of Physiology. Heart and Circulatory Physiology*. 287(2), H728-H734.

Gutierrez, J., Santiesteban, R., Garcia, H., Voustianiouk, A., Freeman, R., Kaufmann, H. (2002). High blood pressure and decreased heart rate variability in the Cuban epidemic neuropathy. *Journal of Neurology Neurosurgery and Psychiatry*. 73(1), 71-72.

Hamilton, L.A., Aliyu, M.H., Lyons, P.D., May, R., Swanson, C.L. Jr., Savage, R., Go, R.C. (2006). African-American community attitudes and perceptions toward schizophrenia and medical research: an exploratory study. *Journal of the National Medical Association*. 98(1), 18-27

Kaufman, C.L., Kaiser, D.R., Steinberger, J., Kelly, A.S., Dengel, D.R. (2007a). Relationships of cardiac autonomic function with metabolic abnormalities in childhood obesity. *Obesity* (Silver Spring). 15(5), 1164-1171.

Kaufman, C.L., Kaiser, D.R., Steinberger, J., Dengel, D.R. (2007b). Relationships between heart rate variability, vascular function, and adiposity in children. *Clinical Autonomic Research*. 17(3), 165-71.

Lucini, D., Guzzetti, S., Casaraghi, S., Pagani, M. (2002). Correlation between baroreflex gain and 24-h indices of heart rate variability. *Journal of Hypertension*. 20 (8), 1625-1631.

Martini, G., Riva, P., Rabbia, F., Molini, V., Ferrero, G.B., Cerutti, F., Carra, R., Veglio, F. (2001). Heart rate variability in childhood obesity. *Clinical Autonomic Research*. 11(2), 87-91.

Matsumoto, T., Miyawaki, T., Ue, H., Kanda, T., Zenji, C., Moritani, T. (1999). Autonomic responsiveness to acute cold exposure in obese and non-obese young women. *International Journal of Obesity and Related Metabolic Disorders*. 23(8), 793-800.

Millis, R.M., Austin, R.E., Bond, V., Faruque, M., Goring, K.L., Hickey, B.M., Blakely, R., DeMeersman, R.E. (2009). Effects of high-carbohydrate and high-fat dietary treatments on measures of heart rate variability and sympathovagal balance. *Life Sciences*. 85(3-4), 141-145.

Millis, R.M., Austin, R.E., Hatcher, M.D., Bond, V., Faruque, M., Goring, K.L., Hickey, B.M., DeMeersman, R.E. (2010). Association of body fat percentage and heart rate variability measures of sympathovagal balance. *Life Sciences*. 86(5-6), 153-157.

Nagai, N., Matsumoto, T., Kita, H., Moritani, T. (2003). Autonomic nervous system activity and the state and development of obesity in Japanese school children. *Obesity Research*. 11(1), 25-32.

Nagai, N., Moritani, T. (2004). Effect of physical activity on autonomic nervous system function in lean and obese children. *International Journal of Obesity and Related Metabolic Disorders*. 28(1), 27-33.

Nagai, N., Sakane, N., Hamada, T., Kimura, T., Moritani, T. (2005). The effect of a high-carbohydrate meal on postprandial thermogenesis and sympathetic nervous system activity in boys with a recent onset of obesity. *Metabolism* 54(4):430-438.

Nagai, N., Sakane, N., Moritani, T. (2006). Impact of aging and beta3-adrenergic-receptor polymorphism on thermic and sympathetic responses to a high-fat meal. *Journal of Nutritional Science and Vitaminology*. (Tokyo) 52(5):352-359.

Narkiewicz, K., Montano, N., Cogliati, C., van de Borne, P.J., Dyken, M.E., Somers, V.K. (1998). Altered cardiovascular variability in obstructive sleep apnea. *Circulation*. 98(20), 1071-1077.

Paolisso, G., Manzella, D., Montano, N., Gambardella, A., Varricchio, M. (2000). Plasma leptin concentrations and cardiac autonomic nervous system in healthy subjects with different body weights. *Journal of Clinical Endocrinology and Metabolism*. 85(5), 1810-1814.

Piccirillo, G., Vetta, F., Viola, E., Santagada, E., Ronzoni, S., Cacciafesta, M., Marigliano, V. (1998). Heart rate and blood pressure variability in obese normotensive subjects. *International Journal of Obesity and Related Metabolic Disorders*. 22(8), 741-750.

Pichon, A.P., De Bisschop, C., Roulaud, M. (2004). Spectral analysis of heart rate variability during exercise in trained subjects. *Medicine and Science in Sports and Exercise*. 36(10), 1702-1708.

Pinna, G.D., Maestri, R., La Rovere, M.T., Gobbi, E., Fanfulla, F. (20060. Effect of paced breathing on ventilatory and cardiovascular variability parameters during short-term investigations of autonomic function. *American Journal of Physiology. Heart and Circulatory Physiology*. 290(1), H424-H433.

Pöyhönen, M., Syväoja, S., Hartikainen, J., Ruokonen, E., Takala, J. (2004). The effect of carbon dioxide, respiratory rate and tidal volume on human heart rate variability. *Acta Anaesthesiologica Scandinavica*. 48(1), 93-101.

Rabbia, F., Silke, B., Conterno, A., Grosso, T., De Vito, B., Rabbone, I., Chiandussi, L., Veglio, F. (2004). Assessment of cardiac autonomic modulation during adolescent obesity. *Obesity Research*. 2003, 11(4), 541-548.

Routledge, H.C., Chowdhary, S., Coote, J.H., Townend, J.N. (2002). Cardiac vagal response to water ingestion in normal human subjects. *Clinical Science* (London). 103(2), 157-162.

Salo, T.M., Jula, A.M., Piha, J.S., Kantola, I.M., Pelttari, L., Rauhala, E., Metsala, T.H., Jalonen, J.O., Voipio-Pulkki, L.M., Viikari, J.S. (2000). Comparison of autonomic withdrawal in men with obstructive sleep apnea syndrome, systemic hypertension, and neither condition. *American Journal of Cardiology*. 85(2), 232-238.

Sanderson, J.E., Yeung, L.Y., Yeung, D.T., Kay, R.L., Tomlinson, B., Critchley, J.A., Woo, K.S., Bernardi, L. (1996). Impact of changes in respiratory frequency and posture on power spectral analysis of heart rate and systolic blood pressure variability in normal subjects and patients with heart failure. *Clinical Science* (London). 91(1), 35-43.

Task Force of the European Society of Cardiology the North American Society. (1996). Heart rate variability, standards of measurement, physiological interpretation, and clinical use. *Circulation*. 93, 1043-1065.

Tentolouris, N., Pavlatos, S., Kokkinos, A., Perrea, D., Pagoni, S., Katsilambros, N. (2008). Diet-induced thermogenesis and substrate oxidation are not different between lean and obese women after two different isocaloric meals, one rich in protein and one rich in fat. *Metabolism*. 57(3), 313-320.

Vanninen E., Tuunainen, A., Kansanen, M., Uusitupa, M., Lansimies, E. (1996). Cardiac sympathovagal balance during sleep apnea episodes. *Clinical Physiology* (Oxford). 16(3), 209-216.

14

Electrocardiographic Analysis of Heart Rate Variability in Aging Heart

Elpidio Santillo[1], Monica Migale[2], Luca Fallavollita[1],
Luciano Marini[1] and Fabrizio Balestrini[1]
[1]*Geriatric-Rehabilitative Department- Italian National Research Centre on Aging - Fermo*
[2]*Internal Medicine Unit "Villa Verde" Clinic – Fermo*
Italy

1. Introduction

Heart rate variability (HRV) is a non-invasive and quantitative marker of cardiac autonomic function that reflects the regulation of the sinoatrial node by the sympathetic and parasympathetic branches of the autonomic system (Task Force of the European Society of Cardiology and the North American Society of Pacing and Electrophysiology, 1996).
The clinical importance of autonomic function became evident when HRV was confirmed to be strong and independent predictor of mortality after acute myocardial infarction (Kleiger RE et al., 1987; Bigger JT et al., 1993; Huikuri HV, 1995; Bigger JT et al., 1997). Recently, in addition to the well-accepted application in cardiology, heart rate variability has also drawn attention in other important application fields as geriatric medicine.
Aim of the chapter is to illustrate the usefulness of electrocardiographic analysis of heart rate variability, focusing on senescent heart. The number of elderly people in western developed countries is rapidly growing-up.
Currently, 31 million people are older than 65 years in the United States, representing 12% of the global population. By 2025 a percentage of 20% of the population will be older than 65 years. The prognostic significance of conventional risk factors applicable to younger ages tends to disappear in old age (Anderson KM et al., 1987; Harris T et al., 1988). So it is important to find prognostic and diagnostic markers to define the risk of death among elderly subjects.
HRV analysis is able to give prognostic information beyond that obtained by traditional risk markers in populations of elderly subjects (Heikki V et al., 1998). Assessment of heart rate variability in older subjects is, however, complicated by changes in the autonomic nervous system that occur with advancing age (O'Brien IAD & O'Hare P, 1986).

2. Measurement of heart rate variability

The employ of high frequency 24-h electrocardiographic Holter recorders for analysis of HRV has provided helpful insight into physiological and pathological conditions and risk stratification in different cardiac diseases.
There are many commercial accessible automated HRV measurement devices utilizing variety of methods, providing cardiologists, internists and geriatricians with a seemingly simple tool for both research and clinical studies.

In 1996, time and frequency domain parameters for the assessment of the autonomic regulation was established (Task Force of the European Society of Cardiology and the North American Society of Pacing and Electrophysiology, 1996). Variations in heart rate may be evaluated by a number of methods including:

- time-domain analysis,
- frequency domain analysis
- non linear analysis

2.1 Time-domain analysis

When heart rate variability is assessed by time-domain indices (Table 1), in a continuous electrocardiographic record, each QRS complex is detected, and the so-called normal-to-normal (NN) intervals (that is all intervals between adjacent QRS complexes resulting from sinus node depolarizations), or the instantaneous heart rate is calculated (Figure 1, Figure 2). Simple time–domain variables that can be obtained include the mean NN interval, the mean heart rate, the difference between the longest and shortest NN interval, the difference between night and day heart rate, etc.

Other time–domain measurements that can be used are: variations in instantaneous heart rate secondary to respiration, tilt, Valsalva manoeuvre, or secondary to phenylephrine infusion. These differences can be described as either differences in heart rate or cycle length. Time-domain analysis of HRV can be performed using both statistical and

Time-Domain Measures of HRV			
Statistical Measures		***Geometric Measures***	
SDNN	Standard deviation of all NN intervals.	**HRV triangular index**	Total number of all NN intervals divided by the height of the histogram of NN intervals measured on a discrete scale with bins of 7·8125 ms (1/128 s).
SDANN	Standard deviation of the averages of NN intervals in all 5 min segments of the entire recording.		
RMSSD	The square root of the mean of the sum of the squares of differences between adjacent NN intervals.	**TINN**	Baseline width of the minimum square difference of the triangular interpolation of the highest peak of the histogram of all NN intervals.
SDNN index	Mean of the standard deviations of all NN intervals for all 5 min segments of entire recording.		
SDSD	Standard deviation of differences between adjacent NN intervals.	**Differential index**	Difference between the widths of the histograms of differences between adjacent NN intervals measured at selected heights.
NN50 count	Number of pairs of adjacent NN intervals differing by more than 50 ms in the entire recording.		
pNN50	NN50 count divided by the total number of all NN intervals.	**Logarithmic index**	Coefficient φ of the negative exponential curve $k \cdot e^{-\varphi t}$ which is the best approximation of the histogram of absolute differences between adjacent NN intervals.

Table 1. Time-Domain measures of HRV

geometrical methods. From a series of instantaneous heart rates or cycle intervals, particularly those recorded over longer periods, traditionally 24 h, complex statistical time-domain measures can be calculated. Few studies have fully used the main 4 statistical time domain measures of heart rate variability (HRV):

- the root mean square of the successive normal sinus RR interval difference (rMSSD)
- percentage of successive normal sinus RR intervals >50 ms (pNN50)
- standard deviation of all normal sinus RR intervals during a 24-hour period (SDNN)
- standard deviation of the averaged normal sinus RR intervals for all 5-minute segments (SDANN)

The series of NN intervals can also be converted into a geometric pattern (Figure 3, Figure 4) such as the sample density distribution of NN interval durations, sample density distribution of differences between adjacent NN intervals, Lorenz plot of NN or RR intervals, etc.

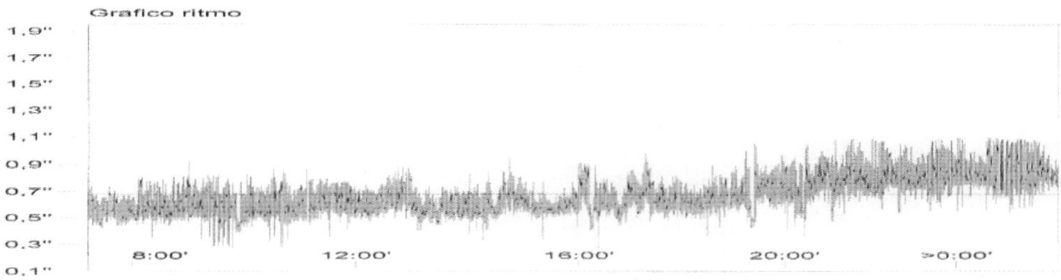

Fig. 1. NN sequences tachogram in a young healthy subject

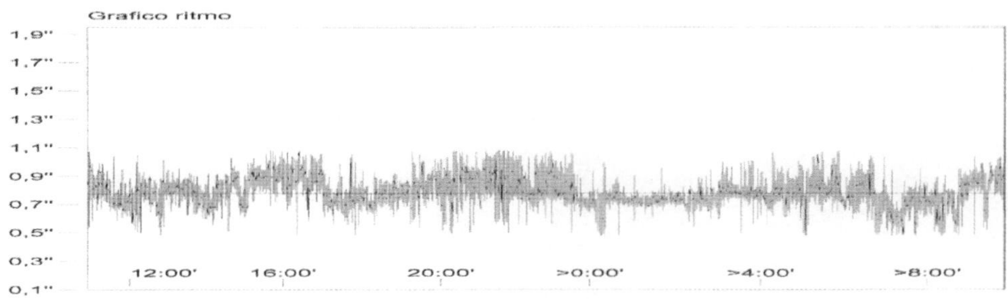

Fig. 2. NN sequences tachogram in an old healthy subject

2.2 Frequency domain analysis

Frequency domain measures of HRV (Table 2) provide information about the frequency distribution of the components of HRV using Power Spectral Density analysis (PSD) (Malliani A et al., 1994). PSD analysis provides the basic information of how power (i.e. variance) distributes as a function of frequency (Figure 5) (Akselrod S et al. 1981). Independent of the method employed, only an estimate of the true PSD of the signals can be obtained by proper mathematical algorithms. Fast Fourier transform, point process, and autoregressive procedures quantify components of HRV that are expressed in 2 main frequency regions or bands (Hz):

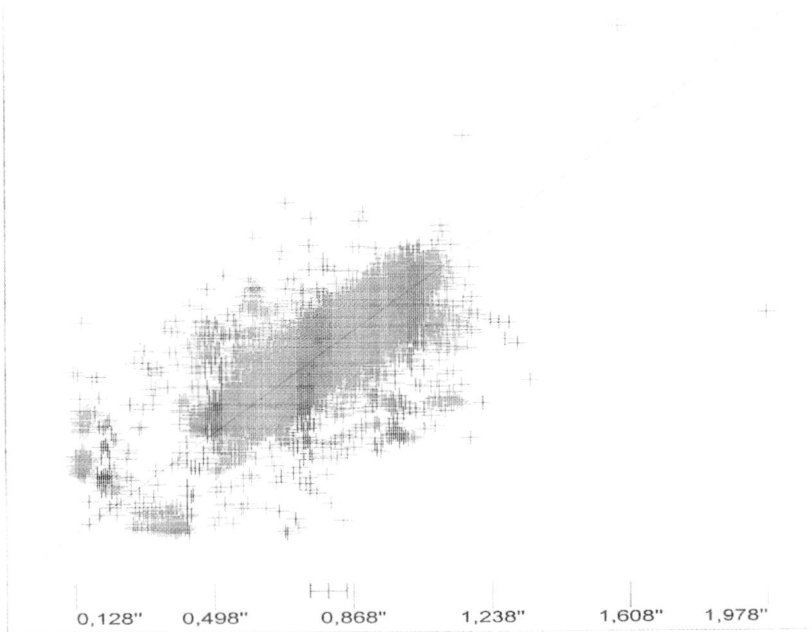

Fig. 3. Scattergram representation of HRV: on X axis the duration of RR sequence, on Y axis the duration of the precedent RR sequence

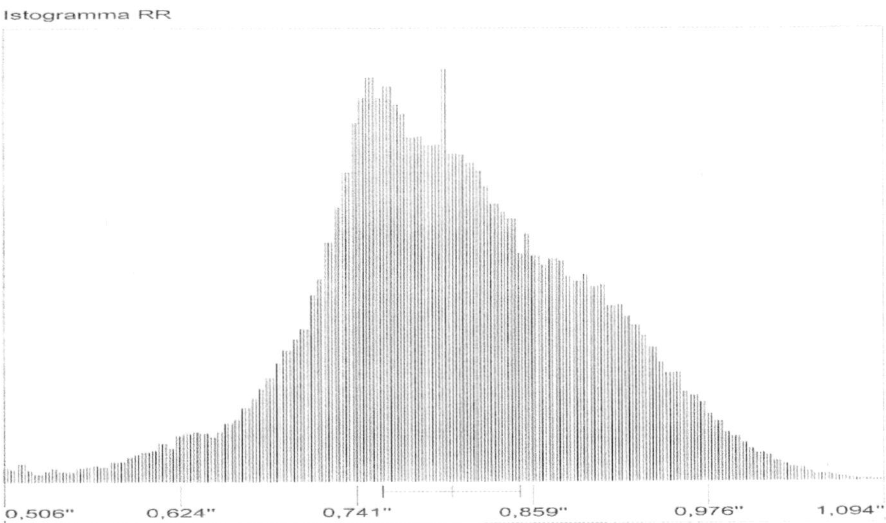

Fig. 4. Histogram representation of HRV: graphic shows the distribution of duration of RR sequences

high-frequency (HF) and low-frequency (LF) power. HF power primarily reflects respiratory-modulated parasympathetic outflow, whereas LF power is subject to both substantial sympathetic influence and varying amounts of parasympathetic contribution. The LF/HF ratio has been proposed, by some investigators, as an index of relative balance of sympathovagal influences on the heart, with higher LF/HF ratios reflecting increased sympathetic activity and/or decreased parasympathetic tone. The origin of very low frequency (VLF) oscillations in the power spectra of HRV is controversial with possible mechanisms involving thermoregulation and/or renin-angiotensin-aldosterone system. When spectral analysis is used to analyse the sequence of NN intervals in the entire 24-h period the result include an ultra-low frequency component (ULF), in addition to VLF, LF and HF components. Methods for the calculation of PSD are generally classified as non-parametric and parametric.

Frequency-Domain Measures of HRV			
Short-term recordings		***Analysis of 24 hh***	
Variable	**Description**	**Variable**	**Description**
5 min total power (ms^2)	The power of NN intervals over the temporal segment	**Total power (ms^2)**	Variance of all NN intervals
VLF (ms^2)	Power in very low frequency range	**ULF (ms^2)**	Power in ultra low frequency range
LF (ms^2)	Power in low frequency range	**VLF (ms^2)**	Power in very low frequency range
LF norm	LF power in normalised units LF/(Total Power-VLF)X100	**LF (ms^2)**	Power in low frequency range
HF (ms^2)	Power in high frequency range	**HF (ms^2)**	Power in high frequency range
HF norm	HF power in normalised units HF/(Total Power-VLF)X100	**α**	Slope in the linear interpolation of the spectrum in a log-log scale
LF/HF	Ratio LF [ms^2]/HF [ms^2]		

Table 2. Frequency-Domain measures of HRV

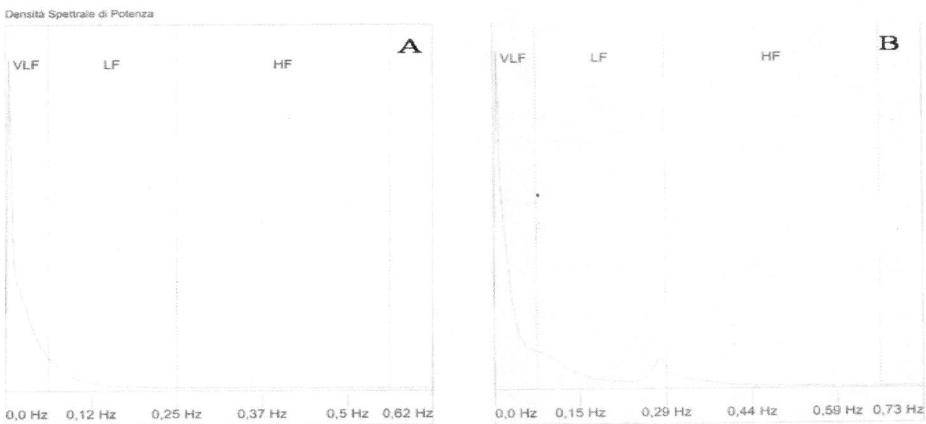

Fig. 5. Power spectral density analysis (A) in an old and (B) in a young subject

2.3 Non linear analysis

Cardiovascular signals have been largely analyzed using traditional time and frequency domain measures. However, such measures fail to account for important properties related to multi-scale organization and nonequilibrium dynamics.

In recent years there has been increasing evidence that HRV may reflect a much more complex phenomenon representing the nonlinear fluctuations of cardiac-autonomic outflows in a fractal or entropic, perhaps chaotic way (Perkiomaki JS et al., 2005). The chaotic vs. fractal/entropic/stochastic descriptions of HRV present a dilemma in interpreting its power spectrum (Watanabe MA, 2003). Definitive testing of these divergent characterizations is key to unrevealing the physiologic mechanisms underlying HRV, which is critical to its proper use as a noninvasive marker for cardiac mortality risk assessment and stratification in chronic heart failure and other cardiac diseases (Mäkikallio TH et al., 2002).

Non-linear phenomena are determined by complex interactions of haemodynamic, electrophysiological and humoral variables, as well as by autonomic and central nervous regulations. It has been speculated that analysis of HRV based on the methods of non-linear dynamics might elicit valuable information for the physiological interpretation of HRV and for the assessment of the risk of sudden death (Mansier P et al., 1996).

3. Heart rate turbolence

In 1999, the analysis of the heart rate turbulence (HRT) was introduced. Heart rate turbolence describes the fluctuations of the RR interval after ventricular premature beats expressing the residual ability of the sympathetic nervous system to adapt itself to instantaneous pressure variations and to adjust cardiac frequency to sudden and unexpected flow reductions (Francis J et al., 2005; Klingenheben T et al., 2008). Ventricular extrasystole induces a modification of the ventricular contraction axis, causing a reduction of the cardiac flow which is proportional to the previous beat and to its point of origin.

A reduction of the cardiac flow brings about an immediate decrease of the cerebral flow, followed in a few seconds by a stimulation of the aortic baroreceptors and a subsequent neurovegetative cardiac stimulation according with a frequency reduction. However, this reflex occurs in patients with a normal sympathetic-vagal balance.

HRT is usually expressed by two parameters, the turbulence onset and the turbulence slope. The turbulence onset describes the difference between the mean of the two sinus RR intervals before and the first two sinus RR intervals after the ventricular premature depolarization divided by the mean of the last two sinus RR intervals before the ventricular premature depolarization. The turbulence slope is defined as the highest slope of the regression line over any of the five successive sinus beat RR intervals during first 20 sinus beat RR intervals after a ventricular premature depolarization.

4. Autonomic regulation in senescent heart

It is well known that the anatomy, histology and physiology of the heart changes with age (Klausner SC & Schwartz AB, 1995). Together, age-related structural and functional changes reduce the complexity of physiologic heart rate control, impairing the individual's ability to adapt to stresses such as hypotension.

Aging heart is characterised by peculiar biophysical properties such as increased deposition of collagen and fat. On the electrophysiological level in senescent heart several alterations have been described such as a progressive prolongation of the action potential (explained by a decreasing density of the transient outward potassium current, and a prolongation of the decay time of the L-type calcium current) (Salameh A et al., 2010). Interestingly beat-to-beat fluctuation of heart rate, commonly known as heart rate variability declines steadily with age (Colosimo A et al., 1997). Reduced intrinsic heart rate were also observed in older individuals (Fleg JL & Kennedy HL, 1982). Furthermore it has been described an age-related decline in parasympathetic regulation and greater sympathetic modulation (De Meersman RE & Stein PK, 2007). Studies have demonstrated a decline in sino-atrial node parasympathetic activity and an increase in sympathetic activity in the heart with aging (Eckberg DL et al., 1971). The impairment of cardiac-vagal neurons appears to be the major determinant of changes in the control of heart rate that come with aging, since aging reduces the tachycardia that may be induced by atropine in humans and animals (Ferrari AU et al., 1991). The age-related increases in sympathetic nervous system activity under resting conditions seem to be related mainly to a primary increase in central sympathetic nerve discharge (Esler M et al., 2002).

Functional changes in elderly populations include a gradual increase in basal and stimulated plasma noradrenaline concentrations, altered adrenoceptor function and diminished responsiveness to adrenergic agonists and antagonists (Rubin PC et al., 1982; Xiao RP et al., 1998).

5. Frailty and heart rate variability

The age-related changes in the "complexity" of cardiovascular dynamics reflect the breakdown and decoupling of integrated physiologic regulatory systems occurring with senescence (Goldberger AL, 1996) .

Results from the Cardiovascular Health Study (CHS), confirmed an impairment in cardiovascular ability to adapt to external and internal perturbations with advancing age. The Cardiovascular Health Study (CHS) was a population based study of risk factors for cardiovascular disease (CVD) and stroke, enrolling 5,888 community-dwelling subjects aged ≥65 years. Authors found that cardiac autonomic function, assessed by frequency-domain HRV, declines most at 65–70 and levels off at age >75. The decline was independent of CVD risk or change in CVD risk (Stein PK et al., 2009).

Frailty is a biological syndrome typical of old persons, characterized by low reserve and resistance to stressors. It has been suggested that frailty may result from cumulative declines across multiple physiological systems that cause vulnerability to adverse outcomes. Fried et al. proposed a phenotype of frailty involving at least three of five components: unintentional weight loss, self-reported low energy level, weak grip strength, slow walking speed and low level of physical energy (Fried LP et al., 2001). Using a frailty index based on this phenotype, researchers have reported its association with falls, hospitalization, disability and death (Bandeen-Roche K et al., 2006; Boyd CM et al., 2005; Cawthon PM et al., 2007; Ensrud KE, et al., 2008). Recently a study showed that in old women, decreased HRV indices were associated with an increased risk of frailty (Varadhan et al., 2009). Similarly in Women's Health and Aging Study I, a community-based observational study that enrolled 389 community-dwelling women aged 65 years and older with moderate to severe disability, frailty was consistently associated with lower HRV as assessed using time and frequency-domain indices (Chaves PHM et al., 2008).

Both studies supports the notion that less physiological complexity marks frailty and provides an empirical basis to the concept of frailty as a syndrome of homeostatic impairment.
Congruent with this theory are the results of a cross-sectional study of HRV of 344 healthy subjects, (10 to 99 years old) which assessed the relation between autonomic function and longevity. Authors evidenced that a persistently high HRV in the elderly represents a marker predictive of longevity (Zulfiqar U et al., 2010). Another study (Chiang JK et al., 2011) evaluated the association between frequency domain heart rate variability and the risk of unplanned readmission in hospital in total of 78 geriatric patients. Frequency domain heart rate variability indices measured on admission were significantly associated with increased risk of unplanned readmission that was significantly higher in patients with lower levels of total power, LF power and HF power.
All these evidences suggest that healthy longevity could depend on preservation of autonomic function, in particular, HRV parasympathetic function, despite the early age-related decrease.

6. Heart rate variability and mortality in elderlies

Reduced HRV variability is commonly found in older people (Colosimo A et al., 1997) and has been linked to increased risk for morbid and fatal outcomes (Tsuji H et al., 1996).
Framingham Heart Study participants, in a closely monitored community-based study, underwent a routine biennial examination including 2-hour ambulatory ECG recordings to evaluate the prognostic implications of heart rate variability. Results, based on 2-hour monitoring, demonstrated that reduced heart rate variability predicts mortality in a population based sample of elderly subjects (Tsuji H et al., 1994).
UK-HEART, a prospective study powered for mortality, examined the value of heart rate variability measures as independent predictors of death in old patients with heart failure. In UK-HEART study were recruited 433 outpatients 62±9.6 years old with heart failure. Concordant to the above, a reduced HRV identified patients at high risk of death. Interestingly reduced HRV was a better predictor of death due to progressive heart failure than other conventional clinical measurements (Nolan J et al., 1998).
In another study of 347 subjects of ≥65 years of age (mean, 73± 6 years) HRV gave prognostic information beyond that obtained by traditional risk markers (Heikki V et al., 1998). In particular, after a 10-year follow-up, among all analyzed variables, a steep slope of the power-law regression line of HRV was the best predictor of all-cause mortality.
Interestingly in the Rotterdam Study, a population-based cohort study of 2,088 men and 3,184 women aged ≥55 years (mean follow-up: 4 years), increased heart rate variability resulted an even stronger indicator of cardiac mortality than decreased heart rate variability (de Bruyne MC et al., 1999). The authors examined the association between heart rate variability on a standard 10-second electrocardiogram and cardiac and all-cause mortality. In subjects in the highest quartile of SDNN (a time-domain measure of HRV), a more pronounced risk for cardiac mortality was present. In the Zutphen Study an association of increased HRV with all-cause mortality was observed only in elderly men (Dekker JM et al., 1997). Similarly, in the Bronx Aging Study (Bernstein JM et al., 1997), among men and women aged 75-85 years, no association was found between decreased HRV and cardiac or all-cause mortality, but an association of increased HRV with cardiac events was present in women.

It has been suggested that, increased HRV, unlike decreased HRV, is hardly influenced by the autonomic nervous system. The risk of mortality presumably associated with increased HRV has been reported to sinus node dysfunction.
More recently LILAC study examined 298 people older than 75 years (average age: 79.6 years). One hour of ambulatory ECG recording was obtained during routine medical examination conducted each year in July (mean follow-up time of 1152 days). Authors evidenced that an intermediate-term fractal-like scaling exponent of RR intervals is a better predictor of death than the traditional measures of HRV in elderly community-dwelling people (Hotta N et al., 2005).
Taken together the above data indicate that analysis of heart rate variability can be used to identify older men and women with an increased risk for cardiac mortality.

7. Influences on heart rate variability

Biologically, the physiological outputs of the human body, including heart rate variability, emerge from interactions among a variety of factors, ranging from genes to organs to the environment.
Heart rate variability analysis in elderlies, is influenced by various physiological factors including gender, postural changes, ventilation and time of day. Pathological conditions such as congestive heart failure and diabetic diabetic neuropathy are associated with alterations in heart rate variability.

7.1 Genetic influences on heart rate variability

Recent evidence suggests that genetic factors may contribute to the beat-to-beat variability in heart rate (Singh JP et al., 1999).
Analysis from Framingham study suggested there may be influential genetic regions contributing to HRV on chromosome 15 at 62 cM and on chromosome 2 at 153 cM (Singh JP et al., 2002).
Another study in an Asian population showed genes located on 216 cM region at chromosomes 5 and on 77 cM region at chromosome 18 may be involved in the regulation of heart rate (Gombojav B et al., 2008).
The apolipoprotein-E (APOE) gene has been studied extensively in regard to its relationship to aging-associated medical illness including cardiovascular disease, geriatric cognitive decline and late-onset Alzheimer's disease.
It has been hypothesized that diminished physiological complexity, as measured by heart rate variability, is influenced by polymorphisms in the APOE allele among elderly individuals. In a study, multi-scale entropy (MSE), an analysis used in quantifying complexity for nonlinear time series, was employed to analyze heart-rate dynamics. Reduced physiological complexity, as measured by MSE, was significantly associated with the presence of the APOE ε4 allele in healthy elderly subjects, as compared to APOE ε4 allele non-carriers (Cheng D et al., 2009). This finding suggests a role for the APOE gene in the diminished physiological complexity seen in elderly populations.
Variants in transcription factor 7-like 2 (TCF7L2) gene have been found strongly associated with an increased risk of type 2 diabetes, as well as with an impairment of glucagon-like peptide-1 (GLP-1) signalling chain. It has been shown that TT genotype of rs12255372 and rs7903146 TCF7L2 gene variants are associated with lower insulin secretion and higher

cardiosympathetic activity (Boccardi V et al., 2010). Moreover, such effect is independent of GLP-1 and insulin plasma concentrations suggesting a potential role of such gene variants in increasing cardiovascular risk through enhanced sympathetic nervous system activity.
It has been demonstrated that AKAP10 Val allele, the dual-specific A kinase-anchoring protein 2, predicted greater resting heart rate and diminished HRV suggesting that this variant may modulate the sensitivity of cardiac pacemaker cells to autonomic inputs, possibly conferring risk for arrhythmias and sudden cardiac death (Neumann SA et. al., 2009).
Other evidences support that variation in the choline transporter gene (CHT1), which encodes the choline transporter, may conceivably also account for some portion of interindividual variability in cholinergic transmission, as reflected in HRV phenotypes (Neumann SA et al., 2005). These findings show that polymorphic variation in the CHT1 gene is associated significantly with interindividual variability in HRV indices related to parasympathetic (cholinergic) activity.
All these studies strongly indicate that heart rate is controlled by genes mapped to several loci.

7.2 Environmental and behavioural influences on heart rate variability

Results of several studies support a potential benefit of increasing or maintaining fitness in order to slow the decline of parasympathetic control of heart rate with normal aging.
In a meta-analysis of 13 studies exercise training results in significant increases in RR interval and HF power. These changes are influenced by study population age (Sandercock GR et al., 2005). Other studies have provided inconclusive results regarding the effects of aerobic training on HRV in elderly subjects. The different results from these studies may be due to the different exercise loads (Wichi RB et al., 2009). It is well known that exercise training has direct and reflex sympathoinhibitory beneficial effects in chronic heart failure. The mechanism by which exercise training normalizes autonomic derangement and neurohumoral activation is to elucidate for further development of chronic heart failure-related training programs aimed at maximizing efficacy while minimizing workload.
Animal data support the hypothesis of the alteration of the autonomic nervous system by air pollution. Clinical exposure studies also support these findings (Schneider A et al., 2010). It has been reported that elderly subjects experienced significant decreases in HRV immediately following exposure to concentrated air pollution particles persisting at least 24 hours after exposure for some HRV parameters (Devlin RB et al., 2003).
Various studies with different recording lengths of ECG and different populations evidenced a negative association of smoking with measures of HRV, although significant effects were not always observed for all HRV measures determined or for both sexes, or were not confirmed in multivariable analyses (Hayano J et al., 1990; Kobayashi F et al., 2005).
A recent report from the Whitehall Study (Chandola T et al., 2008) has shown that work stress is associated with decreased heart rate variability. Dietary pattern also could influence HRV.
It has been suggested that higher intake of green leafy vegetables may reduce the risk of cardiovascular disease through favorable changes in cardiac autonomic function in aging heart (Park SK et al., 2009).
Moderate alcohol assumption and intake of omega-3 fatty acids and vitamin D through fish or nut consumption seem also effective approaches for which there is some suggestive evidence linking them to increased HRV (Mozaffarian D et al., 2008).

7.3 Physiologic influences on heart rate variability

Gender is one of the factors that influence HRV (Kuo TB et al., 1999; Ryan SM et al. 1994). Studies involving models of linear analysis showed that women presented higher HRV in the supine position than men of a similar age, indicating that the female population has a higher cardiac vagal modulation and a lower cardiac sympathetic modulation.

Women demonstrate a more appropriate response to a postural change than the men even though women are postmenopausal, suggesting that autonomic heart rate modulation is better preserved in the women's group (Perseguini NM et al., 2011).

Several studies have described a circadian pattern of cardiac autonomic modulation (Malpas SC & Purdie GL, 1990), which can be quantified with a cosine periodic regression model consisting of three cosine function parameters: mean (M), amplitude (Â), and acrophase (θ) (Rodríguez-Colón SM et al., 2010). The cosine function parameter M measures the overall average of a HRV index, the Â measures the amplitude of the oscillation of a HRV index, and the θ measures the clock time when the highest oscillation (amplitude) is reached. Lack of circadian variation of HRV is associated with increased vulnerability to cardiovascular events.

Aging is commonly associated with decreased sleep quality and increased periodic breathing that can influence heart rate variability (Brandenberger G. et al. 2003). Two distinct features depending on respiratory pattern characterize HRV in the elderly during sleep: (1) during periods of normal breathing, there is a large fall in absolute values of HRV indices without any significant sleepstage dependent variation, and a relative increase in sympathetic activity associated with decreased sleep quality, and (2) periodic breathing, that often interrupts normal respiratory patterns in most of the elderly, induces substantial modification in HRV by triggering important oscillations in the VLF range via autonomic efferents. So it is clear that respiration must be considered to correctly interpret HRV in the elderly (Schäfer C et al., 1998).

It is likely that several mechanisms are contributing at some level to the HRV that is observed with respiration (Shields RW, 2009).

Recent studies have shown that ormonal factors such as sex steroid levels, may also influence autonomic functions (Moss AJ, 2004). While physiological levels of androgens seem to be positively related with parasympathetic activity, estrogens appear positively related with sympathetic activity in men. In contrast, decreased androgen levels in aging males have controversial effects on autonomic function (Tolga Doĝru M et al., 2010). Adrenal androgens seem to be more important for cardiac autonomic control.

7.4 Pathologic influences on heart rate variability

Many studies have shown decreased HRV in patients with congestive heart failure. Several reports suggested that the withdrawal of parasympathetic activity and the concomitant increase of sympathetic activity lead to decreased HRV in heart failure patients (Mark AL, 1995; Chattipakorn N et al., 2007). Measures of heart rate variability have been shown to provide independent prognostic information in congestive heart failure patients (Galinier M et al., 2000; La Rovere MT et al., 2003; Sandercock GR & Brodie DA, 2006).

Findings from large, epidemiological studies provide strong evidence that vagal tone, as measured by HRV, is lower in persons with hypertension than in normotensives even after adjustment for a range of covariates. Importantly, these studies suggest that decreases in vagal tone may precede the development of this critical risk factor for cardiovascular disease (Singh JP et al. 1998; Schroeder EB et al. 2003).

The association between diabetes and autonomic nervous system dysfunction is well known to clinicians caring for patients with clinically manifest autonomic neuropathy (Lefrandt JD et al., 2010). Recently it has been documented that even minor degrees of glucose intolerance are associated with abnormalities of autonomic balance. Homeostasis model assessment of insuline-resistance (HOMA-IR) has been applied to quantify insuline-resistance in people with or without glucose intolerance, and it has been a reliable tool in the evaluation of insuline-resistance, especially before the clinical diagnosis of type 2 diabetes. Several epidemiological studies have shown that individuals with insuline-resistance, hyperinsulinemia or increased fasting glucose have increased heart rate and reduced HRV (Galinier M et al., 1999).

In communities study, a consistent association between, metabolic syndrome and impaired cardiac autonomic modulation has been reported (Liao D et al., 1998; Park SK et al., 2006). People with metabolic syndrome tend to have a greater percentage of adipose, atherogenic dyslipidemia, hypertension, and a higher proinflammatory and prothrombotic state, all of which are associated with decreased parasympathetic and increased sympathetic tone.

In chronic obstructive pulmonary disease (COPD) patients, functional and structural changes of the respiratory system deeply influence cardiovascular function. Cardiac autonomic dysfunction, in COPD patients, is important in the development of arrhythmias.

It has been suggested that in COPD patients, combination of HRV and HRT analysis may improve risk stratification leading to a more accurate identification of high risk patients, more aggressive treatment toward preventing sudden death and/or preventing progression of disease to mortality (Gunduz H et al., 2009).

A study in COPD patients (Antonelli-Incalzi R et al., 2009) found that autonomic control deteriorates as COPD worsens. It would be plausible that the diffuse cerebral metabolic impairment well documented in COPD patients, might induce, among others, lesions to functional connection of the insular cortex. The right anterior insula has a role in modulation of sympathetic tone and is implicated in the sympathetic arousal associated with mental tasks.

Major depression and depressive symptoms are associated with decreased HRV, both in patients with coronary heart disease (Carney et al., 2001; Vigo et al., 2004) and in community subjects (Udupa et al., 2007; van der Kooy et al., 2006). Depression has been associated with increased risk of morbidity and mortality in patients with coronary artery disease (Lett et al., 2004). Dysregulation of the autonomic nervous system has been proposed as a plausible explanation (Carney et al., 2005). Results from a recent study (Kop WJ et al., 2010) confirmed that the long-term adverse cardiovascular consequences of depression may be partially explained by autonomic nervous system dysfunction and inflammation. In particular depression was associated with selected indices of autonomic nervous system dysfunction and inflammation markers (white blood cell count and fibrinogen) in individuals >65 years of age free of clinical cardiovascular diseases.

Recently authors have suggested that association between depressive symptoms with decreased HRV is due, in large part, to a shared genetic effect (Su S et al., 2010).

Autonomic dysfunction can occur in all common dementias in older people, but is a particularly common feature of Lewy body dementia and Parkinson disease dementia (Allan LM et al., 2007). Cholinergic dysfunction has been discussed as a potential cause of autonomic failure in patients with dementia, and may be particularly important in Lewy body dementia and Parkinson disease dementia, where cholinergic deficits are especially pronounced, and where the disease pathology involves the dorsal vagal nucleus.

8. Conclusions

Since reduced HRV is associated with higher cardiovascular morbidity and mortality rates, it has an important clinical impact on the elderly. The age-related changes in HRV and their implications for mortality suggest that periodic HRV monitoring of the elderly could help predict and promote longevity. Further studies are needed to clarify what different HRV measures reflect physiologically and which measure of HRV is more useful. Identifying HRV abnormalities in subjects free from clinically evident mechanical and arrhythmic problems might be a clue to detect timely patients at risk of such diseases. Recognition of the genetic determinants of HRV may provide additional insights into the pathophysiology of the autonomic nervous system and offer clues to its modulation.

The intensified research about correlations between heart rate variability and pathologies with a variety of methods (in particular from nonlinear dynamics) will not only increase our knowledge about the complex autonomic regulation but will lead us to an enhanced diagnostics and therapy for older patients. Future research will determine whether noninvasive measures of physiological complexity underlying heart rate dynamics might be useful for screening and monitoring of clinical vulnerability in older adults. Research will be needed also to identify behavioural strategies of favorably modulating autonomic function that improve outcomes in the clinic and among large populations.

9. References

Allan LM, Ballard CG et al. (2007). Autonomic dysfunction in dementia. *J Neurol Neurosurg Psychiatry*;78:671–677.

Anderson KM, Castelli WP et al. (1987). Cholesterol and mortality: 30 years of follow-up from the Framingham study. *JAMA*. 1987;257:2176 –2182.

Antonelli- Incalzi R, Corsonello A et al. (2009). Heart rate variability and drawing impairment in hypoxemic COPD. *Brain and Cognition* 70 163–170

Akselrod S, Gordon D et al. (1981); Power spectrum analysis of heart rate fluctuation: a quantitative probe of beat-to-beat cardiovascular control. *Science*. 213:220-222.

Bandeen-Roche K, Xue QL et al. (2006). Phenotype of frailty: Characterization in the Women's Health and Aging Studies. *J Gerontol A Biol Sci Med Sci*; 61A: 262–266.

Bernstein JM, Frishman WH et al. (1997). Value of ECG P-R and Q-Tc interval prolongation and heart rate variability for predicting cardiovascular morbidity and mortality in the elderly: The Bronx Aging Study. *Cardiol Elderly*. 5: 31-41.

Bigger JT Jr, Fleiss JL et al. (1993); Frequency domain measures of heart period variability to assess risk late after myocardial infarction. *J Am Coll Cardiol*. 21:729-736.

Bigger JT, Fleiss LF et al. (1995). RR variability in healthy, middle-aged persons compared with patients with chronic coronary heart disease or recent acute myocardial infarction. *Circulation*. 91: 1936 –1943.

Boccardi V, Ambrosino I et al. (2010). Potential role of TCF7L2 gene variants on cardiac sympathetic/parasympathetic activity. *Eur J Hum Genet*. 18, 1333–1338.

Boyd CM, Xue QL et al. (2005). Frailty, hospitalization, and progression of disability in a cohort of disabled older women. *Am J Med*; 118: 1225– 1231.

Brandenberger G, Viola AU et al. (2003) . Age-related changes in cardiac autonomic control during sleep. *J. Sleep Res*. 12, 173–180.

Carney RM, Blumenthal JA et al. (2001). Depression, heart rate variability, and acute myocardial infarction. *Circulation*; 104:2024–2028.

Carney RM, Freedland KE et al. (2005). Depression, the autonomic nervous system, and coronary heart disease. *Psychosomatic medicine*; (67 Suppl 1):S29–S33.

Cawthon PM, Marshall LM et al. (2007). Frailty in older men: Prevalence, progression, and relationship with mortality. *J Am Geriatr Soc*; 55:1216– 1223.

Chandola T, Britton A et al. (2008). Work stress and coronary heart disease: what are the mechanisms? Eur Heart J;29:640–8.

Chattipakorn N, Incharoen T et al. (2007). Heart rate variability in myocardial infarction and heart failure. *Int J Cardiol*. 3;120(3): 289-96.

Chaves PHM, Varadhan R et al. (2008). Physiological Complexity Underlying Heart Rate Dynamics and Frailty Status in Community-Dwelling Older Women. *J Am Geriatr Soc*. 56: 1698–1703.

Cheng D, Tsai SJ et al. (2009). Reduced Physiological Complexity in Robust Elderly Adults with the APOE e4 Allele. *PLoS ONE*. 4 (11): e7733.

Chiang JK, Fu CH et al. (2011). Association between Frequency Domain Heart Rate Variability and Unplanned Readmission to Hospital in Geriatric Patients. *BMC Public Health*. 11:137.

Colosimo A, Giuliani A et al. (1997). Estimating a cardiac age by means of heart rate variability. *Am J Physiol.*; 273 (4 Pt 2):H1841-7.

de Bruyne MC, Kors JA et al. (1999). Both Decreased and Increased Heart Rate Variability on the Standard 10-Second Electrocardiogram Predict Cardiac Mortality In the Elderly The Rotterdam Study. *Am J Epidemiol*. 150: 1282-8.

Dekker JM, Schouten EG et al. (1997). Heart rate variability from short electrocardiographic recordings predicts mortality from all causes in middle-aged and elderly men: The Zutphen Study. *Am J Epidemiol*. 145: 899-908.

De Meersman RE, Stein PK. (2007). Vagal modulation and aging. *Biological Psychology*. 74: 165–173.

Devlin RB, Ghio AJ et al. (2003). Elderly humans exposed to concentrated air pollution particles have decreased heart rate variability. *Eur Respir J Suppl*, 40:76s-80s.

Eckberg DL, Drabinsky M et al. (1971). Defective cardiac parasympathetic control in patients with heart disease. *N Engl J Med.*;285: 877-83.

Ensrud KE, Ewing SK et al. (2008). Comparison of 2 frailty indexes for prediction of falls, disability, fractures, and death in older women. *Arch Intern Med*;168: 382–389.

Esler M, Hastings J et al. (2002).The influence of aging on the human sympathetic nervous system and brain norepinephrine turnover. *Am J Physiol Regul Integr Comp Physiol.*;282: R909-16.

Ferrari AU, Daffonchio A et al. (1991). Differential effects of aging on the heart rate and blood pressure influences of arterial baroreceptors in awake rats. *J Hypertens*. 9: 615-21.

Fleg JL, Kennedy HL. (1982). Cardiac arrhythmias in a healthy elderly population: detection by 24-hour ambulatory electrocardiography. *Chest*. 81: 302-7.

Francis J, Watanabe MA et al. (2005). Heart rate turbulence: a new predictor for risk of sudden cardiac death. *Ann Noninvasive Electrocardiol*; 10 (1): 102–109.

Fried LP, Tangen CM et al. (2001). Frailty in older adults: evidence for a phenotype. *J Gerontol A Biol Sci Med Sci* . 56: M146 – M156.

Galinier M, Fourcade J et al. (1999). Hyperinsulinism, heart rate variability and circadian variation of arterial pressure in obese hypertensive patients. *Arch Mal Coeur Vaiss*, 92:1105-1109.

Galinier M, Pathak A et. al. (2000) Depressed low frequency power of heart rate variability as an independent predictor of sudden death in chronic heart failure. *Eur Heart J*;21:475–482.

Goldberger AL (1996). Non-linear dynamics for clinicians: chaos theory, fractals, and complexity at the bedside. *Lancet* 347: 1312–1314.

Gombojav B, Park H et al. (2008). Heritability and linkage study on heart rates in a Mongolian Population. *Exp Mol Med*. 40 (5), 558-564.

Gunduz H, Talay F et al. (2009). Heart rate variability and heart rate turbulence in patients with chronic obstructive pulmonary disease. *Cardiol J*; 16, 6: 553–559.

Harris T, Cook EF, et al (1988). Proportional hazard analysis of risk factors for coronary heart disease in individuals aged 65 or older. *J Am Geriatr Soc.*;36:1023–1028.

Hayano J, Yamada M et al. (1990). Short- and long-term effects of cigarette smoking on heart rate variability. *Am J Cardiol*; 65:84–8.

Heikki V, Huikuri HV et al. (1998). Power-Law Relationship of Heart Rate Variability as a Predictor of Mortality in the Elderly. *Circulation*; 97: 2031-2036.

Hotta N, Otsuka K et al. (2005). Fractal analysis of heart rate variability and mortality in elderly community-dwelling people - Longitudinal Investigation for the Longevity and Aging in Hokkaido County (LILAC) study. *Biomed Pharmacother*.59 (Suppl 1): S45-8

Huikuri HV. (1995). Heart rate variability in coronary artery disease. *J Intern Med*. 237: 349 - 357.

Klausner SC, Schwartz AB. (1995). The aging heart. *Clin Geriatr Med*; 1: 119-141.

Kleiger RE, Miller JP et al. (1987). The Multicenter Post-infarction Research Group. Decreased heart rate variability and its association with increased mortality after acute myocardial infarction. *Am J Cardiol*. 59:256-262.

Klingenheben T, Ptaszynski P et al. (2008). Heart rate turbulence and other autonomic risk markers for arrhythmia risk stratification in dilated cardiomyopathy. *J Electrocardiol*. 41(4): 306-11.

Kobayashi F, Watanabe T et al. (2005). Acute effects of cigarette smoking on the heart rate variability of taxi drivers during work. *Scand JWork Environ Health*;31: 360–6.

Kop WJ, Stein PK et al, (2010). Autonomic Nervous System Dysfunction and Inflammation Contribute to the Increased Cardiovascular Mortality Risk Associated With Depression. *Psychosom Med*. September ; 72(7): 626–635.

Kuo TB, Lin T, et al. (1999). Effect of aging on gender differences in neural control of heart rate. *Am J Physiol*.; 277: H 2233-9.

La Rovere MT, Pinna GD et al.(2003) Short-term heart rate variability strongly predicts sudden cardiac death in chronic heart failure patients. *Circulation*;107:565–570.

Lefrandt JD, Smit AJ et al. (2010). Autonomic dysfunction in diabetes: a consequence of cardiovascular damage. *Curr Diabetes Rev*. 6(6): 348-58.

Lett HS, Blumenthal JA et al. (2004). Depression as a risk factor for coronary artery disease: Evidence, mechanisms, and treatment. *Psychosom Med*; 66:305–315.

Liao D, Sloan RP et al. (1998). Multiple metabolic syndrome is associated with lower heart rate variability. The Atherosclerosis Risk in Communities Study. *Diabetes Care* 21:2116–2122.

Mäkikallio TH, Tapanainen JM et al. (2002). Clinical applicability of heart rate variability analysis by methods based on nonlinear dynamics. *Card Electrophysiol Rev.*;6(3):250-5.

Malliani A, Lombardi F. (1994). Power spectrum analysis of heart rate variability: a tool to explore neural regulatory mechanisms. *Br. Heart J.* 71: 1–2.

Malpas SC, Purdie GL. (1990) Circadian variation of heart rate variability. *Cardiovasc Res*, 24: 210-213.

Mansier P, Clairambault J et al. (1996). Linear and non-linear analyses of heart rate variability: a minireview. *Cardiovasc Res Mar*; 31 (3): 371-379.

Mark AL. (1995). Sympathetic dysregulation in heart failure: mechanisms and therapy. *Clin Cardiol*;18 (3 Suppl I): I3-8.

Moss AJ. (2004). Modulating effects of sex hormones on cardiac function. *Ann Noninvasive Electrocardiol*;9:99-100.

Mozaffarian D, Stein PK et al. (2008). Dietary fish and omega-3 fatty acid consumption and heart rate variability in US adults. *Circulation* 2008;117:1130–7.

Neumann SA, Lawrence EC et al. (2005). Heart Rate Variability Is Associated With Polymorphic Variation in the Choline Transporter Gene. *Psychosom Med.* 67(2): 168–171.

Neumann SA, Tingley WG et al. (2009). AKAP10 (I646V) functional polymorphism predicts heart rate and heart rate variability in apparently healthy, middle-aged European-Americans. *Psychophysiology*. 46 (3): 466–472.

Nolan J, Batin PD et al. (1998). Prospective Study of Heart Rate Variability and Mortality in Chronic Heart Failure Results of the United Kingdom Heart Failure Evaluation and Assessment of Risk Trial (UK-Heart). *Circulation*. 98: 1510-1516.

O'Brien IAD, O'Hare P. (1986). Heart rate variability in healthy subjects: effect of age and the derivation of normal ranges for tests of autonomic function. *Br Heart* J; 55: 348-54.

Park SK, Schwartz J et al. (2006). Low-Level Lead Exposure, Metabolic Syndrome, and Heart Rate Variability: The VA Normative Aging Study. *Environ Health Perspect* 114:1718–1724.

Park SK, Tucker KL et al. (2009). Fruit, vegetable, and fish consumption and heart rate variability: the Veterans Administration Normative Aging Study *Am J Clin Nutr*; 89:778–86.

Perkiomaki JS, Makikallio TH et al. (2005) Fractal and complexity measures of heart rate variability. *Clin Exp Hypertens* 27: 149–158.

Perseguini NM, Takahashi ACM et al. (2011) Spectral and symbolic analysis of the effect of gender and postural change on cardiac autonomic modulation in healthy elderly subjects. *Braz J Med Biol Res*. Jan;44(1): 29-37.

Rodríguez-Colón SM , Li X et al. (2010). Insulin resistance and circadian rhythm of cardiac autonomic modulation. *Cardiovascular Diabetology* 9:85.

Rubin PC, Scott PJ et al. (1982). Noradrenaline release and clearance in relation to age and blood pressure in man. *Eur J Clin Invest*; 12: 121-5.

Ryan SM, Goldberger AL et al. (1994). Gender and age-related differences in heart rate dynamics: are women more complex than men? *J Am Coll Cardiol.*;24(7): 1700- 7.

Salameh A, Dhein S et al. (2010). The aging heart: Changes in the pharmacodynamic electrophysiological response to verapamil in aged rabbit hearts. *J Physiol Pharmacol*, 61, 2:141-151.

Sandercock GR, Bromley PD et al. (2005). Effects of exercise on heart rate variability: inferences from meta-analysis. *Med Sci Sports Exerc.* Mar; 37 (3):433-9.

Sandercock GR, Brodie DA. (2006) The role of heart rate variability in prognosis for different modes of death in chronic heart failure. *Pacing Clin Electrophysiol.*29(8): 892-904.

Schäfer C, Rosenblum MG et al. (1998). Heartbeat synchronized with ventilation. Nature.;392(6673):239-40.

Schneider A, Hampel R et al. (2010). Changes in deceleration capacity of heart rate and heart rate variability induced by ambient air pollution in individuals with coronary artery disease. *Particle and Fibre Toxicology,* 7:29.

Schroeder EB, Liao D et al. (2003). Hypertension, blood pressure, and heart rate variability: the Atherosclerosis Risk in Communities (ARIC) study. *Hypertension;* 42:1106–11.

Shields RW. (2009) Heart rate variability with deep breathing as a clinical test of cardiovagal function .*Cleveland Clinic Journal of Medicine*; 76: S37-40.

Singh JP, Larson MG et al. (1998). Reduced heart rate variability and new-onset hypertension: insights into pathogenesis of hypertension: the Framingham Heart Study. *Hypertension*; 32:293–7.

Singh JP, Larson MG et al. (1999). Heritability of Heart Rate Variability: The Framingham Heart Study. *Circulation*; 99: 2251-2254.

Singh JP, Larson MG et al. (2002). Genome scan linkage results for heart rate variability (the Framingham Heart Study). *Am J Cardiol.* 90,(12) :1290-1293.

Stein PK, Barzilay JI et al. (2009). Heart rate variability and its changes over 5 years in older adults. *Age and Ageing*; 38: 212–218.

Su S, Lambert L et al. (2010) Common Genes Contribute to Depressive Symptoms and Heart Rate Variability: The Twins Heart Study *Twin Res Hum Genet.* February ; 13(1): 1–9.

Task Force of the European Society of Cardiology and the North American Society of Pacing and Electrophysiology. Heart rate variability. (1996) Standards of measurement, physiological interpretation, and clinical use. *Eur Heart J.*;17(3):354-81.

Tolga Doĝru M, Murad Başar M et al (2010). The relationship between serum sex steroid levels and heart rate variability parameters in males and the effect of age. *Arch Turk Soc Cardiol.* 38(7):459-465.

Tsuji H, Venditti FJ Jr et al. (1994). Reduced heart rate variability and mortality risk in an elderly cohort. The Framingham Heart Study. *Circulation.* 90: 878-883.

Tsuji H, Larson MG et al. (1996). Impact of reduced heart rate variability on risk for cardiac events. *Circulation.* 94:2850–2855.

Udupa K, Sathyaprabha TN et al. (2007). Alteration of cardiac autonomic functions in patients with major depression: A study using heart rate variability measures. *Journal of Affective Disorders*;100:137–141.

van der Kooy KG, van Hout HP et.al. (2006). Differences in heart rate variability between depressed and non-depressed elderly. *International Journal of Geriatric Psychiatry*;21:147–15.

Varadhan R, Chaves PHM et al. (2009). Frailty and Impaired Cardiac Autonomic Control: New Insights From Principal Components Aggregation of Traditional Heart Rate Variability Indices. *J Gerontol A Biol Sci Med Sci*. Vol. 64A, No. 6, 682–687.

Vigo DE, Nicola Siri L et al. (2004). Relation of depression to heart rate nonlinear dynamics in patients ≥60 years of age with recent unstable angina pectoris or acute myocardial infarction. *Am J Cardiol*;93:756–776.

Watanabe MA. (2003). Heart rate turbulence: a review. *Indian Pacing Electrophysiol J*; 3(1): 10–22.

Wichi RB, De Angelis K et al. (2009). A brief review of chronic exercise intervention to prevent autonomic nervous system changes during the aging process. *Clinics.*;64 (3):253-8.

Xiao RP, Tomhave ED et al. (1998). Age-associated reductions in cardiac β1 and β2-adrenoceptor responses without changes in inhibitory G proteins or receptor kinases. *J Clin Invest* 15; 101(6): 1273–1282.

Zulfiqar U, Jurivich DA et al. (2010). Relation of High Heart Rate Variability to Healthy Longevity. *Am J Cardiol*; 105: 1181–1185.

15

Changes of Sympathovagal Balance Measured by Heart Rate Variability in Gastroparetic Patients Treated with Gastric Electrical Stimulation

Zhiyue Lin and Richard W. McCallum
Northwestern University and Texas Tech University
USA

1. Introduction

Gastroparesis, a gastric motility disorder characterized by delayed gastric emptying without evidence of mechanical obstruction (Nilsson, 1996), clinically presents as nausea, vomiting, abdominal pain, with a compromised nutritional state. Gastroparesis has multiple etiologies but the dominant ones are diabetes (DM), idiopathic (ID) and post-surgical (P-S). Frequent hospital admissions, and severe symptoms make gastroparesis patients socially restricted (Soykan et al., 1998). Approximately one third of gastroparesis cases are caused by diabetes mellitus. Diabetic gastroparesis may be attributed to impaired motor activity involving gastric hypomotility and unpropagated contractions (lack of peristalsis) and/or impaired myoelectrical activity explained by abnormal frequency of the gastric slow wave (dysrhythmia), low amplitude and/or uncoupling of slow waves (You et al., 1980; Telander et al.,1978; Geldof et al.,1986; Chen et al., 1992).

The most common treatment for gastroparesis is the use of prokinetic agents, such as metoclopramide, erythromycin and domperidone. However, only two agents are currently available in the USA, metoclopramide and erythromycin. Side effects from these agents result in up to 40% of patients being unable to tolerate chronic use (Sturm et al., 1999). Those who are refractory or intolerant to prokinetic agents often undergo abdominal surgery for the placement of a feeding jejunostomy tube which is only for nutritional support and does not improve gastric motility (Reardon et al., 1989; Ejskjaer et al., 1999).

Gastric electrical stimulation (GES) is an emerging therapy for refractory gastroparesis. Currently two types of GES have been investigated for treatment of gastroparesis: (i) long-pulse or high energy with low frequency stimulation and (ii) short-pulse or low energy with high frequency stimulation. Gastric electrical stimulation (GES) with short pulses and low energy (Enterra Device) was FDA approved in 2000 as a therapeutic option in the management of refractory gastroparesis (Familoni et al., 1997; Forster et al., 2001; Abell et al., 2002, 2003). Long-pulse and high energy stimulation, another approach to GES, achieves gastric pacing and represents a promising new treatment for gastric motility disorders (Hocking et al., 1992; McCallum et al., 1998; Lin et al., 1998). In this method, the electrical stimulus is composed of repetitive single pulses with a pulse width in the order of milliseconds (10-600 ms), and a stimulation frequency in the vicinity of the physiological frequency of the gastric slow wave. Single-channel GES with a pair of electrodes located in the mid-body of the stomach and using long pulses is able to normalize gastric dysryhthmia (Hocking et al., 1992; McCallum et al., 1998; Lin et al., 1998; Qian et al., 1999) and improve gastric emptying in both patients with gastroparesis and animal models of gastroparesis (McCallum et al., 1998; Bellahsene et al., 1992). Recently, two or four-channel GES with long pulses has been investigated and the preliminary results from several studies in both healthy and diseased canine models are promising (Song et al., 2005; Chen et al., 2005; Xu et al., 2008). Compared with single-channel GES, multi-channel GES is substantially more effective in entraining gastric slow waves and accelerating gastric emptying. However, the mechanisms underlying symptomatic improvement by GES remain unclear. Animal studies have shown that GES with high frequency and low energy parameters affects autonomic function. The aims of this chapter were to evaluate the effect of GES on autonomic function in patients with gastroparesis and identify possible mechanisms that could help explain how GES is effective in treating nausea and vomiting associated with refractory gastroparesis.

2. Methods

2.1 Subjects

Twenty nine gastroparetic patients were enrolled in two studies. Study I was performed in 10 gastroparetic patients (2 men and 8 women; mean age, 44 years; range, 20-58 years) with severe gastroparesis (7 diabetic, 3 idiopathic) refractory to standard medical therapies treated with short-pulse GES using an implantable neurostimulator (ENTERRA™ Therapy System, Medtronic, Minneapolis, MN). Nineteen diabetic gastroparetic patients (8M, 11F, mean age: 41 years, range: 26-60) refractory to standard medical therapy were included in Study II and they were treated with long-pulse GES using an external multi-channel pulse stimulator (GI Stimulation Inc., Charlottesville, VA).

The entry criteria included 1) delayed gastric emptying of a solid meal (>60% gastric retention at 2 hours and >10% at four hours after eating) using a standardized 4-hour scintigraphic method (Tougas et al., 2000); 2) more than 7 episodes of vomiting and/or nausea per week; 3) symptoms of gastroparesis for longer than one year; 4) refractoriness or intolerance to 2 of 3 classes of prokinetic drugs (cholinergic agonists, motilin receptor agonists, and dopamine receptor antagonists) and 2 of 3 classes of antimetics (anticholinergics/antihistamines, serotonin receptor antagonists, and dopamine receptor antagonists). Patients with documented organic or intestinal pseudo-obstruction, primary eating or swallowing disorders, chemical dependency, a diagnosis of active malignancy, positive pregnancy test or psychogenic vomiting were excluded. The study protocol was approved by the Human Subjects Committee at University of Kansas Medical Center, Kansas City, Kansas and written consent forms were obtained from all subjects before the study.

2.2 Study design

Each study consisted of a baseline, within two weeks before surgery for implantation of GES system, and follow-up sessions 6 weeks after GES therapy was initiated. In each session, a total symptom score (TSS) derived from 7 upper GI symptom sub-scores using a 5-point scale was assessed and electrocardiogram (ECG) were measured for 30 min in the fasting state and for 60 min after a caloric liquid meal (240 kcal). Autonomic activity was assessed by spectral analysis of the heart rate variability.

2.3 Surgical and GES techniques

The GES system for Enterra therapy used in study I consisted of 3 components: a battery-powered implantable pulse generator (Medtronic Model 3116, Medtronic), 2 intramuscular electrodes (Model 4300, Medtronic) (Figure 1) and an external programmer (Medtronic N'Vision clinician programmer 8840) to adjust the output parameters of the pulse generator. One pair of permanent electrodes (about 1 cm apart) was inserted during laparotomy into the muscularis propria layer on the greater curvature at 9.5 and 10.5 cm proximal to the pylorus. The electrodes were secured to the serosa of the stomach using 5-0 silk sutures and plastic disks. The other end of each electrode was connected to the pulse generator which was positioned in a subcutaneous pocket in the abdominal wall to the right of the umbilicus. The load impedance of the circuit was checked both before and after the GES device was placed in the pocket using the external programmer. The pulse generator was usually activated in the operating room or within 48 hours after surgery and initially programmed to standardized parameters: pulse width, 330 μs; (current) amplitude, 5 mA; frequency, 14 Hz; cycle ON: 0.1 seconds; cycle OFF, 5.0 seconds. At various intervals of follow-up after the implant, those parameters can be adjusted based on patient's symptomatic status or changes in impedance reading.

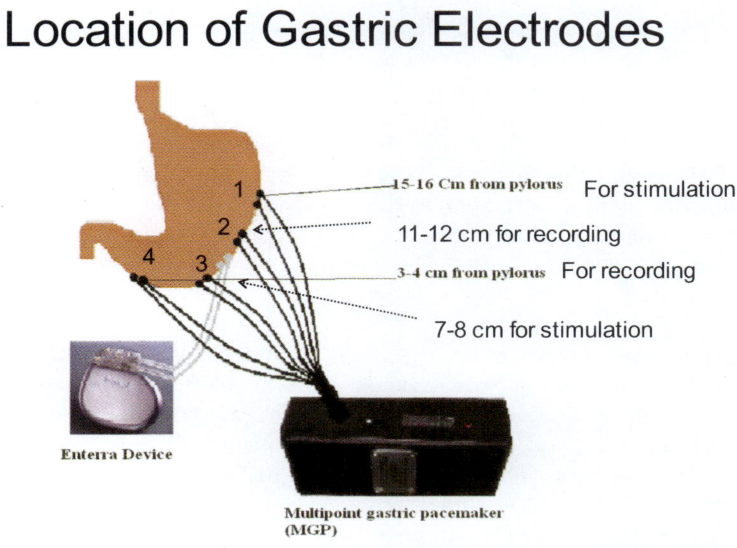

Fig. 1. The location of permanent electrodes for implantable Enterra device and temporary electrodes for external stimulation by a multi-channel gastric pulse generator (MGP). During laparotomy to place a permanent gastric neurostimulator, a pair of intramuscular electrodes were implanted into the gastric muscle at 9 and 10 cm from the pylorus on the greater curvature of the stomach and connected to the Enterra device. Then 4 pairs of serosal electrodes for gastric pacing were sewed on the serosa of the greater curvature of the stomach. The electrodes utilized for stimulation where at 15-16 and 7-8 cm from the pylorus whereas the electrodes for recordings the signal were located at 11-12 and 3-4 cm from the pylorus.

After laparotomy for implantation of permanent electrodes and pulse generator for the Enterra Therapy, four pairs of bipolar temporary electrodes used for gastric pacing in Study II were sewed on the serosa of the greater curvature of the stomach with an inter-electrode distance of 1 cm using a previously published method (McCallum et al., 1998; Lin et al., 1998). These four pairs of electrodes were TPW62 multifilament surgical steel temporary cardiac pacing wires (Ethicon, Inc, Somerville, NJ, USA). The most distal pair of electrodes was positioned 3-4 cm above the pylorus and the most proximal one, 15-16 cm above. The interval between two pairs of electrodes was 4 cm (Figure 1). The first pair (the most proximal pair) and the third pair of electrodes at 7 to 8 cm proximal to the pylorus were for electrical stimulation. The second and the fourth pairs at 11 to 12 cm and at 3 to 4 cm proximal to the pylorus respectively were for recording of gastric electrical activity. Wires from the electrodes were brought out through the abdominal wall percutaneously and placed under a sterile dressing to be connected to an external pulse generator for the study. Four to five days after surgery the function of the electrodes was validated by 4 channel-serosal recordings and the optimal pacing parameters for entrainment of gastric slow waves in each patient were identified using a newly developed external multi-channel pulse generator (GI Stimulation Inc., Charlottesville, VA) (see Figure 1). Before being sent home with a portable multi-channel pulse generator, the patient was trained on how to connect the electrodes to the external pulse generator, activate and care for the device. The patients were asked to place the device in a fanny pack for protection during the day and to self-administer GES 30 minutes before each meal, during the meal and 4 hours after each meal and to disconnect the pulse generator from the electrodes and charge the battery at night. The parameters utilized were determined by optimization session outlined above: two-channel pacing at 1.1 times the intrinsic frequency ranging from 3 to 3.5 cpm, a pulse width of 10 to 300 ms and the amplitude of 0.5 to 3 mA. The phase shift of electrical stimuli between the first and third stimulation channels was adjusted to be the same as the intrinsic phase shift calculated from the baseline slow wave recording and varied from 8 to 10 seconds. Enterra device was turned OFF and kept inactivated for the duration of the study II.

2.4 Recording and analysis of Heart Rate Variability (HRV)

After the patient fasted for at least 12 hours, one-channel ECG was measured for at least 30 minutes using the UFI Bio-Amplifier (UFI, Morro Bay, CA). Prior to the attachment of electrodes (BioTac, Graphic Controls Corporation, Buffalo, NY), the chest where the electrodes were to be positioned was shaved if applicable (in males) and cleaned with sandy skin-prep paste to reduce the impedance. Three electrodes were placed on the chest for recording ECG. To avoid motion artifact, the patients were asked to lie quietly in supine position on the bed and try to be as still as possible during the recording period. Analysis of autonomic function was accomplished through power spectral analysis of heart rate variability (HRV) (Figure 2). The following parameters were computed from the ECG recordings using a validated program (Wang & Chen, 2000; Oppenheim, A.V. & Schafer, 1975): (a) average and standard deviation of the heart rate, (b) spectral components of HRV in low frequency band (PL: 0.04 – 0.15 Hz) and in high frequency band (PH: 0.15 – 0.4 Hz), (c) the percentage of power in low frequency band, P1= (PL/(PL+PH) %) and the percentage of power in high frequency band, P2= (PH/(PL+PH) %) and (d) PL/PH, which measures sympathovagal balance, with higher values indicating greater overall sympathetic dominance.

2.5 Assessment of upper GI symptoms

Each patient completed a self assessment Symptom Interview Form at baseline and after 6 weeks of active GES. This form assessed the symptoms of gastroparesis occurring during the 2 weeks before the interview and the two last weeks of a total 6 weeks of GES therapy for severity of vomiting, nausea, early satiety, bloating, postprandial fullness, epigastric pain, and epigastric burning. The severity of each symptom was graded by the patients as 0 = absent, 1 = mild (not influencing the usual activities), 2= moderate (diverting from, but not urging modifications, of usual activities), 3 = severe (influencing usual activities, severely enough to urge modifications) and 4 = extremely severe (requiring bed-rest). The sum of the severity ratings of the 7 symptom sub-scores comprised the overall total symptom score (TSS) for severity.

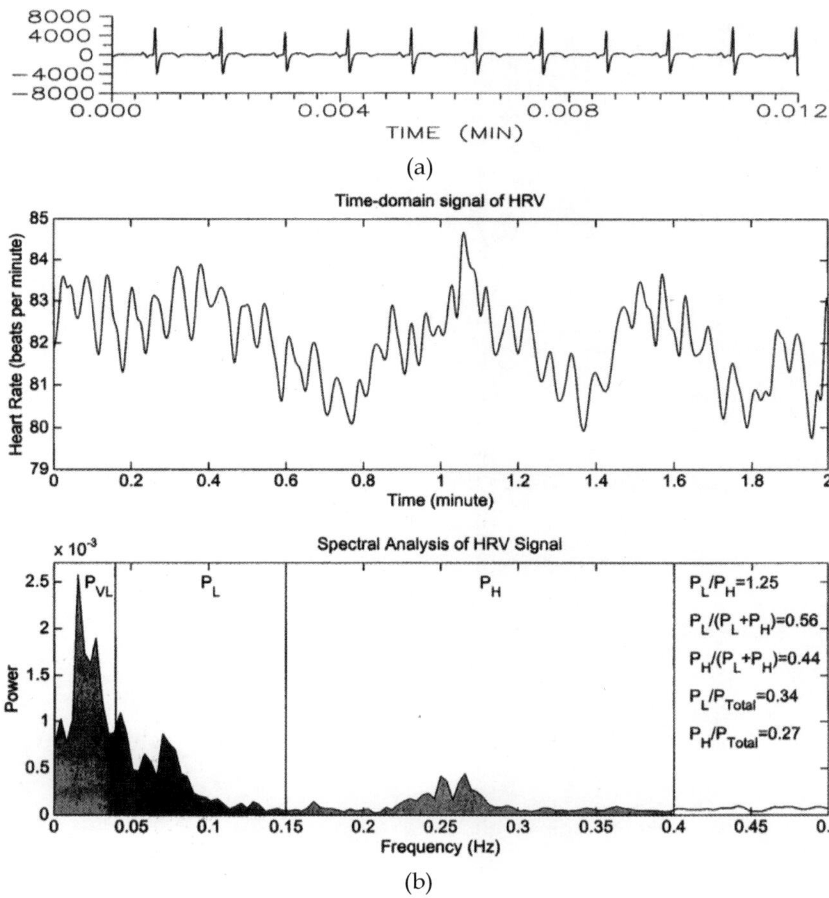

Fig. 2. Examples of (a) electrocardiogram recording, (b) time-domain signal of heart rate variability (HRV) (upper panel) and spectral analysis of heart rate variability signal (lower panel). P_L: power in low frequency band; P_H: power in high frequency band; P_{VL}: power in very-low frequency band; P_{TOTAL}: total power.

2.6 Statistical analysis

All data are expressed as mean ± SD. Analysis of variance (ANOVA) and paired t-test were used to determine significant difference between baseline and follow-up visit (Microsoft Excel, Redmond, WA). Statistical significance was assigned for P<0.05.

3. Results

Similar results were observed in these two studies.

In study I, the results of heart rate (HR), power in the low frequency band (0.04-0.15 Hz), power in the high frequency band (0.15-0.4 Hz) and power ratio (P_L/P_H) are summarized in Table 1. Figure 3 shows (a) individual percentages of power in the low-frequency band and (b) in high-frequency band derived from heart rate variability before and after Enterra GES. The sympathovagal balance (P_L/P_H) was significantly decreased after Enterra GES therapy with low energy and high frequency parameters (2.2±0.6 vs. 0.5±0.2), indicating a significant increase in vagal activity during Enterra GES. Severity of nausea and vomiting and TSS was significantly reduces after GES therapy (see table 2). The mean symptom reduction in TSS was substantially greater in 7 patients who had a decrease in the sympathovagal balance than that in 3 patients who had an increase in the sympathovagal balance (59% vs. 26%).

	Mean HR (beats/min)	SD	P1 (%)	P2 (%)	P_L/P_H
Before GES	98.7	60.1	69	31	2.2
During GES	88.2	40.0	34	66	0.5
P values (t-test)	NS	NS	NS	0.04	0.04

Table 1. Comparison of heart rate variability (HRV) before and during gastric electrical stimulation (GES). Note: HR, heart rate; SD, standard deviation; P1, the percentage of power in low frequency band; P2, the percentage of power in high frequency band; P_L, power in high frequency band; P_H, power in high frequency band. NS, not significant.

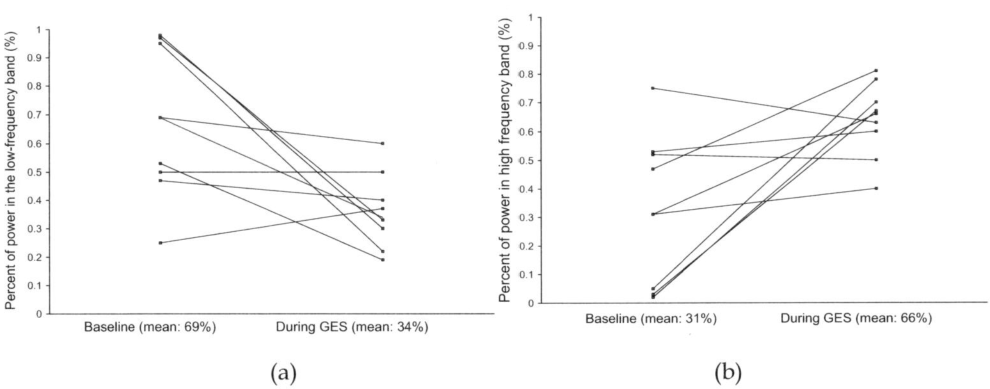

Fig. 3. (a) Individual percentages of power in the low-frequency band and (b) in high-frequency band derived from heart rate variability before and during gastric electrical stimulation (GES) (Mean data also included for comparison).

	Before GES	During GES	P value (t-test)
Nausea score (0-4)	3.8±0.1	1.7±0.4	<0.05
Vomiting score (0-4)	2.2±0.4	1.8±0.5	<0.05
TSS in severity (0-28)	23.1±0.8	11.5±2.6	<0.01

Table 2. Results of gastroparetic symptom responses in Study I. Note: TSS (Total Symptom Score) derived from 7 upper GI symptom sub-scores (vomiting, nausea, early satiety, bloating, postprandial fullness, epigastric pain and burning) using a 5-point scale (0=none, 4=extremely severe) before and after initiation of GES (Gastric Electrical Stimulation).

In study II, the P_L/P_H was significantly decreased from 0.45±0.05 at baseline to 0.28±0.04 after 6 weeks of two-channel GES with high energy and low-frequency parameters. Figure 4 shows the effect of the two-channel gastric pacing on the spectral components of HRV. Severity for each GP symptom (nausea, vomiting, early satiety, bloating, postprandial fullness, epigastric pain, and epigastric burning) was significantly reduced after 6 weeks of two-channel gastric pacing (P<0.01, Figure 5). Therefore, the significant reduction of TSS from 21.3±1.1 at baseline to 7.0±1.5 after 6 weeks of two-channel gastric pacing was observed.

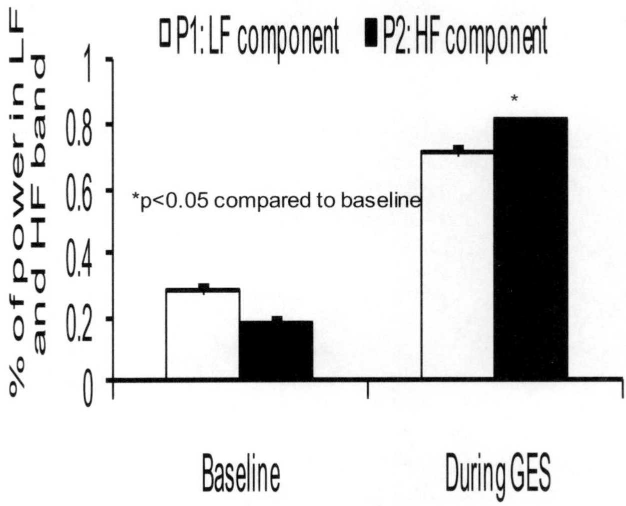

Fig. 4. Effect of two-channel gastric pacing on the spectral components of the HRV. Comparing to baseline, the high frequency component of the HRV increased significantly during two-channel gastric pacing. P1, the percentage of power in low frequency band; P2, the percentage of power in high frequency band.

4. Discussion and conclusion

This study identifies significantly enhanced vagal activity during chronic GES with both Enterra therapy and two-channel gastric pacing while significantly improving upper GI symptoms. These observations augment previous reports on the purported mechanisms of high-frequency GES therapy (Tougas & Huizinga, 1998; Tack et al., 1999; Al-Jubiri et al., 2001; Wang et al., 2001; Liu et al., 2004; Luo et al., 2005; Lin et al., 2004, 2008; McCallum et al., 2010).

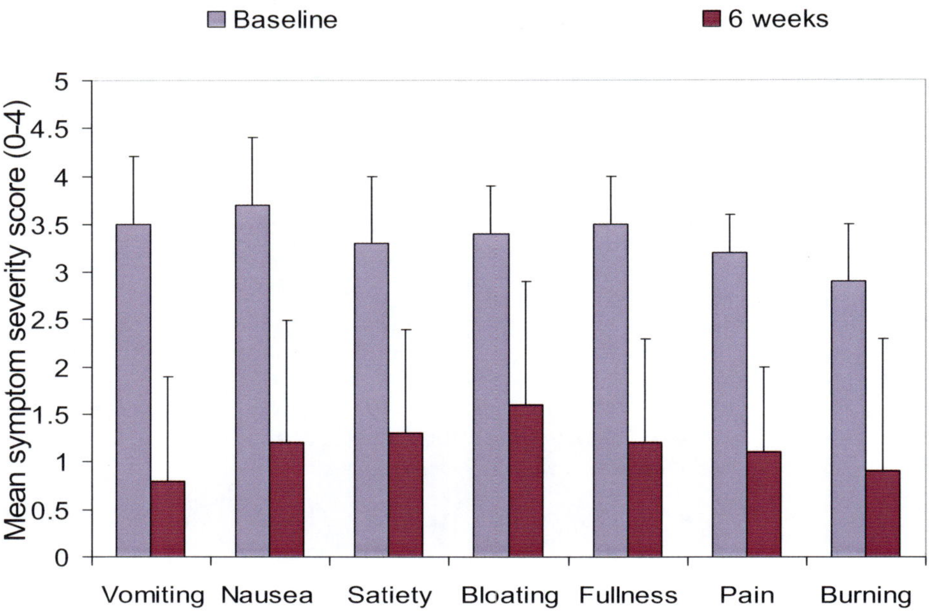

Fig. 5. Comparison of individual upper gastrointestinal symptoms (vomiting, nausea, early satiety, bloating, postprandial fullness, epigastric pain and epigastric burning) using a severity grading scale of 0 to 4 with a maximum of 28 points between baseline and after 6 weeks of Multi-channel Pulse Generator (MPG) gastric pacing. There was a significant reduction in all symptoms ($P<0.01$) after 6 weeks of GES.

The most common symptoms of gastroparesis patients are vomiting and nausea. In our study, we proved that GES with both Enterra device and two-channel gastric pacing significantly reduced voniting and nausea of gastroparesis patients. This would be a reliable evidence to demonstrate significant benefits for GES in the treatment of refractory gastroparesis. A certain number of studies investigated the mechanism of high-frequency GES to improve symptoms of gastroparesis, which included adrenergic and cholinergic functions (Luo et al., 2005), fundic relaxation (Tack et al., 1999), GI hormones (Al-Jubiri et al., 2001) and afferent brain stem pathways (Tougas & Huizinga, 1998), improvement of gastric emptying (Lin et al., 2008), activation of vagal afferent pathways to influence CNS control mechanisms for nausea and vomiting, and decreasing gastric sensitivity to volume distention which enhanced postprandial gastric accommodation (McCallum et al., 2010).

The autonomic nervous system (ANS) is involved in the modulation of normal gastrointestinal function. It consists of extrinsic control exerted by the parasympathetic and sympathetic nervous system (Thumshirn & Camilleri, 2004). A number of methods have been developed to assess specific aspects of autonomic nervous function. In recent years the development of techniques based on the autonomic modulation of heart rate function have largely replaced other methods because of their simplicity and validity as markers of vagal as well as sympathetic function (Tougas et al., 1997; Tougas, 2000). The power spectral analysis of the heart rate variability (HRV) derived from the electrocardiogram now provides a simple and accurate measure of the respective outflow of the vagal and sympathetic branches of the ANS (Kamath & Fallen, 1993). Preliminary studies in animals using spectral analysis of HRV have shown that short-pulse GES significantly increased vagal activity at a frequency four times the intrinsic slow-wave frequency and is mediated via the vagal efferent pathway (Liu et al., 2004; Wang et al., 2001). These short-pulse and high-frequency stimulation parameters have been used in previous clinical trials (Familoni et al., 1997; Forster et al., 2001; Abell et al., 2002, 2003) and in clinical practice. In this current study, we used power spectral analysis of heart rate variability derived from raw ECG recordings to assess the effect of GES on autonomic function and found that the sympathovagal balance (power in the low frequency band/power in high frequency band) was significantly decreased during GES therapy with both Enterra therapy and two-channel gastric pacing, attributing to an increase in vagal activity. To our knowledge, this is the first study to demonstrate that these stimulation parameters would evoke a similar change in vagal activity in humans as previously observed in the dog (Liu et al., 2004; Wang et al., 2001).

In conclusion, GES with Enterra therapy and two-channel gastric pacing in patients with severe gastroparesis results in a decrease in the sympathovagal balance (power in the low frequency band/power in high frequency band), indicating a significant increase in vagal activity while significantly improving upper GI symptoms. These findings are one explanation for the significant symptomatic improvement induced by GES in these patients with refractory gastroparesis.

5. Acknowledgment

The authors would like to acknowledge the following individuals for their contributions: Jameson Forster, Irene Sarosiek, Katherine Roeser, Pernilla Foran, Teri Lavenbarg and Irene King as well as faculty, fellows and nursing staff in the Division of Gastroenterology at University of Kansas Medical Center, Kansas City, Kansas, USA.

6. References

Abell, T.L.; Cutsem, E.V.; Abrahamsson, H.; Huizinga, J.D.; Kontruek, J.W.; Galmiche, J.P.; Voeller, G.; Filez, L.; Everts, B.; Waterfall, W.E.; Domschke, W.; des Varanbes, S.B.; Familoni, B.O.; Bourgeois, I.M.; Janssens, J. & Tougas, G. (2002) Gastric electrical stimulation in intractable symptomatic gastroparesis. Digestion, Vol. 66, pp. 204-212

Abell, T.; McCallum, R.W.; Hocking, M.; Koch, K.; Abrahamssion, H.; LeBlang, I.; Lindberg, G.; Konturek, J.; Nowak, T.; Quigley, E.M.M.; Tougas, G. & Starkebaum, W. (2003). Gastric electrical stimulation for medically refractory gastroparesis. Gastroenterology, Vol.125, pp. 421-428

Al-Jubiri, A.; Luo, J.; Rashed H. et al. (2001). Gastric electrical stimulation is associated with increased pancreatic synthetic function when compared to normals and medical controls (abstract). Gastroenterology, Vol. 120, pp. A647

Bellahsene, B.E.; Lind, C.D.; Schirmer, B.D. et al. (1992). Acceleration of gastric emptying with electrical stimulation in a canine model of gastroparesis. American Journal of Physiology, Vol. 262, pp. G826–834

Chen, J. & McCallum, R.W. (1992). Gastric slow wave abnormalities in patients with gastroparesis. American Journal of Gastroenterology, Vol.87, pp. 477-482

Chen, J.D.Z.; Xu, X.; Zhang, J. et al. (2005). Efficacy and efficiency of multi-channel gastric electrical stimulation. Neurogastrology and Motility, Vol. 17, pp. 878-882

Ejskjaer, N.T.; Bradley, J.L. & Buston-Thomas, M.S. et al. (1999). Novel surgical treatment and gastric pathology in diabetic gastroparesis. Diabetic Med Vol. 16, pp. 488-495

Familoni, B.O.; Abell, T.L.; Nemoto, D.; Voeller, G.; Salem, A. & Gabor, O. (1997). Electrical stimulation at a frequency higher than basal rate in human stomach. Digestive Diseases and Sciences, Vol. 42, pp. 885-891

Forster, J.; Sarosiek, I.; Delcore, R; Lin, Z.Y.; Raju, G.S. & McCallum, R.W. (2001). Gastric pacing is a new surgical treatment for gastroparesis. American Journal of Surgery, Vol. 182, pp. :676-681

Geldof, H.; van der Schee; E.J.; Van Blankenstein; M. & Grashius, J.L. (1986). Electrogastrographic study of gastric myoelectrical activity in patients with unexplained nausea and vomiting. Gut, Vol.26, pp. 799-808

Hocking, M.P.; Vogel, S.B. & Sninsky, C.A. (1992). Human gastric myoelectrical activity and gastric emptying following gastric surgery and with pacing. Gastroenterology, Vol. 103, pp. 1811-1816

Kamath, M.V. & Fallen, E.L. (1993). Power spectral analysis of heart rate variability: a non-invasive signature of cardiac autonomic function. Critical Review in Biomedical Engineering, Vol.21, pp. 245-311

Lin, Z.Y.; McCallum, R.W.; Schirmer, B.D.; Chen, J.D.Z. (1998). Effects of pacing parameters in the entrainment of gastric slow waves in patients with gastroparesis. American Journal of Physiology, Vol.274, pp. G186-G191

Lin, Z.; Forster, J.; Sarosiek, I. & McCallum, R.W. (2004). Effect of high-frequency electrical stimulation on gastric myoelectric activity in gastroparetic patients. Neurogastroenterology and Motility, Vol.16, pp. 205-212

Lin, Z.; Hou, Q.; Sarosiek, I. et al. (2008). Association between changes in symptoms and gastric emptying in gastroparetic patients treated with gastric electrical stimulation. Neurogastroenterology and Motility, Vol.20, pp. 464-470

Liu, J.; Qiao, X. & Chen, J.D.Z. (2004). Vagal afferent is involved in short-pulse gastric electrical stimulation in rats. Digestive Diseases and Sciences, Vol.49, pp. 29-737

Luo, J.; Rashed, H.; Eaton, P. et al. (2005). Long-term treatment of gastric electrical stimulation is associated with autonomic and enteric nervous system changes(abstract).Digestive Diseases and Sciences, Vol.45, pp. 1244

McCallum, R.W.; Chen, J.D.Z.; Lin, Z.Y.; Schirmer, B.D.; Williams, R.D. & Ross, R.A. (1998). Gastric pacing improves emptying and symptoms in patients with gastroparesis. Gastroenterology, Vol.114, pp. 456-61

McCallum, R.W.; Dusing, R.W.; Sarosiek, I.; Cocjin, J.; Forster, J. & Lin, Z. (2010). Mechanisms of symptomatic improvement after gastric electrical stimulation in gastroparetic patients. Neurogastroenterology and Motility, Vol.22, pp. 161-167

Nilsson, P.H. (1996). Diabetic gastroparesis: A review. Journal of Diabetes and its Complications, Vol.10, pp. 113-122

Oppenheim, A.V. & Schafer, R.W. (1975). Digital Signal Processing, Englewood Cliffs, NJ: Prentice Hall

Qian, L.; Lin, X. & Chen, J. D. Z. (1999). Normalization of atropine-induced postprandial dysrhythmias with gastric pacing. American Journal of Physiology, Vol. 276, pp. G387-G392

Reardon, T.M.; Schnell, G.A. & Smith, O.J. & Schubert, T.T. (1989). Surgical therapy of diabetic gastroparesis. Journal of Clinical Gastroenterology, Vol. 11, pp. 204-207

Song, G.Q.; Hou, X.H.; Yang, B. et al. (2005). Two-channel gastric electrical stimulation accelerates delayed gastric emptying induced by vasopressin. Digestive Diseases and Sciences, Vol.50, pp. 662-668

Soykan, I.; Sivri, B.; Sarosiek, I. et al. (1998). Demography, clinical characteristics, psychological and abuse profiles, treatment, and long-term follow-up of patients with gastroparsis. Digestive Diseases and Science, Vol. 43, pp. 2398-2404

Sturm, A.; Holtmann, G.; Goebell, H. & Gerken, G. (1999). Prokinetics in patients with gastroparesis: A systematic analysis. Digestion, Vol. 60, pp. 422-427

Tack, J.; Coulie, B.; Van Cutsem, E. et al. (1999). The influence of gastric electrical stimulation on proximal gastric motor and sensory function in severe idiopathic gastroparesis (abstract). Gastroenterology, Vol.116, G4733

Telander, R.L.; Morgan, K.G.; Kreulen, D.L.; Schemalz, P.F.; Kelly, K.A. & Szurszewki, J.H. (1978). Human gastric atony with tachygastria and gastric retention. Gastroenterology, Vol.75, pp. 495-5

Thumshirn, M. & Camilleri, M. (2004). Evaluation of gastrointestinal autonomic function. In: Gastrointestinal Function in Diabetes Mellitus, Horowitz, M. and Samsom, M. (Ed.), 323-337, John Wiley & Sons Ltd.

Tougas, G.; Kamath, M.; Watteel, G. et al. (1997). Modulation of neurocardiac function by esophageal stimulation in humans. Clinical Sciences, Vol.92, pp. 167-174

Tougas, G. & Huizinga, J.D. (1998). Gastric pacing as a treatment for intractable gastroparesis: shocking news? Gastroenterology, Vol.114, pp. 598-601

Tougas, G.; Eaker, E.Y.; Abell, T.L. et al. (2000). Assessment of gastric emptying using a low fat meal: Establishment of international control values. American Journal of Gastroenterology, Vol.95, pp. 1456-146

Tougas, G. (2000). The autonomic nervous system in functional bowel disorders. Gut, Vol.(Suppl IV)47, pp. iv78-iv80

Wang, Z.S. & Chen, J.D.Z. (2000). Robust ECG R-R wave detection using evolutionary-programming-based fuzzy inference system (EPFIS), and application to assessing brain-gut interaction. IEE Proc. Scientific Measurement Technology Vol.147, pp. 351-356

Wang, Z.S.; Xu, X.H.; Ueno, T. et al. (2001). Effects and mechanisms of forward and backward gastric electrical stimulation with pulse train. Gastroenterology, Vol.120, pp.A2348.

Xu, J.; Ross, R.A.; McCallum, R.W. & Chen, J.D.Z. (2008). Two-channel gastric pacing with a novel implantable gastric pacemaker accelerates glucagons-induced delayed gastric emptying in dogs. American Journal of Surgery Vol.195, pp. 122-129

You, C.H.; Lee, K.Y.; Chey, W.Y. & Menguy, R. (1980). Electrogastrographic study of patients with unexplained nausea, bloating and vomiting. Gastroenterology, Vol.79, pp. 311-314

Part 5

ECG Signal Processing

An Analogue Front-End System with a Low-Power On-Chip Filter and ADC for Portable ECG Detection Devices

Shuenn-Yuh Lee[1], Jia-Hua Hong[1], Jin-Ching Lee[2] and Qiang Fang[3]
[1]*Department of Electrical Engineering, National Chung-Cheng University, Taiwan*
[2]*Department of Biotechnology, College of Life Science, Kaohsiung Medical University,*
[3]*Department of Electrical and Computer Engineering, RMIT University,*
[1,2]*Taiwan*
[3]*Australia*

1. Introduction

Medical diagnostic instruments can be made into portable devices for the purpose of home care, such as the diagnosis of heart disease. These assisting devices are not only used to monitor patients but are also beneficial as handy and convenient medical instruments. Hence, for reasons of both portability and durability, designers should reduce the power consumption of assistant devices as much as possible to extend their battery lifetime. However, achieving the low power requirement of the ECG sensing and the processing board for the ECG with commercial discrete components (A21-0003) is difficult because the low power consumer electronics for ECG acquisition systems are not yet available. With the help of the integrated circuit technology, the power-saving requirement of portable and durable equipment gives circuit designers the impetus to reduce the power consumption of analogue front-end circuits in ECG acquisition systems. In addition, the analogue front-end circuits, which are the interface between physical signals and the digital processor, must be operated at a low-supply voltage to be integrated into the low-voltage system-on-a-chip (SOC) system (Eshraghian, 2006). Therefore, the chapter will present two design examples of low-voltage (1 V) and low-power (<1 μW) on-chip circuits including a low-pass filter (LPF) and an analogue-to-digital converter (ADC) to demonstrate the possibility of developing the low-voltage low-power ECG acquisition SOC.

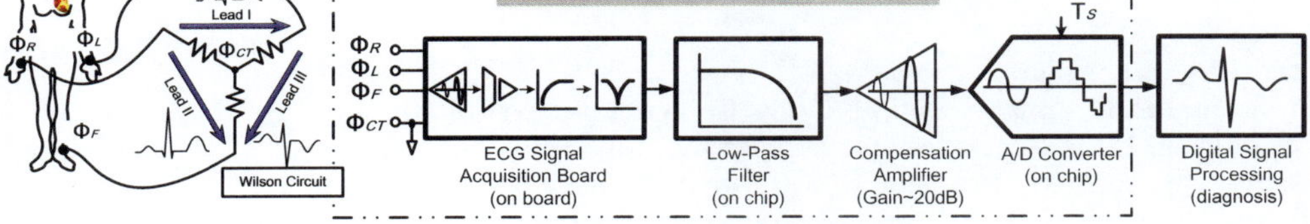

Fig. 1. An analog front-end system for portable ECG detection devices

In clinical electrocardiogram (ECG) acquisition, several leads combined with signals from different body parts (i.e., from the right wrist and the left ankle) are utilised to trace the electric activity of the heart. In this system, as shown in Fig. 1, the ECG acquisition board translates the body signal to six leads and processes the signal using a low-pass filter (LPF) and a successive-approximation analogue-to-digital converter (SAADC). The acquisition board is composed of some discrete components including an instrumentation amplifier, a high-pass filter, a 60-Hz notch filter, and a common-level adjuster. The main function of the acquisition board is to pre-amplify the weak ECG signal whose amplitude is between 100 μV and 4 mV (Webster, 1995). The range of the ECG signal means that this system requires a signal-to-noise and distortion-ratio (SNDR) of at least 32 dB (that is, 6 bits) to detect heart activities precisely. There is more than one sensing channel on the board, and thus this system suffers from some problems such as crosstalk, settling time, and dispensable switch-induced noise (Olsson et al., 2005). The frequency range of the ECG signal is between 0.1 Hz to 250 Hz. Therefore, an on-chip low-power LPF behind the acquisition board provides a low cut-off frequency (250 Hz) to decrease the out-of-band high-frequency noise. On the other hand, the noise under 0.1 Hz will be eliminated by a high-pass filter on the acquisition board. To compensate for the in-band signal attenuation in the LPF, an adjustable compensation amplifier located between the filter and the SAADC was designed. It can decrease the influence of the switch-induced noise caused by the sampling behaviour of the SAADC. Because the total power of the ECG acquisition board will be dominated by the high-order LPF and ADC integrated by off-chip components, in this chapter, low-power integrated-circuit design techniques are proposed and adopted to implement these two chips under the 0.18-μm TSMC CMOS process. It reveals that the low-power miniature ECG acquisition system is realisable, and it can be integrated into wearable devices for ECG signal acquisition.
The whole analogue front-end system will be introduced in detail. First, a multi-function acquisition board for the ECG signal and a low-power anti-aliasing operational transconductance amplifier-C (OTA-C) filter without the off-chip capacitors under low-frequency operation are described in Section 2. Furthermore, the design and utilisation of the low-power SAADC are also presented in Section 2. Finally, the practical human-body measurement results of the whole system and the conclusions are presented in Sections 3 and 4, respectively.

2. Design

2.1 ECG signal acquisition board

Human-body signals are too complex to be directly fed into on-chip analogue circuits including a LPF and a SAADC, and hence the Wilson circuit on board is used to transfer human-body signals to six leads. In addition to the Wilson circuit, other elements including an instrumentation amplifier, an isolator, a high-pass filter, and a 60-Hz notch filter on the acquisition board are required to capture the ECG signal, as shown in Fig. 2. They will be introduced in the next subsections.

2.1.1 Wilson circuit

In normal ECG signal detection, the Wilson circuit is commonly used. As shown in the left part of Fig. 1, the electrodes are stuck on the right wrist, left wrist, and left ankle, and each node connects with a resistor to a common node called the Wilson central terminal. The three main leads (Lead I, II, and III) and three minor leads (aV_R, aV_F, and aV_L) are formed by these terminals and some nodes in the circuit.

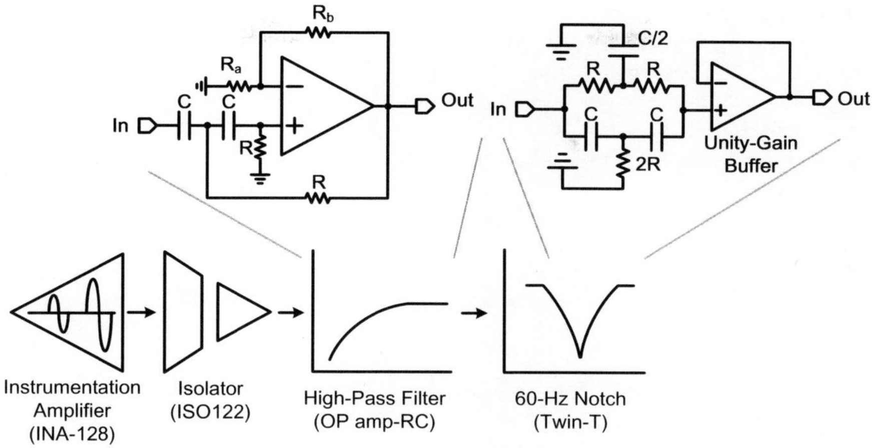

Fig. 2. Analogue blocks on the ECG signal acquisition board and analogue filters implemented by discrete components.

2.1.2 Instrumentation amplifier and isolation circuit

To obtain a high common-mode rejection ratio (CMRR), an instrumentation amplifier is adopted as the preamplifier in the analogue front-end system. In this case, an instrumentation amplifier with chip INA-128 is used. It not only provides a high CMRR (at least 120 dB) but also high precision, low power consumption, and low quiescent current. Aside from these, the gain of this amplifier can be adjusted to an appropriate level to fit the operation condition of the chip. Because the experimentation in this chapter is done on an actual human body, for safety considerations, a high linear isolator with an ISO122 chip is utilised to prevent electric shock.

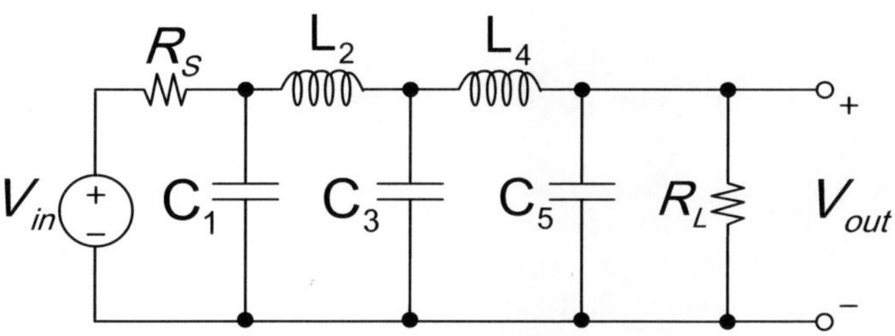

Fig. 3. Ladder type fifth-order passive Butterworth filter

2.1.3 High pass and 60-Hz notch filters

Behind the isolator, a high-pass filter with a cut-off frequency of 0.1 Hz is implemented by an active RC circuit to reject the low-frequency noise. The last stage is a notch filter with a twin-T structure; it protects the circuits against the 60-Hz noise produced by the AC-110V power supply. The realisations of the high-pass filter and notch filter are shown in Fig. 2, respectively.

2.2 Anti-aliasing OTA-C filter

For the long-term physical signal detection and monitor system, the use of a switched capacitor (SC) is a popular technique (Lasanen & Kostamovaara, 2005). However, the low sampling frequency in the kilohertz range will result in leakage, and the power consumption will be increased by the operational amplifiers in the SC circuits. Hence, continuous-time operational transconductance amplifier (OTA)-based filters are preferred in low-frequency applications, and the transistors inside a filter can be operated in the sub-threshold region to save power and to achieve ultra-low transconductance (a Gm of the order of a few nano-amperes per volt to save the capacitive area) (Salthouse & Sarpeshkar, 2003). The performance of the OTA-based filter is dominated by OTA, and the time constant of the OTA-C integrators is determined by the ratio of the capacitor value to the small transconductance.

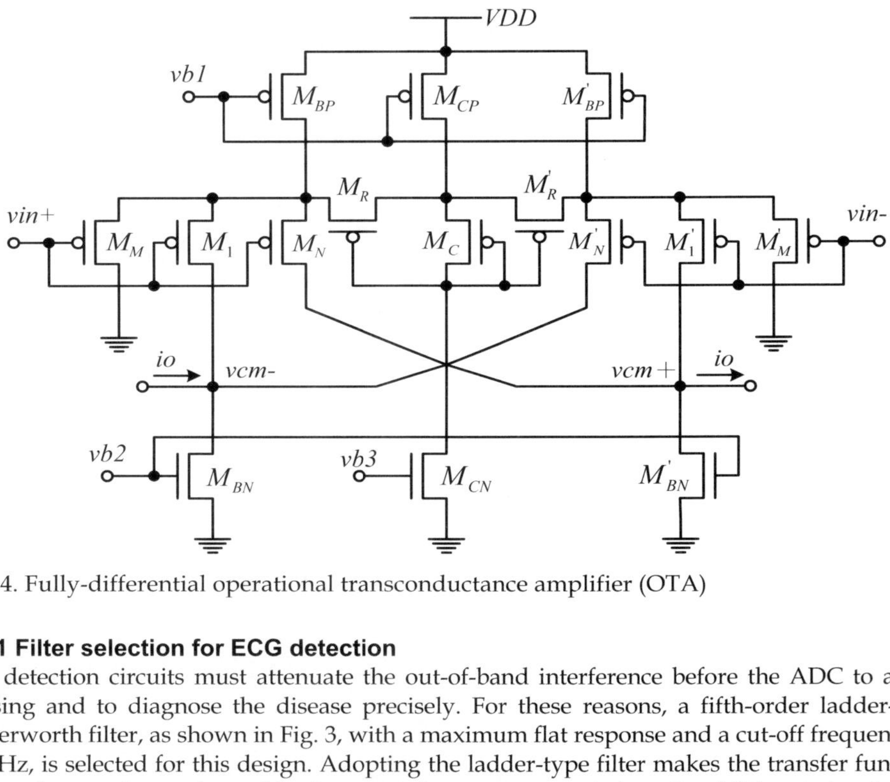

Fig. 4. Fully-differential operational transconductance amplifier (OTA)

2.2.1 Filter selection for ECG detection

The detection circuits must attenuate the out-of-band interference before the ADC to avoid aliasing and to diagnose the disease precisely. For these reasons, a fifth-order ladder-type Butterworth filter, as shown in Fig. 3, with a maximum flat response and a cut-off frequency of 250 Hz, is selected for this design. Adopting the ladder-type filter makes the transfer function more robust and more insensitive in terms of component variations. In addition, to implement the filter with the integrated circuits (ICs), the filter synthesis using the signal flow graph (SFG) mapping method should be applicably used (Schaumann & Valkenburg, 2001).

2.2.2 Nonlinearity and input referred noise of the OTA

An ultra-low-G_m OTA can be implemented as the low-frequency filter with an on-chip capacitor (Bustos et al., 2000). Fig. 4 shows an OTA circuit that uses two techniques to reduce the transconductance, including current cancellation and current division.

Furthermore, the fully differential structure provides a higher capability in terms of common-mode rejection and an increase of 3 dB in the dynamic range rather than the single-end structure. In addition, all transistors in the OTA are operated in sub-threshold region to save the power consumption.
According to the analysis of the nonlinearity and input referred noise of this filter (Lee & Cheng, 2009), the dominated third harmonic distortion (*HD3*) caused by the device M_R can be expressed as

$$HD3 \cong \frac{\gamma \cdot v_{SD}^2}{96(v_{SG} - V_{th})(2\phi_F - v_{SB})^{3/2}} \tag{1}$$

where ϕ_F represents the Fermi potential. In this design, HD3 is to be suppressed below -50 dB with a differential input level of 100 mV. Second harmonic distortion (HD2) is almost cancelled by using a fully differential structure. As previously mentioned, the system detecting the ECG signal should possess an SNDR greater than 32 dB. Because the distortion is below 50 dB (that is, it is sufficient), the other issues in terms of equivalent input noise should be considered in the filter design.
By selecting the PMOS as the input stage of Fig. 4, the flicker noise should be low. Given this, the required input referred noise of the filter can be expressed as

$$Noi_{in,ref}(rms) = V_{in,rms} \Big/ 10^{SNR(dB)/20} \tag{2}$$

According to the description, with an SNR of 42 dB (7 bits), the input referred noise must be less than 560 μV_{rms} for an input voltage of 100 mV_{rms}.

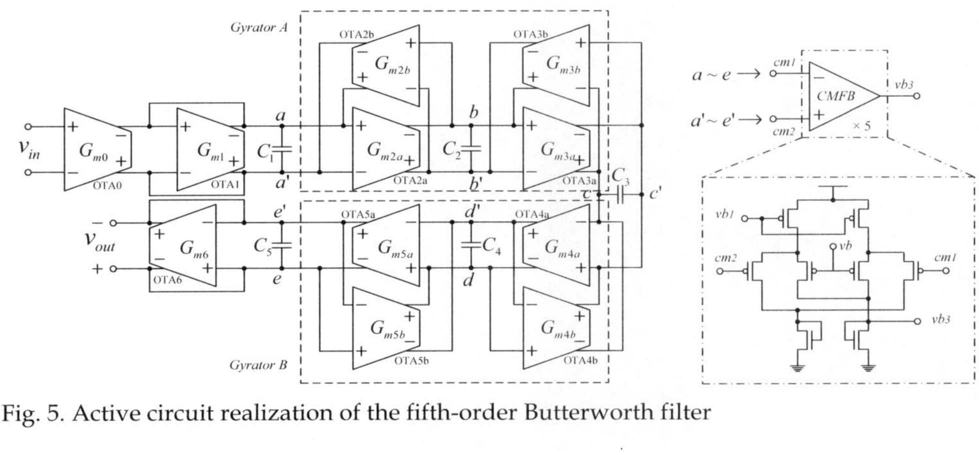

Fig. 5. Active circuit realization of the fifth-order Butterworth filter

2.2.3 Fifth-order OTA-C low-pass filter

The realisations of the fifth-order OTA-C filter with common-mode feedback (CMFB) circuits are illustrated in Fig. 5. To contrast with the ladder type, the overall circuit is composed of two grounded resistors G_{m0} and G_{m6}, two gyrators A and B, which implement the equivalent inductors L_2 and L_4, respectively, and five capacitors C_1~C_5. To reduce the power consumption, five common-mode feedback circuits are shared by the eleven OTAs of the filter. The common-mode feedback circuits provide sensing of the common output voltages on nodes *a~e* to control the bias voltage vb3 of the OTA.

2.3 Low-power successive approximation ADC

For the required performance of ECG signals with an amplitude between 100 μV and 4 mV (Webster, 1995), the resolution of the ADC with analogue filter in this ECG signal processing system usually only has to be between 6 to 8 bits. In this chapter, a low-power SAADC with 8-bit resolution and 10-KHz sampling frequency is designed. It is not only applied to the ECG signal, but also used for other physical signals, such as Electroneurography (ENG). The basic architecture of a SAADC is illustrated in Fig. 6. The converter consists of a sample/hold (S/H) circuit, a comparator, a successive approximation register (SAR) controller, and an 8-bit digital-to-analogue converter (DAC). Using a binary searching algorithm, the input sample voltage can be successively approximated by the DAC output voltage. For a N-bit SAADC, N cycles are required to convert the analogue signals into digital codes. Obviously, the DAC dominates the accuracy and the speed of the SAADC. To conform to the system specifications, a low-power, opamp-free, capacitor-based DAC with an 80-kHz sampling rate is implemented. The sub-circuit design of the SAADC will be described in the following subsections in detail.

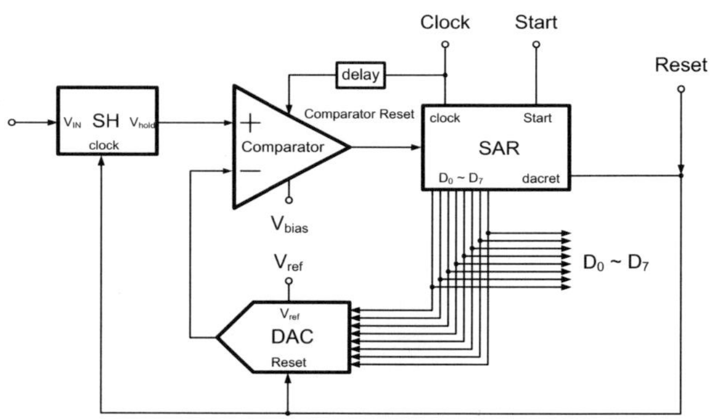

Fig. 6. Block diagram of a successive approximation ADC.

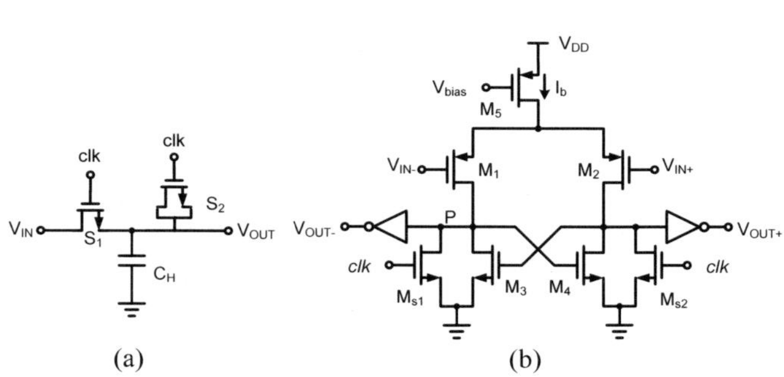

Fig. 7. (a) Passive S/H circuit with dummy switch, and (b) Comparator circuit

2.3.1 Sample/hold circuit

To decrease the power consumption of the SAADC, a passive S/H circuit illustrated in Fig. 7(a) is adopted. It consists of the NMOS switch S_1 and the sampling capacitor C_H. A dummy switch S_2 is adopted to circumvent the problem of the charge injection and the clock feedthrough and to compensate for the charge error. It will meet the requirements of 8-bit resolution.

2.3.2 Comparator circuit

The comparator used in the SAADC is illustrated in Fig. 7(b); it is a track-and-latch stage. Because the accuracy of the comparator plays a critical role in the SAADC, the transistors M_{s1} and M_{s2} are included to avoid hysteresis or delayed response when resetting the phase. The operational principle is as follows. When the clock is high, the comparator is operated in the resetting mode, and both outputs (V_{OUT+} and V_{OUT-}) are pulled to V_{DD} (high). On the other hand, when the clock is low, the circuit will execute the comparison of differential input, and the outputs level (V_{OUT+} or V_{OUT-}) of the comparator will depend on the difference between V_{IN+} and V_{IN-}.

The design of the bias current I_b is critical for the performance of the comparator, including speed, noise, and power consumption. For speed considerations, the frequency response of the comparator depending on the dominant pole should be analysed. The dominated pole of the comparator is located at node P and can be described as follows:

$$\omega_P = \frac{g_{m1}}{C_P}\ , \quad C_P = C_{gs3} + C_{db2} + C_{db4} + C_{db\_s2} + C_{buffer} \tag{3}$$

where C_p is the total capacitance at node P. To fit the 10 kS/s sampling rate of the 8-bit SAADC, the speed of the comparator must be operated at no less than 80 kHz. However, for settling within the 0.1% accuracy, the required unity-gain bandwidth of the comparator must satisfy seven times its time constant. Therefore, a comparator with a unity-gain bandwidth of 1 MHz is implemented. Hence, a comparing time of less than 1 μs can be achieved.

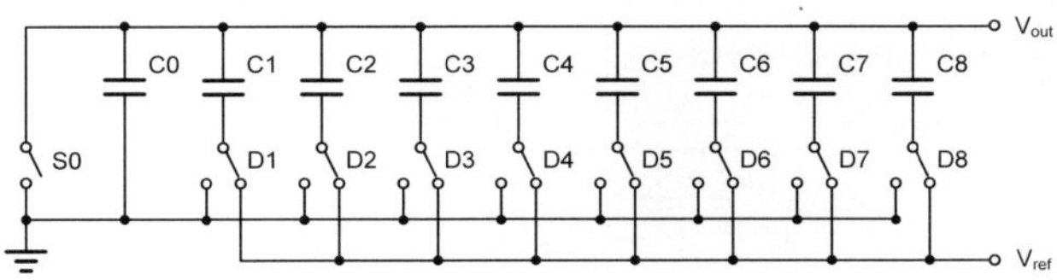

Fig. 8. Architecture of an 8-bit capacitor-based DAC.

Because the operational speed of the comparator is at a low frequency, flicker noise will dominate the input-referred noise. Hence, a low bias current with large channel width is appropriate to decrease power consumption. In this chapter, a bias current with only 400 nA is adopted to let the comparator operate in the sub-threshold region under the 8-bit and 10-kHz requirements.

2.3.3 Capacitor-based DAC

There are various structures, including resistor strings, the current-mode approach, and capacitor arrays, that can be adopted to implement the internal DAC in the SAADC. Among these, the capacitor-array structure is most suitable for the low-power approach (Hong &

Lee, 2007). Therefore, in this chapter, an opamp-free, capacitor-based approach, as shown in Fig. 8, is used to implement the DAC. Based on the binary-weighted capacitor array, the output voltage of the DAC can be described as follows:

$$V_{out} = V_{ref} \frac{C_i + \sum_{j=i+1}^{8} D_j C_j}{C_{total}} \tag{4}$$

where C_{total} is the total capacitance of the DAC, and the value of i is from 0 to 7.
The power source of the above mentioned passive capacitor array is dominated by the reference voltage, V_{ref}. It can be analysed by calculating the required charge of all the capacitors during charging and discharging periods (Hong & Lee, 2007). A relative equation described below can be used to estimate the power:

$$P_{Vref} = \frac{f_{clk}}{9} 2^8 C_0 \left(\frac{5}{6} V_{DD}{}^2 - \frac{1}{2} V_{in}{}^2 \right) \tag{5}$$

where f_{clk} is the operational frequency of the DAC, V_{in} is the sampling voltage of the S/H circuit, and C_0 is the unity capacitor. According to (5), a smaller capacitor, C_0, can reduce power consumption. However, it will also contribute to an increase in thermal noise (KT/C), which degrades the resolution of the DAC. In this chapter, a metal-insulator-metal (MIM) capacitor of 24 fF is implemented in a TSMC 0.18-μm 1P6M CMOS process to trade off between power consumption and the noise contribution.

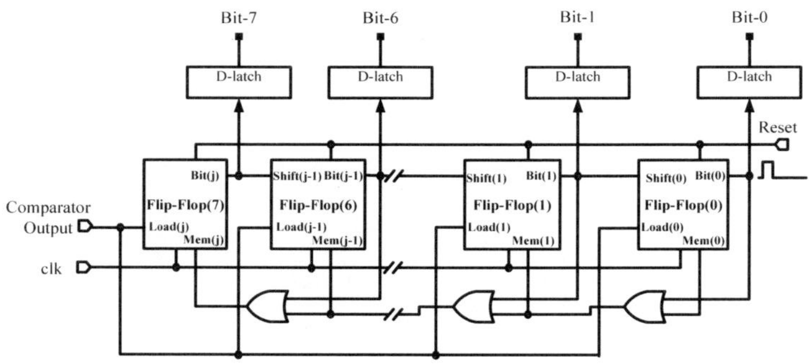

Fig. 9. N-bit SAR controller based on the non-redundant structure.

Moreover, the matching and noise in the capacitor array will dominate the accuracy of the DAC. However, the process variation resulting in matching error commonly plays a more important role compared with the thermal noise. Hence, the layout of the capacitor array based on the common-centroid structure is adopted to protect against the matching error.

2.3.4 SAR Controller

For a N-bit SAR, two sets of registers are required in the binary search algorithm. One is used for storing the conversion results, and the other is used for estimating the results. A non-redundant structure, as illustrated in Fig. 9, is adopted to reduce the usage of the registers; the result is to reduce power consumption (Rossi & Fucili, 1996). In this structure, a finite state machine (FSM) is used to generate the control signal. At the beginning of conversion, the most significant bit (MSB) is set to one, whereas the remaining bits are set to zero. The initial value of the DAC output is then set to 0.5 V (1/2 full scale). If the comparator output is low, the MSB will be set to 0 and saved in the output of the SAR. If the output is high, the MSB will remain 1. The residue bits will be processed in the same operations until the least significant bit (LSB) is determined.

3. Experimental results

The three main elements introduced above were integrated to a low-power analogue front-end system on a detection board; the measured analogue front-end system was set up as shown in Fig. 10. The picture also shows the practical measurement conditions: the electrodes are stuck on both wrists and both ankles. The circuits of the OTA-C filter and SAADC were fabricated in a 0.18-μm TSMC process with metal-insulator-metal (MIM) capacitors. The die area of the OTA-C filter and SAADC are 0.135 mm^2 and 0.12 mm^2, respectively. Figure 10 also shows the microphotographs of the two chips.

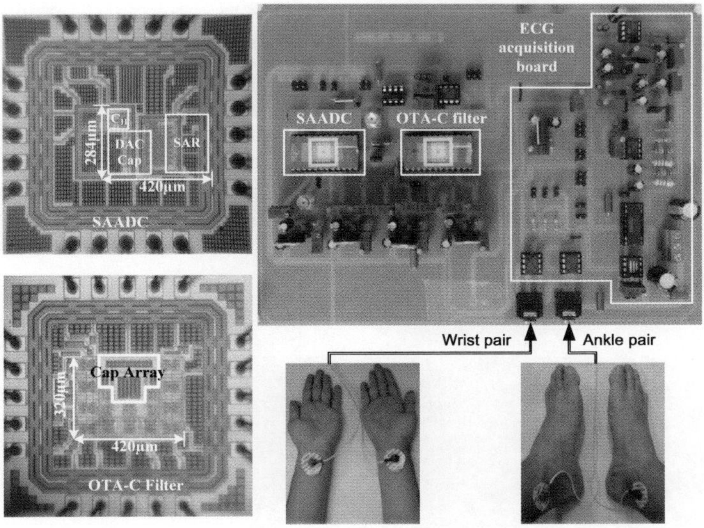

Fig. 10. Chip-microphotographs of an OTA-C filter and SAADC, respectively, and the measurement setup of an analog front-end ECG detection system

3.1 Filter measurement

A differential sinusoidal wave with a magnitude of 100 mV_{PP} is fed into the chip to measure the frequency response and the power spectrum with an input frequency of 50 Hz. Referring to Fig. 11(a), the -3 dB frequency is around 240 Hz, where the inband gain degradation (from -6 dB to -10 dB) arises from the finite-gain effect of the OTA. The measured third harmonic distortion (HD3) in Fig. 11(b) is well below -49 dB, which is close to the simulation estimation. In addition, the integrated input referred noise from 1 - 250 Hz is 340 μV_{rms}. The power consumption is 453 nW at a supply voltage of 1 V.

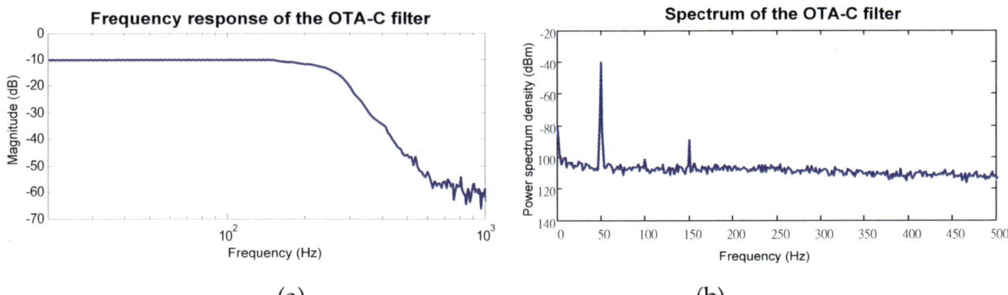

Fig. 11. Measurement of the OTA-C filter. (a) Frequency response. (b) Output power spectrum density.

3.2 SAADC measurement

The 1-kHz input signal with a 500-mV_{pp} full-swing magnitude sinusoidal wave is fed into the SAADC to measure integral nonlinearity (INL) and differential nonlinearity (DNL). Moreover, the sampling rate is 10 kHz. Fig. 12 shows the maximum DNL is +0.38/-0.41 LSB, whereas the maximum INL is +0.6/-0.89 LSB. Moreover, a full-scale 100-Hz sine-wave spectrum measured at a 1-kHz sampling rate is illustrated in Fig. 13 to demonstrate the low-frequency performance. The signal-to-noise distortion ratio (SNDR) in the ECG bandwidth (250 Hz) is 48.46 dB, and the spurious free dynamic range (SFDR) is 57 dB. Meanwhile, the effective number of bits (ENOB) defined as follows is 7.76 bits:

$$ENOB = \frac{SNDR - 1.76}{6.02} \tag{6}$$

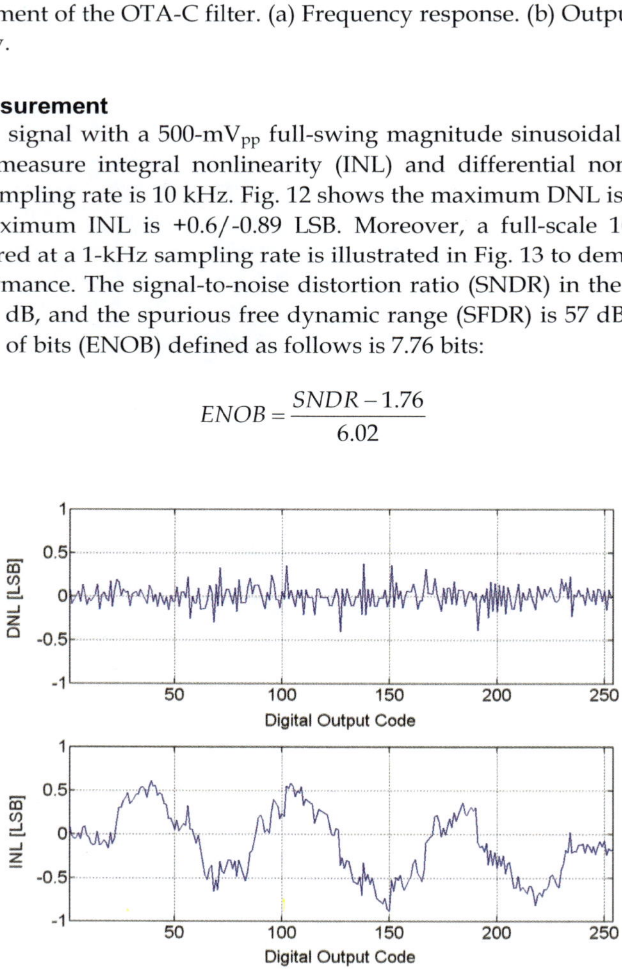

Fig. 12. Measured DNL and INL of the SAADC

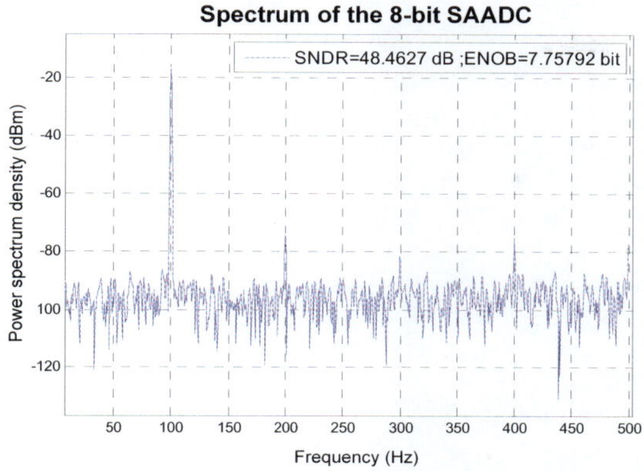

Fig. 13. Measured output spectrum at 100Hz input frequency and 1 kHz sampling rate.

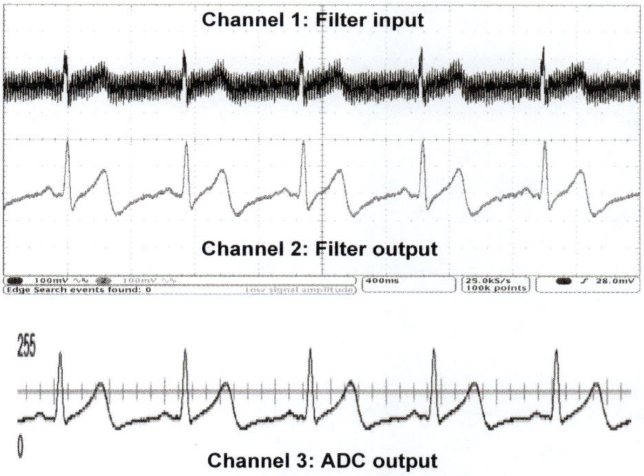

Fig. 14. Measurement results of the ECG analog front-end system

3.3 Real ECG signal testing

Corresponding to the system shown in Fig. 1, the measurement results are also illustrated in Fig. 14. They are measured from each output node of the three main partitions on the system, including (a) the ECG acquisition board, (b) the OTA-C filter, and (c) the SAADC. We can observe the relations and functions between each output. Channel 1 in Fig. 14 is the initial pre-amplified ECG signal with obvious high-frequency noise generated by the human body. Because some tiny physical waves are covered, this kind of ECG signal is inconvenient for the diagnosis of heart disease. With the help of the low-pass OTA-C filter, the high frequency noise can be significantly attenuated, and the tracing signal with a clear baseline is shown in channel 2. To demonstrate the operation of the SAADC, the waveform view showing in the logic analyser is adopted to present the conversion result. Channel 3 in Fig. 14 shows the real-time human-body digital ECG waveform reconstructed by the 8-bit decimal codes of the SAADC. Similarly, a clear baseline is observed in this graph, and the 8-bit digital codes can be accepted by the post digital processor to diagnose the abnormal heart activities precisely.

4. Conclusions

A low-power analogue front-end system for ECG detection consisting of an acquisition board and two low-power on-chip components is presented. The design issues including an off-chip ECG signal acquisition board, an on-chip analogue filter, and an on-chip ADC are introduced in this chapter. The result reveals that developing an ultra low-power ECG acquisition SOC is possible. In the future, the entire elements of these three partitions will be integrated into a single chip to save area and achieve a fully low-voltage and low-power ECG acquisition SOC for wearable applications.

5. Acknowledgment

The authors would like to thank the Chip Implementation Center (CIC), the National Science Council (NSC) of Taiwan, R. O. C. under Grant NSC 99-2628-E-194-032, NSC 99-2220-E-194-001, and NSC 99-2220-E-194-006, the Australian Research Council, Australia for their support of this work, and the help of CBIC Laboratory members, Yu-Cheng Su, Chih-Jen Cheng, Kun-Min Huang, and Wei-Chun Kao.

6. References

A21-0003. ECG acquisition board. http://www.icci.com.tw

Bustos S. S., Martinez J. S., Maloberti F., Sinencio E. S., (2000). A 60-dB dynamic-range CMOS sixth-Order 2.4Hz low-pass filter for medical application. *IEEE Trans. Circuits Syst. II: Analog and Digital Signal Processing,* Vol. 47. No.12, (2000), pp. 1391–1398, ISSN 1057-7130.

Eshraghian K. (2006). SoC emerging technologies. *Proc. IEEE,* Vol. 94, No. 6, (2006), pp. 1197-1213, ISSN 0018-9219.

Hong H. C., Lee G. M. (2007). A 65-fJ/conversion-step 0.9-V 200-kS/s rail-to-rail 8-bit successive approximation ADC. *IEEE J. Solid-State Circuits,* Vol. 42, No. 10, (2007), pp. 2161-2168, ISSN 0018-9200.

Lasanen K., Kostamovaara J. (2005). A 1-V analog CMOS front-end for detecting QRS complexes in a cardiac signal. *IEEE Trans. Circuits Syst. I: Regular Papers,* Vol. 52, No. 12, (2005), pp. 2584-2594, ISSN 1057-7122.

Lee S. Y., Cheng C. J. (2009). Systematic design and modeling of a OTA-C filter for portable ECG detection. *IEEE Trans. Biomed. Circuits Syst.,* Vol. 3, No. 1, (2009), pp. 53-64, ISSN 1932-4545.

Olsson R. H., Buhl D. L., Sirota A. M. Guzsaki G., Wise K. D. (2005). Band-tunable and multiplexed integrated circuits for simultaneous recording and stimulation with microelectrode arrays. *IEEE Trans. Biomed. Eng.,* Vol. 52, No. 7, (2005), pp. 1303-1311, ISSN 0018-9294.

Rossi A., Fucili G. (1996). Nonredundant successive approximation register for A/D converters. *Electronics Letters,* Vol. 32. No. 12, (1996), pp. 1055-1056, ISSN 0013-5194.

Salthouse C.D., Sarpeshkar R. (2003). A practical micropower programmable bandpass filter for use in bionic ears. *IEEE J. Solid-State Circuits,* Vol. 38, No. 1, (2003), pp. 63-70, ISSN 0018-9200.

Schaumann R., Valkenburg M. E. V. (2001). *Design of Analog Filters.* New York: Oxford.

Webster J. G. (1995). *Design of Cardiac Pacemakers.* Piscataway, NJ: IEEE Press.

17

Independent Component Analysis in ECG Signal Processing

Jarno M.A. Tanskanen and Jari J. Viik
Tampere University of Technology and Institute of Biosciences and Medical Technology
Finland

1. Introduction

Electrocardiogram (ECG) signal processing aims basically 1) at artifact reduction to make the ECG signals cleaner and better interpretable by human or machine observers, 2) at revealing aspects not immediately observable in plain measured ECG signals even after artifact reduction, or 3) at diagnostics decision support and automated ECG signal interpretation, including classification of ECG signals into different classes associated with normal or pathological heart function. Thus, sports related applications aside, body surface ECG signal processing aims at enhancing ECG based diagnostics. In this Chapter, we review and demonstrate a statistical signal processing approach, independent component analysis (ICA), which is inherently very suitable for ECG signal processing regarding the aims 1) and 2) above, and also equally applicable as a component in systems aimed at accomplishing the aim 3). For more on general ECG signal processing, the reader is directed to the textbook written by Sörnmo & Laguna (2005), and for a thorough treatment of ICA to the Hyvärinen's book (Hyvärinen et al., 2001). A concise review on ICA in ECG signal processing has been presented by Castells et al. (2007a). In this Chapter, we describe and illustrate several widely adopted applications of ICA in ECG signal processing, and discuss associated practical aspects, some of which are not generally found in the literature. The treatment of the matter is aimed at conceptual and practical understanding, leaving the mathematical derivations and proofs far mostly for the interested reader to find in the references.

ICA (Castells et al., 2007a; Comon, 1994; Hyvärinen et al., 2001; Hyvärinen & Oja, 2000; Naik & Kumar, 2011) is a statistical signal processing method for decomposing a set of signals into a set of mutually independent component signals. In general, in the applications of ICA, including in ECG signal processing, the objective is that the resulting independent component signals are the original source signals. Since ICA operates purely based on the input signals and a few assumptions, ICA belongs to the class of methods called blind source separation methods. For ICA, a source signal is called an independent component (IC). The terms 'IC' and 'source signal' are here used interchangeably. For ECG, the source signals are the bioelectrical signals generated by the heart, and all the possible artifact signals.

Generally, ICA input signals are the observed signals, which may be measurement time series, such as sampled voltage values in time as in the case of ECGs, image pixel values, or basically any sets of values fulfilling the assumptions of ICA. In the sequel, the term 'measured signals' refers to a set of simultaneously measured digital discrete-time signals with constant interval between the measured signal samples. All signals are assumed to be sampled at the same time instances.

ICA is realized by an iterative numerical algorithm, several of which exist. In Section 2 of this Chapter, we first introduce the basics of ICA, review ICA estimation principles and note a few commonly used available ICA methods. Thereafter, the specific applications of ICA in ECG signal processing are described and illustrative examples are given. Internet addresses of a few ICA related web sites and ICA program packages are given in the Appendix.

For simplicity of presentation and the ease of reproducibility of the results shown in this Chapter, all the ICA calculations have been performed using FastICA (Aalto University [Aalto], 2005; Hyvärinen, 1999) with the default parameters. Note that for this kind of statistical signal processing software the results will differ from one run to another, but the conclusions should remain unaltered. Also, as usual with signals of biological origin, an ICA algorithm may or may not converge, and if not, further ICA input signal preprocessing may be necessary. For some ECG signals ICA just might not succeed. In the examples given in this Chapter only minor preprocessing has been applied, if any (possible preprocessing has been described in conjunction with the examples).

In Section 2.1, we introduce the basic concepts of ICA and illustrate its functioning with a toy example. ICA estimation principles and the ICA package employed in the examples in this Chapter, FastICA (Aalto, 2005), and a few other popular ICA methods are mentioned in Section 2.2. In Section 2.3, practical aspects and reliability of the ICA results are discussed. The conceptual differences between ICA and principal component analysis (PCA) are outlined in Section 2.4, and common ICA related misconceptions in the literature are discussed in Section 2.5. Common ECG artifacts are shortly reviewed in Section 3.1 before proceeding to describe the applications of ICA in ECG signal processing in Sections 3.2 through 3.5. In Section 3, also illustrative examples are presented. In Section 4, usage of ICA as a part of diagnostic systems is discussed, and finally, concise conclusions on ICA in ECG signal processing are given in Section 5.

2. Basics of ICA

2.1 The basic concepts of ICA

ICA requires the fulfillment of two assumptions: 1) the measured signals are linear combinations of independent source signals, and 2) the independent source signals are nongaussian. Fulfillment of the first assumption can usually be assessed based on the knowledge of the signal sources and the measurement setup with respect to the sources. Naturally, should there exist no source signals which were independent of each others, ICA would make no sense. To an approximation, the assumption of linear combinations of sources can be taken to be valid for ECG signals and most artifacts. The nature of the different artifacts is discussed in Section 3.1. The fulfillment of the second assumption cannot in general be known, unless an appropriate source signal model exists or the properties of the source signals can be otherwise assessed. For example, Rieta et al. (2004) conclude that during atrial arrhythmia episodes, atrial activity and ventricular activity are generated by independent generators, whose amplitude distributions are nongaussian. Shkurovich et al. (1998) show also nongaussian amplitude distributions of sinus rhythm and atrial fibrillation measured during defibrillator implantation. The first assumption would be clearly fulfilled if we considered the heart as one or several point sources and the possible electromyogram (EMG) and other artifacts as other point sources. Even though such a model might not exactly describe reality, ICA has been demonstrated to be feasible and useful in several ECG applications. Also, even if there is no knowledge on the fulfillment of the second assumption, ICA may be attempted. Please, see also Section 2.3 on practical considerations and ICA reliability.

In the context of ECG signal processing, ICA assumes that the measured possibly artifact containing ECG signals are linear combinations of source signals. This is indicated by the mixing model

$$\mathbf{Y} = \mathbf{AX}, \tag{1}$$

where the voltage signal samples measured over a limited period of time are in the rows of the measurement matrix **Y**, the source signals are in the rows of **X**, and **A** is the mixing matrix. For ICA of ECGs, signal samples measured during a short period of time via one ECG lead form one row of **Y** (1). For a standard 12-lead ECG measurement, **Y** is thus a matrix of $L = 12$ rows and N columns, with N being the number of signal samples taken to be processed by ICA at one time from each ECG lead signal. N may in general be decided according to the ECG sampling rate and the phenomena of interest, e.g., to span one or several cardiac cycles. Let us denote one measured ECG signal sample by $y(l,n)$, where $n = 1, \ldots, N$ is the discrete time index, and $l = 1, \ldots, L$ is the ECG lead index. ICA can naturally be performed in a running window, but here we always consider running ICA once for one measured ECG signal segment. Writing (1) out with signal samples, we get

$$\begin{bmatrix} y(1,1) & \cdots & y(1,N) \\ \vdots & \ddots & \vdots \\ y(L,1) & \cdots & y(L,N) \end{bmatrix} = \begin{bmatrix} a(1,1) & \cdots & a(1,L) \\ \vdots & \ddots & \vdots \\ a(L,1) & \cdots & a(L,L) \end{bmatrix} \begin{bmatrix} x(1,1) & \cdots & x(1,N) \\ \vdots & \ddots & \vdots \\ x(L,1) & \cdots & x(L,N) \end{bmatrix}. \tag{2}$$

For performing the matrix multiplication (2), see (5). After successful ICA, the rows of the matrix **X** contain the ICs. In general, the aim of applying ICA is that each IC carried a signal generated by a single physiological or physical source, such as a signal generated by the heart or its individual structure, possible additive noise, or other artifact, such as EMG artifact. The mixing matrix **A** describes how the source signals are weighted as they are conducted from the respective generators to the electrode sites and summed at each ECG electrode on the body surface, i.e., how the measurements are linear combinations of the sources.

ICA can find at maximum as many ICs are there are ICA input signals. In (1) and (2), we have assumed that there are equally many ICs in **X** than there are input signals in **Y**. In the case that there are more measurements than actual sources, the resulting **X** has fewer ICs than there are measured signals in **Y**, and correspondingly the mixing matrix **A** is not a square matrix. Given L measured signals and L' true sources, and $L > L'$, upon successful ICA, **X** will be of size L'-by-N, and **A** of size L-by-L'. On the other hand, in the case of more actual sources than measurements, $L < L'$, the sizes of the matrixes are as shown in (2), but the system is underdetermined, and the true ICs appear mixed in unknown fashion in ICs in **X**, if the ICA algorithm converges. These cases are illustrated with a toy example in Fig. 1.

From (1) and (2), we also see a common application of ICA: measurement reconstruction with only the ICs carrying desired information. First, calculating ICA on **Y**, if successful, yields both **A** and **X**. Thereafter, the ICs in **X** can be analyzed to determine which ICs carry noise or artifacts and which carry contributions from the actual ECG. To reconstruct the ECG without the noise and artifacts, the corresponding rows of **X** are set to zero in (2), and **Y** is calculated according to (2) without altering **A**. This completely removes the contributions of the zeroed ICs. This is the basis of several ECG applications of ICA.

Due to the nature of the mixing model (1), ICA has three ambiguities: 1) signs of the ICs are arbitrary, 2) energies of the ICs are arbitrary, and 3) the order in which the ICs appear in **X** (1) is arbitrary. The ambiguities of **X** are facilitated by the corresponding changes in the mixing matrix **A** in (1). With an arbitrary nonzero real constant c, (1) can be written as

$$\begin{aligned}\mathbf{Y} &= \mathbf{AX} \\ &= \begin{bmatrix} a(1,1) & \cdots & a(1,L) \\ \vdots & \ddots & \vdots \\ a(L,1) & \cdots & a(L,L) \end{bmatrix} \begin{bmatrix} x(1,1) & \cdots & x(1,N) \\ \vdots & \ddots & \vdots \\ x(L,1) & \cdots & x(L,N) \end{bmatrix} \\ &= \begin{bmatrix} -a(1,1) & \cdots & a(1,L) \\ \vdots & \ddots & \vdots \\ -a(L,1) & \cdots & a(L,L) \end{bmatrix} \begin{bmatrix} -x(1,1) & \cdots & -x(1,N) \\ \vdots & \ddots & \vdots \\ x(L,1) & \cdots & x(L,N) \end{bmatrix} \\ &= \begin{bmatrix} \frac{1}{c}a(1,1) & \cdots & a(1,L) \\ \vdots & \ddots & \vdots \\ \frac{1}{c}a(L,1) & \cdots & a(L,L) \end{bmatrix} \begin{bmatrix} cx(1,1) & \cdots & cx(1,N) \\ \vdots & \ddots & \vdots \\ x(L,1) & \cdots & x(L,N) \end{bmatrix},\end{aligned} \tag{3}$$

which means that for the same set of measured signals **Y** (3), the signs and amplitudes of the ICs are arbitrary, as accommodated by the corresponding changes in **A** (3). Similarly, the indeterminate order of ICs in **X** is seen from (4).

$$\mathbf{Y} = \begin{bmatrix} a(1,2) & a(1,1) & a(1,3) & \cdots & a(1,L) \\ a(2,2) & a(2,1) & a(2,3) & \cdots & a(2,L) \\ \vdots & \vdots & \vdots & \ddots & \vdots \\ a(L,2) & a(L,1) & a(L,3) & \cdots & a(L,L) \end{bmatrix} \begin{bmatrix} x(2,1) & x(2,2) & \cdots & x(2,N) \\ x(1,1) & x(1,2) & \cdots & x(1,N) \\ x(3,1) & x(3,2) & \cdots & x(3,N) \\ \vdots & \vdots & \ddots & \vdots \\ x(L,1) & x(L,2) & \cdots & x(L,N) \end{bmatrix} \tag{4}$$

Let us present a toy example to illustrate the workings of ICA, alike it can be expected to operate with biomedical signals. The same example will be used also to illustrate the difference between ICA and PCA in Section 2.4. Denote a measured ECG lead signal by $y_l = [y(l,1) \ldots y(l,N)]$, $l = 1, \ldots, L$, and a source signal by x_l analogously. Note that the independence of the sources in this example has not been confirmed, alike usually is the case in the analysis of biomedical signals. Let us consider $L = 4$ simulated measured signals, and denote ICA calculated with input signals y_1 and y_2 by ICA(y_1,y_2), and the ICA of other input signal combinations analogously. In Fig. 1A are shown $L' = 3$ simulated source signals x_1, x_2, and x_3, which are linearly combined to form the simulated measured signals according to $y_1 = 0.7x_1 + 0.2x_2$, $y_2 = 0.6x_1 + 0.7x_2$, $y_3 = 0.9x_1 + 0.2x_2 + 0.4x_3$, and $y_4 = 0.5x_2 + 0.2x_3$. In ECG measurements, this would correspond to the weighted summation of the source signals at the ECG electrodes. In reality the weights are dictated by the electrical conduction paths from the sources to the electrodes, including the electrode-skin contacts. The four simulated measured signals are seen in Fig. 1B. In Fig. 1C, the results of ICA on all the subsets of at least two simulated measurements are shown, displaying the ICs from one ICA calculation in each column.

In the results of ICA(y_1,y_2), IC_{11} and IC_{12} in the first column of the subfigures in Fig. 1C, correspond quite well to the source signals x_1 and x_2, as expected, since the simulated measurements y_1 and y_2 are composed only of these two sources. The results of ICA(y_1,y_3), ICA(y_2,y_3), and ICA(y_3,y_4), in Fig. 1C, illustrate one type of possible cases encountered in biomedical signal processing, including in ECG signal processing: the simulated measurements are composed of a larger number of sources than there are measured signals as ICA input. In these cases, the ICs are inhabited by the sources in an arbitrary manner, as clearly illustrated by the ICs resulting from ICA(y_2,y_3) and ICA(y_3,y_4). The results of ICA(y_1,y_3) may seem to display fairly clean source signals, but the contribution of the source

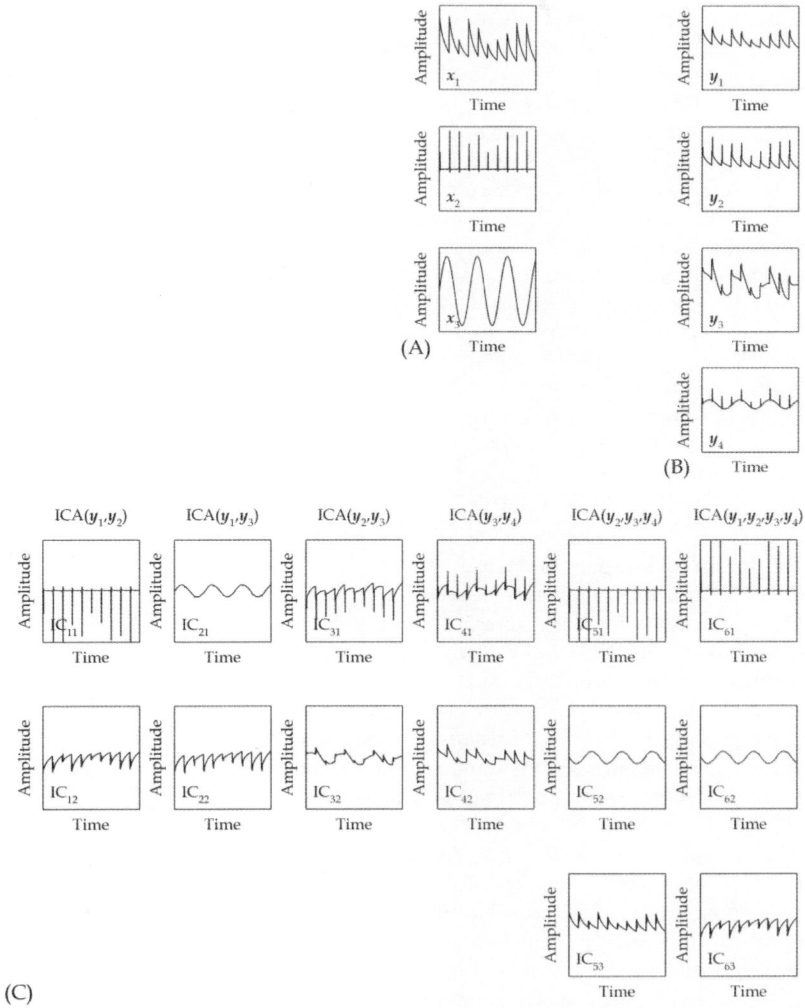

Fig. 1. (A) The three simulated original sources, i.e., the desired results of ICA. (B) The four simulated measured signals, constructed as linear combinations of the sources as $y_1 = 0.7x_1 + 0.2x_2$, $y_2 = 0.6x_1 + 0.7x_2$, $y_3 = 0.9x_1 + 0.2x_2 + 0.4x_3$, and $y_4 = 0.5x_2 + 0.2x_3$. (C) The results of ICAs, with the results from one ICA calculation presented in each column. Note the arbitrary sign of the ICs, e.g., comparing IC_{53} and IC_{63}. Units of amplitude are arbitrary in all (A), (B), and (C), and the time span is equal in all subfigures. Adapted from (Tanskanen et al., 2005).

x_2 is still buried in an unknown manner in the ICs. For ICA(y_2,y_3,y_4), there are equally many ICA input signals as there are original sources and ICA succeeds well in separating the sources, as expected. Due to the numerical nature of ICA calculations, and the fact that we did not ensure independence of the original sources, the ICs may not be exactly clear of the contributions from the other sources. The same holds for ICA(y_1,y_2,y_3,y_4) (Fig. 1C) where we also see the inherent property of ICA to determine the true number of ICs in an overdetermined case: even though there are four simulated measurements as ICA inputs, ICA correctly produces only three ICs. Such an observation is highly desirable also in practice in biomedical signal processing, since is it allows us to determine the true number of the sources (down to a numerical approximation). Note that in the examples shown in Figs. 3 and 6, there are eight measured ECG leads and one calculated lead, and thus ICA can find at maximum eight ICs since the calculated lead does not contribute new independent information. Such dimension reduction does therefore not indicate that the true number of sources would be indicated by the number of ICs.

Let us note that in ECG measurements, artifacts quickly increase the number of the true sources. Given too few measured ECG leads as ICA input signals, this may render the results of ICA useless, since the artifacts may populate most of the ICs, thus possibly causing the separation of the desired sources fail. This may be alleviated by increasing the number of ICA input ECG leads, and by general preprocessing of the ECG signals such as noise alleviation filtering, line interference alleviation, and baseline wander reduction. On the other hand, if the artifacts are well separated by ICA in the ICs of their own, they may be easily removed, as illustrated in Section 3. For example, the fist clenching artifact seen in Fig. 3A was removed easily with ICA (Fig. 3C).

2.2 ICA estimation principles and algorithms

In this Section, we bring into attention the multiplicity of ICA approaches without going into details or mathematics. The general ICA estimation principles (Hyvärinen et al., 2001) are: 1) Nonlinear decorrelation: the components are independent if they are uncorrelated *and* their appropriately chosen nonlinear transformations are uncorrelated. The appropriate nonlinear functions can be found using estimation and information theories. 2) Maximization of component nongaussianity. Intuitively, since central limit theorem states that summing nongaussian random signals yields signals that are closer to gaussian than the original signals, decomposing such sums of signals into the components maximizing the nongaussianity of the components results in ICs.

ICA has been realized by numerous methods including nongaussianity maximization, maximum likelihood estimation (Pham & Garat, 1997), mutual information minimization, tensorial methods, nonlinear decorrelation, and nonlinear PCA (Stamkopoulos et al., 1998). One practical difference between the methods is that several methods estimate all the ICs simultaneously, whereas, for example, nongaussianity maximization can be used to estimate a single IC at a time or all the ICs simultaneously. All the mentioned methods have been discussed by Hyvärinen et al. (2001), and several comparisons of ICA algorithms have been published, including a more general comparison by Giannakopoulos et al. (1999), comparison of different ICA methods for arrhythmia analysis (Llinares & Igual, 2009), atrial fibrillation analysis (Vayá et al., 2007), fetal ECG extraction in (Hild et al., 2007; Parmar Sargam & Sahambi, 2004), and movement artifact removal (Milanesi et al., 2008).

There exist numerous ICA software packages implementing different ICA algorithms. Web addresses of several ICA web sites and program packages are listed in the Appendix at the end of the Chapter. In the examples presented in this Chapter, we have applied FastICA (Aalto, 2005; Hyvärinen, 1999; Hyvärinen et al., 2001) version 2.5 using its default parameters. FastICA is an iterative numerical algorithm, which has been developed by Hyvärinen (1999), giving also instructions for parameter selection. FastICA runs in Matlab (The MathWorks, Inc., Natick, MA, USA) and is available also for a few other environments. FastICA package includes both a command line function and a graphical user interface. The program also automatically performs signal preprocessing in order to greatly ease the ICA calculations. The preprocessing steps are mean removal and PCA, or more exactly, whitening (Hyvärinen et al., 2001). Whitening the data makes the ICA input signals uncorrelated and of unit variance. PCA also provides for possible dimension reduction prior to ICA.

Since the ICA algorithms are necessarily numerical and generally iterative, the independence can be achieved only down to an error. According to our experience, the FastICA default parameters are usually appropriate. By default, FastICA strives to estimates all true ICs and possible further dimension reduction can be set by the user. For example, leaving out the most insignificant PCs in the preprocessing phase results in fewer ICA input signals. For this, the eigenvalues of the PCs can be observed also graphically. Furthermore, the nonlinear function to be used in the ICA can be selected from the given choices, with general selection criteria stated in (Hyvärinen, 1999). That said, according to our experience, the default parameters are a very good starting point for most experimentations with ICA. Should FastICA fail to converge, one can resort to the parameter settings, to the practical considerations described in the next Section, or finally to another ICA algorithm. Finally, for some specific ECG signals ICA just might not succeed.

2.3 Practical considerations and reliability of ICA results

In general, biomedical signals are stochastic random signals by nature, and the fulfillment of the ICA assumptions, especially regarding nongaussianity cannot be guaranteed. An appropriate model or measurement analysis may naturally shed light on the matter. In any case, ICA may be attempted. On the other hand, failing ICA with the specific input signals and using one algorithm with certain parameters, may not mean that the data at hand was unfit for ICA in general. Specifically in the case in which we can assume that the ICA assumptions should be sufficiently fulfilled, but ICA algorithm tends to fail, achieving convergence can attempted by changing number of ICA input samples, i.e., the length of the ECG signal segment used as input to ICA at one time, or by changing the number of ICA input ECG lead signals, input signal bandwidth and sampling rate, or ICA parameters. Also different ICA algorithms may yield different performances.

Due to the stochastic nature of the ECG measurements and the properties of ICA estimation algorithms, the ICA results can vary from one run to another. This raises the question of ICA reliability, which should be assessed at least in critical applications. At simplest, ICA reliability assessment can be approached by running ICA several times on the same data, and for example also on slightly time shifted data. First and foremost, the ICA results should naturally result in the same final conclusions regarding the original hypothesis. Secondly, the ICA results should greatly resemble each other from run to run. Note that the signs, amplitudes, and the order of appearance of the ICs may vary from one run to another; this does not constitute a reliability issue but is expected behavior, which is to taken into consideration by the biomedical algorithm developer. Another approach is to resample the same data in a few different ways, calculate ICA on the differently sampled data, and use the average of the resulting ICs as ICA results. Further methods for reliability assessment have been devised, for example, by Meinecke et al. (2002), and Icasso: software for investigating the reliability of ICA estimates by clustering and visualization developed by Himberg et al. (2004) (c.f. the Appendix for the Internet address).

2.4 ICA vs. PCA

PCA (Hyvärinen et al., 2001; Jolliffe, 2002) employs the same mixing model (1) as ICA, but the resulting components are fundamentally different. Whereas ICA yields components, which are mutually statistically independent, PCA yields principal components (PCs), which are mutually statistically uncorrelated. Uncorrelatedness is a much weaker requirement than independence; independent signals are also uncorrelated, but uncorrelatedness does not imply independence. Thus, also the aims of applying PCA and ICA are partially different. One of the applications in which both PCA and ICA have been successfully applied is noise reduction by excluding noise carrying components from the reconstruction. However, due to the different nature of the components resulting from PCA and ICA, the basis of noise reduction is different. For PCA in ECG signal processing see, e.g., (Castells et al., 2007b).

The PC found first by a PCA algorithm explains the greatest amount of variance in the measured signals and the last found PC the least. Thus, in practice the last found one or a few PCs may consist of mostly noise, thus PCA has been successfully applied in noise and dimensionality reduction. As the PCs are only statistically uncorrelated, they are in general not directly related to the actual independent physical or physiological sources. Therefore, in contrast with ICA, PCA cannot in general recover the actual source signals. Furthermore, strictly speaking, even if the last found PC may resemble a noise only signal, it may still contain contributions of the actual source signals. Even though such contributions were most probably minor, the ECG information they carry would be lost in noise reduction by PCA. Nevertheless, PCA is a powerful tool for noise reduction if applied appropriately. Also, as noted in Section 2.2, PCA is often used as preprocessing for ICA.

Functioning of PCA is illustrated in Fig. 2. The PCs produced by PCA of the simulated toy measurements shown in Fig. 1B are seen in Fig. 2A. In the toy example, comparing the ICs produced by ICA(y_2,y_3,y_4) or ICA(y_1,y_2,y_3,y_4) in Fig. 1C with the PCs shown in Fig. 2A, it is seen that ICA was able to separate the sources whereas PCA was clearly not. In Fig. 2B are shown the results of PCA applied on the eight-lead ECG measured on the abdominal region of a pregnant mother. The corresponding original measured signals are shown in Fig. 4A. Maternal ECG contributions are seen in PC_7 and PC_8 in Fig. 2B and fetal ECG is evident at least in PC_2 and PC_3. Results of ICA calculated on the same data are shown in Fig. 4B. Comparing Figs. 2B and 4B, the inability of PCA to separate the different sources is not obvious to the eye, but the effects of PCA vs. the effects of ICA are expected to be similar to those seen in the toy example. The PCs in Fig. 2 were produced with FastICA using the command line option which yields only PCs, or more precisely, components which are zero-mean and white, meaning that in addition to being uncorrelated they are of unit variance.

2.5 Common misconceptions in the biomedical ICA literature

The main misconception appearing in the biomedical ICA and PCA literature is that of ICA vs. PCA, especially regarding their capabilities to separate sources. As already noted, ICA yields independent components, whereas PCA yields merely uncorrelated components. Thus, PCA is incapable of separating the independent sources.

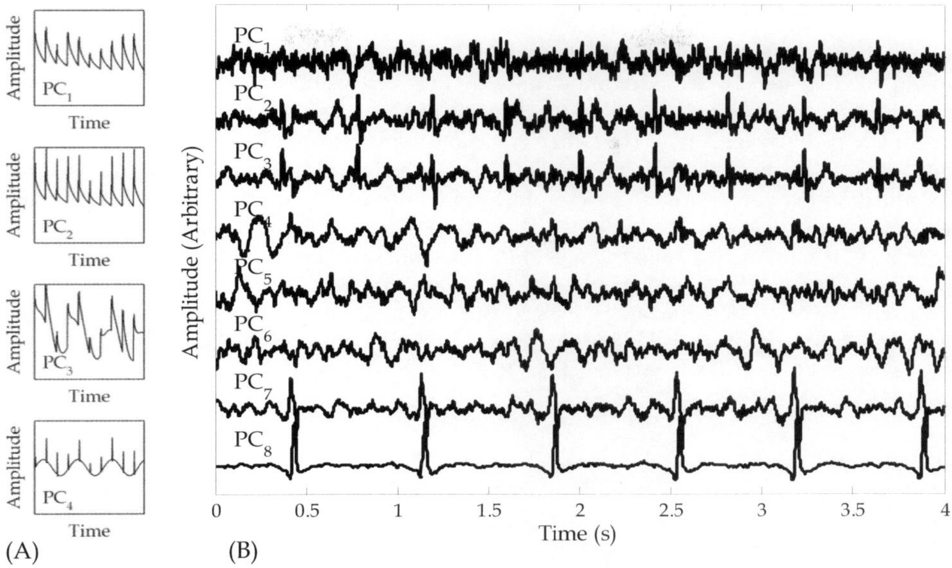

Fig. 2. (A) The results of PCA of all four simulated signals in the toy example seen in Fig. 1B. The corresponding ICA results are those of ICA(y_2,y_3,y_4) and ICA(y_1,y_2,y_3,y_4) seen in Fig. 1C. (B) The results of PCA of the eight-lead maternal ECG seen in Fig. 4A. The results of ICA calculated on the same data are shown in Fig. 4B. Units of amplitude are arbitrary in (A) and (B). The time span in (A) is the same as in all the subfigures in Fig. 1.

Reconstructing ECG lead signals from the ICs excluding also one or several ICs carrying ECG activity can be a hazardous practice. Whereas the resulting ECG signal reconstructions are cleaned of the noise and other artifacts carried in the excluded ICs, such reconstruction may yield ECG signals whose morphology may have been altered, or some waves may have disappeared altogether or appear with changed relative amplitudes.

An expected IC not appearing in the results of ICA is sometimes claimed to be due to the IC being minor in amplitude and buried in noise, and thus not separable. On the contrary, ICA is often very powerful in separating weak ICs whose contributions cannot be observed directly in the original measured ECG signals. Rather, the explanation is likely to be either one or several of the following: there may be an insufficient number of measured ECG leads, i.e., less measured ECG lead signals have been used as input to ICA than there are sources. As a consequence, the expected IC may be buried in a mixture of sources in the ICs. Noise or artifacts not independent of the expected IC, which thus are not separable by ICA. For example, respiration and blood pressure are known to modulate ECG (Sörnmo & Laguna, 2005), although it is unknown if these contributions were actually able to mask expected ICs. The expected IC may also have fallen victim of dimension reduction by PCA in signal preprocessing, if the information of the expected IC was contained in PCs whose eigenvalues were below the threshold for inclusion. Still, as discussed in Section 2.3, it is not impossible that the results of ICA have not been sufficiently reliable, and may thus be false. In this case, the precautions noted in the Section 2.3 are recommended.

3. ICA in ECG signal processing

Basically, many ICA based ECG processing techniques work similarly: After ICA, the unwanted ICs in (2) are identified and set to zero, and the measured signals are reconstructed using (2), thus yielding reconstructed signals clean from the artifacts contained in the zeroed ICs. The other common application is ECG beat classification, in which the ICA results are used as features based on which the beats are classified. Classification may be desired, for example, to indentify pathological beats and subsequently determine the pathology.

Whereas ICA is usually applied to a set of a few concurrently measured ECG signals, such as 12-lead ECG, ICA based methods for single-channel ECG signals have also been proposed, e.g., by de Chazal et al. (2003) and Mijović (2010). The other extreme is represented by ICA of high-density ECG measurements with tens (Zhu et al., 2008) or even hundreds of ECG lead signals used as ICA input to achieve enhanced level of source separation.

3.1 ECG artifacts

In this Section, the artifacts generally encountered in ECG signals (Sörnmo & Laguna, 2005) are shortly reviewed and discussed in the view of the ICA assumptions. In all cases in which ICA can be expected to work, a sufficient number of measured ECG leads must be provided for efficient artifact signal separation and removal.

In most environments, electrical devices and wiring can be found in the vicinity of the ECG measurement equipment and wiring, and 50/60 Hz power line frequency artifact can be easily introduced to the measured ECG signals. Power line frequency artifact is clearly independent from the ECG signals and often well-separable and removable by ICA.

EMG artifacts generated by muscles other than the heart muscle are generally independent of ECG signals. However, in principle, EMG represents a distributed source and cannot be immediately assumed to originate from a single or a small number of discrete sources comparative to the number of ECG leads. Nevertheless, separating EMG artifacts may well be attempted and can be successful in practice (c.f., the fist clenching example in Fig. 3). A usual application of ICA is also the removal of ECG artifacts from EMG or electroencephalogram (EEG) signals, as e.g., proposed in (Jung et al., 2000).

Baseline wander is a usual artifact seen in ECG signals. It is clearly an independent effect, which may be seen in only one or a few ECG lead signals. It may also appear totally different in different leads and can easily be generated by applying slowly changing pressure to an ECG electrode, among other reasons. In general, the effect is well separable and removable. ECG baseline wander removal by ICA has been proposed by Barati & Ayatollahi (2007), for example.

Limb movement, couching, and general restlessness among other similar activities represent a more complex class of artifacts, which may include EMG artifacts and other artifacts due to the movement of wires and stresses on ECG electrode contacts, and maybe other artifacts as well. Removal of such complex artifacts may be attempted but in general the success cannot be predicted a priori. Shoulder movement artifact removal was successfully performed in (Milanesi et al., 2008).

Holding hands together or grasping hospital bed metal side railings with both hands may effectively bring the two wrist electrodes to a nearly equal potential, thus making the signals of the standard ECG leads II and III almost equal, and lead III signal may nearly disappear.

Such an effect is not caused by an independent source of interference, and cannot be expected to be removable by ICA.

3.2 ICA for noise and artifact removal

As described earlier, the basic approach to noise and artifact removal is to perform ICA followed by ECG reconstruction using (2) with the noise and artifact carrying ICs set to zero. Here, a crucial step is the recognition of the ICs carrying the artifacts. This may be achieved, e.g., by different statistical or waveform classification methods in time domain or in frequency domain, or by more advanced methods as described, e.g., by He et al. (2006) who also give several illustrative examples. Note that in the examples in (He et al., 2006) the artifacts and noise to be removed are contained in ICs which seemingly do not carry ECG contributions, thus yielding correct ECG reconstruction which does not alter the actual ECG waveforms. In this Chapter, recognition of the ICs carrying atrial fibrillation is considered in the example shown in Fig. 6, whereas otherwise IC classification has been performed by visual observation only. ICA can also be successfully applied, for example, to ECG baseline wander (Barati & Ayatollahi, 2007) and motion artifact removal (Milanesi et al., 2008).

In Fig. 3A, a standard ECG is shown with an artifact caused by the subject clenching his left fist. The artifact is evident in all leads except in the lead II. The measurements were performed with NeuroScan (SynAmp by Compumedics NeuroScan, El Paso Texas, USA) with the reference on the left ankle. The standard chest ECG leads in Fig. 3A have been determined using Wilson's central terminal.

In Fig. 3B, ICs resulting from ICA calculated on the ECG signals seen in Fig. 3A, are shown. Since the lead III in Fig. 3A has been calculated from the leads I and II, there are only eight actual measurements in the nine ICA input signals. Accordingly, ICA found only eight ICs (Fig. 3B), as it could at maximum. In Fig. 3B, the left fist clenching artifact is nicely contained in IC_4, although here the artifact has been detected by visual assessment only, and it is hard to exclude the possibility of artifact contributions in the other ICs. At least IC_1, IC_2, IC_3, IC_5, IC_6, and IC_7, can be seen to carry ECG information. IC_7 might be taken to display contributions from T wave in addition to some other ECG contributions during QRS complex, but this is only speculative. IC_8 may be noise and carry also minor ECG information (noise is comparative to the possible ECG information). In Fig. 3C, the ECG reconstructed without IC_4 is shown. In visual inspection, the fist clenching artifact has been removed, and for the second heart beat shown, the T wave morphology in the lead I′ and the details of the QRS complex morphology in the lead II′, both of which are unobservable in Fig. 3A, have been recovered in Fig. 3C. A reconstructed lead is denoted with a prime in the lead name, also in the sequel.

3.3 ICA for ECG feature extraction

ECG feature extraction using ICA (Huang et al., 2010; Hyvärinen et al., 2001; Jiang et al., 2006) generally includes preprocessing the ECG signals by mean removal and dimension reduction. In dimension reduction, the original large data set is reduced to a smaller number of signals, also decreasing noise. The resulting data set is input to ICA, whose output is the set of features, or basis functions. Thereafter, ECG data to be classified, e.g., according to pathology, is then classified based on the basis functions. For example, Jiang et al. (2006) classified heart beats into 14 classes of arrhythmia types, including normal beats. Heart beat classification using ICA has also been considered in several other publications, e.g., in (Chou & Yu, 2007; Herrero et al., 2005; Ye et al., 2010).

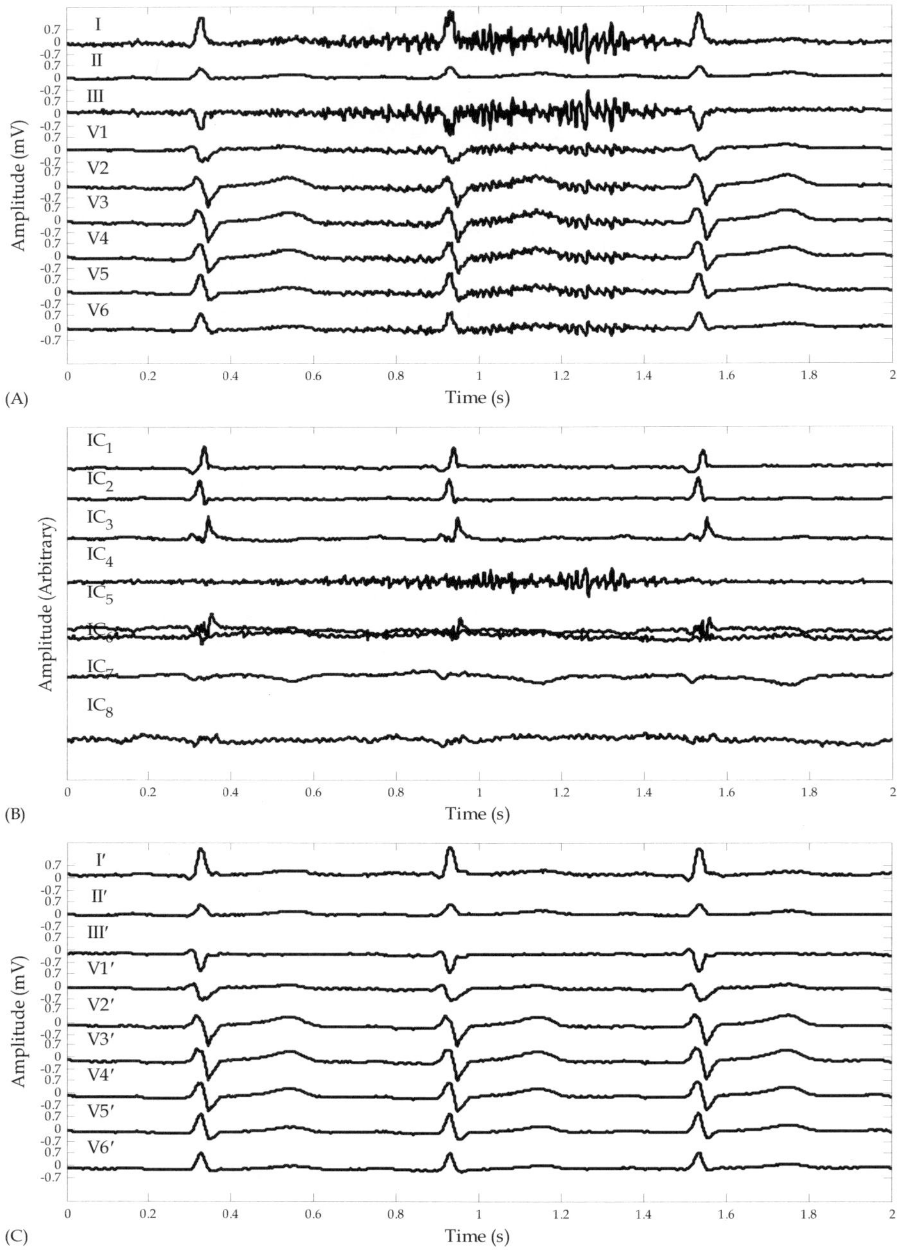

Fig. 3. (A) ECG with left fist clenching artifact visible in all leads but II. (B) Results of calculating ICA on the signals in (A). Fist clenching artifact has been separated into IC_4. (C) ECG signals reconstructed using all the ICs except IC_4.

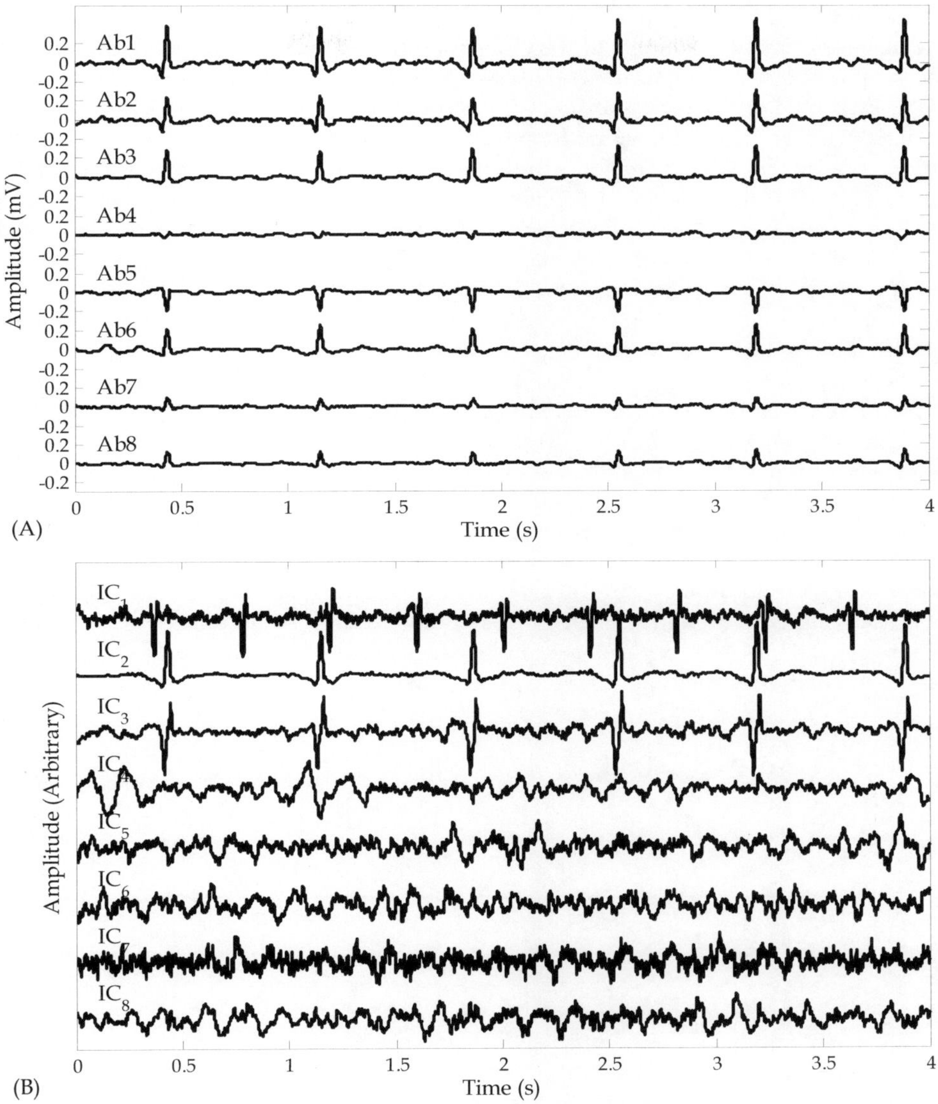

Fig. 4. (A) Eight-lead ECG measured on the abdominal region (leads Ab1 though Ab8) of a pregnant mother[1]. Maternal heart beats are clearly recognizable but fetal ECG cannot be visually observed. (B) Results of ICA on the data seen in (A). It can be clearly seen that IC_1 exhibits fetal ECG, whereas IC_2 and IC_3 carry maternal ECG.

---

[1]The data used in this example was obtained from The Open-Source Electrophysiological Toolbox, http://www.oset.ir/, Shiraz University, Shiraz, Iran, to where the data was provided by Dr. A. Tokarev, Biomedical Signal Processing Laboratory, National Aerospace University, Kharkov, Ukraine. The data was offered for download and usage under the GNU General Public License.

3.4 ICA for fetal ECG extraction

ECG signals originating from the hearts of the mother and the fetus are clearly independent of each other and they can be efficiently separated using ICA, thus providing for extraction of fetal ECG (Lee et al., 2005; Martín-Clemente et al., 2011; Sameni et al., 2006; Zarzoso & Nandi, 2001). The approach is to perform ICA on a set of ECG leads, which includes leads measured on the abdominal region of the mother and possibly also other leads, such as chest ECG leads. The abdominal lead signals are expected to carry both fetal and maternal ECGs. Upon successful ICA, recognizing the ICs containing fetal ECG is generally straight forward based on the different heart rates. Thereafter, fetal ECG can be reconstructed from the recognized ICs carrying fetal ECG information, if desired. A simple method to determine which ICs carry fetal or maternal ECG, is to perform beat detection, e.g., by highpass filtering followed by peak detection by thresholding, and subsequently calculating the heart rates for every IC carrying ECG information. If the ICA source separation is successful, ICs with two distinct heart rates can be recognized, with the ICs with the faster heart rate belonging to the fetal ECG. An eight-lead ECG measured from the abdominal region of a 25-year old mother in the 33rd week of pregnancy is shown in Fig. 4A. In Fig. 4B, are shown the ICs resulting from ICA on the signals shown in Fig. 4A. Fetal heart rate can be easily assessed from IC_1 in Fig. 4B, where as fetal ECG is not directly observable in the original measured ECG signals (Fig. 4A). In Fig. 5 are shown the fetal ECG signals reconstructed for all the abdominal leads using only IC_1 (Fig. 4B). Comparing Figs. 4A and 5, it is seen that even though no fetal ECG is visually observable in the original abdominal measurements (Fig. 4A), every abdominal lead carried fetal ECG information and even some fetal heart beat morphology can be observed from the reconstructions (Fig. 5).

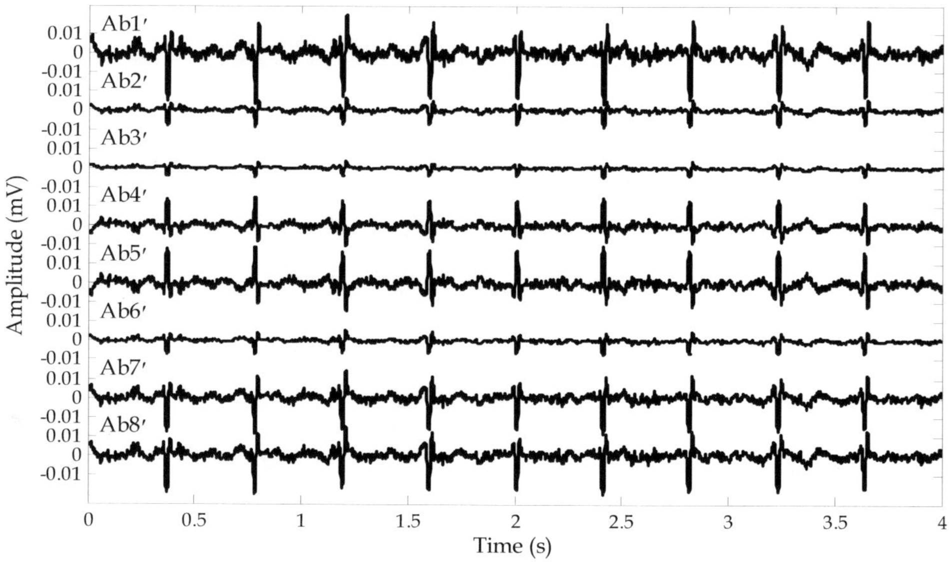

Fig. 5. Fetal ECG reconstructed for all the abdominal leads shown in Fig. 4A using only IC_1 seen in Fig. 4B.

Before ICA, baseline wander was removed from the measured signals by highpass filtering with an equiripple FIR filter of length 916, satisfying passband cutoff frequency of 5 Hz at -3 dB, stopband attenuation of at least -80 dB below 2 Hz, and passband ripple less than 1 dB. Note that this filter was not optimized to maximally remove baseline wander, but only to provide for the convergence of ICA. With original unfiltered measured signals FastICA did not converge. Note that ICA of maternal and fetal ECG does not always succeed. This may be due to either the general facts regarding ICA of biomedical signals discussed in Section 2.3, or due to too few ECG lead signals available. Considering that abdominal ECG leads also record the mother's abdominal EMG and the EMG of the fetus, the ECG lead count must be sufficiently high for the separation to succeed.

3.5 ICA of amplitude parameterized ECG

Diagnostics based on amplitude parameterized ECG is common practice. By ECG amplitude parameterization, we mean construction of a new set of signals from the signal amplitudes at some defined fiducial points of the ECG, such as R peak or ST60 amplitudes (amplitudes 60 ms after the start of the ST segments), or from time averages of delineated ECG segments. ICA of parameterized ECG has been proposed, e.g., by Chawla (2007) and Tanskanen et al. (2006a, 2006b). In this Section, we explicitly show that such ECG signal parameterizations in fact fulfill the assumption of linearly combined components. Related to parameterized ECG and more generally to the ECG wave delineation problem (Sörnmo & Laguna, 2005), an ICA based method for locating R peaks have been proposed by Chawla et al. (2008).

From (2) it can be seen that the mixing matrix **A** remains unchanged for a new set of ICA input signals formed by picking individual columns from **X** (samples measured at the same time instances from all the measured signals). This means that we may freely choose the ICA input samples in time as long as all the ECG leads are sampled at the same time.

One ECG sample (2) measured at time n via the lead l is given by

$$y(l,n) = \sum_{k=1}^{L} a(l,k)x(k,n), \tag{5}$$

where L is the number of ECG leads. Time average of M samples of the lth measured lead, starting from the sample number n_0, is given by

$$y_{av}(l,n_0) = \frac{1}{M}\sum_{n=n_0}^{M+n_0-1} y(l,n). \tag{6}$$

Inserting (5) into (6) we get

$$\begin{aligned} y_{av}(l,n_0) &= \frac{1}{M}\sum_{n=n_0}^{M+n_0-1}\sum_{k=1}^{L} a(l,k)x(k,n) = \sum_{k=1}^{L} a(l,k)\cdot\frac{1}{M}\sum_{n=n_0}^{M+n_0-1} x(k,n) \\ &= \sum_{k=1}^{L} a(l,k)x_{av}(k,n_0), \end{aligned} \tag{7}$$

which means that time averaging measured signals does not invalidate the assumption of the linearly combined ICs. From (7) we see that time averaged measured signals are linear combinations of correspondingly time averaged source signals, and that the separation matrix remains unaltered.

A word of warning is in place regarding time averaging. An assumption of ICA is that the ICs are nongaussian. According to the central limit theorem, a sum of nongaussian random signals is closer to gaussian than the original signals. Here, it means that time averaged ICs might be theoretically forbidden. Nevertheless, running ICA on averaged measurements may be attempted with due consideration given to the reliability of the results, as discussed earlier. Amplitude parameterization without averaging is naturally free of such concerns.

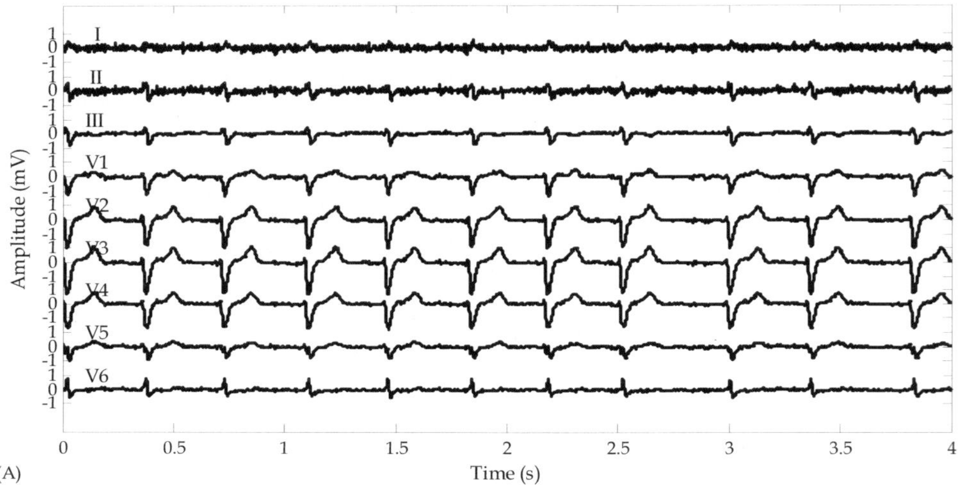

(A)

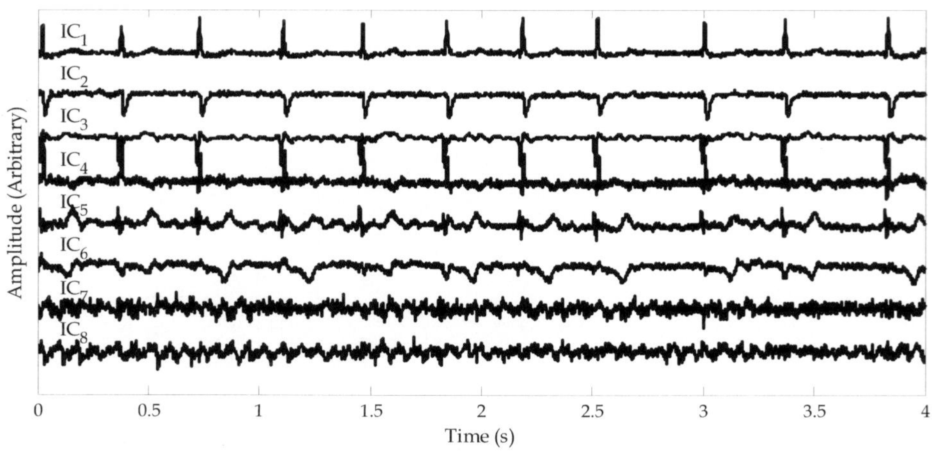

(B)

Fig. 6. (A) ECG measured from a patient with atrial fibrillation during exercise stress test. (B) Results of ICA on the signals in (A). Atrial fibrillation is detectable in IC_7 and IC_8.

4. ICA in ECG based diagnostics

ICA has found several applications in signal processing systems aimed at aiding in diagnostics. ECG based diagnostics applications in which ICA has been utilized include, e.g., classification of ECG beats (Chou & Yu, 2007; Huang, et al., 2010), analysis of parameterized ECG signals (Chawla, 2007; Tanskanen et al., 2006a, 2006b), heart rate variability analysis (Zhangyong et al., 2005), arrhythmia estimation (Castells et al., 2005; Jiang et al., 2006; Llinares & Igual, 2009), and atrial fibrillation extraction and analysis (Rieta et al., 2004; Stridh & Sörnmo, 2001; Zarzoso & Comon, 2010). A nice diagram of an atrial source separation system has been presented by Castells et al. (2005). Analyzing sub-signals in heart rate variability, Zhangyong et al. (2005) proposed to approach analysis of the effects of the autonomic nervous system. For a general description of the effects of blood pressures and respiration, see the book by Sörnmo & Laguna (2005). As mentioned, several proposed ECG analysis systems employ ICA as one system component, e.g., as in the heart beat classification system by Herrero et al. (2005), in which ICA based feature extraction is employed in combination with preprocessing, time-frequency feature extraction, and neural network based classifiers.

As mentioned earlier, 12-lead ECG may sometimes be insufficient for efficient ICA based analysis of the phenomenon of interest. For example, Zhu et al. (2008) analyzed 72-lead and 98-lead ECG measurements using ICA and were able to separate the P wave, QRS complex, and T wave. Thus, with high-density ECG measurements and ICA based analysis more detailed diagnostics applications might be realizable.

In Fig. 6A, ECG measured from a patient with atrial fibrillation during exercise stress test is shown. In Fig. 6B, the results of ICA on the signals in Fig. 6A are shown. In Fig. 6B, atrial fibrillation can be identified in IC_7 and IC_8. For both IC_7 and IC_8, power spectrum estimation using Welch method (Sörnmo & Laguna, 2008) reveals a clear peak around 6–7 Hz, which translates to the fibrillation rate of 360–420 beats per minute. Corresponding power spectral peaks are not found for the other ICs seen in Fig. 6B. Thus, in this case power spectral peak detection can also be used to recognize the ICs carrying atrial fibrillation information.

5. Conclusions

The numerous features making up the measured ECG signals originate largely from independent sources, whose contributions are linearly combined at the ECG electrodes. These sources are artifacts, such as muscle generated electric signals, and actual ECG generator signals originating from the operation of the heart itself. Also within the heart, a few independent signal generators can be identified. Due to the inherent independent component nature of the measured ECG signals, they lend themselves to be effectively processed with ICA, given the proper precautions outlined in this Chapter. Thus, ICA has been widely applied to enhance the ECG signals or their specific features to provide for enhanced diagnostic value. ICA has also been employed as a component in several proposed signal processing system aimed at diagnostics decision support. In this Chapter, several of these aspects were reviewed and practical illustrations were provided. To get the reader started on ICA of ECG signals, notes on popular available ICA program packages were made and the list of references was designed to widely cover the associated fields. We sincerely hope that this Chapter provides valuable practical insight into ICA and to the nature of the ECG signals with regard to processing them using ICA, and promotes novel ideas for enhancing ECG based diagnosis with the aid of this powerful statistical signal processing method.

6. Acknowledgment

The work of J. M. A. Tanskanen was funded by Academy of Finland (decision numbers 135220 and 122947). We thank Dr. Pasi Kauppinen, Dept. of Biomedical Engineering, Tampere University of Technology, Finland, for the help with the ECG artifact measurements using Neuroscan and for insightful comments.

7. Appendix

In this Appendix, Internet addresses of some ICA related web sites and program packages are given. There exist numerous ICA related sites and ICA software packages and scripts available in the Internet, and the list provided here is far from exhaustive. The list is intended to serve as a starting point for research using ICA. Although some of the listed web sites and ICA program packages are concerned with EEG processing, they are nevertheless excellent sources of ICA related information and programs.

ICA Central

Signal and Image Processing Department, Télécom ParisTech, France
http://www.tsi.enst.fr/icacentral/

Independent Component Analysis (ICA) and Blind Source Separation (BSS)

Including:

- FastICA
- Icasso (software for investigating the reliability of ICA estimates by clustering and visualization)

Department of Information and Computer Science, Aalto University, Finland
http://research.ics.tkk.fi/ica/

ICA - CNL Overview

The Computational Neurobiology Laboratory, Salk Institute for Biological Studies, CA, USA
http://cnl.salk.edu/~tewon/ica_cnl.html

RobustICA

Laboratoire d'Informatique, University of Nice - Sophia Antipolis, France
http://www.i3s.unice.fr/~zarzoso/robustica.html

EEGLAB

Swartz Center for Computational Neuroscience, University of California San Diego, CA, USA
http://sccn.ucsd.edu/eeglab/

ICALAB Toolboxes

Laboratory for Advanced Brain Signal Processing, RIKEN Brain Science Institute, Japan
http://www.bsp.brain.riken.jp/ICALAB/

Mutual Information Least-dependent Component Analysis

UCL Institute of Neurology, UK
http://www.klab.caltech.edu/~kraskov/MILCA/

8. References

Aalto University, Department of Information and Computer Science. (2005). *The FastICA package for Matlab*, May 5, 2011, Available from http://research.ics.tkk.fi/ica/fastica/

Barati, Z. & Ayatollahi, A. (2007). Baseline wandering removal by using independent component analysis to single-channel ECG data, *Proceedings of International Conference on Biomedical and Pharmaceutical Engineering*, pp. 152–156, ISBN 978-981-05-79, Singapore, December 11-14, 2006, Available from http://ieeexplore.ieee.org/stamp/stamp.jsp?tp=&arnumber=4155882

Castells, F., Cebrián, A. & Millet, J. (2007a). The role of independent component analysis in the signal processing of ECG recordings. *Biomedizinische Technik/Biomedical Engineering*, Vol. 52, No. 1, (February 2007), pp. 18–24, ISSN 0013-5585, Available from http://dx.doi.org/10.1515/BMT.2007.005

Castells, F., Laguna, P., Sörnmo, L., Bollmann, A. & Roig, J. M. (2007b). Principal component analysis in ECG signal processing. *EURASIP Journal on Advances in Signal Processing*, Vol. 2007, 21 pgs., ISSN 1110-8657, Available from http://dx.doi.org/10.1155/2007/74580

Castells, F., Rieta, J. J., Millet, J. & Zarzoso, V. (2005). Spatiotemporal blind source separation approach to atrial activity estimation in atrial tachyarrhythmias. *IEEE Transactions on Biomedical Engineering*, Vol. 52, No. 2, (February 2005), pp. 258–267, ISSN 0018-9294, Available from http://dx.doi.org/10.1109/TBME.2004.840473

Chawla, M. P. S. (2007). Parameterization and R-peak error estimations of ECG signals using independent component analysis. *Computational and Mathematical Methods in Medicine*, Vol. 8, No. 4, (December 2007), pp. 263–285, ISSN 1748-6718, Available from http://dx.doi.org/10.1080/17486700701776348

Chawla, M. P. S., Verma, H. K. & Kumar, V. (2008). A new statistical PCA–ICA algorithm for location of R-peaks in ECG. *International Journal of Cardiology*, Vol. 129, No. 1, (September 2008), pp. 146–148, ISSN 0167-5273, Available from http://dx.doi.org/10.1016/j.ijcard.2007.06.036

Chou, K.-T. & Yu, S.-N. (2007). Classifying ECG beats using ICA features and probabilistic neural network, *IFMBE Proceedings, World Congress on Medical Physics and Biomedical Engineering*, pp. 1013–1016, ISSN 1680-0737, ISBN 978-3-540-36839-7, Vol. 14, Part 8, Seoul, Korea, August 27-September 1, 2006, Available from http://dx.doi.org/10.1007/978-3-540-36841-0_241

Comon, P. (1994). Independent component analysis, a new concept? *Signal Processing*, Vol. 36, No. 3, (April 1994), pp. 287–314, ISSN 0165-1684, Available from http://dx.doi.org/10.1016/0165-1684%2894%2990029-9

de Chazal, P., Heneghan, C., Sheridan, E., Reilly, R., Nolan, P. & O'Malley, M. (2003). Automated processing of the single-lead electrocardiogram for the detection of obstructive sleep apnoea. *IEEE Transactions on Biomedical Engineering*, Vol. 50, No. 6, (June 2003), pp. 686–696, ISSN 0018-9294, Available from http://dx.doi.org/10.1109/TBME.2003.812203

Giannakopoulos, X., Karhunen, J. & Oja, E. (1999). An experimental comparison of neural algorithms for independent component analysis and blind separation. *International Journal of Neural Systems*, Vol. 9, No. 2, (April 1999), pp. 99–114, ISSN 0129-0657, Available from http://dx.doi.org/10.1142/S0129065799000101

He, T., Clifford G. & Tarassenko, L. (2006). Application of independent component analysis in removing artefacts from the electrocardiogram. *Neural Computing & Applications*, Vol. 15, No. 2, (April 2006), pp. 105–116, ISSN 0941-0643, Available from http://dx.doi.org/10.1007/s00521-005-0013-y

Herrero, G. G., Gotchev, A., Christov, I. & Egiazarian, K. (2005). Feature extraction for heartbeat classification using independent component analysis and matching pursuits, *Proceedings of 2005 IEEE International Conference on Acoustics, Speech, and Signal Processing*, March 18-23, 2005, ISSN 1520-6149, ISBN 0-7803-8874-7, pp. iv/725–iv/728, Philadelphia, PA, USA, Available from http://dx.doi.org/10.1109/ICASSP.2005.1416111

Hild, K. E., Alleva, G., Nagarajan, S. & Comani, S. (2007). Performance comparison of six independent components analysis algorithms for fetal signal extraction from real fMCG data. *Physics in Medicine and Biology*, Vol. 52, No. 2, (January 2007), pp. 449–462, ISSN 0031-9155, Available from http://dx.doi.org/10.1088/0031-9155/52/2/010

Himberg, J., Hyvärinen, A. & Esposito, F. (2004). Validating the independent components of neuroimaging time series via clustering and visualization. *NeuroImage*, Vol. 22, No. 3, (July 2004), pp. 1214–1222, ISSN 1053-8119, Available from http://dx.doi.org/10.1016/j.neuroimage.2004.03.027

Huang, H. F., Hu, G. S. & Zhu, L. (2010). Sparse representation-based heartbeat classification using independent component analysis. *Journal of Medical Systems*, (September 2010), 13 pgs., ISSN 0148-5598, Available from http://dx.doi.org/10.1007/s10916-010-9585-x

Hyvärinen, A. & Oja, E. (2000). Independent component analysis: algorithms and applications. *Neural Networks*, Vol. 13, No. 4-5, (June 2000), pp. 411–430, ISSN 0893-6080, Available from http://dx.doi.org/10.1016/S0893-6080%2800%2900026-5

Hyvärinen, A. (1999). Fast and robust fixed-point algorithms for independent component analysis. *IEEE Transactions on Neural Networks*, Vol. 10, No. 3, (May 1999), pp. 626–634, ISSN 1045-9227, Available from http://dx.doi.org/10.1109/72.761722

Hyvärinen, A., Karhunen, J. & Oja, E. (2001). *Independent Component Analysis*, John Wiley & Sons, ISBN 978-0-471-40540-5, New York, NY, USA, Available from http://dx.doi.org/10.1002/0471221317

Jiang, X., Zhang, L., Zhao, Q. & Albayrak, S. (2006). ECG arrhythmias recognition system based on independent component analysis feature extraction, *Proceedings of IEEE Region 10 Conference*, 4 pgs., ISBN 1-4244-0548-3, Hong Kong, November 14-17, 2006, Available from http://dx.doi.org/10.1109/TENCON.2006.343781

Jolliffe, I. T. (2002). *Principal Component Analysis*, Springer, ISBN 0-387-95442-2, New York, NY, USA, Available from http://dx.doi.org/10.1007/b98835

Jung, T.-P., Makeig, S., Humphries, C., Lee, T.-W., McKeown, M. J., Iragui, V. & Sejnowski, T. J. (2000). Removing electroencephalographic artifacts by blind source separation. *Psychophysiology*, Vol. 37, No. 2, (March 2000), pp. 163–178, ISSN 1469-8986, Available from http://dx.doi.org/10.1111/1469-8986.3720163

Lee, J., Park, K. L. & Lee, K. J. (2005). Temporally constrained ICA-based foetal ECG separation. *Electronics Letters*, Vol. 41, No. 21, (October 2005), pp. 1158–1160, ISSN 0013-5194, Available from http://dx.doi.org/10.1049/el:20052235

Llinares, R. & Igual, J. (2009). Application of constrained independent component analysis algorithms in electrocardiogram arrhythmias. *Artificial Intelligence in Medicine*, Vol. 47, No. 2, (October 2009), pp. 121–133, ISSN 0933-3657, Available from http://dx.doi.org/10.1016/j.artmed.2009.05.006

Martín-Clemente, R., Camargo-Olivares, J. L., Hornillo-Mellado, S., Elena, M. & Román, I. (2011). Fast technique for noninvasive fetal ECG extraction. *IEEE Transactions on Biomedical Engineering*, Vol. 58, No. 2, (February 2011), pp. 227–230, ISSN 0018-9294, Available from http://dx.doi.org/10.1109/TBME.2010.2059703

Meinecke, F., Ziehe, A., Kawanabe, M. & Müller, K.-R. (2002). A resampling approach to estimate the stability of one-dimensional or multidimensional independent components. *IEEE Transactions on Biomedical Engineering*, Vol. 49, No. 12, (December 2002), pp. 1514–1525, ISSN 0018-9294, Available from http://dx.doi.org/10.1109/TBME.2002.805480

Mijović, B., De Vos, M., Gligorijević, I., Taelman, J. & Van Huffel, S. (2010). Source separation from single-channel recordings by combining empirical-mode decomposition and independent component analysis. *IEEE Transactions on Biomedical Engineering*, Vol. 57, No. 9, (September 2010), pp. 2188–2196, ISSN 0018-9294, Available from http://dx.doi.org/10.1109/TBME.2010.2051440

Milanesi, M., Martini, N., Vanello, N., Positano, V., Santarelli, M. F. & Landini, L. (2008). Independent component analysis applied to the removal of motion artifacts from electrocardiographic signals. *Medical and Biological Engineering and Computing*, Vol. 46, No. 3, (March 2008), pp. 251–261, ISSN 0140-0118, Available from http://dx.doi.org/10.1007/s11517-007-0293-8

Naik, G. R. & Kumar, D. K. (2011). An overview of independent component analysis and its applications. *Informatica*, Vol. 35, No. 1, (March 2011), pp. 63–81, ISSN 0350-5596, Available from http://www.informatica.si/PDF/35-1/10_Naik%20-%20An%20Overview%20of%20Independent%20Component%20Analysis%20and%20Its%20Applications.pdf

Parmar Sargam, D. & Sahambi, J. S. (2004). A comparative survey on removal of MECG artifacts from FECG using ICA algorithms, *Proceedings of International Conference on Intelligent Sensing and Information Processing*, pp. 88–91, ISBN 0-7803-8243-9, Chennai, India, January 4-7, 2004, Available from http://dx.doi.org/10.1109/ICISIP.2004.1287630

Pham, D. T. & Garat, P. (1997). Blind separation of mixture of independent sources through a quasi-maximum likelihood approach. *IEEE Transactions on Signal Processing*, Vol. 45, No. 7, (July 1997), pp. 1712–1725, ISSN 1053-587X, Available from http://dx.doi.org/10.1109/78.599941

Rieta, J. J., Castells, F., Sánchez, C., Zarzoso, V. & Millet, J. (2004). Atrial activity extraction for atrial fibrillation analysis using blind source separation. *IEEE Transactions on Biomedical Engineering*, Vol. 51, No. 7, (July 2004), pp. 1176–1186, ISSN 0018-9294, Available from http://dx.doi.org/10.1109/TBME.2004.827272

Sameni, R., Jutten, C. & Shamsollahi, M. B. (2006). What ICA provides for ECG processing: application to noninvasive fetal ECG extraction, *Proceedings of 2006 IEEE International Symposium on Signal Processing and Information Technology*, pp. 656–661, ISBN 0-7803-9753-3, Vancouver, BC, Canada, August 27-30, 2006, Available from http://dx.doi.org/10.1109/ISSPIT.2006.270882

Shkurovich, S., Sahakian, A. V. & Swiryn, S. (1998). Detection of atrial activity from high-voltage leads of implantable ventricular defibrillators using a cancellation technique. *IEEE Transactions on Biomedical Engineering*, Vol. 45, No. 2, (February 1998), pp. 229–234, ISSN 0018-9294, Available from http://dx.doi.org/10.1109/10.661270

Stamkopoulos, T., Diamantaras, K., Maglaveras, N. & Strintzis, M. (1998). ECG analysis using nonlinear PCA neural networks for ischemia detection. *IEEE Transactions on Signal Processing*, Vol. 46, No. 11, (November 1998), pp. 3058–3067, ISSN 1053-587X, Available from http://dx.doi.org/10.1109/78.726818

Stridh, M. & Sörnmo, L. (2001). Spatiotemporal QRST cancellation techniques for analysis of atrial fibrillation. *IEEE Transactions on Biomedical Engineering*, Vol. 48, No. 1, pp. 105–111, (January 2001), ISSN 0018-9294, Available from http://dx.doi.org/10.1109/10.900266

Sörnmo, L. & Laguna, P. (2005). *Bioelectrical Signal Processing in Cardiac and Neurological Applications*, Elsevier Academic Press, ISBN 0-12-437552-9, London, UK, Available from http://www.sciencedirect.com/science/book/9780124375529

Tanskanen, J. M. A., Mikkonen, J. E. & Penttonen, M. (2005). Independent component analysis of neural populations from multielectrode field potential measurements. *Journal of Neuroscience Methods*, Vol. 145, No. 1-2, (June 2005), pp. 213–232, ISSN 0165-0270, Available from http://dx.doi.org/10.1016/j.jneumeth.2005.01.004

Tanskanen, J. M. A., Viik, J. J. & Hyttinen, J. A. K. (2006a). Independent component analysis of parameterized ECG signals, *Proceedings of 28th Annual International Conference of the IEEE Engineering in Medicine and Biology Society*, pp. 5704–5707, ISBN 1-4244-0032-5, ISSN 1557-170X, New York City, NY, USA, August 30–September 3, 2006, Available from http://dx.doi.org/10.1109/IEMBS.2006.260345

Tanskanen, J. M. A., Viik, J. J. & Hyttinen, J. A. K. (2006b). Independent component analysis of parameterized electrocardiogram signals, *Proceedings of 7th Nordic Signal Processing Symposium*, pp. 230–233, ISBN 1-4244-0412-6, Reykjavik, Iceland, June 7-9, 2006, Available from http://dx.doi.org/10.1109/NORSIG.2006.275230

Vayá, C., Rieta, J. J., Sánchez, C. & Moratal, D. (2007). Convolutive blind source separation algorithms applied to the electrocardiogram of atrial fibrillation: study of performance. *IEEE Transactions on Biomedical Engineering*, Vol. 54, No. 8, (August 2007), pp. 1530–1533, ISSN 0018-9294, Available from http://dx.doi.org/10.1109/TBME.2006.889778

Ye, C., Coimbra, M. T. & Vijaya Kumar, B. V. K. (2010). Arrhythmia detection and classification using morphological and dynamic features of ECG signals, *Proceedings of 2010 Annual International Conference of the IEEE Engineering in Medicine and Biology Society*, pp. 1918–1921, ISSN 1557-170X, ISBN 978-1-4244-4123-5, Buenos Aires, Argentina, August 31-September 4, 2010, Available from http://dx.doi.org/10.1109/IEMBS.2010.5627645

Zarzoso, V. & Comon, P. (2010). Robust independent component analysis by iterative maximization of the kurtosis contrast with algebraic optimal step size. *IEEE Transactions on Neural Networks*, Vol. 21, No. 2, (February 2010), pp. 248–261, ISSN 1045-9227, Available from http://dx.doi.org/10.1109/TNN.2009.2035920

Zarzoso, V. & Nandi, A. K. (2001). Noninvasive fetal electrocardiogram extraction: blind separation versus adaptive noise cancellation. *IEEE Transactions on Biomedical Engineering*, Vol. 48, No. 1, (January 2001), pp. 12–18, ISSN 0018-9294, Available from http://dx.doi.org/10.1109/10.900244

Zhangyong, L., Biao, L. & Zhengxiang, X. (2005). Extracting and analyzing sub-signals in heart rate variability. *Colloids and Surfaces B: Biointerfaces*, Vol. 42, No. 2, (May 2005), pp. 131–135, ISSN 0927-7765, Available from http://dx.doi.org/10.1016/j.colsurfb.2005.01.014

Zhu, Y., Shayan, A., Zhang, W., Chen, T. L., Jung, T.-P., Duann, J.-R., Makeig, S. & Cheng, C.-K. (2008). Analyzing high-density ECG signals using ICA. *IEEE Transactions on*

Biomedical Engineering, Vol. 55, No. 11, (November 2008), pp. 2528–2537, ISSN 0018-9294, Available from
http://dx.doi.org/10.1109/TBME.2008.2001262

18

Customized Heart Check System by Using Integrated Information of Electrocardiogram and Plethysmogram Outside the Driver's Awareness from an Automobile Steering Wheel

Motohisa Osaka
Nippon Veterinary and Life Science University, Japan

1. Introduction

1.1 Sudden cardiac death of drivers

The annual number of sudden cardiac deaths is increasing in Japan, and is estimated to be more than 50,000 on the basis of findings from the multicenter research group (Toyoshima et al., 1996). In the United States, sudden cardiac death is the greatest cause of natural death, causing more than 400,000 adult fatalities each year (Zipes & Wellens, 1998) and it is the most common lethal manifestation of heart disease (Bauer et al., 2006). The high incidence makes sudden cardiac death a major challenge in public health. In most cases, the mechanism is abrupt occurrence of ventricular tachyarrhythmia, rapidly progressing to ventricular fibrillation and causing cardiac pump failure with unconsciousness. It is supposed that sudden cardiac death sometimes occurs while the subject is driving an automobile. A Japanese newspaper (March 29, 2010) reported, "While a bus driver (65 years old) was driving a bus, he suffered severe chest pain and gave up steering so that the bus ran in a zigzag and crashed into a wall to be on fire. " Although such cases can easily be found on web sites, there has been little reported study. Lam and Lam reported that among older drivers aged 60 or above in New South Wales, Australia from 1996 to 2000, 409 (1.1%) of 36,595 were recognized as having suffered a sudden illness immediately prior to a crash, and that 254 (0.7%) of those episodes resulted in the driver's death and injury in the crash (Lam & Lam, 2005). According to "Suicide and Natural Deaths in Road Traffic – Review" from Accident Research Centre of Monash University, the percentages of natural driver deaths out of all vehicle deaths were reported to vary from 0.2% to 19% in 10 studies (Routely et al., 2003). The Review listed 19 studies in total in the Appendix. It was reported that the percentages of cardiovascular disease in drivers who met natural deaths were from 68% to 97%. We speculated, on examination of a summary of those studies, that the total number of natural driver deaths and the number of natural driver deaths due to cardiac events were, respectively, 5 -10% and about 5% as percentages of all vehicle deaths. There may also be cases in which a patient receives a warning from his own heart of imminent sudden cardiac death, and is able to survive, or at least to prevent injury to others.

1.2 Is there any precursor of sudden cardiac death?

Is it possible to predict sudden cardiac death a few hours in advance of its occurrence? The mechanism is abrupt occurrence of ventricular tachyarrhythmia or complete atrioventricular block. It was noted on analyses of ambulatory 24-hour electrocardiogram recordings (Holter recordings) that some measures of heart rate variability may change about 1 hour before the onset of sustained or nonsustained ventricular tachycardia (Huikuri et al., 1993). No reliable precursor of sudden cardiac death, however, had yet been discovered.

Muller et al. reported that there were two peaks of the frequency of circadian variation of sudden cardiac death at 11 am and 6 pm (Muller et al., 1987). Particularly, the highest peak was about 3 hours after awakening. These results suggested that there might be the relationship between the occurrence of sudden cardiac death and the intrinsic circadian rhythm of autonomic nervous system and/or endocrine system. We analyzed ambulatory 24-hour electrocardiogram (ECG) recordings of 24 patients who were hospitalized due to leg fracture. We calculated the low-frequency component (LF: 0.04-0.15Hz), the high-frequency component (HF: 0.15-0.4Hz) of RR intervals (ms), and the ratio LF/HF, which are recognized as measures of combined sympathetic and parasympathetic activity,

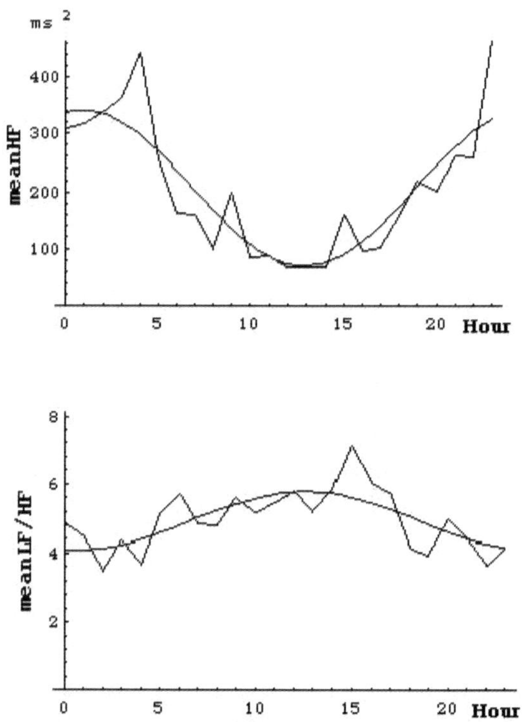

Fig. 1. Circadian variation of autonomic activity. LF (unit, ms^2), the low-frequency component of RR intervals (ms); HF (unit, ms^2), the high frequency component; LF/HF (no unit), the ratio of LF to HF.

parasympathetic activity, and sympathetic activity, respectively (Berger et al., 1989; Osaka et al., 1993; Task Force of the European Society of Cardiology and the North American Society of Pacing and Electrophysiology, 1996). Since those patients were lying still on bed during the recordings, the variations of HF and LF/HF represents intrinsic circadian rhythm of parasympathetic and sympathetic activity, respectively. Figure 1 shows that the peak of LF/HF and the nadir of HF are around noon, and that the increase of LF/HF and the decrease of HF begin around awakening. Thus, these findings suggest that the predominance of sympathetic activity over parasympathetic activity may trigger the cardiac event about 3 hours after awakening.

Experimentally, Schwartz et al. demonstrated that autonomic stress could trigger lethal ventricular arrhythmias in dogs with myocardial infarction (Schwartz et al., 1988). Their observation was made in an animal model for sudden cardiac death. According to their article, dogs with healed anterior myocardial infarctions perform an exercise stress test, toward the end of which a 2-minute myocardial ischemia is created by occluding the left circumflex coronary artery. This clinically relevant combination of transient myocardial ischemia at the time of physiologically elevated sympathetic activity results in ventricular fibrillation in almost 60 per cent of the animals. The outcome during the exercise and ischemia test identifies and defines two groups of animals according to the occurrence of ventricular fibrillation or survival –"susceptible" and "resistant", respectively. Although the former group tends to show a further increase in the already elevated heart rate, the latter group tends to show a decrease. This heart rate reduction is prevented by atropine and clearly reveals the presence of powerful vagal reflexes. Such a behavior of heart rate could be taken to suggest the presence of a relative sympathetic dominance among susceptible animals and of a relative parasympasthetic dominance among resistant animals.

Clinically, analysis of Holter recordings was the basis for our previous report that heart rate and LF/HF increase steadily with the decrease of HF from 45 minutes before the onset of nonsustained ventricular tachycardia until the actual onset (Osaka et al., 1996). This suggested that increased sympathetic activity and decreased parasympathetic activity may trigger nonsustained ventricular tachycardia, and also indicated that trends in autonomic activity may be useful for detecting any precursor of a cardiac event that is triggered or worsened by autonomic imbalance.

It has been known for some time that the power spectra of heart rate from healthy individuals exhibit a *1/f*-like pattern ($Power = C f^{b}$, where $b \approx -1$ and C is a proportionality constant) in the low-frequency range ($f < 0.1$Hz) (Kobayashi & Musha, 1982; Peng et al., 1993). This is reflected in the fractal nature of HR. Loss of multifractality is closely correlated with prognosis and severity of heart disease (Ivanov et al., 1999). Hence, we presumed that the low-frequency component would be strongly correlated with prognosis. Experimentally, we showed that sympathetic activity strongly correlates with heart rate and blood pressure at both 0.05Hz and 0.80Hz in conscious rats and that this correlation is baroreflex-independent (Sakata et al., 2002). This was consistent with the finding that that the low-frequency component (<0.1Hz) of the transfer function between blood pressure and heart rate is baroreflex-independent in normotensive humans (Taylor & Eckberg, 1996). Hence, we presumed that the low-frequency component of sympathetic activity may play a key role in triggering lethal tachyarrhythmias, and that characteristic changes in sympathetic activity might occur before a cardiac event.

1.3 V-shaped trough in autonomic activity as a possible precursor

We aimed at finding a consistent precursor of a lethal cardiac event by examining Holter recordings in which such a spontaneous event was recorded. Holter recordings of 34 patients experiencing a cardiac event (Event-group, 20 deaths) were compared with 191 controls (NoEvent-group) (Osaka et al., 2010). The Event-group included 25 patients with ventricular fibrillation or acute myocardial infarction, and 9 with cardiac arrest due to complete atrioventricular block. We calculated logarithms of the moving average of 5 successive values for the low-frequency component (LF), the high-frequency component (HF), and the ratio LF/HF of heart rate variability: ln(LF), ln(HF) and ln(LF/HF). A V-shaped trough appeared in the curve of ln(LF/HF) [sV-trough] or ln(HF) [pV-trough] before such an event in 31 patients of the Event-group. The V-trough was marked by a small variation lasting 2 hours, an abrupt descent lasting 30 minutes, and a sharp ascent for 40 minutes. Figure 2a-e shows a representative case in the Event-group. The patient (male, 72 years old) suffered from acute myocardial infarction and died of ventricular fibrillation during the recording. Figure 2a shows progression from regular sinus rhythm to ventricular fibrillation with sporadic short runs of ventricular tachycardia. In Figure 2b sustained ST elevation appears at 21:50, indicating the occurrence of acute myocardial infarction. It is noted that thereafter slow oscillations of HR seem to disappear with their variability depressed (Figure 2c). The variation of ln(LF/HF) decreases from 20:00 to 22:00, and lies approximately within the mean±SD which was calculated as described below (Figure 2d). This decrease appears before ST elevation. Next, ln(LF/HF) falls steeply and then rises sharply. Figure 2d shows a V-shaped trough in sympathetic activity, which is referred to subsequently in the manuscript simply as "V-trough." Although such a sharp rise of ln(LF/HF) and a simultaneous decrease of ln(HF) (Figure 2e) would normally be expected to accompany an increase of HR, there is instead a decrease in heart rate which is accompanied by a reduction in variability (Figure 2c). Slow ventricular tachycardia appeared at 0:30 and ceased at 0:50, then ventricular fibrillation appeared at 1:27 terminating in cardiac standstill at 1:55 (data not shown).

Figure 3a-d shows another representative case in the Event-group. The patient (male, 74 years old) suffered from complete atrioventricular block and died during the recording. ST elevation appeared at 10:56, indicating the occurrence of acute myocardial infarction. Figure 3a shows that complete atrioventricular block, which was induced by acute myocardial infarction, causes a compensatory atrioventricular rhythm at 11:00 and finally, cardiac arrest at 11:10. Heart rate decreases during sleep from 23:00 to 6:00 (Figure 3b). The variation of ln(HF) decreases from 2:00 to 4:00, which is approximately within the mean±SD (Figure 3c). Then ln(HF) declines quickly, but suddenly reverses direction and shows a striking increase, although it might normally be expected to fall after rising so abruptly. These changes are characteristic of a V-trough in parasympathetic activity. In spite of the predominance of changes in ln(HF) as compared with ln(LF/HF), heart rate increases abruptly at 7:20, and fails to react normally to the predominance of parasympathetic activity vs. sympathetic activity.

From the finding that a V-shaped trough was observed preceding the event in almost all patients of the Event-group, we defined the criteria for a V-trough in sympathetic activity (sV-trough) as indicated in Figure 4. To characterize the time series of ln(LF/HF), we calculated the mean±SD of consecutive values of ln(LF/HF), which corresponded to a

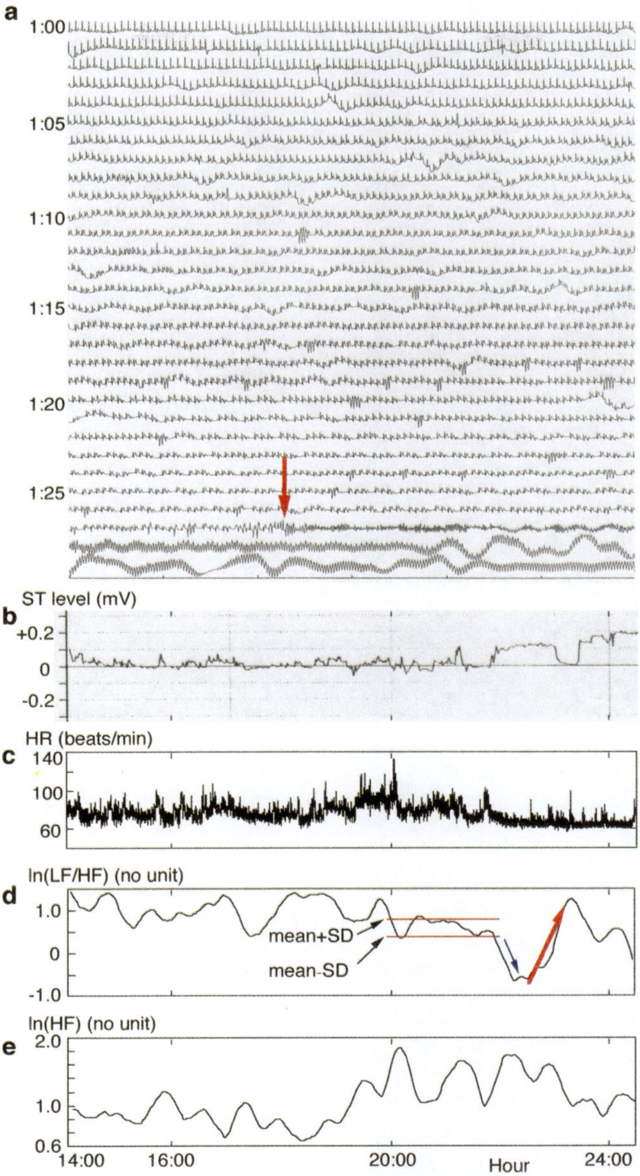

a. Holter recording before the occurrence of ventricular fibrillation (starting from the red arrow). b. ST level up to the time of onset of slow ventricular tachycardia (0:30). c. Tachogram of heart rate (HR). d. Tachogram of the logarithm of the ratio of the low-frequency component to the high-frequency component, ln(LF/HF). The two red horizontal lines represent mean±SD for 120 minutes. e. Tachogram of the logarithm of the high-frequency component, ln(HF). From (Osaka et al., 2010).

Fig. 2. V-trough of sympathetic activity in a representative case from the Event-group.

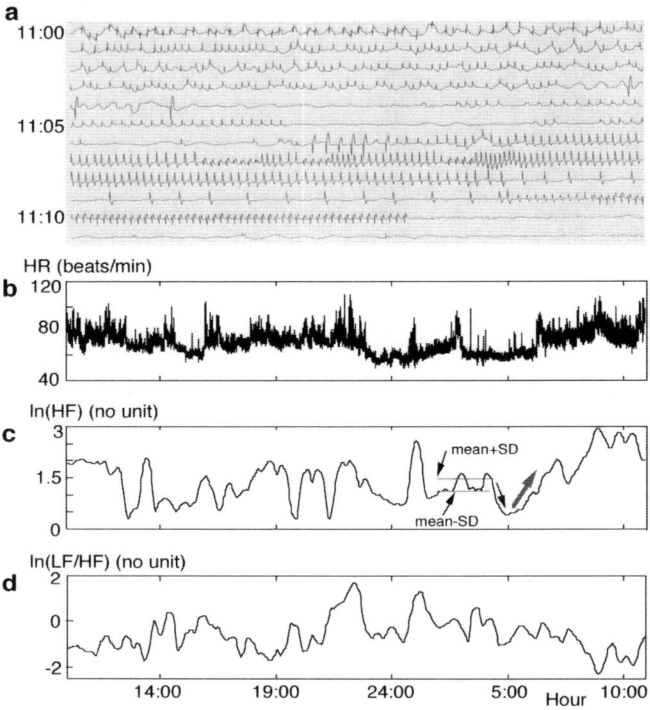

a. Holter recording displaying a compensatory atrioventricular rhythm which is induced by complete atrioventricular block at 11:00, followed by cardiac arrest. b. Tachogram of heart rate (HR). c. Tachogram of ln(HF). d. Tachogram of ln(LF/HF). From (Osaka et al., 2010).

Fig. 3. V-trough of parasympathetic activity in a representative case from the Event-group.

baseline period of 120 min. The criteria included four necessary conditions, the first that ln(LF/HF) fluctuate approximately within a narrow range between mean±SD for 120 minutes, and the second that ln(LF/HF) must increase sharply for a period of 40 minutes (ascent period) after an abrupt descent lasting 30 minutes (descent period). These necessary conditions were as follows:

R is defined as (mean + SD) of ln(LF/HF) in each of the consecutive baseline periods (Figure 4). Slope 1 is defined as a slope of 3SD of ln(LF/HF) per the baseline period of BL minutes (BL = 120). Slope 2 is defined as a slope of a straight line fitted into values of ln(LF/HF) during the ascent period.

T is defined as total time, in which mean – SD ≤ ln(LF/HF) ≤ mean + SD.

Figure 4 shows such an example that $T = T_1 + T_2 + T_3$.

Necessary condition 1: If R ≥ 1.5, T ≥ BL×(3/4) min, and if not, T ≥ BL×(2/3) min.

Necessary condition 2: Slope 2 > Slope 1.

Necessary condition 3: The lower end of Slope 2 < mean – 3SD.

Necessary condition 4: HR decreases, while ln(LF/HF) increases sharply for a period of 40 minutes.

It may be noted that larger values of mean and SD for ln(LF/HF) are associated with stricter conditions (Figure 4). V-troughs of ln(HF) were used in place of ln(LF/HF) as an index of parasympathetic activity (pV-trough). The necessary condition 4 was also replaced with that HR increases, while ln(HF) increases sharply for a period of 40 minutes. We examined all the recordings automatically using this algorithm. An sV-trough was observed in 22 patients before the onset of ventricular fibrillation or acute myocardial infarction. A pV-trough was observed in all 9 patients before the onset of complete atrioventricular block. In the NoEvent-group, an sV-trough and a pV-trough were observed in 10 (5%) and 20 (10%) subjects, respectively. The positive predictive accuracy of an sV-trough for ventricular fibrillation or acute myocardial infarction and that of a pV-trough for complete atrioventricular block was 88% and 100%, respectively. We reported that the hemodynamics consisting of heart rate, sympathetic activity and blood pressure is modeled excellently by modification of a known chaotic electrical circuit, Chua circuit (Osaka & Watanabe, 2004). A V-trough of sympathetic activity appears by increasing the resistive element between sympathetic activity and blood pressure in the circuit, which corresponds to the impaired regulation of blood pressure by sympathetic activity (Osaka, in press). This finding is consistent with an acknowledged finding that the depressed baroreflex (reflex of blood pressure by sympathetic activity) may trigger a lethal arrhythmia (Schwartz et al., 1988).

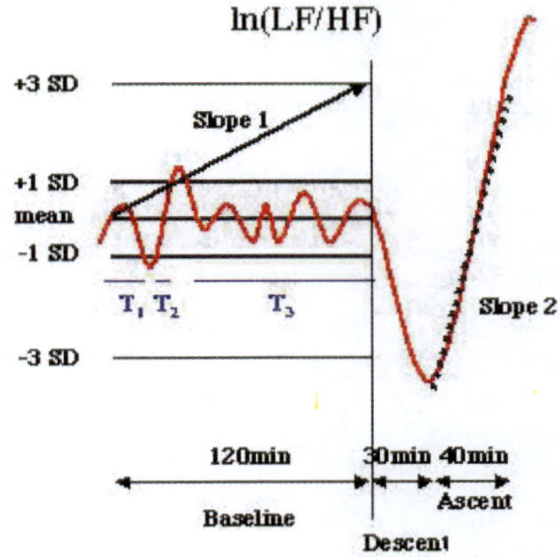

Fig. 4. Criteria for V-trough of ln(LF/HF). From (Osaka et al., 2010).

2. Recording of ECG outside the driver's awareness

2.1 Inevitable noise of ECG

Although there were some trials monitoring the ECG of drivers (Jeong et al., 2007), no automobile equipped with such a system has never been marketed, as a result of the fact that the ECG was largely contaminated by noise. Therefore, we developed new electrodes for installation on a steering wheel, through which an ECG limb lead could be recorded with suppression of noise (Osaka et al., 2008). However, some artifacts were still present as a result of the physical movements accompanying the handling of a steering wheel and as a result of jolts due to road conditions. Such artifacts are inevitable, because drivers sitting in the driver's seat do not remain still, as they might during the recording of a standard ECG. At the present time we have not yet succeeded in recording the entire PQRST pattern of waves in ECG from a steering wheel (steering-ECG), because of contamination of the baseline by noise. Therefore, the first half of our goals for recording the steering-ECG were in the following: i) confirmation of correctness of steering-ECG, ii) confirmation of correctness of RR intervals of steering-ECG, iii) confirmation of correctness of heart rate variability analysis of steering-ECG, when a driver remains still with gripping a steering wheel by both hands. However, noise unavoidably contaminates the steering-ECG, because the driver is not lying on the bed calmly but is handling the steering wheel. Although an ECG from a chest lead (chest-ECG) was recorded simultaneously as a reference in order to examine the correctness of the steering-ECG, the chest-ECG was also unavoidably contaminated. Hence, it was impossible to continuously find a one-to-one correspondence between the R waves of a steering-ECG and those of a chest-ECG. However, it was possible to observe fluctuations of heart rate variability by neglecting those inevitable artifacts. The second half of our goals was thus to evaluate the fluctuation of autonomic nervous activity from the heart rate variability analysis of steering-ECG in spite of noise. We examined whether fluctuations of sympathetic and parasympathetic nervous activities measured from steering-ECG were consistent with those from chest-ECG.

2.2 Methods for steering-ECG

2.2.1 Subjects

We simultaneously recorded the ECG from a chest lead and, separately, from a steering wheel in each of 10 normal subjects driving an automobile for 90 minutes. Then, the subjects sitting in the driver's seat remained still with gripping a steering wheel by both hands during the first minute of the recording.

2.2.2 Steering wheel

We refurbished the steering wheel of an automobile that was on sale by installing a pair of electrodes around the grip site on each side (Figure 5). One electrode of the right pair was a (-) electrode, and the other, an indifferent electrode. One electrode of the left pair was a (+) electrode, and the other, an indifferent electrode. From these electrodes we made ECG recordings which corresponded to the standard ECG of lead I. The electric wires from the installed electrodes were connected to a signal amplifier set up in the front portion of the automobile through a spiral cable within the steering wheel. We carefully kept the horn and an air bag intact for safety purposes. The recorded signals were 1~5mV. These signals were amplified 1,700 times. A bandpass-filter of 0.2~35Hz was used to remove noise. With an AD converter, the signals from the steering wheel lead were sampled at 200Hz. We consecutively searched the R waves of the steering-ECG and chest-ECG visually on a screen. We examined whether the R waves of the steering-ECG corresponded in a regular one-to-one fashion with the R waves of the chest-ECG. The R waves that did correspond to each other in this way were represented as {steering-R_k} and {chest-R_k}. Intervals of {steering-R_k} and {chest-R_k} ({steering-RR_k} and {chest-RR_k}) were measured as the intervals of the QRS waves at a threshold level. The threshold level was manually determined for each record. {steering-RR_k} were compared with {chest-RR_k} to identify errors due to the filtering of steering-ECG. Since each element of {steering-R_k} corresponded to each one of {chest-R_k} in a regular one-to-one fashion, these time series of {steering-R_k} and {chest-R_k} were used to examine the reliability of heart rate variability of steering-ECG. There were 3 chest electrodes served by a (+) electrode on V5 of the left chest, a (-) electrode below the right clavicle, and an indifferent electrode below the left clavicle. This corresponded to lead II of a standard ECG. These electrodes were connected with an electrocardiograph (DPA-250S; Dia

Medical System Co., Tokyo; time constant = 1.5sec, low-pass filter of 0.7 - 30Hz). The signals were transferred to an AD converter and were sampled at 200Hz.

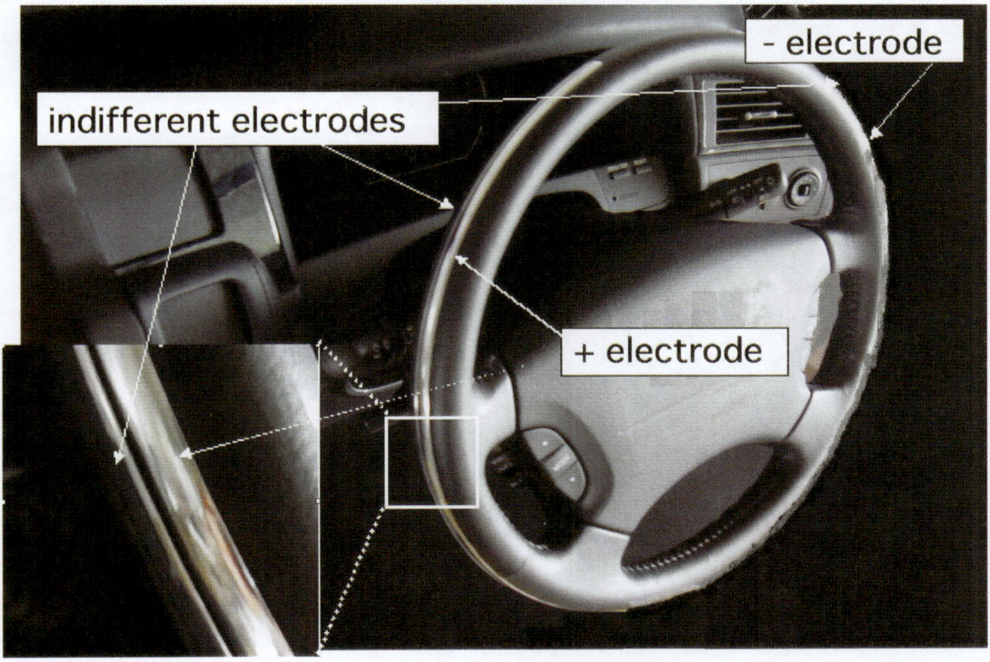

Fig. 5. A steering wheel. One pair of electrodes is installed around the grip site on each side. One of the two electrodes of each side is an indifferent electrode. The installed electrodes are arc-like (length 535mm, width 7mm, thickness 0.5mm) so that a driver can to some degree select a preferred grip site. From (Osaka et al., 2008).

2.2.3 Automated detection of QRS waves and measurement of RR intervals

The QRS waves were detected according to a flow chart, which we proposed newly (Figure 6). In a preliminary study, we examined the reliability of the algorithm by applying it to the electrocardiograms of the PhysioBank (Goldberger et al., 2000), which are freely available and downloadable digitized data (sampling rate 250Hz). Our algorithm could detect not only normal QRS waves but also abnormal QRS waves shown in Figure 7. After detecting QRS waves, the RR intervals, $\{I_n\}$, were measured as the intervals of peaks of two successive QRS waves. As the subjects sitting in the driver's seat did not remain still, outliers of RR intervals were always observed. Outliers were excluded as follows: 1) calculation of the MI and SDI (the mean value and standard deviation of $\{I_n\}$); 2) exclusion of outliers as $I_n > MI + 2SDI$ or $< MI - 2SDI$, and representation of those intervals remaining after exclusion of the outliers as $\{J_n\}$; 3) calculation of the standard deviation of $\{J_n\}$(expressed as the SDJ); 4) calculation of the median, $MedJ_n$, of a set consisting of eleven consecutive intervals, $\{J_{n-5}, J_{n-4}, \ldots, J_n, J_{n+1}, \ldots, J_{n+5}\}$ for each interval (indexed as J_n); 5) consecutive search of outliers as $J_n > MedJ_n + SDJ$ or $< MedJ_n - SDJ$; and 6) replacement of each of the outliers by $MedJ_n$ so that the intervals after the replacement could be regarded as RR intervals, $\{RRI_n\}$.

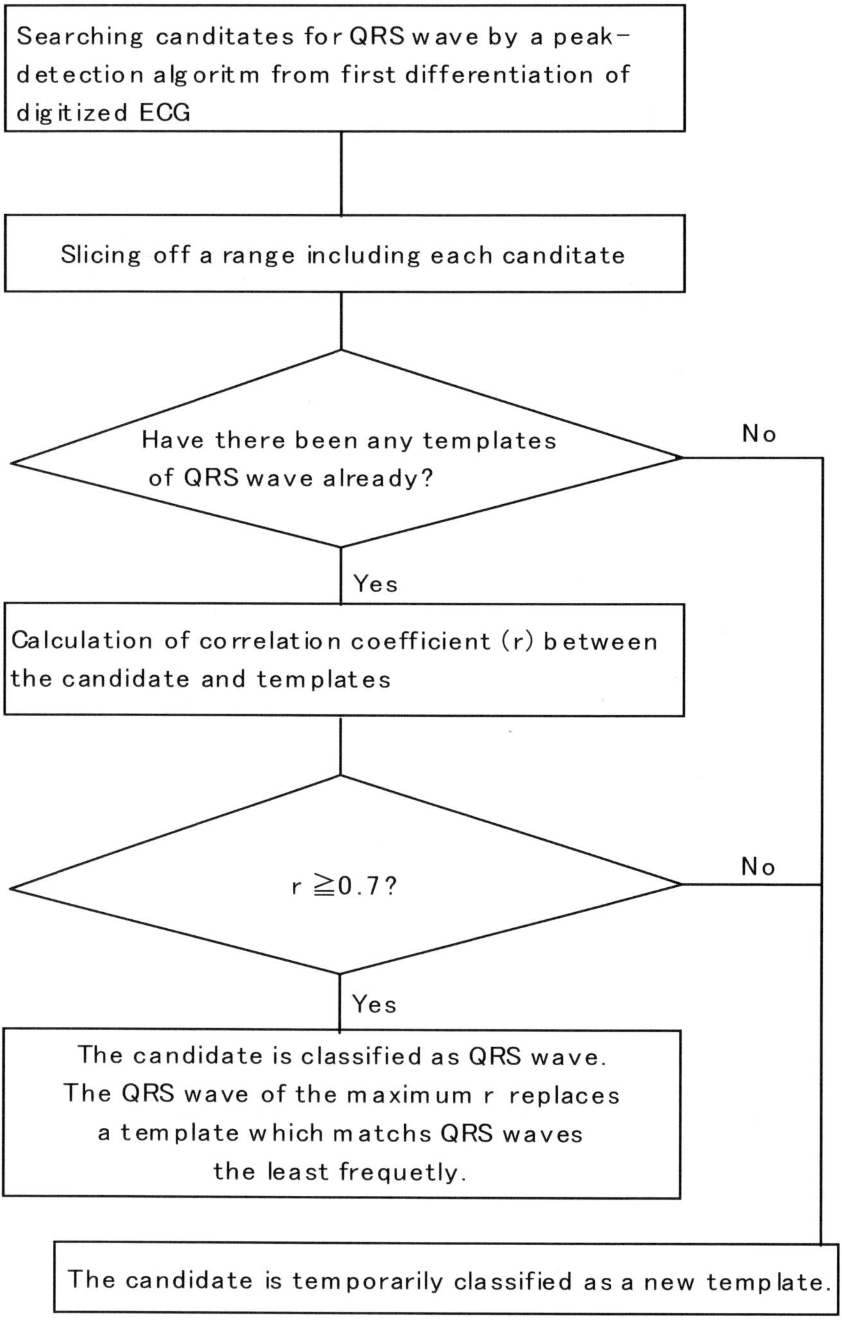

Fig. 6. A flow chart to detect QRS waves. From (Osaka et al., 2008).

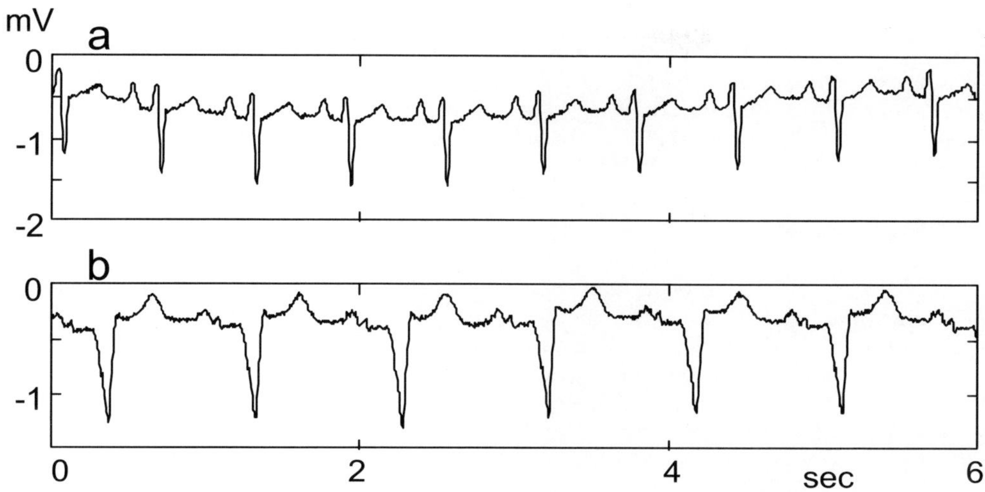

Fig. 7. Samples from the ECG database of PhysioBank. **a**, rS type. **b**, QS type.

2.2.4 Frequency analysis

A smoothed instantaneous heart rate time series was constructed from the RR-intervals and sampled at 8 Hz, according to Berger's method (Berger et al., 1986). The data length of an epoch was 64 sec. The confidence in spectral estimates could be enhanced by dividing the data into 5 epochs and by ensemble averaging of Welch's method (Bendat & Piersol, 1986). To reduce the loss of stability, the data were divided using a 50% overlap. Linear trends were removed from the data, and the data were tapered by use of a Hanning window. Then, a fast Fourier algorithm was used. We calculated the low-frequency component (LF: 0.04 - 0.15Hz) as a parameter of combined sympathetic and parasympathetic activity, the high-frequency component (HF: 0.15 - 0.40Hz) as that of parasympathetic activity, the ratio LF/HF as that of sympathetic activity, for each epoch. The natural logarithms of LF, HF, LF/HF, namely, ln(LF), ln(HF), and ln(LF/HF), were used to make these distributions approximate to normal distribution (Berger et al., 1989). The entire length of one record of ECG was 90 min, the data length of one epoch was 64 sec, and 2 consecutive epochs were overlapped by 50%. Hence, the total number of epochs was at most 168 (≈ 90min/32sec).

Since the subjects sitting in the driver's seat did not remain still and sometimes gripped a steering-wheel by only a single hand, more artifacts appeared in the steering-ECG than in the chest-ECG so that normal QRS waves were not recorded frequently. Hence, we took two steps to examine the reliability of heart rate variability of steering-ECG. Firstly, we compared ln(LF), ln(HF), and ln(LF/HF) of {steering-RR_k} with those parameters of {chest-RR_k}, because {steering-R_k} corresponded in a regular one-to-one fashion with {chest-R_k}. Each pair of R_k of {chest-R_k} and {steering-R_k} was consecutively searched visually on a screen. We would able to examine the reliability of the hardware system by the first step. The correlation coefficients between chest-ECG and steering-ECG for each parameter were calculated. The correlation coefficients were considered significant at $P<0.05$. Secondly, it was necessary to examine the reliability of the automated detection of QRS waves and measurement of RR intervals for practical use of our present system. According to the algorithm, the outliers in $\{I_n\}$ of steering-ECG were more frequently replaced by $MedJ_n$ than those in $\{I_n\}$ of chest-ECG. We examined whether ln(LF), ln(HF), and ln(LF/HF) of steering-ECG were reliable in spite of such a disadvantage. We calculated the moving average of subsequent 5 epochs for ln(LF), ln(HF), and ln(LF/HF), and instantaneous heart rate (HR): m-ln(LF), m-ln(HF), m-ln(LF/HF), and m-HR. We constructed a time series of 4 parameters for chest-ECG and steering-ECG.

2.2.5 Mutual information

We drew graphs of fluctuations of m-ln(LF), m-ln(HF), m-ln(LF/HF), and m-HR for chest-ECG and steering-ECG. In order to compare the fluctuation of each parameter of steering-ECG with that of chest-ECG, we calculated the mutual information between them. This mutual information method was used to gauge the likeness between them. We calculated mutual information values, according to an algorithm proposed by Fraser and Swinney (Fraser & Swinney, 1986) and our previous study (Osaka et al., 1998). For a couple of time series, {x(t)} and {y(t)}, we measured how dependent the values of y(t) were on the values of x(t). We made the assignment [s,q] = [x(t), y(t)] to consider a general coupled system (S,Q). For example, {x(t)} was the time series of moving averages of m-ln(LF) for chest-ECG and {y(t)} was the time series of moving averages of m-ln(LF) for steering-ECG. Mutual information is defined as the answer to the question, "Given a measurement of *s*, how many bits on the average can be predicted about *q*?":

$$I(S,Q) = \int P_{sq}(s,q)\, log[P_{sq}(s,q)/(P_s(s)P_q(q))]dsdq,$$

where i) S and Q denote the systems, ii) $P_s(s)$ and $P_q(q)$ are the probability densities at s and q, respectively, and iii) $P_{sq}(s, q)$ is the joint probability density at s and q. The data length is 2^n. The algorithm is as follows: 1) an x-y plot is normalized into a square: each value W_i (= x(t) or y(t)) was replaced by an integer N_i; $1 \leq N_i \leq 2^n$; if $W_i < W_j$, $N_i < N_j$; if $W_i = W_j$ and $i < j$, $N_i < N_j$, so that each of the values of {x(t)} and {y(t)} is one to one replaced by an integer from 1 to 2^n, 2) it is successively divided into smaller squares, 3) a value for the dependence of y(t) on x(t) is calculated in each square, and 4) mutual information is the average of those values weighted by respective areas. Even if there is no significant correlation in the entire square, any significant correlation in smaller squares is taken into the final correlation by weighting by the respective areas. Therefore, mutual information is considered to be applicable more generally than a correlation coefficient of regression analysis. The larger is the value of mutual information for (S,Q), the stronger is the mutual dependence between S and Q. The data length was 2^7 (= 128). If S = Q, the correlation between them should be perfect. Then, I(S,Q) = n, where the data length is 2^n, because the algorithm is developed to the discrete case (Fraser & Swinney, 1986). The mutual information value between the same two time series is n. Hence, mutual information values were normalized by n, that is, these values were divided by n, resulting in values between 0 and 1. If the mutual information value was larger than or equal to 0.047, the correlation was taken to be strongly correlated on the basis of our previous report (Osaka et al., 1998).

2.3 Results

2.3.1 Results on the hardware system

Although small high-frequency noise still contaminated the baseline, the reproduced signals demonstrated the characteristics of P, R, and T waves well (Figure 8)). Each steering-ECG R

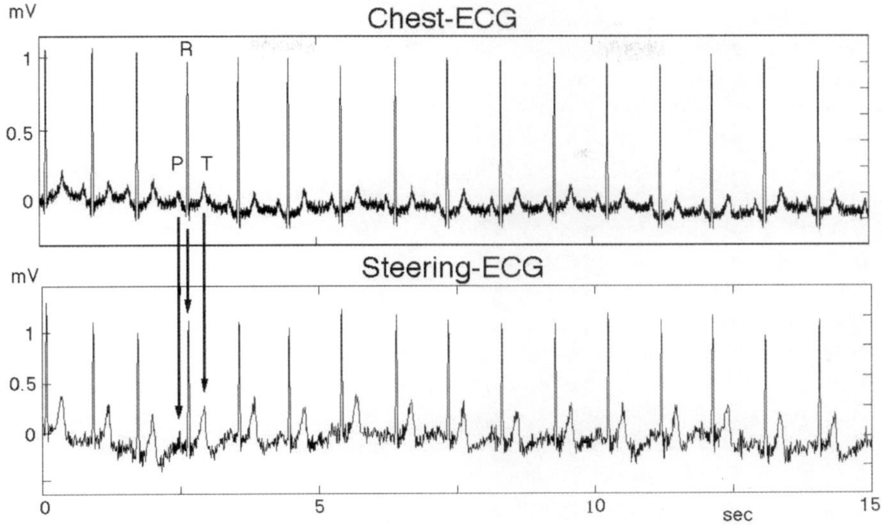

Fig. 8. Comparison of the electrocardiogram recorded from a steering wheel (steering-ECG) with that from a chest lead (chest-ECG). From (Osaka et al., 2008).

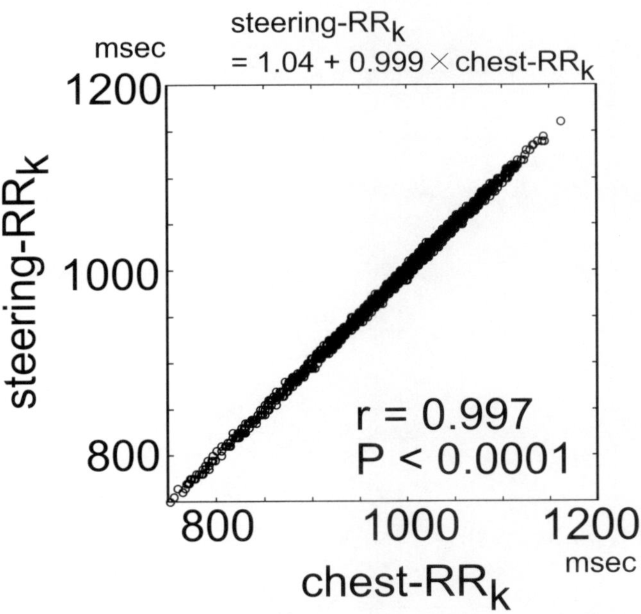

Fig. 9. A regression graph of steering-RR_k to chest-RR_k in the same subject as in Figure 8. Each element of {steering-R_k} corresponds to each one of {chest-R_k} in a regular one-to-one fashion by consecutively searching the R waves of the steering-ECG and chest-ECG visually on a screen. From (Osaka et al., 2008).

wave showed time-consistency with the respective R wave of the chest-ECG during the handling of a steering wheel as well as during the sitting still in the driver's seat. Figure 9 shows a regression graph of steering-RR_k to chest-RR_k in one of the subjects: steering-RR_k = 1.04 + 0.999×chest-RR_k (r = 0.997, P<0.0001). Hence, {steering-RR_k} was almost perfectly consistent with {chest-RR_k}. Similarly, the other subjects showed such a perfect consistency. For each parameter of ln(LF), ln(HF), and ln(LF/HF), a regression graph of steering-ECG (Y) to chest-ECG (X) was in the following: Y = a + b×X ($-0.012 \leqq a \leqq 0.043$, $0.997 \leqq r \leqq 1.000$, P<0.0001) in all the subjects. ln(LF), ln(HF), and ln(LF/HF) of steering-ECG were almost perfectly consistent with those of chest-ECG.

2.3.2 Results on the software system

Figure 10 shows RR intervals from steering-ECG and from chest-ECG for the same subject as in Figure 8. When the driver moved his (her) upper body abruptly, the baseline of the chest-ECG fluctuated so that, intermittently, the R waves could not be detected. Hence, rather long erroneous RR intervals sometimes appeared in the tachogram of the chest-ECG as well as the steering-ECG. Longer RR intervals were observed more frequently in the tachogram of steering-ECG. This occurred because the driver sometimes gripped only one side of the steering wheel with a single hand. Since more long erroneous RR intervals were deleted in

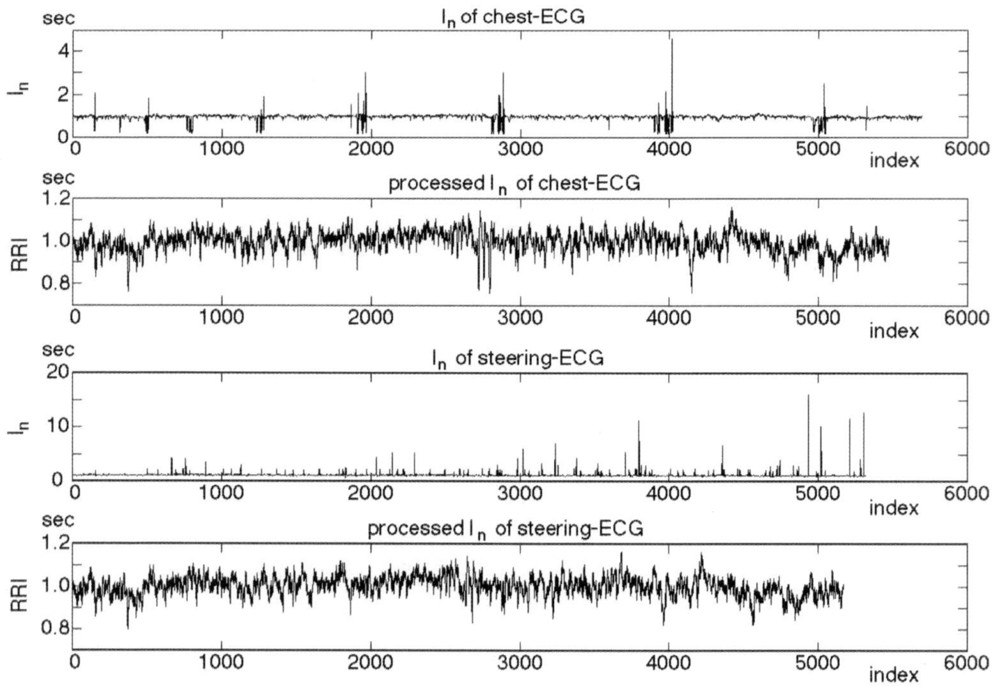

Fig. 10. RR intervals from steering-ECG and from chest-ECG for the same subject as in Fig. 8. {I_n}: intervals of peaks of two successive QRS waves. {RRI_n}: intervals regarded as RR intervals after the processing of outliers from {I_n} by the algorithm. From (Osaka et al., 2008).

the steering-ECG than in the chest-ECG, the last index number of processed I_n of steering-ECG, {steering-RRI_n}, was smaller than that of processed I_n of chest-ECG, {chest-RRI_n} (Figure 10). Hence, each element of {steering-RRI_n} did not correspond in a regular one-to-one fashion with that of {chest-RRI_n} so that {steering-RRI_n} and {chest-RRI_n} could not be compared by the regression analysis. Figure 11 shows that the fluctuation from the steering-ECG resembled that from the chest-ECG for each parameter of the same subject as in Figure 8. Particularly, most of upslopes and downslopes of each parameter of steering-ECG corresponded one to one with those of chest-ECG. These findings were seen in the other subjects, when mutual information values were larger than 0.047. Figure 12 shows that mutual information of each parameter was larger than 0.047 with 95% confidence. Hence, it indicated that the fluctuation of each parameter of steering-ECG significantly resembled that of chest-ECG. However, the mutual information of m-ln(HF) in one subject and that of m-ln(LF/HF) in another were both 0. Mutual information values were all larger than 0.047 except for these 2 values.

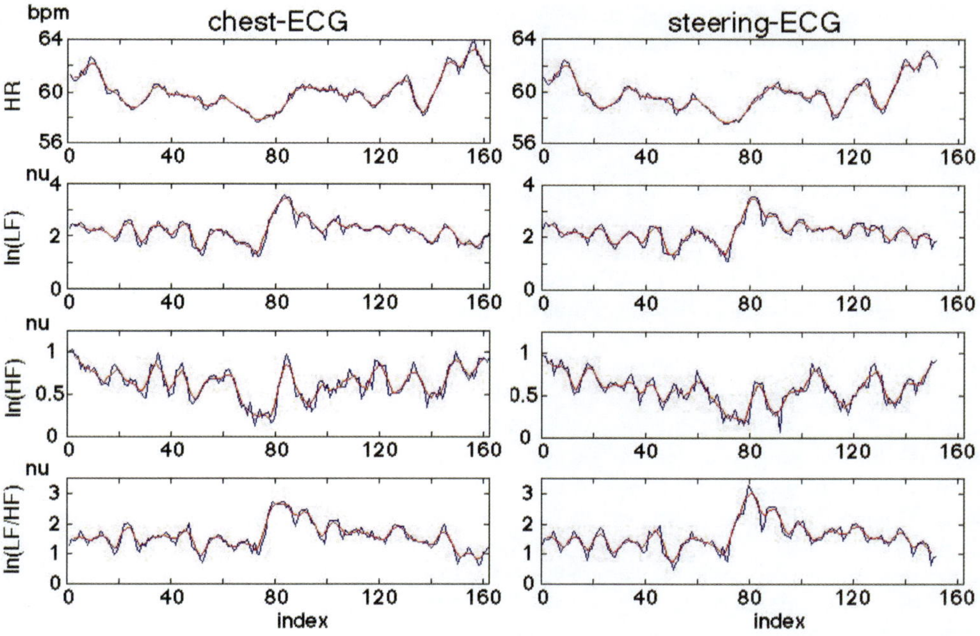

Fig. 11. Comparison of a fluctuation from steering-ECG with that from chest-ECG for each parameter of the same subject as in Figure 8. Red lines show the moving averages of blue lines. Mutual information values are 0.225, 0.223, 0.209, and 0.184 for m-HR, m-ln(LF), m-ln(HF), and m-ln(LF/HF). HR, heart rate; LF, low-frequency component (0.04 - 0.15Hz); HF, high-frequency component (0.15 - 0.40Hz); LF/HF, the ratio of LF to HF. ln(LF), ln(HF), and ln(LF/HF): natural logarithms of LF, HF, and LF/HF. m-HR, m-ln(LF), m-ln(HF), and m-ln(LF/HF): moving averages of HR, ln(LF), ln(HF), and ln(LF/HF). From (Osaka et al., 2008).

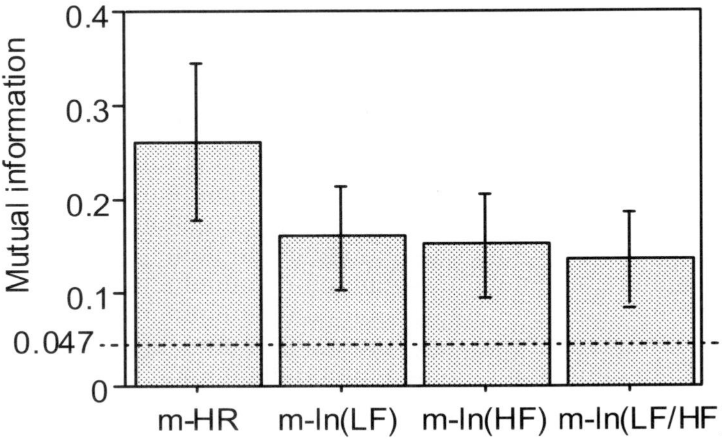

Fig. 12. Mean and 95%-confidence error bar of mutual information of m-HR, m-ln(LF), m-ln(HF), and m-ln(LF/HF). Threshold of significance: 0.047. HR, heart rate; LF, low-frequency component (0.04 - 0.15Hz); HF, high-frequency component (0.15 - 0.40Hz); LF/HF, the ratio of LF to HF. ln(LF), ln(HF), and ln(LF/HF): natural logarithms of LF, HF, and LF/HF. m-HR, m-ln(LF), m-ln(HF), and m-ln(LF/HF): moving averages of HR, ln(LF), ln(HF), and ln(LF/HF). From (Osaka et al., 2008).

2.4 Confirmation of correctness of steering ECG

The waves of P, Q, R, S, and T are generally visible clearly in a standard ECG, while a subject lies on the supine position. In the present study, the waves of P, R, and T could be recorded clearly in steering-ECG (Figure 8). {steering-RR_k} was almost perfectly consistent with {chest-RR_k} in all the subjects. Similarly, ln(LF), ln(HF), and ln(LF/HF) of steering-ECG were almost perfectly consistent with those of chest-ECG. Hence, the first half of our goals was achieved, using the following technical measures. The long indifferent electrodes were installed into both sides of the steering wheel so as to work without fail even if the driver's hands should move on the steering wheel. The electrodes installed into the steering wheel were made of plating to increase electrical conductivity. A bandpass filter of 0.2 ~35Hz was used for steering-ECG. It may be compared with the generally used bandpass filter of an electrocardiograph. Hence, the waves P, R, and T of the steering-ECG rather resembled those of chest-ECG. Small high-frequency noise contaminated not only the baseline of the steering-ECG but also that of the chest-ECG (Figure 8), indicating that it is difficult to record noise-free ECG in an automobile. This contaminating noise resulted from alternating current, making the ST-segment of the ECG unclear. Generally, small P waves, flat T waves, and small inverted T waves may be invisible by the contaminating noise. In order to detect ischemic attacks, namely, angina pectoris and acute myocardial infarction, it is necessary to eliminate that noise. We will endeavor to reduce noise in a further study.
After detecting QRS waves by our algorithm shown in Figure 6, we measured RR-intervals by using a peak-detection algorithm. In the preliminary study, we examined the reliability of this algorithm by applying to the ECG database of PhysioBank. It was applicable to the ECG of patients with abnormal Q waves in lead I, usually observed in broad anterior myocardial infarction or dilated cardiomyopathy (Figure 7) as well as the ECG of normal

subjects. When a driver moved his or her upper body abruptly and/or gripped only one side of the steering wheel with a single hand, normal R waves could intermittently not be detected, and long erroneous RR intervals appeared. Heart rate variability mainly results from the pacemaker sinus node rhythm, which is under the control of the autonomic nervous system. Therefore, a time series including frequent noisy RR intervals, for example, in subjects at high risk of lethal arrhythmia who have frequently premature beats, atrial tachyarrhythmia such as atrial fibrillation, or pace maker implantation is unsuitable for heart rate variability analysis. Practically, arrhythmias such as premature beats sometimes appear in even normal subjects, which cause erroneous RR intervals. Although the Task Force of the European Society of Cardiology and the North American Society of Pacing and Electrophysiology published a report about standards of measurement for heart rate variability in 1996, no standard for how to deal with such noisy RR intervals was included in the report. In subjects with frequent premature beats, the values of LF, HF, and LF/HF are rather inaccurate for data epochs including more premature beats. Thus, we presume that a method of dividing the data into 5 epochs with a 50% overlap and ensemble averaging is useful to enhance the confidence of those values, according to Welch's method (Bendat & Piersol, 1986).

Rather long or short RR intervals were excluded as outliers: I_n > MI + 2SDI or < MI - 2SDI. Consequently, about 5% of all the intervals I_n were excluded. These outliers resulted from artifacts due to abrupt body movement and/or gripping only one side of the steering wheel. More long erroneous RR intervals appeared in steering-ECG than in chest-ECG, and more outliers were excluded in steering-ECG. The number of RR intervals was less in steering-ECG than in chest-ECG (Figure 10). Each element of {steering-RRI_n} did not correspond in a regular one-to-one fashion with that of {chest-RRI_n} so that {steering-RRI_n} and {chest-RRI_n} could not be compared by the regression analysis. Hence, we needed the mutual information method as an alternative one in order to compare heart rate variability of {steering-RRI_n} and {chest-RRI_n}.

We aimed at drawing a reliable graph following a fluctuation of autonomic nervous activity. Mutual information of each parameter was larger than 0.047 with 95% confidence. This indicated statistically that the fluctuation of each parameter of steering-ECG significantly resembled that of chest-ECG. In detail, all but 2 mutual information values were larger than 0.047: mutual information of ln(HF) in one subject and that of ln(LF/HF) in another were 0. When these values of mutual information were 0, the fluctuations of steering-ECG did not seem to resemble the respective fluctuations of chest-ECG, since the steering-ECG was noisy due to the frequent gripping of a steering wheel by a single hand. We succeeded in demonstrating a fluctuation in autonomic nervous activity from steering-ECG, which was statistically consistent with that of chest-ECG. It is possible for a driver to observe a fluctuation of sympathetic nervous activity by ln(LF/HF) and a fluctuation of parasympathetic nervous activity by ln(HF). Hence, drivers can detect their own autonomic stress continuously. Atrial or ventricular premature beats can be detected by the present algorithm.

3. Addition of information from plethysmogram

Although the chest-ECG was recorded simultaneously as a reference in order to examine the correctness of the steering-ECG, the chest-ECG was also unavoidably contaminated. Hence, it was impossible to continuously find a one-to-one correspondence between the R waves of a steering-ECG and those of a chest-ECG. We recorded plethysmogram as well as ECG from the steering wheel in order to compromise such missing recordings of ECG. Blood pressure is also very important information on physiological conditions. We examined whether various cardiac abnormalities could be detected reliably by ECG and plethysmogram recorded from the steering wheel. We aimed at making a robust system for monitoring a driver's physical conditions against noise and providing reliable information to the driver by integrating information from the steering-ECG and that from the plethysmogram for safety driving.

3.1 Subjects & methods

Forty-six subjects were evaluated: 9 normal volunteers and 37 patients (hypertension (N = 7), cardiomyopathy (N = 7), atrial fibrillation (N = 7), myocardial infarction (N = 6), valvular disease (N = 6), angina pectoris (N = 4)). Of these subjects, 8 showed ST depression, 4 left bundle block, 4 right bundle block, 4 low voltage, and 2 pacing rhythm of a implanted pacemaker.

We installed a sensor of a transmitted green photoelectric plethysmogram to detect the variation of arterial concentration of hemoglobin by reflection (bandpass-filter 0.2 ~ 5 Hz with reduction of 3 dB, sampling rate 1 kHz) into the steering wheel. Since the absorption rate of green by hemoglobin was higher than that of infra-red, which is used generally, the signal-to-noise ratio (S/N ratio) of the former was better than the latter so that plethysmogram could be recorded at the palm near the right thumb. The sensor was set up to touch the palm near the right thumb naturally, while the driver grips the steering wheel into which the electrodes for ECG were installed. To compare with those recordings from the steering wheel, we recorded ECG from a chest lead and plethysmogram directly from a finger simultaneously while they were sitting on the driving seat of the simulator for 10 minutes (Figure 13). We calculated the second derivative of plethysmogram as the

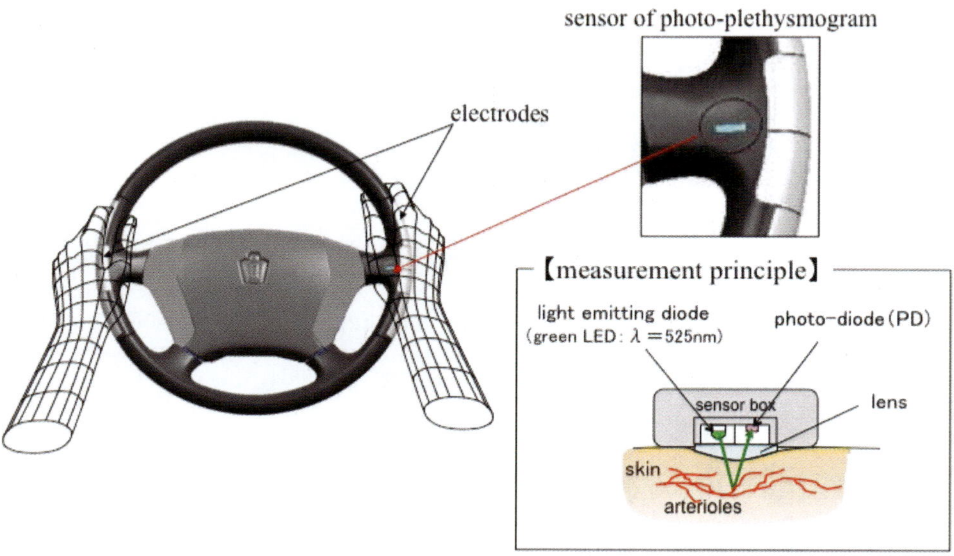

Fig. 13. Electrodes for electrocardiogram & a sensor for photo-plethysmogram.

acceleration of pulse wave. The positive component (a-wave) and the following negative component (b-wave) represent the forward component of systolic blood pressure (Figure 14) (Chua et al., 2010). Therefore, we presumed that the total amplitude of a-wave and b-wave reflects the strength of ejection in systole. The data of ECG and plethysmogram recorded from the steering wheel were stored in a hard disk, which were analyzed to obtain RR intervals and the second derivative of plethysmogram.

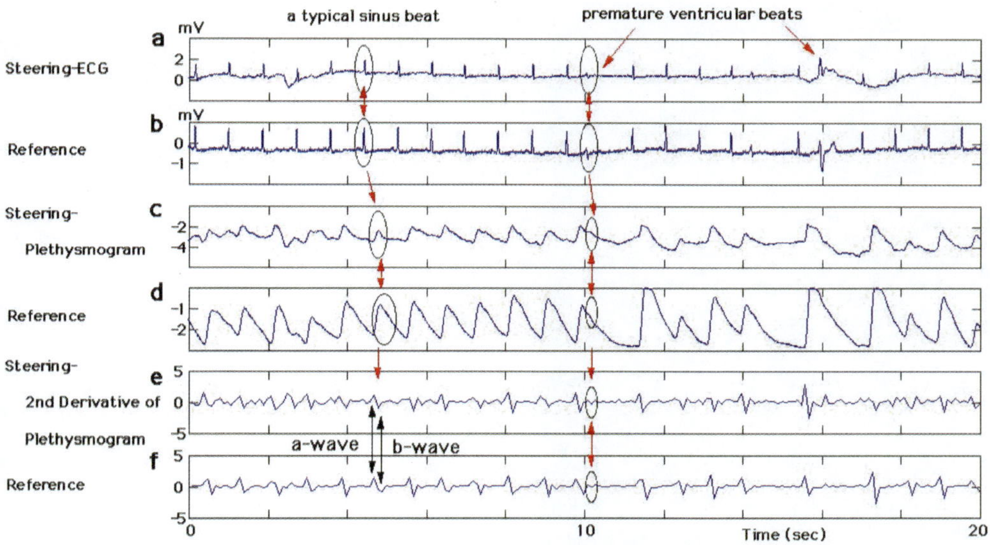

Fig. 14. An example of steering-electrocardiogram and plethysmogram.

3.2 Results

Figure 14 shows an example of steering-ECG, steering-plethysmogram and steering-second derivative of plethysmogram, comparing with the reference recordings. Each of QRS wave of the steering-ECG was consistent with that of the reference. Each of pulse wave of the steering-plethythmogram was consistent with that of the reference. Similarly, each pair of a-wave and b-wave of the steering-second derivative of plethysmogram was consistent with that of the reference. We could discriminate sinus bradycardia, sinus tachycardia, and atrial fibrillation by measuring RR-intervals. We could also discriminate premature ventricular beats and premature atrial beats by measuring the timing and width of QRS and by plethysmogram, which was particularly useful because premature ventricular beats caused only a minute pulse wave (Figure 14c, d) and premature atrial beats caused almost normal pulse waves. Since only a minute blood volume is outputted by premature ventricular beats, a-wave and b-wave did not appear (Figure 14e, f). When a subject did not grip the steering wheel normally, the recordings of ECG were sometimes contaminated by noise, such as a fluctuation of the baseline. Figure 15 shows that beat-to-beat intervals can be calculated from the steering-plethysmogram and/or the steering-second derivative of it, in case a large fluctuation of the baseline hinders the calculation of RR intervals. If plethysmogram was recorded normally, such missing RR intervals of the steering-ECG could be replaced by peak intervals of plethysmogram. Figure 14 shows that ST depression can be observed in the steering-ECG like the reference. Thus, ST changes could be detected without such a large fluctuation of the baseline.

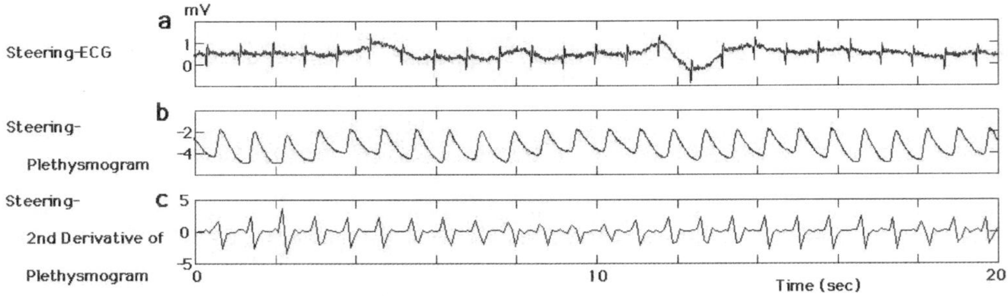

Fig. 15. An example of fluctuaion of the baseline of steering-electrocardiogram.

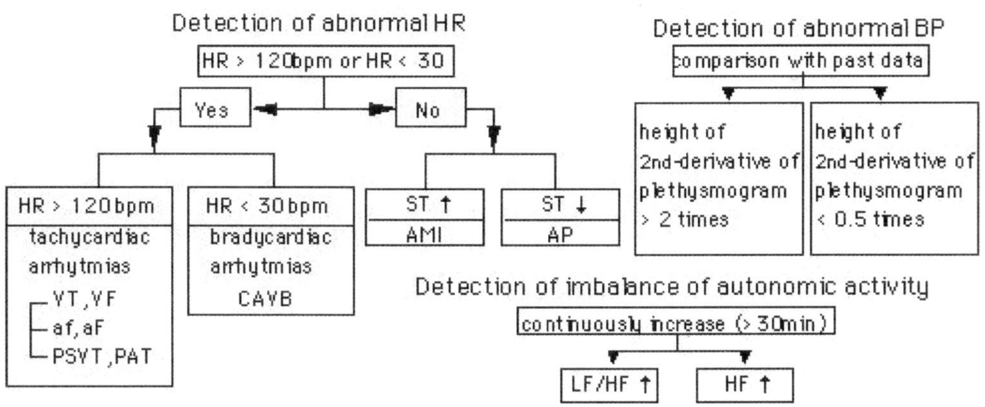

Fig. 16. Flow chart to detect abnormal physiological conditions. HR, heart rate; bpm, beats per minute; BP, blood pressure; VT, ventricular tachycardia; VF, ventricular fibrillation; af, atrial fibrillation; aF, atrial flutter; PSVT, paroxysmal supraventricular tachycardia; PAT, paroxysmal atrial tachycardia; CAVB, complete atrioventricular block; AMI, acute myocardial infarction; AP, angina pectoris; LF, low-frequency component of heart rate variability; HF, high-frequency component.

4. Conclusion

In order to improve the reliability of the system to detect abnormal physiological conditions while driving and make it more applicable, we installed the sensor of photo-plethysmogram besides the electrodes of ECG into the steering wheel. We demonstrated that RR intervals calculated from the steering-ECG and the graph following a fluctuation of autonomic activity were consistent with those obtained from the reference-ECG. It is possible for a driver to observe a trend of heart rate, a fluctuation of sympathetic activity by ln(LF/HF), and a fluctuation of parasympathetic activity by ln(HF) on a monitor of navigation. Hence, drivers can check whether arrhythmia appears or not, and their own autonomic stress continuously and easily. Similarly, we showed that the plethysmogram of the steering wheel and the second derivative of it were consistent with those from the reference. In a stable condition such as sitting on a driving seat, HR > 120 beats/min (bpm) and HR < 30 bpm are considered to be abnormal so that the driver is possibly at risk from causing a traffic accident (Figure 16). When the height of a-wave plus b-wave of the second derivative of plethysmogram is >2 times larger than the mean value of it for the previous 30 minutes or <0.5 times smaller, blood pressure is considered to increase or decrease abruptly. When LF/HF or HF is increasing steadily for >30 minutes, it will indicate that sympathetic activity may predominate over parasympathetic activity excessively or vise versa (Figure 16). If these abnormalities are detected, a message of inquiring of the driver, "Are you all right?" will be delivered in our system. If the driver needs any help, some of the nearest hospitals will be displayed on the screen of the navigation system. This hospital-referring system has already installed into automobiles of a high grade of TOYOTA MOTOR CORPORATION. A network system by which the data is continuously transferred to a center and monitored by medical doctors will be made in the near future. We will call it the human-machine talking system. We propose such a new system by which it is monitored whether physiological conditions are within a normal state of the driver or not. To decide it, the present data of heart rate, the height of a-wave plus b-wave, LF/HF and HF are continuously compared with those parameters from the past data of the driver. Hence, we call it a customized heart check system. Feedback of information to the driver on autonomic stress and the appearance of premature beats will improve safety. Our system will open doors to new strategies to minimize driver's risk by making available the relevant data during the actual process of driving. We reported that a V-shaped trough in autonomic activity is a possible precursor of life-threatening cardiac events (Osaka et al., 2010). The V-trough including the small variations that precede it spans approximately 190 minutes. Hence, a necessary condition for the detection of the precursor with our algorithm is that the time from the start of recording to an event must exceed 190 minutes. Thus the somewhat lengthy recording time required is a potential shortcoming of the system. Therefore, the detection of the V-shaped trough is considered to be useful for subjects who drive for long hours, especially professional drivers of bus, taxi, and truck. This system will be also useful to monitor physiological conditions of a man or woman at home as well as an inpatient, for example if the system is installed into the bed. If it is installed into a toilet stool, physiological conditions will be easily checked up daily.

5. Acknowledgement

This study was done in cooperation with Minoru Makiguchi (TOYOTA MOTOR CORPORATION), Tsuyoshi Nakagawa, Taiji Kawachi, Kazuhiro Sakai and Shinya

Matsunaga (DENSO), Hiroshi Hayashi, M.D., Hiroshige Murata, M.D., and Takao Katoh, M.D. (Nippon Medical School).

6. References

Bauer, A.; Kantelhardt, J.W.; Barthel, P.; Schneider, R.; Mäkikallio, T.; Ulm, K.; Hnatkova, K.; Schomig, A.; Huikuri, H.; Bunde, A.; Malik, M. & Schmidt, G. (2006) Deceleration capacity of heart rate as a predictor of mortality after myocardial infarction: cohort study. *Lancet*, Vol.367, pp. 1674-1681

Bendat, J.S. & Piersol, A.G. (1986) *Random Data Analysis and Measurement Procedures* (2nd edition), Wiley, New York

Berger, R.D.; Akselrod, S.; Gordon, D. & Cohen, R.J. (1986) An efficient algorithm for spectral analysis of heart rate variability. *IEEE Transactions of Biomedical Engineering,* Vol.33, pp. 900-904

Berger, R.D.; Saul, J.P. & Cohen, R.J. (1989) Transfer function analysis of autonomic regulation I. Canine atrial rate response, *American Journal of Physiology (Heart Circulation Physiology)* Vol.256, pp. H142-H152

Chua, E.C., Redmond, S.J., McDarby, G. & Heneghan, C. (2010) Towards using photo-plethysmogram amplitude to measure blood pressure during sleep. *Annals of Biomedical Engineering*, Vol.38, pp. 945-954.

Fraser, A.M. & Swinney, H.L. (1986) Independent coordinates for strange attractors from mutual information. *Physical Review A*, Vol.33, pp. 1134-1140

Goldberger, A.L.; Amaral, L.A.N.; Glass, L.; Hausdorff, J.M.; Ivanov, P.C.; Mark, R.G.; Mietus, J.E.; Moody, G.B.; Peng, C.K. & Stanley, H.E. (2000) PhysioBank, PhysioToolkit, and PhysioNet: Components of a New Research Resource for Complex Physiologic Signals. *Circulation,* Vol.101, pp. e215-e220

Huikuri, H.V.; Valkama, J.O.; Airaksinen, K.E.; Seppanen, T; Kessler, K.M.; Takkunen, J.T. & Myerburg, R.J. (1993) Frequency domain measures of heart rate variability before the onset of nonsustained and sustained ventricular tachycardia in patients with coronary disease. *Circulation,* Vol.87, pp. 1220-1228

Ivanov, P.C.; Amaral, L.A.; Goldberger, A.L.; Havlin, S.; Rosenblum, M.G. Struzik, Z.R. & Stanley, H.E. (1999) Multifractality in human heartbeat dynamics, *Nature* Vol.399, pp. 461-465

Jeong; Lee, I.C.; Park, D.H.; Ko, S.W.; Yoon, J. & Ro, H. (2007) Automobile driver's stress index provision system that utilizes electrocardiogram, In: *Intelligent Vehicles Symposium*, pp. (652-656) IEEE, Istanbul, Turkey

Kobayashi, M. & Musha, T. (1982) 1/f fluctuation of heartbeat period. *IEEE Transactions of Biomedical Engineering* Vol.29, pp. 456-457

Lam, L.T. & Lam, M.K.P. (2005) The association between sudden illness and motor vehicle crash mortality and injury among older drivers in NSW, Australia. *Accident Analysis and Prevention,* Vol.37, pp. 563-567

Muller, J.E.; Ludmer, P.L.; Willich, S.N.; Tofler, G.H.; Aylmer, G.; Klangos, I. & Stone, P.H. (1987) Circadian variation in the frequency of sudden cardiac death. *Circulation,* Vol.75, pp131-138

Osaka, M.; Saitoh, H.; Atarashi, H. & Hayakawa, H. (1993) Correlation dimension of heart rate variability: a new index of human autonomic function, *Frontiers of Medical and Biological Engineering,* Vol.5, pp. 289-300

Osaka, M.; Saitoh, H.; Sasabe, N.; Atarashi, H.; Katoh, T.; Hayakawa, H. & Cohen, R.J. (1996) Changes in autonomic activity preceding onset of nonsustained ventricular tachycardia, *Annals of Noninvasive Electrocardiology,* Vol..1, pp. 3-11

Osaka, M.; Yambe, T.; Saitoh, H.; Yoshizawa, M.; Itoh, T.; Nitta, S. & Hayakawa, H. (1998) Mutual information discloses relationship between hemodynamic variables in artificial heart-implanted dogs. *American Journal of Physiology,* Vol.275, pp. H1419-H1433

Osaka, M. & Watanabe, M.A. (2004) A modified Chua circuit simulates *1/f*-fluctuation of heartbeat interval. *International Journal of Bifurcation and Chaos,* Vol.14, pp. 3449-3457

Osaka, M.; Murata, H.; Fuwamoto, Y.; Nanba, S.; Sakai, K. & Katoh, T. (2008) Application of heart rate variability analysis to electrocardiogram recorded outside the driver's awareness from an automobile steering wheel. *Circulation Journal,* Vol.72, pp. 1867-73

Osaka, M.; Watanabe, E.; Murata, H.; Fuwamoto, Y.; Nanba, S.; Sakai, K. & Katoh, T. (2010) V-Shaped Trough in Autonomic Activity is a Possible Precursor of Life-Threatening Cardiac Events. *Circulation Journal*, Vol.74, pp. 1906-1915

Osaka, M. (in press) A modified chua circuit simulates a v-shaped trough in autonomic activity as a precursor of sudden cardiac death. *International Journal of Bifurcation and Chaos*

Peng, C-K.; Mietus, J.; Hausdorff, J.M.; Havlin, S.; Stanley, H.E. & Goldberger, A.L. (1993) Long-range anticorrelations and non-Gaussian behavior of the heartbeat, *Physical Review Letters,* Vol.70, pp. 1343-1346

Routley, V.; Staines, C.; Brennan, C.; Haworth, N. & Ozanne-Smith, J. (2003) Suicide and Natural Deaths in Road Traffic – Review. *Monash University Accident Research Centre Report,* Vol.216

Sakata, K.; Kumagai, H.; Osaka, M.; Onami, T.; Matsuura, T.; Imai, M. & Saruta, T. (2002) Potentiated sympathetic nervous and renin-angiotensin systems reduce nonlinear correlation between sympathetic activity and blood pressure in conscious spontaneously hypertensive rats. *Circulation,* Vol.106, pp. 620-625

Schwartz, P.J.; Vanoli, E.; Stramba-Badiale, M.; De Ferrari, G.M.; Billman, G.E. & Foreman, R.D. (1988) Autonomic mechanisms and sudden death. New insights from analysis of barorecepor reflexes in conscious dogs with and without a myocardial infarction. *Circulation,* Vol.78, pp. 969-979

Task Force of the European Society of Cardiology and the North American Society of Pacing and Electrophysiology. (1996) Heart rate variability: Standards of measurement, physiological interpretation, and clinical use. *Circulation,* Vol.93, pp. 1043-1065

Taylor, J.A. & Eckberg, D.L. (1996) Fundamental relations between short-term RR interval and arterial pressure oscillations in humans. *Circulation,* Vol.93, pp. 1527-1532

Toyoshima, H.; Hayashi, S.; Tanabe, N.; Miyanishi, K.; Satoh, T.; Aizawa, Y. & Izumi, T. (1996) Sudden death of adults in Japan. *Nagoya Journal of Medical Science,* Vol.59, pp. 81-95

Zipes, D.P. & Wellens, H.J. (1998) Sudden cardiac death, *Circulation*, Vol.98, pp. 2334-2351

19

Electrocardiogram in an MRI Environment: Clinical Needs, Practical Considerations, Safety Implications, Technical Solutions and Future Directions

Thoralf Niendorf, Lukas Winter and Tobias Frauenrath
Berlin Ultrahigh Field Facility (B.U.F.F.)
Max Delbrueck Center for Molecular Medicine, Berlin,
Germany

1. Introduction

Magnetic Resonance Imaging (MRI) has been listed as the single most important medical innovation, on par with CT scanning (Fuchs & Sox 2001). In current clinical MRI ECG is being using for three major purposes. Firstly, heart motion, blood flow and blood pulsation are commonly dealt with using electrocardiogram (ECG) for synchronization of MR data acquisition with the cardiac cycle (Lanzer et.al. 1984) to address or compensate for cardiac activity related motion artifacts which is of paramount importance for an ever growing portfolio of cardiovascular MR (CMR) and neurovascular MR (NVMR) applications (Assomull et.al. 2007, Kelle et.al. 2008, Kramer et.al. 2008, Kwong & Korlakunta 2008, Niendorf et.al. 2006, Niendorf & Sodickson 2008, Niendorf & Sodickson 2006, Niendorf et.al. 2010, Pennell et.al. 2004, Schwitter 2008). Secondly, ECG is widely used to simultaneously register cardiac activity with MRI; for example to eliminate physiological fluctuations from brain activation maps derived from functional MRI studies (Purdon & Weisskoff 1998). Thirdly, there are an increasing number of clinical applications that require ECG monitoring prior to/after the MR examination while the patient is still in the MR environment but outside of the MR scanners bore using ECG devices as a patient emergency indicator.

ECG waveform acquisitions, ECG co-registration and ECG monitoring during MRI pose technical challenges and requires safety measures that will not be familiar to users of other conventional ECG technologies. For all those reasons, the basic principles of using ECG in an MRI environment and their implications for clinical MRI and MRI research are provided in this chapter. Key concepts, technical solutions, practical considerations and safety implications for cardiac gated MRI using electrocardiograms are outlined. Unsolved technical problems and unmet clinical needs are also considered carefully, in an attempt to stimulate the community to throw further weight behind the solutions of remaining issues. Driven by the limitations and motivated by the challenges of ECG, the need for novel cardiac gating/triggering technology is discussed. Current trends, such as the trend towards wireless techniques and the move to acoustic cardiac gating techniques, and their implications for daily routine MR applications are surveyed. Demonstrable progress in gating/triggering technology and methodology is shown to provide further encouragement for the imaging community to tackle solutions of the outstanding issues. A concluding section of the presentation explores future directions fueled by a set of alternative gating/triggering techniques.

2. Clinical needs for ECG in MRI

MRI is not a real time imaging modality. In day-to-day clinical routine MRI data acquisition is commonly propagated over a series of cardiac cycles. Consequently, cardiac activity can degrade image quality, particularly when motion suppression techniques are unavailable, unsuccessful or not utilized. The challenge of synchronization of data acquisition with the cardiac cycle constitutes a practical impediment of MRI so that MRI of the heart, large vessels and other organs experiencing motion related to cardiac activity requires speed and efficiency due to cardiac motion and flow constraints, which dictate the viable window for data acquisition.

The need for speed and efficiency prompted the development of various cardiac motion compensation and cardiac motion synchronization techniques. Cardiac motion has been addressed by synchronization strategies exploiting (i) finger plethysmography (Lanzer et.al. 1984), (ii) cardiac activity related esophageal wall motion (Brau et.al. 2002), (iii) invasive left ventricular blood pressure gating (Pattynama et.al. 1994), (iv) Doppler ultrasound (Rubin et.al. 2000), (v) motion induced changes in the impedance match of RF-coils (Buikman et.al. 1988), (vi) self gating techniques (Buehrer et.al. 2008, Crowe et.al. 2004, Larson et.al. 2005, Larson et.al. 2004, Nijm et.al. 2008), (vii) finger pulse oximetry (POX) triggering/gating techniques and optic acoustic methods (Rengle et.al. 2007) including human and animal studies.

In current clinical MR practice, cardiac motion is commonly dealt with using electrocardiographic (ECG) gating/triggering techniques (Chia et.al. 2000, Fischer et.al. 1999, Lanzer et.al. 1985) to synchronize data acquisition with the cardiac cycle. For this purpose, prospective triggering and retrospective gating regimes have been established as summarized in Figure 1. Both triggering/gating regimes share the principle, that only portions of the data needed to form the final image are acquired per cardiac cycle. This data acquisition approach is called segmentation, with the full MR data set being acquired segment by segment over a series of consecutive R-R intervals.

Prospective triggering is used to position the data acquisition window into a specific cardiac phase as demonstrated in Figure 1. Commonly, prospectively triggered MR data acquisition is conducted during the cardiac rest period at mid-diastole to avoid cardiac motion artifacts as illustrated in Figure 1. For this purpose acquisition windows ranging from 50 ms to 200 ms duration are usually applied. If data acquisition is performed during cardiac phases other than the cardiac rest period image quality can be heavily diminished due to cardiac motion effects. For example, Figure 1 shows images of the right coronary artery (RCA) derived from MR angiography (MRA) using acquisition windows placed around systole. For acquisition windows placed at 265 ms and 432 ms in the cardiac cycle, MRAs of the RCA show severe degradation in image quality due to cardiac and coronary artery motion throughout the course of the acquisitions window.

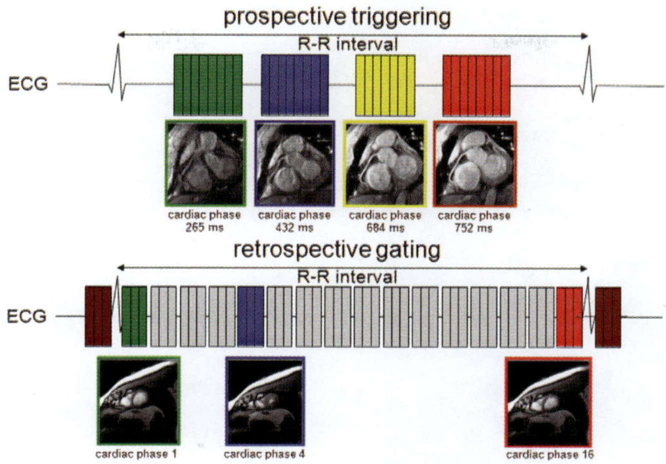

Fig. 1. Basic scheme of prospective triggering and retrospective gating in cardiac MRI using the electrocardiogram.

For retrospective gating data acquisition windows - each covering a specific cardiac phase of limited duration - are spread equidistantly across the entire R-R interval. This approach affords retrospective reconstruction of a series of images of the heart, which form a CINE movie. These movies are used to track myocardial contraction and relaxation for the goal of myocardial (dys)function assessment or cardiac chamber quantification. If the acquisition windows are kept short (20 ms to 50 ms) image quality is free of motion artifacts while long acquisition windows (larger than 50 ms) may hamper image quality due to cardiac motion effects; in particular at systole as illustrated in Figure 2.

To summarize, prospective triggering and retrospective gating regimes require a reliable tracking and monitoring of the cardiac cycle. The quality and stability of the QRS complex detection throughout the exam will dictate the efficiency of scanning and the overall image quality of scans. Mis-detection or mis-registration of the ECG's R-wave can corrupt image quality severely.

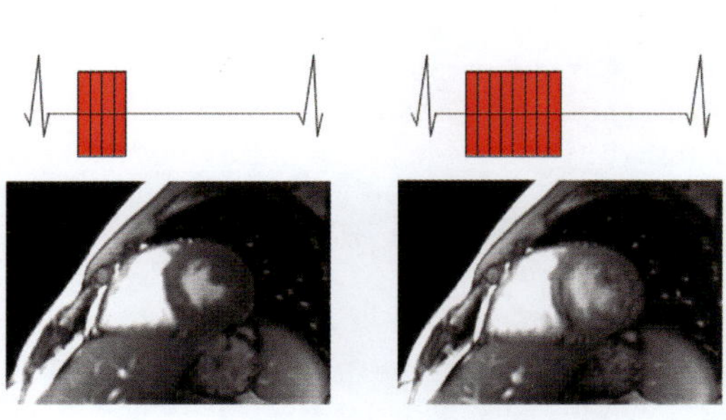

Fig. 2. Short axis views of the heart derived from CINE MRI illustrating the impact of cardiac motion on image quality. Two different durations for the acquisition window were used: (left) short acquisition window (50 ms, marked in red), (right) long acquisition window (200 ms, marked in red).

3. Practical considerations

In current clinical MR practice, MR scanners are equipped with extra hardware for ECG signal detection and processing. The basic setup for ECG monitoring in a clinical MRI environment is shown in Figure 3. This includes (i) ECG electrodes, leads and short high impedance cables, (ii) signal preamplifier and converter box, (iii) optical-fiber or wireless connections used for ECG signal transfer, (iv) physiological monitoring unit for signal processing and trigger generation. The signal flow in Figure 3 is from the left (signal collection using ECG-electrodes), through the middle (signal processing), to the right (input to the MR-systems internal ECG circuitry).

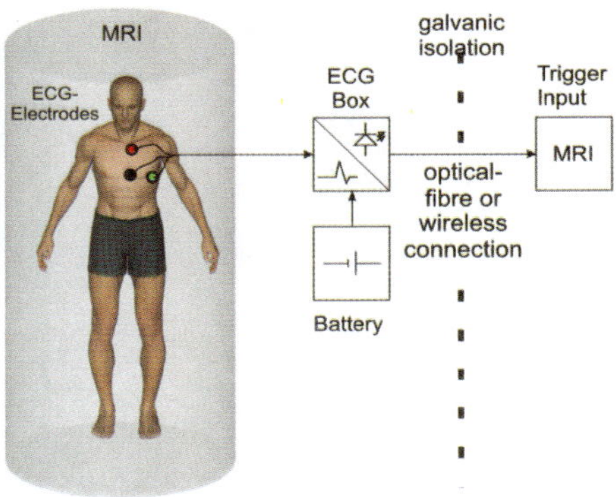

Fig. 3. Basic setup for ECG monitoring in a clinical MRI environment.

Patient preparation such as skin preparation, electrode and lead positioning are of profound importance for any successful ECG monitoring in an MRI environment. Careful skin preparation includes (i) removal of chest hair by shaving, if applicable, (ii) cleaning of the skin with special abrasive skin prepping gel and (iii) the use of a clean gauze pad to thoroughly dry the skin area where the surface electrodes will be positioned. Typical placement of ECG surface electrodes in an MRI environment might differ from ECG electrode positioning commonly used in conventional ECG monitoring. Admittedly, a stronger signal can be achieved from widely spaced electrodes. However, this approach can induce artifacts in the ECG trace in an MRI environment. Consequently, in an MRI environment ECG electrodes are placed relatively close to each other on the left hand side of the upper torso as illustrated in Figure 4. Obtaining a good ECG signal requires the lead alignment with the strongest ECG vector and a good adhesion between the ECG electrode and the patient's skin. It is highly recommended to use electrodes before their expiration date only since old electrodes can be dried out, which will result in bad electrical contact.

The ECG signal transferred into the scanners internal circuitry interfaces is used for gating and triggering of MR acquisitions. For this purpose different parameters can be modified on the scanners user interface to time MR imaging. Those parameters include a trigger delay to place the data acquisition at any phase in the cardiac cycle, the number of cardiac phases to be imaged and a trigger window to allow changes in the heart rate of 10%-20% during the course of segmented MR acquisitions. If changes in the heart rate exceed the duration of the trigger window, arrhythmia rejection will be applied. This means that MR data acquired during cardiac cycles with a duration shorter or longer than the predefined range will be discarded and re-acquired. Of course, this approach increases the scan time. Hence a very limited number of arrhythmia rejections are accepted for breath-held scans.

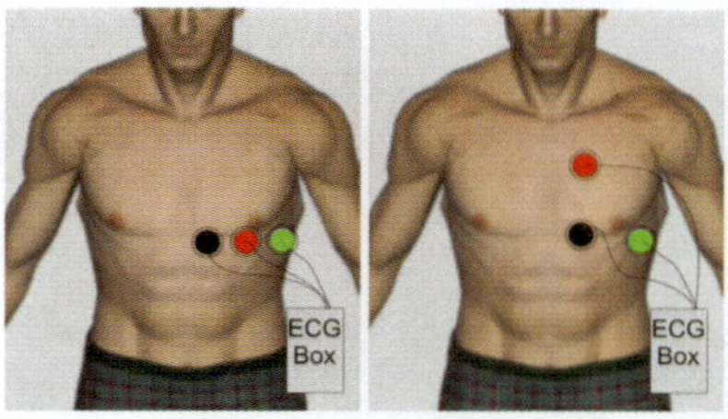

Fig. 4. Typical placement of ECG surface electrodes in an MRI environment. (left) placement in a parallel order which is beneficial for ultra high magnetic fields and (right) the traditional placement of ECG electrodes at field strengths of 1.5 T, which is used by the majority of clinical MR scanner.

4. Safety implications and safety measures

Conventional ECG electrodes are not classified as being MR-safe due to the use of low impedance conductors or ferromagnetic components. ECG, being an inherently electrical measurement with electrically active components (Lanzer et.al. 1985), does carry a risk of surface heating of patients' skin and even of skin burns resulting from induction of high voltages in ECG electrodes or ECG cables due to interactions with RF fields used in MRI (Health 2010, Kugel et.al. 2003, Lange & Nguyen 2006, Shellock & Crues 2004, Shellock & Kanal 1996). The use of non MR safe ECG hardware has even caused an incident in the MR bore, where high-voltage induction in ECG wiring caused a fire (Kugel et.al. 2003).

Various safety measures and technologies have been implemented on clinical MR scanners to safeguard patients with the ultimate goal of avoiding disasters and injuries due to ECG hardware and it's interaction with electromagnetic fields. If electrical ECG leads are used they should not be allowed to form loops which otherwise bear the potential to serve as an RF antenna which might result in burning hazards. Safety measures also involve the use of ECG electrodes being classified as MR-safe. Consequently, user manuals of clinical scanners outline explicitly that MR-safe electrodes which are made available through the MR vendor's accessories catalogue must be used.

Safety measures also recommend the use of high impedance leads instead of conventional low impedance leads. Figure 5 demonstrates how a low impedance wire increases the Rf power deposition inside the human body. Keeping ECG leads as short as possible is essential. In the ideal case ECG leads shorter than the radio-frequency (RF) wave length need to be employed. For this reason the user manuals of clinical MR systems emphasize or even dictate that only ECG cables and ECG equipment provided by the MR vendor must be used. To keep ECG leads short, fiber optic leads or wireless connections are used in modern systems for signal transfer between the battery powered ECG converter box and the MRI system.

The clinical need of ECG monitoring prior/after MRI examinations bears the risk of leading to RF induced skin burns since patients might undergo an MRI scan without removing conventional ECG electrodes commonly used in the telemetry unit. The FDA's MAUDE data base reports several skin burns in for the period 2005-2010 due to induction of high voltages in ECG hardware due to interaction with RF fields (Health 2010), the main cause being that conventional ECG leads used for patient monitoring were not removed or replaced prior to the MR scan.

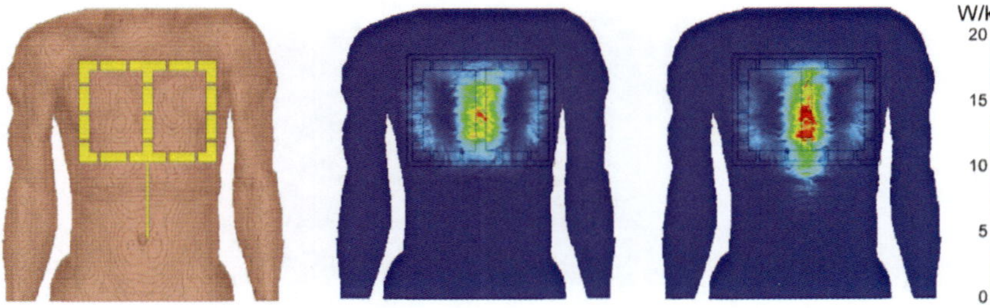

Fig. 5. Signal absorption rate (SAR) simulations which demonstrate the impact of low impedance ECG leads in a human voxel model (left). For this purpose a 4 channel transmit/receive cardiac RF coil was used. The lead positioning mimics the clinical situation where ECG leads are positioned between the coil and the surface of the anterior chest. Point SAR simulations of the cardiac coil at 7T without the lead (middle) and with the lead (right) are shown. RF power deposition is pronounced in the presence of the leads.

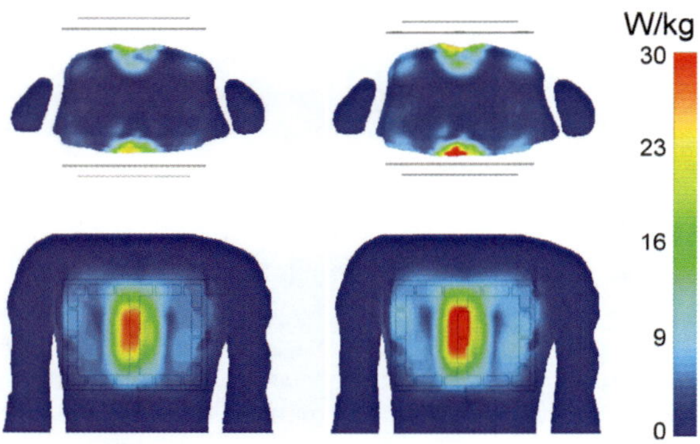

Fig. 6. Axial and coronal views of the upper torso derived from signal absorption rate (SAR_{10g}) simulations. The simulations demonstrate the impact of extra padding for the purpose of keeping RF coils in a safe distance from ECG electrodes. For padding an extra layer with a thickness of 1cm was inserted between the anterior and posterior section of the coil and the anterior and posterior upper chest. For the simulations a 4 channel transmit/receive RF cardiac coil was used together with an accepted power of 30 W without padding (left) and with padding (right). With padding a maximum local SAR_{10g} value of 18.1 W/kg is reached. Without padding the maximum local SAR_{10g} value increased to 21.2 W/kg. This value would exceed the IEC safety guidelines of 20 W/kg.

The manufacturer's user manuals for RF coils advice the use of extra padding for keeping RF coils in a safe distance from ECG electrodes being mounted to the chest. This measure has been implemented to avoid ECG electrodes being positioned in areas of high local electromagnetic (EM) fields caused by the RF coil's. The influence of extra padding on the SAR distribution can be seen in Figure 6.

5. Interference of ECG with magnetic fields

Electrocardiograms acquired in the MR environment are not a patient emergency condition indicator due to ECG waveform distortions. If brought into a magnetic field ECG being an electrical measurement is corrupted by interference with electromagnetic fields and by magneto-hydrodynamic (MHD) effects (Frauenrath et.al. 2009, Stuber et.al. 2002, Togawa et.al. 1967). MHD potential is induced when a conductive fluid travels through a magnetic field. The interference between the magnetic field and the conductive fluid generates a voltage perpendicular to the magnetic field lines and the direction of the fluid flow (Togawa et.al. 1967). The MHD voltage (V) can be described by:

$$V=\int_0^L u \times B \ dL \tag{1}$$

where **B** is the magnetic flux density (T) , **u** is the velocity of the fluid (m/s) , and **dL** is the distance vector between electrodes (Togawa et.al. 1967).

In the clinical setting the MHD effect creates voltages related to blood flow which are superimposed to the ECG potential as surveyed in Figure 7. The MHD effect is pronounced during cardiac phases of systolic aortic flow, which results in a severe distortion of the ECG's S-T segment. The susceptibility to electromagnetic field (EMF) interference manifests itself in ECG waveform distortions already apparent in ECG traces acquired in clinical 1.5 T MR scanners (Becker et.al. 2009). As high and ultrahigh field MR becomes more widespread, the propensity of ECG recordings to MHD effects is further pronounced (Brandts et.al. 2010, Frauenrath et.al. 2009, Snyder et.al. 2009) as demonstrated in Figure 7. Figure 7 shows ECG traces obtained at magnetic field strengths of 1.5 T, 3.0 T and 7.0 T which were acquired simultaneously to prospectively cardiac gated 3D phase contrast MR angiography acquisitions. At 3.0 T severe distortions were detected for cardiac phases around the S-T segment. At 7.0 T the MHD contributions gain amplitudes which are in the order of magnitude of or even larger than the amplitude of the ECG's R-wave.

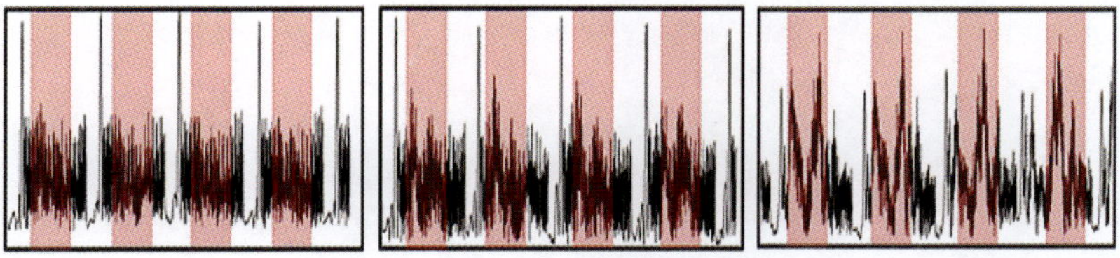

Fig. 7. Unfiltered electrocardiograms (ECG) obtained at magnetic field strengths of 1.5 T (left), 3.0 T (middle) and 7.0 T (right). ECG waveforms were susceptible to T-wave elevation and other waveform distortions shaded in red which increased with field strengths and were pronounced at 7.0 T.

Artifacts in the ECG trace and severe T-wave elevation might be mis-interpreted as R-waves resulting in misdetection of cardiac activity or erroneous cardiac gating together with motion corrupted image quality. These artifacts render MHD effects detrimental for a reliable synchronization of MRI or registration of MRI data with the cardiac cycle and constitute a practical impediment as outlined in Figure 8. Figure 8 shows mid-ventricular, short axis views of the heart together with whole R-R interval time series of one-dimensional projections along the profile (dotted line) marked in the short axis view (top), trigger detection tickmarks used for synchronization of MR imaging with the cardiac cycle which were obtained from a single subject over 18 cardiac cycles after temporal realignment using cross correlation and reassignment (middle) and ECG signal waveforms obtained from the same single subject over 18 cardiac cycles (bottom). In spite of ECG's severe signal distortion faultless ECG triggering was observed for the example shown on the left hand side of Figure 8. In this example of correct recognition of the onset of cardiac activity, ECG gated 2D CINE MRI was found to be immune to the effects of cardiac motion as demonstrated by the sharp delineation between blood and myocardium throughout the entire cardiac cycle. An example of

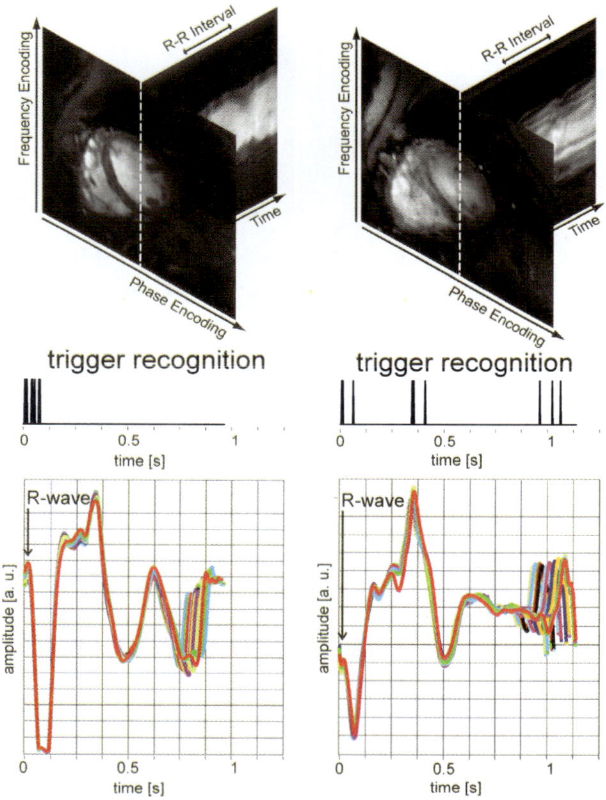

Fig. 8. Top) Mid-ventricular, short axis views of the heart together with whole R-R interval time series of one-dimensional projections along the profile (dotted line) marked in the short axis view. (Middle) Trigger recognition tick marks. Bottom) ECG waveforms obtained from a single subject over 18 cardiac cycles. (Left) Faultless Gating: Clinically acceptable image quality because of the absence of cardiac motion induced blurring; (Right) Erroneous ECG Gating, which diminished the image quality due to cardiac motion induced image blurring.

erroneous ECG trigger detection is shown on the right hand side of Figure 8. Here ECG gated 2D CINE MRI was prone to severe cardiac motion artifacts due to R-wave mis-registration which induced reduction in myocardium/blood contrast and image sharpness. To this end, R-wave mis-registration has been consistently reported for ECG triggered CMR at 7.0 T (Brandts et.al. 2010, Maderwald et.al. 2010). In one report 20% of the healthy subjects needed to be excluded from left ventricular function assessment (Brandts et.al. 2010). In another study 80% of the acquisitions were gated using pulse oximetry due to MHD artifact induced ECG-triggering problems (Maderwald et.al. 2010).

6. Patient monitoring in the fringe field of a MR scanner

Although ECG is known to be non-diagnostic within the bore of any clinical MR system due to magneto-hydrodynamic (MHD) effects, there are an increasing number of clinical indications that require ECG monitoring prior to/after the MR scan or in the MR scanner room using conventional 12 leads ECG devices as a patient emergency indicator (Cheng et.al. 2003, Lubbers et.al. 2011, Paetsch et.al. 2004, Wahl et.al. 2004). For example, in addition to continuous monitoring during stress testing which is commonly used in cardiovascular MRI, ECG monitoring should resume as quickly as possible after post stress MR imaging - ideally while the patient is still on the MRI table or in the fringe magnetic field of the MR scanner as outlined by Jekic et.al. (Jekic et.al. 2010). This monitoring approach requires the ECG signal to stay within the accuracy limits defined by the guidelines of the American Heart Association (AHA) for automated electrocardiography (Bailey et.al. 1990). These guidelines outline that deviation of the real ECG trace due to magneto-hydrodynamic effects from the true, uncompromised waveform taken outside of the MR environment may not exceed 0.025 mV or 5%, whichever is greater. A recent publication reported that this threshold can be achieved in the fringe field of an MRI system for stray magnetic field strengths lower than 70 mT (Jekic et.al. 2010). Also, the clinical need of ECG monitoring prior/after MRI bears the risk of leading to RF induced skin burns since patients might undergo an MRI scan without removing conventional ECG electrodes commonly used in the telemetry unit.

7. ECG alternatives for cardiac gated/triggered MRI

Various approaches have been proposed to cancel, correct for, bypass or extract MHD blood flow potential induced artifacts from the surface electrocardiogram. These efforts include optimization of ECG electrode placement (Dimick et.al. 1987), R-wave detection algorithm based on the vector cardiogram (Fischer et.al. 1999), and sophisticated ECG signal processing (Nijm et.al. 2008).

Realizing the constraints of conventional ECG, a MR-stethoscope has been proposed for the pursuit of robust and safe clinical cardiac gated/triggered MRI (Frauenrath et.al. 2008, Niendorf et.al. 2010). In contrast to ECG-triggering the MR-stethoscope employs acoustic instead of electrical signals. For cardiac gating/triggering, the first heart tone of the phonocardiogram, which marks the onset of the acoustic cardiac cycle, is selected. The acoustic gating device meets the following criteria:

- free of interference with electromagnetic fields
- immunity to magneto-hydrodynamic effects at 1.5 T, 3.0 T and 7.0 T
- compliance with the safety regulations on medical devices defined by the CE and FDA
- support of prospective- and retrospective cardiac gating/triggering regimes

As shown by the block diagram in Figure 9, the acoustic gating device comprises three main components: (i) an acoustic sensor, (ii) a signal processing unit and (iii) a coupler unit to the MRI system (Frauenrath et.al. 2008). Like the chest piece of a common stethoscope, the acoustic sensor, located on the patient's chest, registers the heart sounds. The signal processing unit detects the first heart sound and transforms it into a trigger signal, which mimics the basic waveform of the ECG. The MR-Stethoscope is compatible with common MRI scanners and does not require any hardware or software changes. It should be noted that the R-wave which marks the electrophysiological onset of the cardiac cycle and the 1st heart tone which represents the onset of the acoustic cardiac cycle are separated by a physiological delay of Δt=30 ms (Rangayyan & Lehner 1987). However, it was found that the delay between ECG and the phonocardiogram is heart rate independent (Frauenrath et.al. 2008).

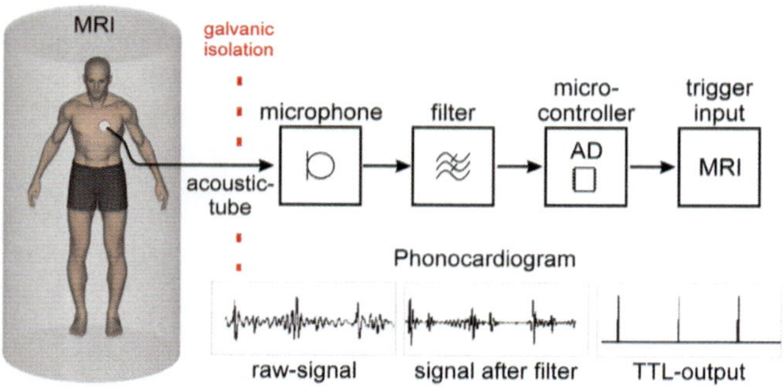

Fig. 9. Block diagram of acoustic cardiac triggering (ACT). ACT is free of interferences from electromagnetic fields and magneto-hydrodynamic effects, and provides a reliable trigger signal free of jitter even in the presence of free breathing.

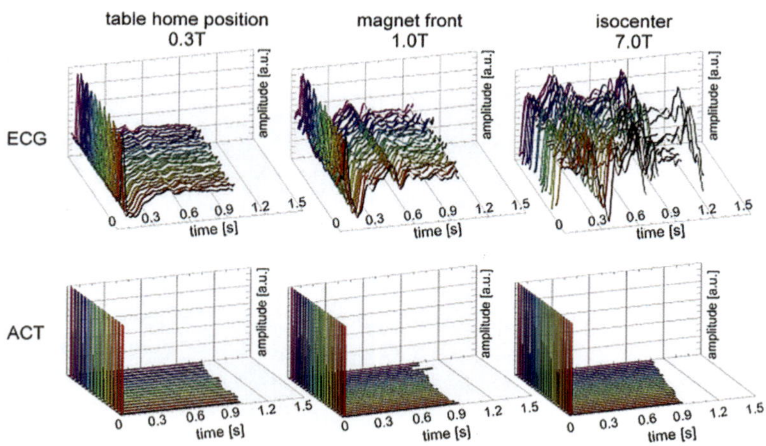

Fig. 10. ECG (top) and acoustic trigger signal (bottom) traces acquired at three different field strengths using the MRI scanners internal physiological signal processing unit. Severe signal distortion occurred in the ECG signal obtained at the magnet's isocenter, whereas the trigger signal derived from ACT remains undistorted

The use of the MR stethoscope substantially reduces the complexity of patient preparation for an MR examination by obviating the need to set up ECG-electrodes and position ECG-leads. Even more, the acoustic triggering (ACT) approach offers suitability for all magnetic field strengths (Frauenrath et.al. 2009, Frauenrath et.al. 2010) as indicated in Figure 10. ACT presents immunity to electromagnetic interference and magneto-hydrodynamic effects as demonstrated in Figure 10 (Frauenrath et.al. 2009, Frauenrath et.al. 2010) which helps to reduce - if not to eliminate - the effect of R-wave mis-registration which is frequently encountered in ECG-triggered acquisitions, in particular at high and ultrahigh magnetic field strengths (Brandts et.al. 2010, Brants et.al. 2010, Maderwald et.al. 2010).
Examples of cardiac images derived from ECG and ACT gated/triggered MR imaging are shown in Figure 11 including retrospective gating and prospective triggering regimes. For retrospective gating Figure 11 shows four chamber views of the heart derived from cardiac gated 2D CINE MRI. ECG gated 2D CINE MRI was prone to severe cardiac motion artifacts if R-wave mis-registration occurred, which resulted in cardiac motion induced blurring. Unlike ECG, ACT gating produced images free of cardiac motion artefacts as illustrated in Figure 11. For prospective triggering examples derived from free breathing coronary artery MR imaging, an application which exhibits pronounced sensitivity to cardiac motion are depicted in Figure 11. For example, the displacement of the right coronary artery (RCA) is in the order of 3 cm to 4 cm throughout the course of cardiac cycle. Mis-triggering due to distortions in the ECG-trace resulted in image blurring embodied by reduced RCA vessel sharpness and diminished RCA vessel delineation. Robust and reliable triggering using ACT revealed excellent image quality for CAI, which is free of motion artifacts.

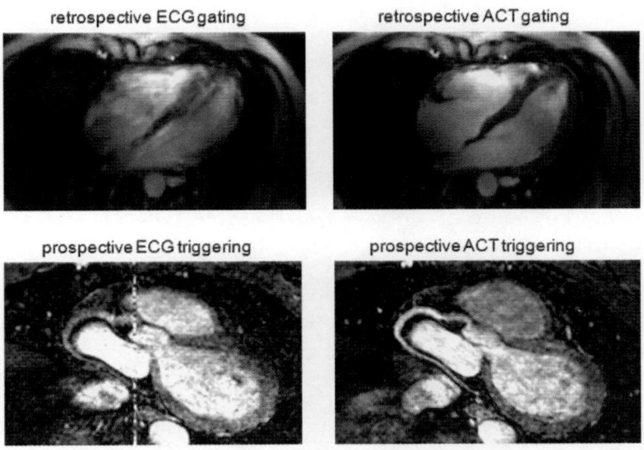

Fig. 11. Top: Four chamber views of the heart derived from ECG (left) and ACT (right) gated 2D CINE MRI at 7.0 T. Unlike ECG which caused mis-triggering ACT gated acquisitions provided a reliable trigger signal together with sharp images. Bottom: Maximum intensity projections (MIP) obtained from free breathing, cardiac gated CAI using ECG triggering (left) and ACT triggering (right) at 1.5 T. Mis-triggering due to distortions in the ECG-trace resulted in image blurring embodied by reduced vessel sharpness and diminished vessel delineation. The DC-offset seen in the centre line of the ECG-gated images is due to RF interferences with the electronics of the ECG-device's A/D converter, which is battery powered and usually positioned on the anterior chest of the volunteer. Robust and reliable triggering using ACT revealed excellent image quality for CAI, which is free of motion artifacts.

The acoustic approach also appears to be an excellent candidate for gating acquisitions in areas located distant from the heart. In clinical practice, areas of interest are usually positioned at the magnet's isocenter. Consequently, the position of the heart together with the position of the ECG electrodes in non-cardiac studies is off-center, closer to the rear or front end bell of the MR scanner gradient coils, which amplifies changes in dB/dt during gradient coil switching which is used for spatial encoding. This geometrical constraint increases the interference between the electrophysiological signals and electro-magnetic fields generated by the gradients, leading to pronounced distortion of the ECG signal. The capability of local acoustic gating can in principal serve to alleviate substantially the fundamental problem of erroneous ECG-gating for off-center positions of the heart. Fetal cardiovascular MRI is another emerging application (Saleem 2008) which suffers from synchronization problems and hence is a driving force for further advancement of the MR-stethoscope towards capturing fetal phonocardiograms at (ultra)high magnetic fields.

8. Future directions

Demonstrable progress in ECG technology and methodology used in the MRI environment is providing encouragement for the imaging community to tackle the solution of the outstanding issues. This includes the refinement and redesign of ECG hardware and devices used in a MR environment but also the broad move towards alternative cardiac gating/triggering approaches. One important development on the hardware horizon is the advent of acoustic triggering techniques using pressure transducers or optical microphones for signal detections. Future development also involve the development of even more sophisticated ECG signal processing algorithms to compensate for MHD contributions to the ECG signal. Even more, contrary to the common notion that considers MHD being adverse concomitants or detrimental artifacts of traditional ECG acquired in a magnetic field environment it is conceptually appealing to explore the merits of MHD effects for the pursuit of cardiac gated MRI. It has been recently proposed that the MHD effect being inherently sensitive to magnetic flux density, flow, orientation of flow with respect to the magnetic field lines and velocity of an electrical charge carrier such as blood in a magnetic field (Togawa et.al. 1967). These characteristics can be put to use as an alternative approach for registration of cardiac activity and for cardiac gating/triggering (Frauenrath et.al. 2011). Early applications include acquisition of MHD waveforms in surface areas close to the heart and the aortic arch but also in peripheral regions including surface areas close to the right common carotid artery, close to the forearm's ulnar artery and close to the lower leg's posterior tibial artery (Frauenrath et.al. 2011).

In any case, the unmet clinical needs and (un)solved problems of cardiovascular MRI are likely to motivate novel approaches used for the assessment of cardiac activity and for the tracking of cardiac contraction and relaxation. One intriguing development on the methodology horizon is the non-contact detection of myocardium's mechanical activity by ultrawideband RF-radar and its interpretation applying electrocardiography (Thiel et.al. 2009, Thiel et.al. 2009). To drive this approach into a clinical application an understanding of how the myocardiums mechanic is rendered by reflected and post processed UWB radar signals is essential (Thiel et.al. 2009, Thiel et.al. 2009). To this end, pioneering research is moved forward to correlate the UWB signal with the ECG through simultaneous acquisition and evaluation of radar signals with signals from a high-resolution electrocardiogram (Thiel et.al. 2009, Thiel et.al. 2009).

9. Conclusion

In short, while today's development of ECG techniques remain in a state of creative flux, productive engagement in this area continues to drive further developments with the ultimate goal of enhancing the capabilities of ECG in a modern high and ultrahigh field MR environment for synchronization of MR data acquisition with the cardiac cycle or for co-registration of functional MR mapping techniques with cardiac activity. Such improvements would benefit an ever growing set of indications for cardiovascular and neurovascular MR applications; in particular those which aim for high spatial resolution which can be easily compromised by physiological motion. If practical challenges can be overcome with appropriate hardware and post-processing design, an optimistically-inclined practitioner might envisage ECG technology tailored for MR which might even open the door to patient monitoring in an MR environment. While this is, for the moment, merely a vision, it continues to motivate new basic and clinical research.

10. Acknowledgment

The authors gratefully acknowledge the enthusiastic researchers at the Berlin Ultrahigh Field Facility (B.U.F.F.), Berlin, Germany, who kindly contributed examples of their pioneering work and other valuable assistance.

11. References

Assomull RG; Pennell DJ & Prasad SK. (2007) Cardiovascular magnetic resonance in the evaluation of heart failure. *Heart*; 93:985-992.

Bailey JJ; Berson AS; Garson A, Jr. (1990) Recommendations for standardization and specifications in automated electrocardiography: bandwidth and digital signal processing. A report for health professionals by an ad hoc writing group of the Committee on Electrocardiography and Cardiac Electrophysiology of the Council on Clinical Cardiology, American Heart Association. *Circulation*; 81:730-739.

Becker M; Frauenrath T; Hezel F. (2009) Comparison of left ventricular function assessment using phonocardiogram- and electrocardiogram-triggered 2D SSFP CINE MR imaging at 1.5 T and 3.0 T. *Eur Radiol*.

Brandts A; Westenberg JJ; Versluis MJ. (2010) Quantitative assessment of left ventricular function in humans at 7 T. *Magn Reson Med*.

Brandts A; Westenberg JJ; Versluis MJ. (2010) Quantitative assessment of left ventricular function in humans at 7 T. *Magn Reson Med*; 64:1471-1477.

Brants A; Versluis M; de Roos A. (2010) Quantitative comparison of left ventricular cardiac volume, mass and function obtained at 7 Tesla with "gold standard" values at 1.5 Tesla. *Proc. Intl. Soc. Mag. Reson. Med.*; 18:1299; Stockholm, SE.

Brau AC; Wheeler CT; Hedlund LW. (2002) Fiber-optic stethoscope: a cardiac monitoring and gating system for magnetic resonance microscopy. *Magn Reson Med*; 47:314-321.

Buehrer M; Curcic J; Boesiger P. (2008) Prospective self-gating for simultaneous compensation of cardiac and respiratory motion. *Magn Reson Med*; 60:683-690.

Buikman D; Helzel T & Roschmann P. (1988) The rf coil as a sensitive motion detector for magnetic resonance imaging. *Magn Reson Imaging*; 6:281-289.

Cheng CP; Schwandt DF; Topp EL. (2003) Dynamic exercise imaging with an MR-compatible stationary cycle within the general electric open magnet. *Magn Reson Med;* 49:581-585.

Chia JM; Fischer SE; Wickline SA. (2000) Performance of QRS detection for cardiac magnetic resonance imaging with a novel vectorcardiographic triggering method. *J Magn Reson Imaging;* 12:678-688.

Crowe ME; Larson AC; Zhang Q. (2004) Automated rectilinear self-gated cardiac cine imaging. *Magn Reson Med;* 52:782-788.

Dimick RN; Hedlund LW; Herfkens RJ. (1987) Optimizing electrocardiograph electrode placement for cardiac-gated magnetic resonance imaging. *Invest Radiol;* 22:17-22.

Fischer SE; Wickline SA & Lorenz CH. (1999) Novel real-time R-wave detection algorithm based on the vectorcardiogram for accurate gated magnetic resonance acquisitions. *Magn Reson Med;* 42:361-370.

Frauenrath T; Niendorf T & Kob M. (2008) Acoustic method for synchronization of Magnetic Resonance Imaging (MRI). *Acta Acustica united with Acustica*:148-155.

Frauenrath T; Kozerke S; Henzel F. (2009) The MR-stethoscope: safe cardiac gating free of interference with electro-magnetic fields at 1.5 T, 3.0 T and 7.0 T. *Journal of Cardiovascular Magnetic Resonance;* 11:O78.

Frauenrath T; Hezel F; Heinrichs U. (2009) Feasibility of cardiac gating free of interference with electro-magnetic fields at 1.5 Tesla, 3.0 Tesla and 7.0 Tesla using an MR-stethoscope. *Invest Radiol;* 44:539-547.

Frauenrath T; Hezel F; Renz W. (2010) Acoustic cardiac triggering: a practical solution for synchronization and gating of cardiovascular magnetic resonance at 7 Tesla. *J Cardiovasc Magn Reson;* 12:67.

Frauenrath T; Dieringer M; Patel N. (2011) From Artifact to Merit: Cardiac Gated MRI at 7T and 3T Using Magneto-Hydrodynamic Effects for Synchronization.4611; Montreal.

Fuchs VR & Sox HC, Jr. (2001) Physicians' views of the relative importance of thirty medical innovations. *Health Aff (Millwood);* 20:30-42.

In: U.S. Food and Drug Administration. Center for Devices and Radiological Health. (2010) MAUDE data base reports of adverse events involving medical devices. http://www.accessdata.fda.gov/scripts/cdrh/cfdocs/cfMAUDE/search.CFM. accessed November 15, 2010.

Jekic M; Ding Y; Dzwonczyk R. (2010) Magnetic field threshold for accurate electrocardiography in the MRI environment. *Magn Reson Med*; 64:1586-1591.

Kelle S; Weiss RG & Stuber M. (2008) Coronary magnetic resonance imaging. *Curr Pharm Des;* 14:1778-1786.

Kramer CM; Barkhausen J; Flamm SD. (2008) Standardized cardiovascular magnetic resonance imaging (CMR) protocols, society for cardiovascular magnetic resonance: board of trustees task force on standardized protocols. *J Cardiovasc Magn Reson;* 10:35.

Kugel H; Bremer C; Puschel M. (2003) Hazardous situation in the MR bore: induction in ECG leads causes fire. *Eur Radiol;* 13:690-694.

Kwong RY & Korlakunta H. (2008) Diagnostic and prognostic value of cardiac magnetic resonance imaging in assessing myocardial viability. *Top Magn Reson Imaging;* 19:15-24.

Lange S & Nguyen QN. (2006) Cables and electrodes can burn patients during MRI. *Nursing;* 36:18.

Lanzer P; Botvinick EH; Schiller NB. (1984) Cardiac imaging using gated magnetic resonance. *Radiology;* 150:121-127.

Lanzer P; Barta C; Botvinick EH. (1985) ECG-synchronized cardiac MR imaging: method and evaluation. *Radiology;* 155:681-686.

Larson AC; White RD; Laub G. (2004) Self-gated cardiac cine MRI. *Magn Reson Med;* 51:93-102.

Larson AC; Kellman P; Arai A. (2005) Preliminary investigation of respiratory self-gating for free-breathing segmented cine MRI. *Magn Reson Med;* 53:159-168.

Lubbers DD; Rijlaarsdam-Hermsen D; Kuijpers D. (2011) Performance of adenosine "stress-only" perfusion MRI in patients without a history of myocardial infarction: a clinical outcome study. *Int J Cardiovasc Imaging.*

Maderwald S; Nassenstein K; Orzada S. (2010) MR imaging of cardiac wall-motion at 1.5T and 7T: SNR and CNR comparison. *Proc. Intl. Soc. Mag. Reson. Med.;* 18:1299; Stockholm, SE.

Niendorf T & Sodickson DK. (2006) Parallel imaging in cardiovascular MRI: methods and applications. *NMR Biomed;* 19:325-341.

Niendorf T; Hardy CJ; Giaquinto RO. (2006) Toward single breath-hold whole-heart coverage coronary MRA using highly accelerated parallel imaging with a 32-channel MR system. *Magn Reson Med;* 56:167-176.

Niendorf T & Sodickson DK. (2008) Highly accelerated cardiovascular MR imaging using many channel technology: concepts and clinical applications. *Eur Radiol;* 18:87-102.

Niendorf T; Sodickson DK; Krombach GA. (2010) Toward cardiovascular MRI at 7 T: clinical needs, technical solutions and research promises. *Eur Radiol;* 20:2806-2816.

Nijm GM; Swiryn S; Larson AC. (2008) Extraction of the magnetohydrodynamic blood flow potential from the surface electrocardiogram in magnetic resonance imaging. *Med Biol Eng Comput;* 46:729-733.

Nijm GM; Sahakian AV; Swiryn S. (2008) Comparison of self-gated cine MRI retrospective cardiac synchronization algorithms. *J Magn Reson Imaging;* 28:767-772.

Paetsch I; Jahnke C; Wahl A. (2004) Comparison of dobutamine stress magnetic resonance, adenosine stress magnetic resonance, and adenosine stress magnetic resonance perfusion. *Circulation;* 110:835-842.

Pattynama PM; van der Velde ET; Steendijk P. (1994) Cardiovascular MR imaging: pressure-gating using the arterial pressure signal from a conventional ferromagnetic micromanometer-tip catheter. *Magn Reson Imaging;* 12:531-534.

Pennell DJ; Sechtem UP; Higgins CB. (2004) Clinical indications for cardiovascular magnetic resonance (CMR): Consensus Panel report. *Eur Heart J;* 25:1940-1965.

Purdon PL & Weisskoff RM. (1998) Effect of temporal autocorrelation due to physiological noise and stimulus paradigm on voxel-level false-positive rates in fMRI. *Hum Brain Mapp;* 6:239-249.

Rangayyan RM & Lehner RJ. (1987) Phonocardiogram signal analysis: a review. *Crit Rev Biomed Eng;* 15:211-236.

Rengle A; Baboi L; Saint-Jalmes H. (2007) Optical cardiac and respiratory device for synchronized MRI on small animal. *Conf Proc IEEE Eng Med Biol Soc.*:2046-2049.

Rubin JM; Fowlkes JB; Prince MR. (2000) Doppler US gating of cardiac MR imaging. *Acad Radiol*; 7:1116-1122.

Saleem SN. (2008) Feasibility of MRI of the fetal heart with balanced steady-state free precession sequence along fetal body and cardiac planes. *AJR Am J Roentgenol*; 191:1208-1215.

Schwitter J. (2008) Extending the frontiers of cardiac magnetic resonance. *Circulation*; 118:109-112.

Shellock FG & Kanal E. (1996) Burns associated with the use of monitoring equipment during MR procedures. *J Magn Reson Imaging*; 6:271-272.

Shellock FG & Crues JV. (2004) MR procedures: biologic effects, safety, and patient care. *Radiology*; 232:635-652.

Snyder CJ; DelaBarre L; Metzger GJ. (2009) Initial results of cardiac imaging at 7 Tesla. *Magn Reson Med*; 61:517-524.

Stuber M; Botnar RM; Fischer SE. (2002) Preliminary report on in vivo coronary MRA at 3 Tesla in humans. *Magn Reson Med*; 48:425-429.

Thiel F; Hein M; Schwarz U. (2009) Combining magnetic resonance imaging and ultrawideband radar: a new concept for multimodal biomedical imaging. *Rev Sci Instrum*; 80:014302.

Thiel F; Kreiseler D & Seifert F. (2009) Non-contact detection of myocardium's mechanical activity by ultrawideband RF-radar and interpretation applying electrocardiography. *Rev Sci Instrum*; 80:114302.

Togawa T; Okai O & Oshima M. (1967) Observation of blood flow E.M.F. in externally applied strong magnetic field by surface electrodes. *Med Biol Eng*; 5:169-170.

Wahl A; Paetsch I; Roethemeyer S. (2004) High-dose dobutamine-atropine stress cardiovascular MR imaging after coronary revascularization in patients with wall motion abnormalities at rest. *Radiology*; 233:210-216.

Part 6

ECG Data Management

20

Broadening the Exchange of Electrocardiogram Data from Intra-Hospital to Inter-Hospital

Shizhong Yuan[1,2], Daming Wei[1,2,3] and Weimin Xu[2]
[1]*Biomedical Information Technology Laboratory, University of Aizu*
[2]*School of Computer Engineering and Science, Shanghai University*
[3]*Graduate School of Medicine, Tohoku University*
[1,3]*Japan*
[2]*China*

1. Introduction

An electrocardiogram (ECG) is a commonly used clinical tool to diagnose cardiac diseases. In most clinical practice, to improve ECG diagnosis accuracy, cardiologists not only determine the abnormal conditions of the current ECG, but also examine the serial changes in reference to the previous ECGs. Expert cardiologists strongly believe that ECG diagnosis is incomplete without a comparison to previous ECGs (Ariet et al., 2005). Obviously, a prerequisite for the clinical practice using serial ECG comparison is the availability of previous ECGs.

For the reason above, it has been a growing interest in medical informatics to improve ease of access to ECG data using information technology. Initially, the computer systems, now referred to as ECG management systems (EMSs), were invented to serve a valuable function for ECG data management (Crevasse & Ariet, 1987). They consisted of a central minicomputer that collected the ECG signals from peripheral electrocardiographs over serial cables, telephone lines or local area network, and provided the power to store and retrieve the collected ECG data. Storage and retrieval of ECG data were organized in the perspective of their future use, particularly for serial comparison, but also for different managerial and research purposes, such as over-reading by physicians, re-analysis by different ECG programs, and statistics for management (Fayn & Rubel, 1991). The EMS solution allows a patient's ECG data accessible throughout the hospital and anywhere outside the hospital through a Web interface.

A major issue in the employment of EMS is the interoperability between electrocardiographs and EMSs, and the interoperability among EMSs. In a major hospital, there are usually a number of electrocardiographs that are from different vendors. These electrocardiographs may use different vendor-proprietary standards for ECG data storage and transmission, but an EMS is developed conformably to only a few vendor-proprietary standards. In order to facilitate the use of electrocardiographs from different vendor, several EMSs that are conformable to different vendor-proprietary standards may coexist in a hospital. As for the issue of the interoperability among the EMSs, some possible solutions have been reported.

Firstly, de Wijs et al. developed the Unified ECG Framework to enable the use of a single viewer for different resting ECG formats (de Wijs et al., 2005). The main part of the Unified ECG Framework is an ECG Toolkit, which provides applications for ECG conversion and viewing (van Ettinger et al., 2008). By using the ECG toolkit all the resting ECGs recorded at the Thoraxcenter can be provided in three open standards: the Standard Communications Protocol for Computer-Assisted Electrocardiography (SCP-ECG) (Association for the Advancement of Medical Instrumentation, 1999), Digital Imaging and Communications in Medicine-Waveform Standard Supplement (DICOM 3.0) (DICOM Standards Committee, 2000), and the HL7 FDA annotated ECG standard (Brown & Badilini, 2005). This solution enables a hospital to be partially or completely manufacturer-independent for resting ECGs. Secondly, the EMS developed by Cho et al. provides the functionality to convert non-DICOM ECG data into DICOM waveform data and act as a DICOM waveform Storage Service Class User (SCU) to send the DICOM waveform data to the Picture Archiving and Communication System (PACS) (Cho et al., 2003). This solution makes the ECG data managed by such EMSs accessible on DICOM workstations. Thirdly, the Retrieve ECG for Display profile proposed by the Integrating Healthcare Enterprise initiative (IHE-ECG profile) (Integrating the Healthcare Enterprise [IHE], 2006) provides a means of ECG data exchange between EMSs. The IHE-ECG profile specifies the Web service interfaces to an EMS for retrieving a list of ECG documents pertaining to a certain patient and retrieving a particular ECG document. The ECG data to be retrieved are converted into the documents in the Adobe Portable Document Format (PDF) or the images in the Adobe Scalable Vector Graphics (SVG) format. Although the ECG data in the PDF format or in the SVG format are not usable any more for further computation, this solution is widely accepted and adopted (Marcheschi et al., 2006).

In addition to the methods and software for the interoperability of an EMS with other EMSs, HL7 interface software have been developed for EMSs to forward their ECG data to hospital information systems for historical record keeping and billing notification.

These facilities mentioned above for intra-hospital exchange of ECG data have significantly improved the ease of access to a patient's ECG data distributed in a hospital. However, the care and treatment of a patient doesn't often take place in a single hospital, and thus a patient's ECG data may distribute across multiple hospitals. This highlights the need for the inter-hospital exchange of a patient's ECG data. Ideally, a patient's historical ECG data should be available anywhere and whenever required.

In this chapter, we report our Web-based system for inter-hospital exchange of ECG data. This system provides a common Web portal for the discovery and retrieval of a particular patient's ECG data distributed across multiple hospitals. We present a metadata model for ECG data discovery and retrieval, and the ECG registry that provides ebXML-based Web services (OASIS, 2005b) for publishing and discovering ECG data using the metadata model. The system also empolyes a Web service framework invented for publishing the ECG data with the ECG registry from a hospital. The framework can interoperate with the disparate ECG data sources in a hospital, and has an access control mechanism to address the privacy and security issues related to the access to the ECG sources.

The chapter is organized as follows. First the system architecture is defined in Section 2 while Section 3 and 4 describe in detail the ECG registry and the Web service framework for the ECG data dissemination from a hospital. Then the performance evaluation results of the system are shown in Section 5. Finally the conclusions are given in Section 6.

2. System architecture

For the ease of access to a patient's ECG data across multiple hospitals, an efficient data discovery mechanism is necessary. Now, a couple of network models can be followed to design such a mechanism. One is the centralized model, which calls for a centralized storage of ECG data from all hospitals involved. Primarily due to the requirement of massive storage to contain all the ECG data and unnecessary bandwidth to upload ECG data from every hospital involved, this model does not scale well. The second model is the distributed model, which leaves the ECG data at their local hospitals and creates an index by collecting and correlating the information about each patient's ECG data from all the ECG data sources involved. The most evident advantages of this model are its performance and scalability. On one hand, all ECG data pertaining to a particular patient is somehow referenced as one of the individual entries in the index. Thus, the discovery process is just a single database query. On the other hand, the only data that needs to be distributed through the network is the indexing data, whose size is very small.

Our system architecture follows the distributed model. As shown in Fig. 1, it has a triangle-like configuration, including the ECG registry, the ECG providers and the ECG querist. The ECG registry is deployed in the Internet and populated with the information about the ECG data from all of the hospitals involved. The ECG providers are deployed in every hospital to populate the ECG registry with the information about the ECG data hold by the hospitals. Then through the ECG querists, which are Web applications, medical and healthcare professionals can search the ECG registry for a patient's ECG data and retrieve the ECG documents from the ECG providers deployed in the hospitals that hold them.

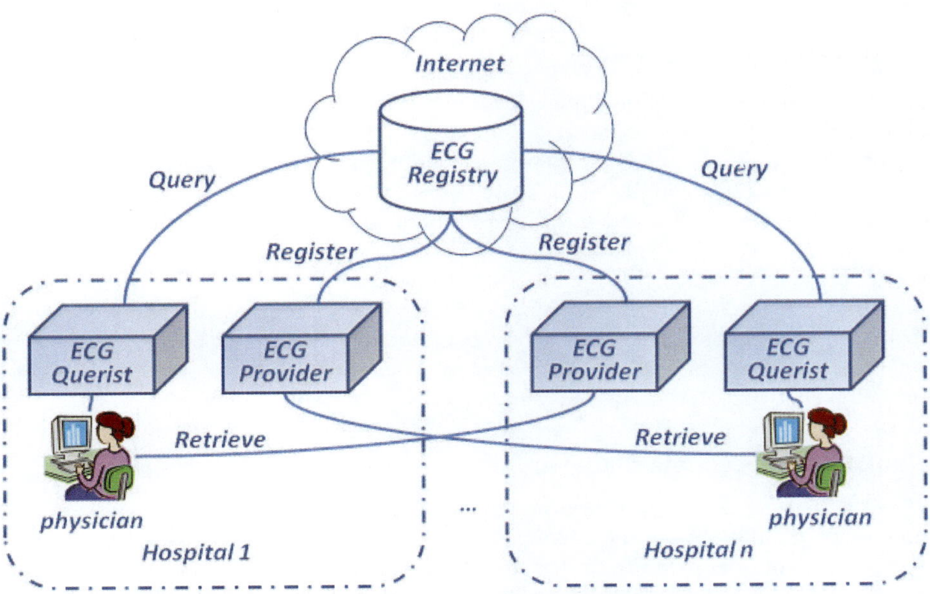

Fig. 1. System architecture for sharing ECG data among multiple hospitals

The key component of this architecture is the ECG registry. It should collect and correlate the information about patients' ECG data in an appropriate way so that patients' ECG data can be indexed for efficient searching. However, ECG data sources in the hospitals involved are mostly autonomous and heterogeneous. The standards they use for ECG storage and interchange may be different. Moreover, over time not only new ECG data sources may be involved, but also existing data sources may request submission of newly-acquired ECG data.

One potential solution to the above problems is to use metadata for enabling interoperability with heterogeneous ECG data sources and indexing ECG data for efficient and effective retrieval. Metadata are usually defined as data about data (Miller, 1996). It is most commonly used to describe an information resource, and consists of a set of attributes or elements necessary to describe that resource (Hillmann, 2000). It has been shown that metadata are not only an effective means for describing schemas in the database community and cataloguing the resources available in the library community, but also a realistic and scalable solution to two main issues pertaining to a resource discovery system: resource discovery and interoperability (Baptista et al., n.d.). Our goal here is to propose a metadata model for facilitating transparent discovery and retrieval of a patient's ECG data across all of the ECG data sources involved.

Fig. 2 presents the metadata model, named MetaEDR. It comprises two types of entities: ECG document that describes an ECG data resource and ECG provider that owns an ECG document. An ECG document must have one and only one ECG provider, and an ECG provider may have many ECG documents.

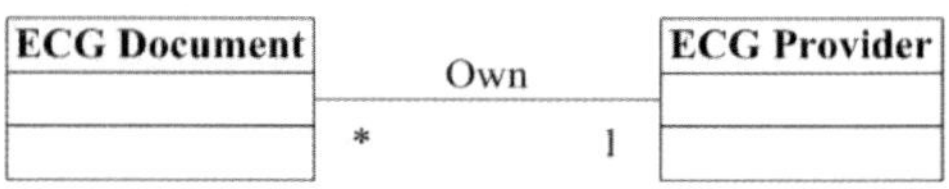

Fig. 2. MetaEDR conceptual schema

The metadata about an ECG document include the properties to enable resource discovery. They consist of three parts: a patient's demographic information such as identifier, name, date of birth, and gender; ECG attribute information such as acquisition date, type of ECG (standard 12-lead ECG, long-term ECG, or stress ECG), and data format (SCP-ECG, HL7 aECG, DICOM, or MFER); and information about technical access method and location URL.

The ECG providers are described using a set of metadata elements to provide the following information: a user-friendly name, an optional description, a global unique identifier, and Web service interfaces for harvesting ECG metadata and retrieving ECG data.

Every MetaEDR entity also has an associated set of administrative metadata, which include information about access control policy and privacy preservation policy.

3. Registry for ECG data discovery

The ECG registry is a Web-services-based platform shared for disseminating and discovering ECG data by means of MetaEDR. It is responsible for the storage of metadata and processing of queries on the metadata. We constructed the ECG registry based on the architecture of the ebXML (Electronic Business that uses eXtensible Markup Language) Registry (OASIS, 2005b).

3.1 Information model

An ebXML Registry is an information system that securely manages any content type and the standardized metadata that describes it. In order to support a wide variety of content, the ebXML Registry is designed with a well-defined information model. The information model of the ebXML Registry provides information on the type of metadata that is stored in the registry as well as the relationships among metadata classes (OASIS, 2005e). The RegistryObject class is an abstract base class used by most classes in the model. It provides minimal metadata for registry objects. Slot instances provide a dynamic way to add arbitrary attributes to RegistryObject instances. An Association class is a RegistryObject instance that is used to associate any two RegistryObject instances. An ExtrinsicObject instance provides metadata that describes submitted content whose type is not intrinsically known to the registry and therefore is described by additional attributes.

We use ExtrinsicObject class to include the MetaEDR information model. Fig. 3 illustrates the MetaEDR information model in the context of the ebXML Registry. ECG Document and ECG Provider in the MetaEDR are mapped into two subclasses of the ebXML ExtrinsicObject, named ECGEntry and ProviderEntry respectively. The association between ECGEntry and ProviderEntry is mapped into the ebXML Association.

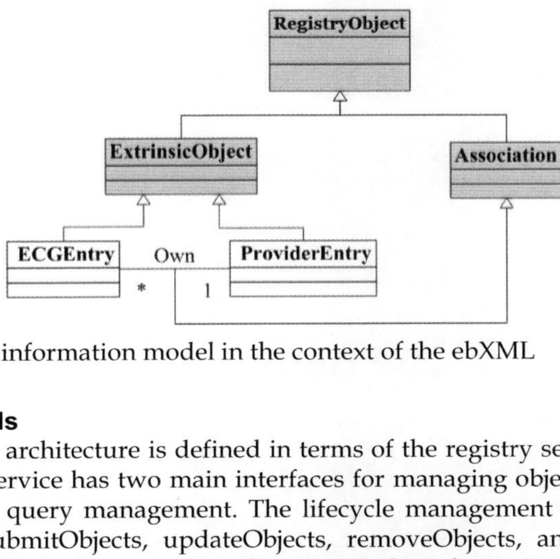

Fig. 3. The MetaEDR information model in the context of the ebXML

3.2 Service protocols

The ebXML Registry architecture is defined in terms of the registry service and the registry client. The registry service has two main interfaces for managing objects in the information model: lifecycle and query management. The lifecycle management interface has abstract methods such as submitObjects, updateObjects, removeObjects, and deprecatedObjects, which are used to submit objects or classifications to the information model. Similarly, the query management interface has interfaces such as submitAdhocQuery, getRegistryObject, and getRepositoryItem, which are used to query the registry itself.

The ECG registry provides two main services that enable the sharing of ECG data in a community of collaborative hospitals:

1. Register

It allows an ECG provider to register ECG data with the ECG registry, by supplying metadata about ECG data to be registered. Each of the ECG metadata will be used to create an instance of ECGEntry in the registry.

2. Query

It allows an ECG querist to query the registry for a particular patient's ECG. In response to this query, the registry returns all the metadata matching the query criteria.

An ECG provider submits a request message to call the "Register" service to register the metadata about ECGs, and the registry issues a response message to report the result status of metadata validation process or the success in creating the instances of ECGEntry for each submitted metadata. In our study, the request message and the response message use the messaging framework of the ebXML service protocol, which is SOAP message with MIME attachments. For the request message, the attachment is the SubmitObjectsRequest message, and for the response message, the attachment is the SubmitObjectsReponse message. The SubmitObjectsRequest message contains the metadata to be submitted, that is, an instance of ECGEntry.

Similarly, the request message submitted by an ECG querist to invoke the "Query" service is the SOAP message, the attachment of which is a standard ebXML AdhocQueryRequest message. In response, the registry returns the SOAP message with an ebXML AdhocQueryResponse message as its attachment. Within the AdhocQueryResponse message there is a list of instances of ECGEntry that contains metadata found to meet the query criteria. Fig. 4 depicts the messaging among the ECG registry, an ECG provider, and an ECG querist.

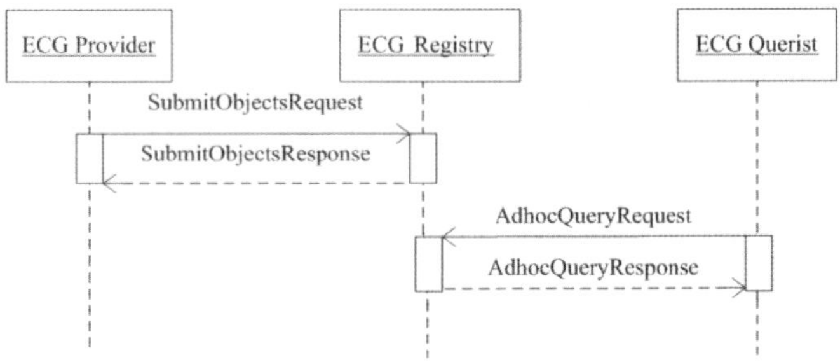

Fig. 4. Messaging between the ECG registry, an ECG provider, and an ECG querist

4. Web service framework for ECG data publishing

In our system, ECG providers are deployed in all the participating hospitals to publish the ECG data resources in every hospital with the ECG registry, and to serve the requests for the retrieval of the published ECG data. An ECG provider is required to be able to register all the ECG data in the ECG sources in a hospital including electrocardiographs, EMSs, and PACSs. However, there exist differences in ECG file formats and information exchange protocols between ECG sources, which conform to different standards. These differences pose the issue of interoperability with various ECG sources. In addition, an ECG provider has an obligation to apply privacy and security control to ECG data access when providing services to ECG retrieval requests.

In this section, we present a framework for ECG data publishing by an ECG provider. The framework specifies a set of functional components for an ECG provider, with the issues, such as the interoperability with various ECG sources, and privacy and security control, taken into account.

4.1 Framework for ECG data publishing

The framework for publishing ECG data is aimed at providing the functionalities of an ECG provider: ECG registration and ECG delivery. The former harvests the metadata about the latest ECG data from the ECG sources, such as an electrocardiograph, an EMS, and a PACS. The letter supports peer-to-peer retrieval of ECG data. When performing these functionalities, an ECG provider has to interact with several different actors for different purposes. One is the ECG registry, with which the ECG provider registers metadata about ECG data to be shared, and one is an ECG querist, to which the ECG provider renders ECG retrieval service. Others can be generalized into an ECG source actor that is simply an electrocardiograph, an EMS, or a PACS, from which the ECG provider acquires ECG data to be published for sharing. Fig. 5 depicts a set of components that accomplish the functionalities which an ECG provider should provide to these actors:

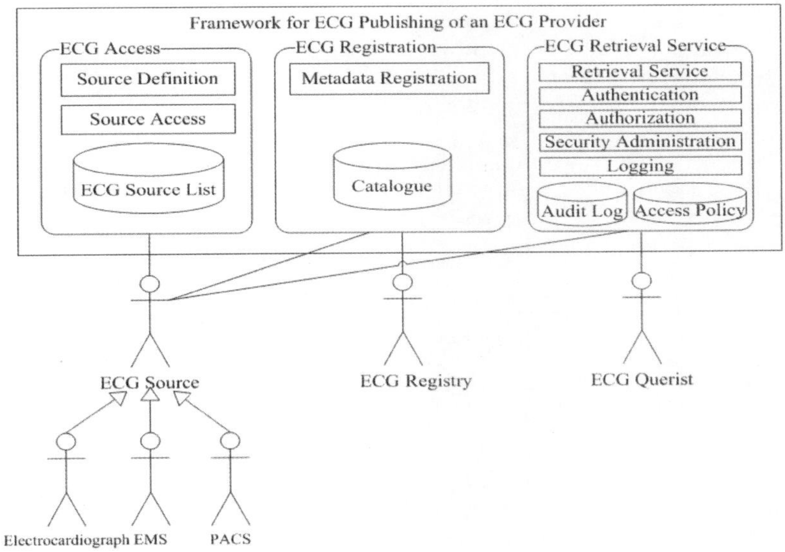

Fig. 5. Functional components of an ECG provider

1. ECG Access

This functionality supports the definition of a set of ECG sources and provides the capability to access ECG data from these ECG sources. It is accomplished by the Source Definition component and the Source Access component. The former aids a system administrator to define a collection of electrocardiographs, EMSs, and PACSs as the ECG sources with the result that each ECG source has an entry in the ECG Source List to record its configuration information, such as source type (electrocardiograph, EMS or PACS), source name, IP address and so on. The later has the capability to access ECGs from a specified ECG source.

2. ECG Registration

This functionality acquires the latest ECG data from the ECG sources, extracts the metadata about these ECG data and registers the metadata with the ECG registry. It is performed by the Metadata Registration component, with each registered ECG data appended to the Catalogue along with its source information required when the ECG data are retrieved.

3. ECG Retrieval Service

This functionality provides a Web service for ECG data retrieval to end users who are authenticated with the corresponding privilege. It is accomplished mainly by the Retrieval

Service component, which transmits the requested ECG data from its source to an end user. The Security Administration component, the Authentication component, the Authorization component, and the Logging component are for the purpose of privacy and access control of ECG resources.

4.2 Interoperability with ECG sources

The processing procedures of the Source Access component and the Metadata Registration component depend on the information exchange protocols and the ECG file formats that the ECG sources adopt. But there are differences in ECG file formats and information exchange protocols between ECG sources which conform to different standards like DICOM and MFER. These differences therefore pose the issue of interoperability with ECG sources. We addressed this interoperability issue through the introduction of Generic ECG Source Layer (GESL) between the two components and ECG sources, as shown in Fig. 6. The GESL is further divided into the Abstract ECG Source (AES) sub-layer and the ECG Source Adaption (ESA) sub-layer. The AES sub-layer provides the two components with ECG source-independent function interface to access ECG files and ECG metadata, and the ESA sub-layer comprises a set of ECG Source Adaptors, such as DICOM-Adaptor, MFER-Adapter and so on, each of which provides an ECG source-specific implementation of the ECG source-independent function interface.

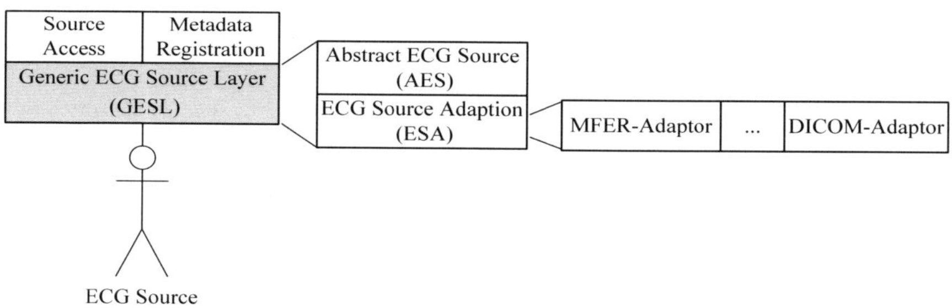

Fig. 6. Generic ECG Source Layer (GESL)

We use Web service technology to build GESL that makes disparate ECG data sources accessible in a uniform manner. Specifically, GESL is a Web service interface that provides operations for extracting metadata about ECG data and retrieving a particular patient's ECG data, and each ECG data source is wrapped with an adaptor that implements GESL by using the data access mechanism specific to the ECG data source.

4.3 Privacy preservation and access control

A patient's ECG data contain his/her sensitive clinical data, so an effective access control mechanism to protect them from disclosure to unauthorized persons is crucial to the successful realization of inter-hospital exchange of ECG data.

The design and implementation of such an access control mechanism can be challenging. On one hand, a user may request access to ECG data in hospitals other than his/her home hospital. The user relevant attributes need to be transferred from his/her home hospital to these hospitals for making a decision about the access request. On the other hand, hospitals may have different authorization policies controlling access to protected health information,

so what user relevant attributes are required for a hospital to evaluate authorization policies in making an access decision may be different among hospitals and unknown to other hospitals. Therefore, the access control mechanism should support authorization policy exchange and authorization determination among hospitals in an interoperable manner.
XACML (OASIS, 2005c), an OASIS standard, defines generic authorization architecture and the constructs for expressing and exchanging access control policy information using XML. SAML (OASIS, 2005a) (OASIS, 2005d), another OASIS standard, is an XML-based framework for communicating user authentication, entitlement, and attribute information among hospitals. XACML complements SAML so that not only policy decisions, as well as the policies themselves, can be exchanged in a standard fashion. Here we present an access control architecture based on XACML and SAML for inter-hospital access to ECG data.

4.3.1 Privacy and security requirements

A patient's ECG data are a kind of protected health information. ECG privacy deals with controlling who is authorized to access a patient's ECG data. It involves two aspects. On one hand, the access to a patient's ECG data is restricted to the individuals who need to access in order to perform their jobs. On the other hand, patients have the rights to create their privacy consent, which defines the rules for sharing and use of their ECG data.
In order to maintain the privacy of a patient's ECG data, the access control to be implemented has to protect a patient's ECG data from accidental or intentional disclosure to both individuals who have no job-related need to access them and individuals who have been denied the privilege to access them by a patient's privacy consent.

4.3.2 Two types of access polices based on the RBAC model

To restrict ECG data accessible to only individuals who have job-related need to access, the Role-Based Access Control (RBAC) model (Sandhu et al., 1996) is adopted. An administrator can create roles representing the job functions in their hospital, such as those defined in (IHE, 2008): Administrative Staff, Dietary Staff, General Care Provider, Direct Care Provider, Emergency Care Provider, and Researcher, Patient or Legal Representative. Each role is associated with an access rule, termed role privilege rule, which grants or denies the role permission to access to patients' ECG data. Individuals in the hospital may be assigned one or more roles representing the job functions they perform.
Patient privacy consent is also based on the RBAC mode. Each patient's ECG data is associated with an access rule, termed privacy consent rule, which defines which roles or which specific individuals may access the ECG data for specific purposes.
So there are two types of access policies in a hospital. One is a set of role privilege rules, which we named role privilege policy. The other is a set of privacy consent rules, which we named privacy consent policy. When an individual from Hospital A requests access to a patient's ECG data in Hospital B, the role privilege policy of Hospital A is first applied to making decision about whether the individual has the privilege to access patients' ECG data. If the access is affirmative, the privacy consent policy of Hospital B is applied to making decision about whether the user is given the permission to access the requested ECG data.

4.3.3 Access control architecture

1. Policy Enforcement

According to the access control framework proposed by XACML (OASIS, 2005c), there should be Policy Enforcement Point (PEP) and Policy Decision Point (PDP) applied along the way from a user to protected resources. PEP is the entry point for an access control mechanism. It receives an access request from a user and inquires of the PDP the access decision about the received request. Then, it permits or denies access to the resource according to the decision rendered by the PDP.

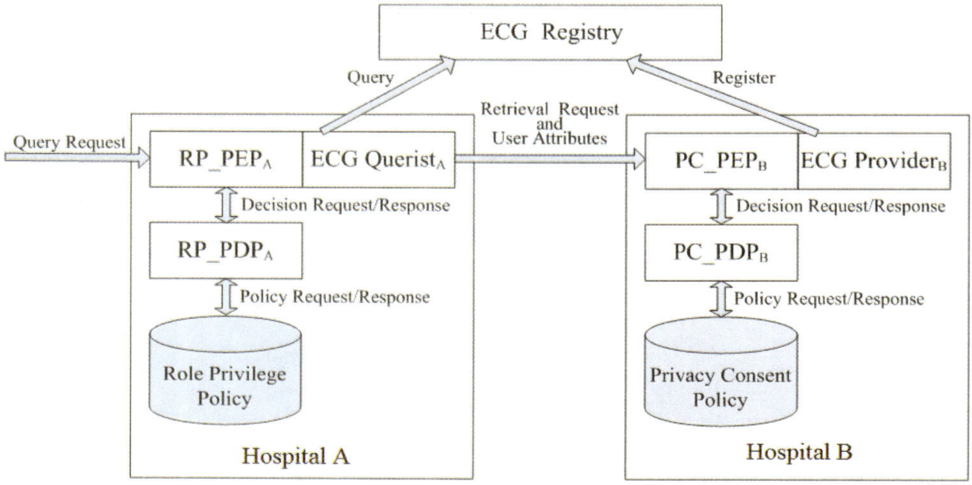

Fig. 7. Proposed access control architecture

As Fig. 7 depicts, our access control architecture employs two PEPs and two PDPs in every participating hospital. The two PEPs are the role privilege policy enforcement point (RP_PEP) and privacy consent policy enforcement point (PC_PEP), and the two PDPs are the role privilege policy decision point (RP_PDP) and privacy consent policy decision point (PC_PDP). Suppose the Hospital A deploys a RP_PEP, named RP_PEP_A, and a PC_PEP, named PC_PEP_A, and also provides an ECG Querist, named ECG $Querist_A$. The RP_PEP_A receives a request from a user of Hospital A, who requests the invocation of the ECG $Querist_A$ to query for a patient's ECG data. The RP_PEP_A sends a decision request to the RP_PDP_A. The RP_PDP_A checks whether the user is allowed to invoke the ECG $Querist_A$ according to the role privilege policy and returns a response of permit or deny. In case of a permit response, the RP_PEP_A invokes the ECG $Querist_A$ for the user. The ECG $Querist_A$ queries the ECG registry and presents the query result on behalf of the user. When the user requests the retrieval of an ECG document in the query result, the ECG $Querist_A$ will forward the retrieval request along with the user relevant attributes required for making a decision about the request to the PC_PEP_B. The PC_PEP_B sends a decision request to the PC_PDP_B. The PC_PDP_B checks whether the user is permitted to access the requested ECG document according to the privacy consent policy and returns a response of permit or deny. In case of a permit response, the PC_PEP_B invokes the ECG $Provider_B$, which is the ECG Provider of Hospital B, to transmit the requested ECG document to the user.

2. User Attributes Transfer for Privacy Consent Policy Decision

The hospital where a user requests the retrieval of an ECG document, like the Hospital A in Fig. 7, and the hospital that holds the ECG to be retrieved, like the Hospital B in Fig. 7, may be different. When the PC_PDP in an hospital makes a decision about a user's request for the retrieval of an ECG document of this hospital, it requires the user relevant attributes to query for a set of applicable privacy consent policies of this ECG document. Because privacy consent policies of different hospitals may be different, the required user relevant attributes may be different. So when the ECG Querist in an hospital forwards a retrieval request from its user to the PC_PEP of the hospital that holds the ECG document to be retrieved, the ECG Querist has to know what user relevant attributes should be passed along with the user request. Our solution to this problem is as follows:

- While the ECG Provider in an hospital registers an ECG document for sharing, the information of what user attributes are required for the privacy consent policy decision on the ECG document is submitted to the ECG registry along with the metadata about the ECG document.
- While the ECG Querist in an hospital queries the ECG registry for a patient's ECG data, the query result from the ECG registry contains not only the metadata about the ECG data which matches the query criteria and the URLs of these ECG data, but also the information of what user attributes are required for making a decision about accessing each ECG document.
- While the ECG Querist in an hospital forwards a user's request for retrieval of an ECG document given in the query result, it inquires the user attributes of the authentication authority and attribute authority of this hospital and passes the user attributes to the PC_PEP of the hospital that holds the ECG document to be retrieved.

5. Experimental evaluation

In this section, we analyze the performance of our system by conducting an experimental evaluation. To evaluate the performance of the ECG registry and the performance of the framework for ECG data dissemination, we constructed an experimental scenario of ECG data sharing across two ECG data sources. One of the two ECG data sources is a collection of recordings of 12-lead ECGs managed using QB-905D ECG Viewer (NIHON KODEN, n.d.), the commercial ECG management software of NIHON KOHDEN Corp. in Japan. The other is a collection of DICOM 12-lead ECGs managed using PACSOne (RainbowFish Software, n.d.), a DICOM-compliant PACS freeware. The data resident in these two ECG data sources were disseminated through the ECG registry and made accessible for the retrieval of an individual's ECG data via a common Web portal.

The experimental scenario is instantiated through deploying the ECG registry, the ECG provider for QB-905D, the ECG provider for PACSOne, and the Web portal on four different machines which all have an Intel Dual-core 2.83GHz CPU and 2G memory, and are accessible to the Internet.

5.1 ECG data publishing

We would like to find the effect of the number of the ECG data published at a time from an ECG data source on the time of publishing the ECG data from its data source to the ECG registry. The publishing-related time types include: 1) the *Extracting Time* ($T_{extract}$), which is equal to the time to read the newly generated ECG data from an ECG data source and to extract the metadata about all the new ECG data, 2) the *Registering Time* ($T_{register}$), which is equal to the time to request registration of the metadata, validate the metadata and store the metadata in the database, and 3) the *Total Time* (T_{total}), which is equal to the time starting from reading the newly generated ECG data from an ECG data source to storing the metadata in the database of the ECG registry, i.e. $T_{total} = T_{extract} + T_{register}$.

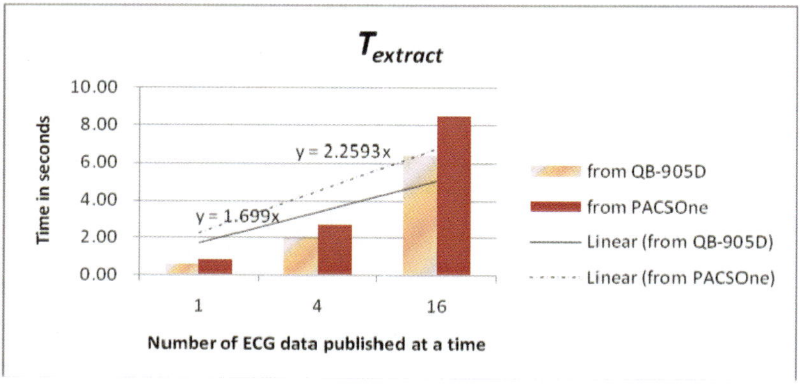

a. Extracting time

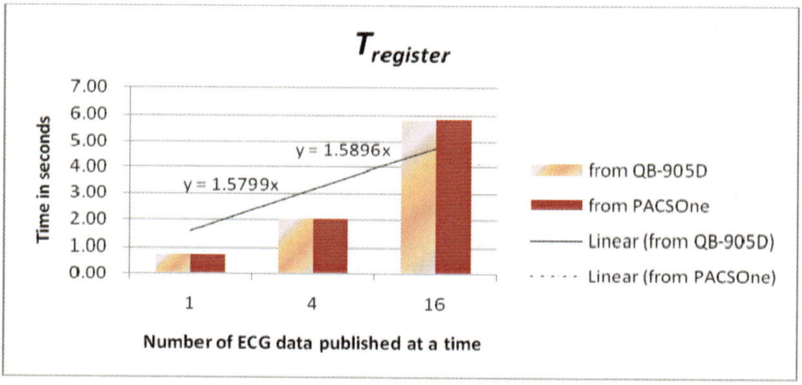

b. Registering time

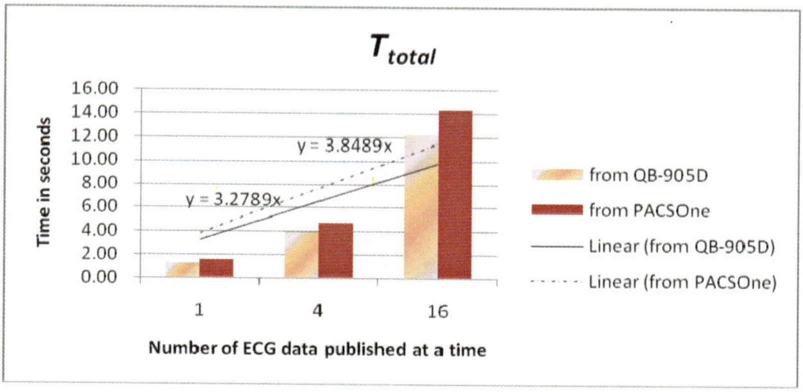

c. Total time

Fig. 8. Publishing time for the different numbers of ECG data published at a time

We measured the time to publish the ECG documents hold in the QB-905D and the time to publish the ECG documents hold in the PACSOne. Table 1 shows the time taken to publish the different numbers (1, 4, and 16) of ECG documents at a time from each of the two ECG data sources. The measurements of publishing time revealed that 1) the extracting time, registering time and total time were larger with increase of the number of ECG data published at a time (Fig. 8), but their ratios of increase were less than that of the number of ECG data published at a time (i.e. 4), 2) the extracting time for different ECG data sources were different due to the different data accessing mechanisms of the ECG data sources, and 3) the registering time for the different ECG data sources were the same, because they only depend on the performance of the ECG registry.

	Number of ECG data published at a time from QB-905D			Number of ECG data published at a time from PACSOne		
	1	4	16	1	4	16
T_{total}	1.29	3.99	12.21	1.54	4.72	14.30
$T_{extract}$	0.58	1.97	6.42	0.83	2.69	8.47
$T_{register}$	0.71	2.02	5.79	0.71	2.03	5.83

Table 1. Publishing time (measured in seconds) for the different numbers of ECG documents published at a time from an ECG data source

5.2 The ECG registry

We would like to find the effect of some factors such as the size of the ECG registry and the distribution of the ECG data that match the query criterion on the time taken to query the ECG registry for a patient's ECG data. The querying time includes the time to request the "Query" service of the ECG registry, the time to validate the query criterion, the time to query the database of the ECG registry, and the time to return the query result.

We collected the time results of performing the queries for patients' ECG data on the different ECG registry sizes. The queries were aimed at the three kinds of patients: 1) whose ECG data that match some query criterion are distributed only in the QB-905D, 2) whose ECG data that match some query criterion are distributed only in the PACSOne, and 3) whose ECG data that match some query criterion are distributed in the QB-905D and in the PACSOne. Table 2 records the time taken to query for those patients's ECG data. As the chart in Fig. 9 shows, the querying time increased as the size of the ECG registry increased, but it was not affected by the distribution of the ECG data that match the query criterion.

Distribution of the ECG data that match the query criteria	Registry size in number of entries				
	1	4	16	64	256
QB-905D only	0.043	0.049	0.059	0.082	0.164
PACSOne only	-	0.048	0.059	0.083	0.167
QB-908D and th PACSOne	-	0.048	0.059	0.082	0.166

Table 2. Querying time (measured in seconds) for patients' ECG data

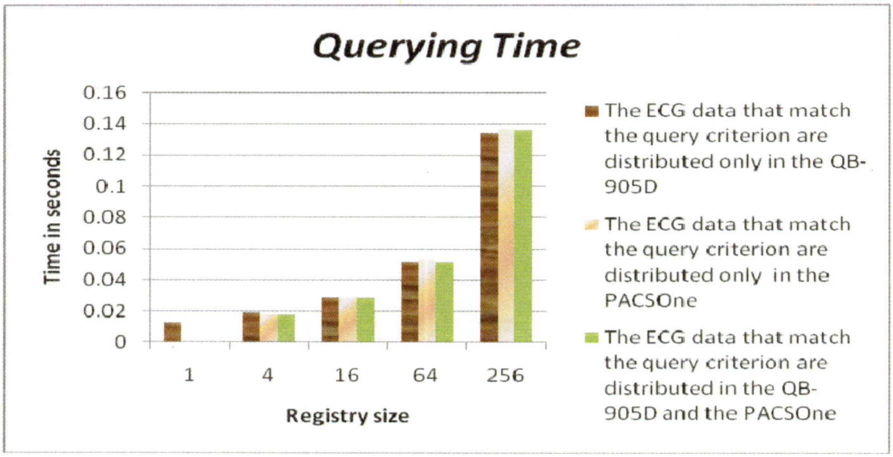

Fig. 9. Querying Time for the different sizes of the ECG registry

6. Conclusions

To broaden the exchange of ECG data from intra-hospital to inter-hospital can improve the ease of access to a patient's previous ECG data, and thus better facilitate serial ECG analysis in clinical practice. We report here a significant effort to provide a platform for inter-hospital exchange of ECG data, i.e., the Web-based system for the search and retrieval of a patient's ECG data across multiple hospitals. We evaluated the performance of the system in an experimental scenario. The experimental results suggest desirable effectiveness and efficiency of the system.

The contributions of this study are: 1) the metadata-based approach to facilitate the ECG data discovery and retrieval, including the metadata conceptual model for ECG data resources, and the ECG registry for disseminating and discovering ECG data based on the metadata conceptual model, 2) the access control mechanism to protect the ECG data in a hospital from disclosure to both the individuals who have no job-related need to access and the individuals who have been denied the privilege to access by a patient's privacy consent.

Future research will focus on the using of the information that has been exchanged across hospitals, and some issues, such as shared data types, terminologies, and coding schemes, will be studied.

7. References

Ariet, M., Zhou, S.H., DeLuca, D.C. & Greenfield, J.C. (2005). Computerized serial comparison of electrocardiograms - program performance in acute myocardial infarction, Computers in Cardiology, 0-7803-9337-6, Lyon, Sept. 2005

Association for the Advancement of Medical Instrumentation. (15 Mar. 1999). Standard communications protocol for computer-assisted electrocardiograph, 25 Mar. 2011, Available from:
http://officemedic.jp/ecgcard/pdf/AAMI.SCPECG.v1.2.pdf

Baptista, C.S., Pinto, F.Q., Kemp, Z. & Ryan, N. (n.d.). MetaCRIS: metadata for research digital libraries, 25 Mar. 2011, Available from: http://kar.kent.ac.uk/22027/1/MetaCRIS_Metadata_for_Research_Digital_Libraries.pdf

Brown, B.D. & Badilini, F. (21 Mar. 2005). HL7 aECG Implementation Guide, 25 Mar. 2011, Available from: http://www.amps-llc.com/website/documents/UsefulDocs/aECG_Implementation_Guide.pdf

Cho, Y.H., Jeon, M.J., Choi, H.S., Kim, I.Y. & Kim, S.I. (2003). Development of ECG management system conformable to DICOM waveform using XML. Journal of Digital Imaging, Vol, 16, No. suppl., (Mar. 2003), pp. (110-112), 0897-1889

Crevasse L. & Ariet M. (1987). Clinical usefulness of computerized ECG systems. Journal of Medical Systems, Vol. 11, No. 1, (Mar. 1987), pp. (21-24), 0148-5598

de Wijs, M.C.J., van Ettinger, M., Meij, S.H. & Nelwan S.P. (2005). Integration of Multiple ECG databases into a unified framework, Computers in Cardiology, 0-7803-9337-6, Lyon, Sept. 2005

DICOM Standards Committee. (26 Sept. 2000). Digital Imaging and Communications in Medicine (DICOM) Supplement 30: waveform interchange, 25 Mar. 2011, Available from: ftp://medical.nema.org/medical/dicom/final/sup30_f2.pdf

Fayn, J. & Rubel, P. (1991). Caviar, a serial ECG management and processing system. Proceedings of the Annual International Conference of the IEEE Engineering in Medicine and Biology Society, Vol. 13, No. 2, (Oct. 1991), pp. (570-571), 0-7803-0216-8

Hillmann, D.I. (16 Jul. 2000). Using Dublin Core, 25 Mar. 2011, Available from: http://dublincore.org/documents/2000/07/16/usageguide/

Integrating the Healthcare Enterprise. (12 Dec. 2008). Appendix P: privacy access policies, In: IHE IT Infrastructure Technical Framework Vol. 1 (ITI TF-1) Integration Profiles, 25 Mar. 2011, Available from: http://www.ihe.net/Technical_Framework/upload/IHE_ITI_TF_5-0_Vol1_FT_2008-12-12.pdf

Integrating the Healthcare Enterprise. (9 June 2006). 5 Retrieve ECG for display (ECG), In: IHE Cardiology Technical Framework Vol. I Integration Profiles, 25 Mar. 2011, Available from: http://www.ihe.net/Technical_Framework/upload/ihe_CARD_tf_vol1_2.pdf

Marcheschi, P., Mazzarisi, A., Dalmiani, S. & Benassi, A. (2006). ECG standards for the interoperability in patient electronic health records in Italy, Computers in Cardiology, 978-1-4244-2532-7, Valencia, Sept. 2006

Miller, P. (11 Sept. 1996). Metadata for the Masses, 25 Mar. 2011, Available from: http://www.ariadne.ac.uk/issue5/metadata-masses/

NIHON KODEN. (n.d.). ECG management and review software QB-905E, 25 Mar. 2011, Available from: http://www.nihonkohden.com/products/type/ecg/qb905e.html

OASIS. (17 Mar. 2005a). Assertions and Protocols for the OASIS Security Assertion Markup Language (SAML), 25 Mar. 2011, Available from: http://docs.oasis-open.org/security/saml/v2.0/ saml-core-2.0-os.pdf

OASIS. (2 May 2005b). ebXML registry services and protocols, 25 Mar. 2011, Available from:

Permissions

The contributors of this book come from diverse backgrounds, making this book a truly international effort. This book will bring forth new frontiers with its revolutionizing research information and detailed analysis of the nascent developments around the world.

We would like to thank Richard M. Millis, PhD, for lending his expertise to make the book truly unique. He has played a crucial role in the development of this book. Without his invaluable contribution this book wouldn't have been possible. He has made vital efforts to compile up to date information on the varied aspects of this subject to make this book a valuable addition to the collection of many professionals and students.

This book was conceptualized with the vision of imparting up-to-date information and advanced data in this field. To ensure the same, a matchless editorial board was set up. Every individual on the board went through rigorous rounds of assessment to prove their worth. After which they invested a large part of their time researching and compiling the most relevant data for our readers. Conferences and sessions were held from time to time between the editorial board and the contributing authors to present the data in the most comprehensible form. The editorial team has worked tirelessly to provide valuable and valid information to help people across the globe.

Every chapter published in this book has been scrutinized by our experts. Their significance has been extensively debated. The topics covered herein carry significant findings which will fuel the growth of the discipline. They may even be implemented as practical applications or may be referred to as a beginning point for another development. Chapters in this book were first published by InTech; hereby published with permission under the Creative Commons Attribution License or equivalent.

The editorial board has been involved in producing this book since its inception. They have spent rigorous hours researching and exploring the diverse topics which have resulted in the successful publishing of this book. They have passed on their knowledge of decades through this book. To expedite this challenging task, the publisher supported the team at every step. A small team of assistant editors was also appointed to further simplify the editing procedure and attain best results for the readers.

Our editorial team has been hand-picked from every corner of the world. Their multi-ethnicity adds dynamic inputs to the discussions which result in innovative outcomes. These outcomes are then further discussed with the researchers and contributors who give their valuable feedback and opinion regarding the same. The feedback is then collaborated with the researches and they are edited in a comprehensive manner to aid the understanding of the subject.

Apart from the editorial board, the designing team has also invested a significant amount of their time in understanding the subject and creating the most relevant covers. They scrutinized every image to scout for the most suitable representation of the subject and create an appropriate cover for the book.

The publishing team has been involved in this book since its early stages. They were actively engaged in every process, be it collecting the data, connecting with the contributors or procuring relevant information. The team has been an ardent support to the editorial, designing and production team. Their endless efforts to recruit the best for this project, has resulted in the accomplishment of this book. They are a veteran in the field of academics and their pool of knowledge is as vast as their experience in printing. Their expertise and guidance has proved useful at every step. Their uncompromising quality standards have made this book an exceptional effort. Their encouragement from time to time has been an inspiration for everyone.

The publisher and the editorial board hope that this book will prove to be a valuable piece of knowledge for researchers, students, practitioners and scholars across the globe.

List of Contributors

Augusta Pelosis
Michigan State University, USA

Jack Rubinstein
University of Cincinnati, USA

Lorenzo Scalise
Dipartimento di Ingegneria Industriale e Scienze Matematiche, Università Politecnica delle Marche, Italy

Cédric Assambo and Martin J. Burke
University of Dublin, Trinity College, Ireland

Michael Scheffer
Maasstad Hospital, Rotterdam, The Netherlands

Berry M. van Gelder
Catharina Hospital, Eindhoven, The Netherlands

Yeon-Sik Noh, Ja-Woong Yoon and Hyung-Ro Yoon
Dept. of Biomedical Engineering, Yonsei University, Republic of Korea

Bojan Vrtovec and Gregor Poglajen
Department of Cardiology, University Medical Center Ljubljana, Slovenia

Srinivasan Jayaraman, Prashanth Swamy, Vani Damodaran and N. Venkatesh
Innovation Labs, Tata Consultancy Services, Bangalore, India

Ryuji Kato, Yoshio Ijiri and Kazuhiko Tanaka
Osaka University of Pharmaceutical Sciences, Japan

James E. Skinner, Daniel N. Weiss and Edward F. Lundy
Vicor Technologies, Inc, USA

Ana Cecilia Vinzio Maggio and Pedro David Arini
Instituto Argentino de Matemática 'A. Calderón', CONICET, Buenos Aires, Argentina

María Paula Bonomini and Pedro David Arini
Instituto de Ingeniería Biomédica, Universidad de Buenos Aires, Buenos Aires, Argentina

Eric Laciar Leber
Gabinete de Tecnología Médica, Universidad Nacional de San Juan, San Juan, Argentina

J.L. Rodríguez-Sotelo
Grupo de Automática, Facultad de Ingeniería, Universidad Autónoma de Manizales, Colombia

G. Castellanos-Domínguez
Grupo de Procesamiento y Reconocimiento de Señales, Universidad Nacional de Colombia, Colombia

C.D. Acosta-Medina
Grupo de Computación Científica y Modelamiento Matemático, Universidad Nacional de Colombia, Colombia

Hasan Ari and Kübra Doğanay
Bursa Postgraduate Hospital, Departments of Cardiology, Bursa, Turkey

Richard M. Millis, Mark D. Hatcher and Rachel E. Austin
Department of Physiology & Biophysics, Howard University College of Medicine, USA

Vernon Bond
Department of Health, Human Performance & Leisure Studies, Howard University Graduate School of Arts & Sciences, USA

Kim L. Goring
Department of Medicine, Howard University Hospital, Washington, DC, USA

Elpidio Santillo, Luca Fallavollita, Luciano Marini and Fabrizio Balestrini
Geriatric-Rehabilitative Department- Italian National Research Centre on Aging - Fermo, Italy

Monica Migale
Internal Medicine Unit"Villa Verde" Clinic - Fermo, Italy

Zhiyue Lin and Richard W. McCallum
Northwestern University and Texas Tech University, USA

Shuenn-Yuh Lee and Jia-Hua Hong
Department of Electrical Engineering, National Chung-Cheng University, Taiwan, Taiwan

Jin-Ching Lee
Department of Biotechnology, College of Life Science, Kaohsiung Medical University, Taiwan

Qiang Fang
Department of Electrical and Computer Engineering, RMIT University, Australia

Jarno M.A. Tanskanen and Jari J. Viik
Tampere University of Technology and Institute of Biosciences and Medical Technology, Finland

Motohisa Osaka
Nippon Veterinary and Life Science University, Japan

Thoralf Niendorf, Lukas Winter and Tobias Frauenrath
Berlin Ultrahigh Field Facility (B.U.F.F.), Max Delbrueck Center for Molecular Medicine, Berlin, Germany

Shizhong Yuan and Daming Wei
Biomedical Information Technology Laboratory, University of Aizu, Japan

Shizhong Yua, Daming Wei and Weimin Xu
School of Computer Engineering and Science, Shanghai University, China

Daming Wei
Graduate School of Medicine, Tohoku University, Japan